Laboratory Medicine/
Urinalysis and Medical Microscopy

Laboratory Medicine/ Urinalysis and Medical Microscopy

Second Edition

JAMES A. FREEMAN, M.D.

Freeman, Gyer, Hemelt & Associates, Inc., Plaquemine, Louisiana; Clinical Professor of Pathology, Louisiana State University Medical Center, New Orleans, Louisiana

MYRTON F. BEELER, M.D.

Professor of Pathology, Louisiana State University Medical Center, New Orleans, Louisiana

Lea & Febiger • *Philadelphia* • *1983*

Lea & Febiger
600 Washington Square
Philadelphia, PA 19106
U.S.A.

Library of Congress Cataloging in Publication Data

Freeman, James A.
Laboratory medicine/urinalysis and medical microscopy.

Rev. ed. of: Laboratory medicine, clinical microscopy. 1974.
Includes bibliographical references and index.
1. Microscopy, Medical. 2. Urine—Examination.
3. Diagnosis, Laboratory. I. Beeler, Myrton F.
II. Title. [DNLM: 1. Microscopy. 2. Diagnosis, Laboratory. QY 4 L1233]
RB43.F85 1983 616.07′5′028 82-17254
ISBN 0-8121-0822-1

PRINTED IN THE UNITED STATES OF AMERICA

Print No. 3 2 1

Preface

During the past century many of the great advances in our understanding of disease and in our ability to diagnose and treat disease effectively have resulted from laboratory investigations later translated into routine patient care resources. Since World War II, the number of medical laboratory tests performed annually in the United States has doubled every 5 years. It has become almost axiomatic that complete good-quality laboratory service enables the physician to recognize the presence of disease earlier, to diagnose it more specifically, and to monitor therapy more effectively.

Every large medical laboratory is subdivided into functional sections. Some of these divisions, like hematology, are named for the specimens analyzed; others, like chemistry, for the type of analyses performed; still others, like bacteriology and virology, for the nature of disease agents studied. One section, involved with the analyses of many body secretions and excretions, particularly urine and feces, has received less recognition than the others; in part, perhaps, because of the unpleasant nature of some of the materials examined, a traditional lack of sophisticated instrumentation and test procedures, limited opportunities, in the past, for adequate quality control, and lack of a sense of identity. In some laboratories this section is relegated to the smallest, least desirable area, and is staffed by the least experienced personnel. The section is sometimes called the "Urinalysis Laboratory," although it might be more appropriately called the "Miscellaneous Laboratory." It is given recognition by the American Board in Pathology, the Registry of Medical Technologists, the Board of Schools, and by many medical laboratories as the "Clinical Microscopy Laboratory." This, too, is something of a misnomer since not all the laboratory procedures include the use of a microscope; but it does, in part, connote a certain air of distinction where it is badly needed.

Some of the analyses performed in the Clinical Microscopy Laboratory also are often performed in physicians' offices. In fact, according to a recent survey, published in Modern Medicine, urinalysis is the one procedure performed in all physicians' office laboratories. Many physicians are attuned to the fact that the presence of increased numbers of white blood cells in the urine suggests the presence of infection, but they may not all appreciate the relationship between proteinuria of various degree accompanied by relatively few white blood cells and chronic renal disease. There also may not be general appreciation of the potential usefulness of results of analysis of urinary calculi. Likewise, they may not all realize that examination of feces of patients with suspected malabsorption may obviate the need for more expensive laboratory diagnostic work. Many are probably not sufficiently familiar with the technical details of the tests.

This book includes consideration of the theory and use of a microscope, fecal analysis, gastric analysis, synovial fluid analysis, semen analysis, urinary stone analysis, cerebrospinal fluid analysis, and pregnancy testing, as well as urinalysis. The theoretical, practical, and definitive aspects of the subjects are covered. Approximately half of the text consists of clinical information useful for proper selection and interpretation of tests. The remainder consists of statements of principles underlying the tests and detailed descriptions of the laboratory procedures. The volume is intentionally didactic, and specific laboratory procedures are described in "cookbook" format for maximal usefulness to the laboratory bench workers. Sophisticated procedures that can be done within the laboratories at most general hospitals with less than 200 beds are reviewed in depth. A number of reproductions of color photographs are included to assist in readily assimilating and understanding the material. Each chapter begins with a historical introduction approached in a spirit of levity. *Mal y soit qui mal y pense.* The chapter on urinalysis includes descriptions of time-honored tests as well as newer, more sophisticated procedures, and comparisons among different methods; for example, specific gravity, refractometry, and osmometry have been included where especially pertinent. The section on fecal analysis includes a description of visual examination, procedures for detection of blood, and a discussion of the tests applicable to the study of malabsorption syndromes. This discussion includes some of the newer test procedures. The section on gastric analysis includes a description of the modern determination of gastric acidity (potentiometry rather than titration) and provides an up-to-date review of the clinical significance of results of gastric analyses. The chapter on pregnancy testing and assay of chorionic gonadotropin includes comparison between newer immunoassay techniques and the older bioassay techniques. The chapter on cerebrospinal fluid testing covers the newest parameters in chemical analysis of this fluid. The chapter on semen analysis includes exclusion of evidence in rape victims. The chapter on synovial fluid testing includes tests for immune deficiency disorders.

The book, therefore, is intended for use by medical laboratory technologists and technicians who will be expressly interested in the procedures; by pathologists interested in procedures and interpretation; and by family practitioners who will be mainly interested in interpretation—both during their educational years and as continuing education in the course of their practice.

Plaquemine, Louisiana JAMES A. FREEMAN
New Orleans, Louisiana MYRTON F. BEELER

Contributors

Myrton F. Beeler, M.D.
Professor of Pathology, Louisiana State University Medical Center, New Orleans, Louisiana

Donald C. Cannon, M.D.
Professional Medical Laboratories, Witchita Falls, Texas

James A. Freeman, M.D.
Freeman, Gyer, Hemelt & Associates, Inc., Plaquemine, Louisiana; Clinical Professor of Pathology, Louisiana State University Medical Center, New Orleans, Louisiana

Meryl H. Haber, M.D.
Executive Vice-President, American Society of Clinical Pathologists, Chicago, Illinois; Professor of Clinical Pathology, Northwestern University Medical School, Chicago, Illinois; Professor of Pathology, Rush Medical College, Chicago, Illinois

Maxine M. Marionneaux, M.T. (ASCP), M.S.
Assistant Professor of Pathology, Louisiana State University Medical Center, New Orleans, Louisiana; Laboratory Manager and Education Coordinator, Earl K. Long Memorial Hospital, Baton Rouge, Louisiana

Alvin J. Mathews, M.D.
Freeman, Gyer, Hemelt & Associates, Inc., New Orleans, Louisiana; Chief of Pathology, Meadowcrest Hospital, Gretna, Louisiana

Robert Morriss, Ph.D.
Professor of Physics, Tulane University, New Orleans, Louisiana

Alfredo Suarez, M.D.
Assistant Professor of Pathology, Louisiana State University Medical Center, New Orleans, Louisiana; Chief of Pathology and Director of Clinical Laboratories, Earl K. Long Memorial Hospital, Baton Rouge, Louisiana

Contents

Chapter 1 Urinalysis

JAMES A. FREEMAN
MERYL H. HABER

In a volume of short stories entitled Seven Gothic Tales, the Danish writer Isak Dinesen relates the musing of an Arab sailing by starlight along the coast of Africa, "What is man when you come to think upon him, but a minutely set, ingenious machine for turning, with infinite artfulness, the red wine of Shiraz into urine?"[1]

The uses of this cleverly altered urine have been so diverse as to include hairdressing among the Eskimos and fire extinguishing among the Lilliputians. There is scarcely a disease that has not been treated by the administration of urine from the time of Pliny (the Elder) even into modern times. The 17th century chemist Robert Boyle is said to have written a volume on the virtues of human urine and its use as a medicinal agent. In France, the wealthy ladies of Boyle's day took urine baths to beautify the skin, while persons in rural communities used urine to soften the hands. In ancient Rome, urine was employed as a mouthwash and prophylactic against dental caries. In ancient China, T'ung pien (boy's urine) was swallowed warm to alleviate sore throat: a practice not so unesthetic perhaps, considering some of the vile tasting mouthwashes used today![2] Before the introduction of yeast, European bakers used urine as a leaven. Until recent times, urine was also used to macerate tobacco leaves in the cigar industry, and to flavor cheese. And today, aging matrons wistfully apply "hormone face cream," unaware that the hormones, in fact, may come from horse urine.[3] For centuries it was considered proper to pause during battle to urinate on a fellow warrior's wounds—neither a more sterile nor a more antiseptic remedy was then available!

By the 14th century, Bernard Gordon is alleged to have declared,

"The science of judging the urine is so easy that all can learn what they wish to know"; this is a remarkable mis-statement, considering that Gordon was a learned physician.[4] Probably the oldest diagnostic test in the history of medicine stemmed from recognition, by the Hindus, of "honey urine," so named after observing the trains of black ants attracted to sweet urine of diabetics. Although it is known that the Egyptians mentioned urine as having an unpleasant odor and referred to it in various diseases of the urinary bladder, none of the papyri mention the diagnostic use of urine. Even William Shakespeare, in the Two Gentlemen of Verona, alluded to uroscopists of the day. Uroscopy, or "water casting" as it was known, was in great vogue in the early 19th century.[5] The urinal actually became the emblem of the medical profession. Physicians were always shown inspecting a urinal (but the urinal was carried in a wicker basket by a servant, as the physician disdained to touch it).

The word "*urine*" is derived from the Latin *urina*, the English usage appearing in the 14th century and remaining in polite circulation today. From the old French word "*pisier*" comes the English word "*piss*" so commonly used by Geoffrey Chaucer and even the Elizabethans, but not much used in polite society after the advent of Cromwellian Puritanism (until very recent times in our more permissive society). The "*piss pot*," often elaborately decorated with flowers and sometimes silver or gold, remained in universal use until the invention of the latrine, about the time of Elizabeth I.[1] Frequently, the pot was emptied out of an upper story window by the chambermaid, who only infrequently uttered a warning—"Lord have mercy on you"—to the dismay of the unwary passerby. This expression eventually gave way to an unintelligible "gardy loo" (derived from the French expression "*gare de l'eau*"—beware of the water).

It was in alchemy that the uses of urine first began to acquire a more scientific cast, the alchemists being concerned with ammonium salts. Urine became a critical commodity when, in the Confederacy during the Civil War, urinary nitrates were reclaimed for manufacture of gunpowder.[1] In fact, a particularly energetic and enthusiastic agent at Selma advertised in the newspaper:

> The ladies of Selma are respectfully requested to preserve the chamber lye collected about the premises for the purpose of making nitre. A barrel will be sent around daily to collect it.
>
> John Harrolson, Agent
> Nitre Mining Bureau

This came to the attention of a poet in the Confederate Army who responded lyrically, as man frequently used to do, thus immortalizing not only the practice, but the ingenious agent as well:

John Harrolson! John Harrolson! You are a wretched creature.
You've added to this bloody war a new and awful feature.
You'd have us think while every man is bound to be a fighter,
The ladies, bless the dears, should save their P for nitre.

John Harrolson! John Harrolson! Where did you get the notion
To send your barrel 'round the town to gather up the lotion?
We thought the girls had work enough making shirts and kissing,
But you have put the pretty dears to patriotic pissing.

John Harrolson! John Harrolson! Do pray invent a neater
And somewhat more modest mode of making your saltpetre;
For 'tis an awful idea, John, gunpowdery and cranky,
That when a lady lifts her shift, she's killing off a Yankee.

The poem was printed on toilet paper, and circulated all over the Confederacy; a copy was smuggled across the line and fell into the hands of an anonymous Yankee poet, who replied with an equally jocular lyric:

John Harrolson! John Harrolson! We've read in song and story
How women's tears through all the years have moistened fields of glory.
But never was it told before amid such scenes of slaughter
Your Southern beauties dried their tears and went to making water.

No wonder that your boys are brave, who wouldn't be a fighter
If every time he fired his gun, he used his sweetheart's nitre;
And vice-versa, what would make a Yankee soldier sadder
Than dodging bullets fired from a pretty woman's bladder?

They say there was a subtle smell that lingered in that powder,
And as the smoke grew thicker and the din of battle louder,
That there was found to this compound one serious objection,
No soldier boy could sniff it without having an erection.

The rediscovery by Thomas Willis (1674) that sugar in the urine of patients with diabetes mellitus could be detected by tasting the urine, has titillated many medical students. Most important was the discovery of urea in urine, and its subsequent synthesis, by Friedrich Wöhler in 1828. This marked the beginning of synthetic biochemistry and an end to the superstitious separation of organic from inorganic chemistry.

There is a notable story of the Dutch scientist who kept an entire population alive, while imprisoned in a Nazi camp in World War II, by using urine (with its content of nitrates) to promote agricultural crop growth for food.

Urine, which commonly inspires men only to contempt and disgust, which is generally ranked amongst the most vile and repulsive of matters, and which is considered a waste (by the uneducated), is actually one of the most useful substances available for laboratory diagnosis in medicine.

SPECIMEN COLLECTION AND PRESERVATION

Because of its nature, urine collection, unlike blood specimen collection, cannot usually be supervised directly by laboratory personnel.

Instead a number of people are involved, including the patient, the nurse or aide, the ward clerk and a human or mechanical conveyance system. Add to this the fact that preoperative urine specimens often arrive in the laboratory late at night, in large numbers, and remain on benches or tables for hours, and one can understand some of the problems involved in the achievement of proper urine analysis and, hence, valid test results.

Collection Containers

Suitable containers are available from many suppliers. For our hospital patients we have used disposable graduated polyethylene 6-oz containers fitted with tight cardboard or polyethylene caps (they cost about $3^1/_2$¢ each) on which is recorded the appropriate identifying information. Other laboratories use heavy glass specimen bottles with sloping sides, graduated to 175 ml and fitted with cardboard caps on which is recorded the appropriate identifying information; they cost about 10¢ each. They are washed and autoclaved prior to reuse. Disposable cardboard containers are also available for a few cents each. We have seen patients use every conceivable container, from perfume bottles to gallon paint buckets. Some women, especially, are ingenious at getting urine into tiny, odiferous perfume bottles. This practice should be condemned, if for no other reason than the resultant chemical contamination of the specimen.

Random Specimens

Probably the best specimen for routine examination is the first morning voiding, fresh, concentrated, with an acid pH. If the urine is dilute, small but pathologic increases in content of protein, sugar, red blood cells, white blood cells, and casts may be missed. Alkalinity and hypoosmolality hasten dissolution of casts and red cells. If specimens cannot be examined immediately, those with specific gravity less than 1.010 should probably be recollected if possible, especially if they are alkaline. First morning specimens also tend to be more uniform, are more likely to reveal impairment of kidney concentrating ability, and to contain pus and mucus in the presence of infection. They are, however, less likely to contain sugar and protein. Most specimens obtained in the practitioner's office are collected from ambulatory patients who have eaten 2 to 3 hours previously. These specimens are more likely to contain protein or reducing substances.

Do not skip lightly over the rather tedious details of proper urine collection and preservation. We sometimes believe it is easier for a camel to get through the eye of a needle than for the patient, nurse, clerk, and messenger to produce an accurately timed, properly collected, and well-preserved urine specimen at the right place and at the proper time! *Neglect of this aspect of the examination frequently renders all subsequent information uninterpretable or useless.*

24-Hour Timed Specimens

Collection of 24-hour urine specimens from hospitalized patients is often started at 7:00 A.M. or 8:00 A.M. All persons instructing patients about 24-hour urine collections should make sure that the patients understand that they must empty the bladder at the time the 24-hour collection is to start and discard this specimen. Nurses and aides should also be warned not to predate and pretime the slips, since it is rare for patients to urinate on the hour. In fact, when laboratory slips accompanying 24-hour urine specimens indicate that collection started and stopped on the hour, to the minute, they should be suspected of being inaccurate. It cannot be stressed enough that the exact time is important, and that it is not important whether this is 9 or 10 minutes more or less than 24 hours, provided that the information is accurate. The patient should, of course, be reminded by someone to try to urinate just at the end of the collection period. Whenever a preservative has to be used, the patient should be warned in advance of any untoward problems that might arise from inadvertent spillage. For instance, patients should be warned of the corrosive nature of hydrochloric acid preservative often used for 24-hour urine collection for vanilmandelic acid

EARL K. LONG MEMORIAL HOSPITAL
CLINICAL LABORATORIES

Instructions for Collecting 24 Hour Urine Specimen

Empty your bladder completely when you awaken in the morning and discard this urine specimen. Save ALL urine specimens passed during the remainder of the day and the night. Also save the first specimen of urine passed the next morning. Pour all urine specimens into the container given to you by the nurse.

It is extremely important that ALL urine be saved and placed in the container. Test results are calculated on the basis of 24 hour output and unless all urine is saved, results will not be accurate. This is most important as the test requested is expensive and complicated and your doctor is depending upon our results to evaluate and treat your condition.

EKLH 411

Fig. 1–1. Label used on a container for 24-hour urine collection at a university hospital. As trite as it may sound, the language used on collection containers should be easily understood by patients. Many patients do not understand what a "specimen" is or what "void" means. Simple terms are absolutely essential for proper understanding. A directive to "piss in the bottle" may be crude, but it may be more meaningful to some patients.

determination. Patients collecting a 24-hour urine sample need to be warned prior to use of bed pans, to urinate before having a bowel movement. Otherwise, they may forget and urinate into the pan while having a bowel movement, spoiling the urine collection.

We attempt to get the nursing staff to apply the above instruction label to the specimen containers for 24-hour collections (Fig. 1–1).

Preservation of Specimens

Ideally, urine should be examined soon enough after voiding (within 2 hours) not to need a preservative. In our laboratories, we prefer to examine the specimen warm, especially for bacteriologic and parasitologic studies. However, if it cannot be examined immediately, refrigeration or preservation is necessary. Many means of preservation have been recommended. We do not recommend any of them for routine urinalysis. There is no universal preservative useful for all tests, and no preservative is as satisfactory as a fresh specimen of urine. The following are commonly used methods of preservation:

1. Refrigeration: This is probably the most satisfactory method of preservation, especially when used in combination with a chemical preservative. (Refrigeration does have its draw-backs, however, such as precipitation of amorphous phosphates and urates, which tends to obscure sediment findings.)
2. Urinary preservative tablets (Metropolitan Life Insurance Co.): Preservative tablets used by insurance companies were originally devised by Francis Kingsbury and are excellent preservatives for routine chemical tests and for formed elements.[5] However, sodium, potassium, and hormone studies are not possible after use of these tablets. The tablets are acid and will adequately buffer all specimens except strongly alkaline urines. In addition, formaldehyde is liberated from the methenamine in the tablets. The tablets do not interfere with analysis for presence of diuretics, especially thiazides, sought by insurance companies. Each tablet will preserve 2 oz. of urine. The tablets are most useful if specimens are to be transported over a long distance.

   The formula of the tablets is:

Constituent	*Content (mg)*
Potassium acid phosphate	100
Sodium benzoate	50
Benzoic acid	65
Methenamine (Urotropin)	50
Sodium bicarbonate	10
Mercuric oxide, red	1
	276 mg

The tablets will affect the specific gravity as follows:

Volume of urine (ml)	*Increase in specific gravity from one tablet*
40	0.003
35	0.004
30	0.005
25	0.006
20	0.007
15	0.009
10	0.013
5	0.025

3. Formalin (40% v/v): This is useful for preservation of the formed elements. An excess should be avoided, otherwise urea will precipitate. Formalin will cause positive Clinitest and Fehling's test results, but not a positive Benedict's test result. One drop (0.05 ml; or 10 ml/24-hour volume) is sufficient.
4. Acidification (pH <3.0): This results in excellent preservation of 24-hour specimens collected for chemical tests in general, provided that the acid does not interfere with the test. It is especially useful for steroid and vanilmandelic-acid determinations. Formed elements are destroyed, and uric acid is precipitated by marked acidity. (10 ml concentrated HCl 24-hour volume or 25 ml 6N HCl 24-hour volume is sufficient.) Since concentrated HCl fumes are dangerous to patients, and because of the old injunction not to add water to acid, it is probably wiser to use the larger volume of about one-third concentrated acid if it is to be added to the container before urine collection, especially for outpatient collections.
5. Thymol: This has been reputed to be a good preservative for most chemical tests. It will cause a false positive reaction for protein with heat and acetic-acid testing, but it does not affect the dipstick tests that depend on the principle of the protein error of indicators. Probably better preservatives are available for most purposes.
6. Boric acid: This delays decomposition of chemical as well as formed elements, but it does not stop the growth of yeast. It also will precipitate uric acid. (5 mg/30 ml is sufficient.)
7. Sodium carbonate: This is useful for preservation of porphyrins and related substances. (5 mg/dl for 2 L of urine will suffice.) This preservative can also be used for 24-hour urine collections for urobilinogen (4 g/24-hour volume).
8. Toluene: This is used for preservation of acetone, diacetic acid, reducing substances, and protein. Toluene excludes air from the specimen, but does not effectively stop the growth of microorganisms. Because of its flammable nature it is more than slightly hazardous! Pipetting through it is difficult and may be hazardous to technologists unless a rubber bulb is used. (Add enough to leave

a layer over the entire surface.) We have never employed toluene for preservation of urine.

9. Chloroform: This is a poor preservative for most chemical tests. It settles to the bottom, interferes with microscopic examination, and reduces Fehling's reagent. The substance, if ingested in large doses, is hepatotoxic. Although it has been recommended, we recommend that it not be used at all.

INDICATIONS FOR URINALYSIS

Except for a hemoglobin or hematocrit determination, urinalysis is the only laboratory test that has been required by the Joint Commission on Accreditation of Hospitals to be performed on all patients at each hospital admission. Additionally, urinalysis is a laboratory procedure generally available 24 hours a day 7 days a week. In a survey (1965) of laboratory procedures performed in the offices of physicians, Modern Medicine reported that urinalysis was the only test performed by 100% of the practitioners returning the questionnaire.

Traditionally, examination of urine and urinary sediment has not been held in high regard. The urinalysis laboratory is more often than not the dingiest, smallest, and least well-equipped section; furthermore, it is often staffed by the most junior bench workers. Benjamin Wells attributed the relatively low prestige rating of the examination of urine to the apparent simplicity of the methods used and the easy availability of specimens, among other things. No less significant in this regard, we believe, is the esthetic unpleasantry of dealing with this material. Examination of the urine, however, when properly performed, can produce a great deal of useful information about metabolic functions, the functional integrity of organs, as well as ingestion of poisons and drugs. Although the study of blood is more direct, this approach offers only an indirect reflection of intracellular metabolic processes. Also, urine is easier to obtain.

The ready availability of urine, according to Benjamin Wells, has led to the practice of "routine" examination en masse. Large numbers of urinalyses are frequently ordered without specific reference to the diagnostic problem at hand; often without subsequent interpretation applied to the individual patient. These circumstances have seriously reduced the effectiveness of this examination in the minds of some clinicians and have created an unwarranted disregard for urinalysis in the minds of the laboratory technologist.

A normal result of urinalysis can be useful. The discovery of pus, red blood cells, protein, and casts is always important. An occasional red blood cell in the urine of a person with an arm fracture would not be given great attention; whereas in a patient suspected of having glomerulonephritis, concentration of the sediment and further examination for red blood cells and casts would be indicated. Certain substances, such as phenylketones, appear in detectable amounts in the urine in pathologic conditions; thus, examination for this "waste product" affords a diagnostic approach in this circumstance. In other conditions, physiologic increases of substances appear during changes in body metabolism, such as gonadotropic hormones during pregnancy, which make examination of urine ideal for detection of this particular physiologic state. As Richard Lippman states, "One may compare the urinary stream to a mountain stream. Arising from a conglomeration of rivulets, water is constantly seeping into its bed, yet simultaneously dissolves a portion of the bed itself, which is carried downstream. Even discrete particles are swept along, and these may be deposited in lower, more general reaches of the river, or they may abrasively erode canyons as they rush on their way. From the study of channels and their structure, from study of the composition of water as it flows downward toward the sea, many inferences may be made concerning mountains in which the stream originated. The urine and its sediment likewise affect their origin, although the changes produced in their miniscule descent possess added complexity since the bed of the urinary stream is composed of living cells."[46]

Urine is a complex mixture of water, electrolytes, body wastes, epithelium desquamated from the genitourinary tract, and debris. Analysis of urine, consequently, is a composite examination. Use of commercially available "dipsticks" for detection of some substances in urine represents a semiautomated procedure instituted before widespread adoption of automation in clinical chemistry or in other phases of laboratory medicine.

ACCURACY, SPECIFICITY, AND SENSITIVITY OF URINALYSIS

The usefulness of a screening test depends in part upon the incidence of the disease it detects in the population tested, as well as on the diagnostic specificity and sensitivity of the test (taken together, its diagnostic accuracy). Diagnostic specificity can be defined as the ability of the test to yield a negative result for patients without the disease. The less specific the test, the greater the percentage of positive test results in patients without the disease. Diagnostic specificity can be expressed quantitatively as follows:

$$\text{Specificity} = \frac{\text{number of negative test results in patients without the disease}}{\text{number of people tested without the disease}} \times 100$$

Thus, if there are no "false positive" test results, the test is 100% specific.

Sensitivity is defined as the ability of the test to yield a positive result for patients with the disease. It can be expressed quantitatively as follows:

$$\text{Sensitivity} = \frac{\text{number of positive test results in patients with the disease}}{\text{number of people tested with the disease}} \times 100$$

If there are no "false negative" test results, the test is 100% sensitive.

Predictive value is defined as the number of true positives divided by the total number of true and false positives. Its formula, then, is as follows:

$$\text{Predictive value} = \frac{\text{number of positive test results in patients with the disease}}{\text{number of positive test results in patients with the disease plus the number of positive test results in patients without the disease}} \times 100$$

Diagnostic accuracy can be defined as the ability of the test to correctly classify the entire population tested for the disease in question. Because most diseases have a low incidence in the population at large, accuracy depends more on specificity than on sensitivity. Thus, the usefulness of a screening test depends on the incidence of the disease in the population screened, as well as on its sensitivity and specificity. The greater the incidence of the disease, the lower the specificity that can economically be accepted; the lower the incidence, the greater the specificity required. Specificity may sometimes be sacrificed for greater sensitivity (the two often tend to be reciprocal) in screening tests, when the penalties for missing the diagnosis are greater than those of falsely suspecting the diagnosis. Reliable data to calculate these parameters for urinalysis are not yet available.

THE ROUTINE URINALYSIS

The "routine urinalysis" is probably the most venerable of the diagnostic laboratory test batteries, although it is seldom considered under the heading "laboratory screening," nor does it appear to have been subjected to the same close scrutiny that the concept of mass screening has been. Urine examination, together with blood hemoglobin or hematocrit, is an examination that has been recommended by the Joint Commission of Accreditation of Hospitals for all patients admitted to hospitals in the United States, as has been mentioned.

Routine urinalysis by conventional wisdom includes examination and notation of:

1. Appearance (color and clarity)
2. pH
3. Solid content (specific gravity, osmolality, refractive index or weight of solids)
4. Presence of protein
5. Presence of glucose or reducing substances
6. Presence of ketone bodies
7. Microscopic examination of (and rough estimate of quantities of) formed elements of sediment

To this, some pathologists and physicians have added the examination for:

1. Hemoglobin
2. Bile
3. Urobilinogen
4. Nitrites
5. Leukocyte Esterases

An intelligent evaluation of this battery still awaits application of general principles outlined elsewhere, as well as other principles of diagnostic laboratory testing. Most components, however, have the sanction of custom, at least. Probably the word "routine" should be dropped, although its use at the time the patient is admitted to the hospital seems justified.

Abnormal test results, as we have said, may reflect not only diseases of the genitourinary tract, but also of remote organs and general metabolic disorders. Many renologists prefer to perform the microscopic examination personally on urine freshly obtained by them from their own patients. We believe that the practice should be encouraged. This is especially true when the clinician is following the course of kidney disease, and it has been recommended by many authorities in the field since Richard Bright, including, notably, Thomas Addis.

To the reader is left the choice from among the procedures described herein. Some of them may have limited usefulness in special circumstances. Recently, some medical centers have begun to screen all newborn or children's urine for aminoacidurias and presence of phenolic substances in abnormal concentrations by chromatographic techniques. We expect the practice to become more widespread.

Because people for whom urinalyses are performed often come from a population in ill health, one expects (and finds) a relatively high incidence of abnormal test results. People having urinalysis as part of the yearly "health check" would be expected to show fewer abnormalities than would hospitalized patients.

COLOR (INTRINSIC AND EXTRINSIC)

The pigments responsible for the normal light straw to dark amber color of urine have not been well characterized, but collectively have been referred to as "urochromes."[6] Dilute urines tend to be light, concentrated urines dark.

Abnormal urinary pigments may color the urine red, orange, brown or black, and include hemoglobin, myoglobin, bile, porphyrins, melanogens, and homogentisic acid.

Many drugs and some food pigments may also cause the urine to be colored abnormally. Some of these are indicators, changing color depending upon pH. Red pigments in an acid urine, turning yellow or colorless with alkalinization, may come from beets or pyridium. The reverse can occur in urine containing PSP (phenolsulfonphthalein), phenolphthalein, congo red, phenindione anticoagulants and santonin. Dyes used in tubeless gastric analysis (Azure B) and methylene blue can color the urine blue or green, depending on concentration and pH.

For a more complete tabulation, see Table 1–1.

CLARITY

Pathologic urines are often turbid, but so are many normal urines. Urates or phosphates may produce cloudiness in normal urine, especially post-prandially. However, this turbidity usually disappears 2 to 3 hours after a meal. When a clear, normal urine stands at room temperature for a few days, a hazy sediment of mucus threads, phosphates, and bacteria may appear in the bottom of the tube. About 200 white cells or 500 red blood cells/mm will cause cloudiness.[3] Mucus threads originate from bladder, prostate, and kidney and are of little significance. There is some evidence that mucus may in part be derived from the kidney and is a Tamm-Horsfall protein product of distal tubular secretion. Cellular contamination in carelessly collected urine samples from female patients is a common cause of turbidity. "Greasy" cloudiness may be caused by large amounts of fat or chyle. (Microscopic examination should be performed in all instances, of course, regardless of clarity or turbidity!)

HYDROGEN ION CONCENTRATION (pH)

Normal pH of a random urine sample ranges from about 4.5 to 8.0, although it generally lies between 5.5 and 6.5. Mean normal value of a 24-hour sample is about 6.0. The pH of urine depends on hydrogen ion secretion by the kidney tubules, titratable acid filtration, ammonia formation, bicarbonate reabsorption, and changes in glomerular filtration rate and renal blood flow. Acids or anions (largely sulfuric and phosphoric acids and ketone bodies) are produced from protein and fat metabolism. The hydrogen normally excreted via the kidney appears

TABLE 1–1. Substances That May "Discolor" Urine.

Color imparted to urine	Drugs and substances responsible
Amber	Normal; urobilin; bilirubin
Nearly colorless	Large fluid intake; reduction of perspiration; chronic nephritis; untreated diabetes mellitus; diabetes insipidus; alcohol ingestion; diuretic therapy; and nervousness
Orange	Concentrated urine; restricted fluid intake; excess sweating; fever; urobilin; small quantities of bile pigments; phenazopyridine and amidopyrine
Orange to orange-red	Ethoxazene (Serenium); phenazophridine (Pyridium)
Orange-red-brown	Rhubarb; senna; verdoglobin
Orange to purple-red	Chlorzoxazone (Paraflex)
Orange-yellow (in alkaline urine)	Salicylazosulfapyridine (Azulfidine); anisindione (Miradon); phenindione (Hedulin)
Rust yellow or brownish	Sulfonamides; nitrofurantoins (Furoxone, Furadantin, etc.)
Pink or red to red-brown	Diphenylhydantoin (Dilantin); phensuximide (Milontin); 1,8-dihydroxyanthraquinone (in Dorbantyl, Doxidan, Modane); Emodin in alkaline urine; phenolphthalein (in Ex-Lax, etc.); phenothiazines (Thorazine, etc.)
Magenta	Phenolphthalein (in Ex-Lax, etc.)
Red	Blood; amidopyrine (Pyramidon) phenazopyridine (Pyridium); neotropin; prontosil; aniline dyes; beet-root; porphyrins, hemoglobin; myoglobin, phenolsulfonphthalein; phenazopyridine (Pyridium)
Purple-red	Phenol red and phenolphthalein in alkaline urine.
Port wine	Porphyrin; mixture of methemoglobin and oxyhemoglobin
Dark brown	Altered blood (methemoglobinuria); phenolic drugs (phenol, cresol); phenylhydrazine; porphyrins; melanin
Brown-black	Much hemoglobin; lysol poisoning; melanin; iron-sorbitol-citric acid complex (Jectofer), homogentisic acid; cascara; rhubarb
Smokey	Red blood cells
Yellow	Riboflavin
Yellow foam	Bilirubin pigments
Green foam	Biliverdin
Green	Biliverdin and other bile pigments; methylene blue; indigocarmine; carbolic acid; guaiacol (in cough remedies); santonin; acriflavine (in bladder irrigants for presurgical skin preparation); methocarbamol (Robaxin) with urine standing a long time
Pale blue fluorescence	Triamterene (Dyrenium)
Blue	Methylene blue; indigo blue
Blue-green	Tolonium (Blutene); methylene blue; amitriptyline (Elavil)

in the urine as ammonium ion, acid phosphate, or undissociated weak organic acids. Excretion of the ammonium ion conserves sodium, potassium, calcium, and magnesium, which are reabsorbed, along with bicarbonate ions. The net result is an acid urine. Hydrolysis of glutamine is a major source of ammonia. Bicarbonate reabsorption aids in determining the rate of acid excretion, particularly in the proximal tubes. Of the H^+ output of the proximal convoluted tubules (about 3500 mEq/day), all but 50 to 100 mEq/day is reabsorbed in the distal tubules. This important function, along with concentrating ability, is one of the earliest physiologic mechanisms lost in a patient with pyelonephritis or with necrosis of the distal tubular epithelium.[7] It should be remembered, however, that urinary pH is a measure of free hydrogen ions and does not reflect the total acid excretion.

Besides being of importance in the early detection of pyelonephritis or tubular necrosis, the determination of urinary pH is important in determining predisposition for type of urinary calculus formation (Table 1–2).[8]

When there is metabolic acidosis, urine tends to become more acid; when there is metabolic alkalosis, more alkaline. Respiratory acidosis and alkalosis tend to be compensated for by appropriate changes in urinary acidity. There may be discrepancies, however, as is the case in renal tubular acidosis, in which urine may be relatively alkaline in the presence of metabolic acidosis, because of inability of kidneys to excrete acid.

More patients with uric acid stones have a consistently acid urine than have an elevated serum uric acid. In acid urine, urates and sulfonamides may precipitate; while in alkaline urine, triple phosphate calculi tend to form. Urine pH is low in patients with metabolic acidosis (diabetes mellitus, starvation, diarrhea), in patients with respiratory acidosis (emphysema, anesthesia, hyperpyrexia, methyl alcohol poisoning), and in patients with certain metabolic diseases (phenylketonuria, alkaptonuria). Patients with uric acid stones, as mentioned previously, may produce persistently acid urines. Fruits and vegetables

TABLE 1–2. Summary of Correlations Between Urinary pH and Stone Constituents.

Acid pH (pH 5.5 to 6.0)	Alkaline pH (pH greater than 7.0)	Acid pH (pH less than 5.5)
Calcium oxalate	Magnesium ammonium phosphate	Uric acid
Apatite	Calcium phosphates (including apatite, calcium dihydrogen phosphate dihydrate, tricalcium phosphate)	Cystine Xanthine

(Freeman, J., and Beeler, M. Courtesy of Postgrad. Med.)

that form bicarbonate in the body (except for cranberries, plums, and foods containing benzoic acid) decrease acidity. Starvation produces ketosis and therefore acidic urine. Persistently alkaline urines may be produced in patients with respiratory and metabolic alkaloses (the latter occur in patients with prolonged gastric suction, intractable vomiting, overdose of alkali, "milk-alkali syndrome," constant diuretic therapy, hyperaldosteronism, Cushing's syndrome), and most commonly in patients with urinary tract infections caused by urea-splitting organisms. Most effective urea-splitting organisms are the proteus species. Dietary protein increases acidity, even though protein metabolism increases ammonia formation. Normally, a "post-prandial alkaline tide" occurs, causing decreased urinary acidity about 1 hour after a meal. Upon standing, as previously mentioned, urine becomes alkaline as bacteria split urea, releasing ammonia. In patients with renal insufficiency, the ability to excrete acid is reduced, chiefly secondary to impairment in ammonia excretion, but the ability to excrete a highly acid urine may be preserved even in frank renal failure. In patients with potassium deficiency, regardless of cause, the pH of urine tends to fall, as hydrogen ions are secreted in exchange for potassium ions, inasmuch as both potassium and hydrogen are excreted by the same mechanism.

In the medical microscopy laboratory, pH or acid excretion can be measured in several ways:

1. Potentiometric determinations (pH meter)
2. Titrametric methods (measure acidity, not pH)
3. Indicator paper methods

Use of the pH meter for the purpose is not practical, although it is an accurate method. Titrametric methods are too time consuming to be practical. Indicator dye methods are widely used because of their rapidity, inexpensiveness, and the useful information gained. Indicators may be regarded as weak organic acids (or bases) whose unionized molecules have one color, but whose anions (or cations, as the case may be) possess a different color.[9] For example:

$$\underset{\text{(color A)}}{[\text{H indicator}]} = \underset{\text{(color B)}}{[\text{indicator}^-] + [\text{H}^+]}$$

in the case of a weak acid. Applying the law of mass action to this ionization of the indicator acid, we get:

$$\frac{[\text{H}^+]\,[\text{indicator}^-]}{[\text{H indicator}]} = \text{K}' \;\; OR \;\; \frac{[\text{H}^+]}{\text{K}'} = \frac{[\text{H indicator}]}{[\text{indicator}^-]}$$

where "K′" is the apparent dissociation constant of the indicator. The color imparted to a solution by the indicator depends upon the relative proportions of the two forms of the indicator present in the solution, and this in turn depends upon the ratio of hydrogen ions to the dissociation constant. Since the K′ is a constant specific for each indicator, the color formed will depend upon hydrogen ion concentration of the solution entirely. In the case of bromcresol green for example, K′ = $10^{-4.7}$; the undissociated molecules are yellow, while the anions are blue. For this indicator, therefore, the following equation may be written:

$$\frac{[H^+]}{10^{-4.7}} = \frac{\text{Yellow molecules}}{\text{Blue ions}}$$

Thus, in solutions having a pH of between 3.8 and 5.4, the indicator exists as a mixture of yellow molecules and blue ions and the relative amounts of each of the substances in the mixture depend entirely on the hydrogen ion concentration. By use of paper strips impregnated with various dyes, the hydrogen ion concentration can be determined by the color of the paper after being dipped in urine. Several dyes are necessary to cover the required range of pH (pHydrion paper, Microessential Laboratories, Brooklyn, N.Y.; nitrazine paper, E.R. Squibb Co., N.Y.; and others).

The pH ranges of indicator dyes, some of which are utilized in these impregnated papers, are indicated in Figure 1–2. Indicator impregnated dye papers are so inexpensive and simple as to warrant their routine use in the clinical laboratory.

CONCENTRATION OF SOLIDS

Although approximately 170 L of fluid, basically an ultrafiltrate of plasma, are formed by the renal glomeruli each day, an average of only 1.5 L is voided as urine. This reduction in volume results from renal tubular activity and from body regulatory systems responsive to changes both in solute concentrations and in fluid volume. Physiologic adjustments result from the level of antidiuretic hormone secretion in turn provoked by osmoreceptors stimulated by increased plasma osmolality. Antidiuretic hormone promotes reabsorption of water from urine in the distal tubules and collecting ducts of the kidney by rendering the epithelium freely permeable to water. Quantity of metabolic products and absorbed foodstuffs and minerals determine the solid content of urine. Increasing protein intake will necessarily increase the urine content of its metabolites, including urea, uric acid, and creatinine. Similarly, increasing intake of salt will necessarily increase the salt content of urine, and increasing the intake of water will normally increase the amount of water in the urine. Because of the normal wide variation in

pH Ranges of Indicators *

Based on data of the Federal Materials Testing and Research Institute, St.Gall, Switzerland

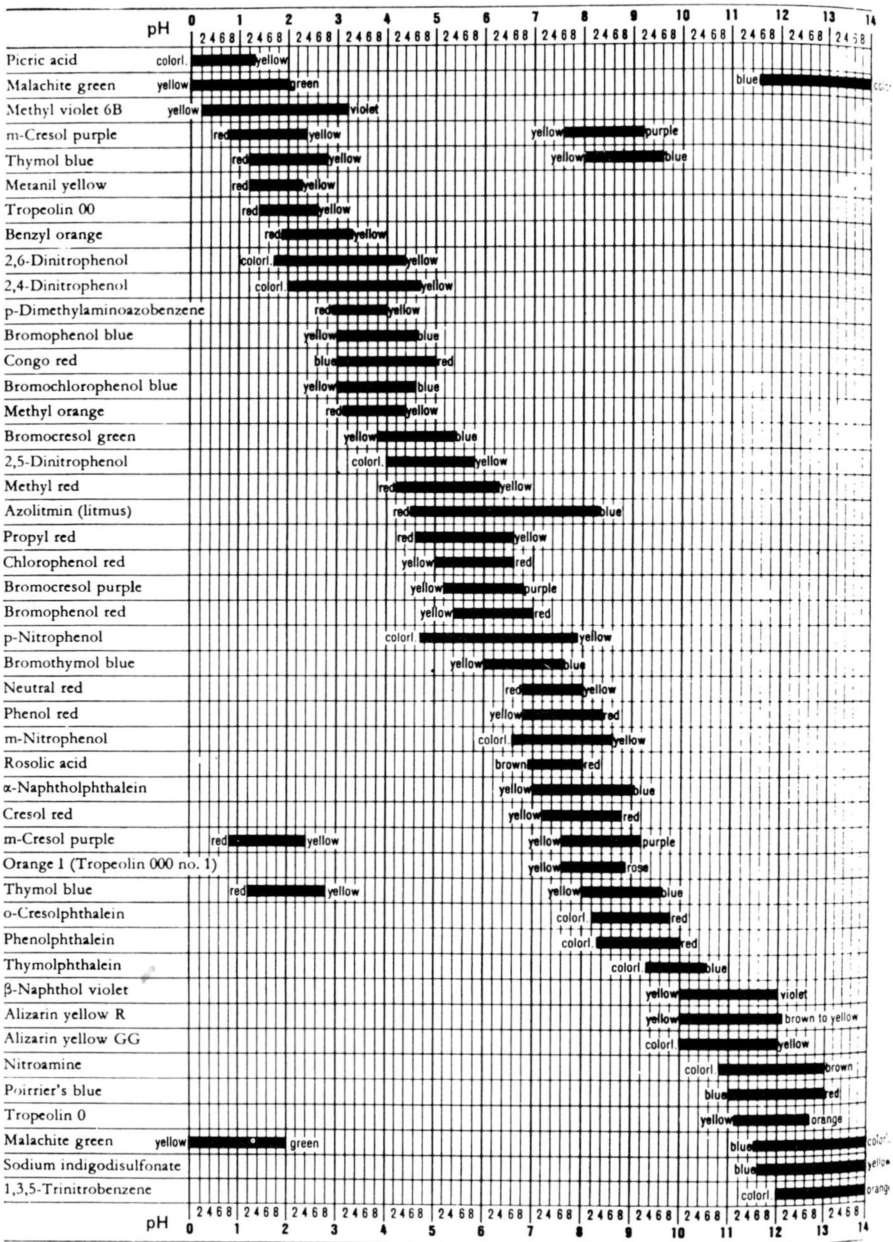

* With acknowledgments to Distillation Products Industries, Rochester, N.Y.

Fig. 1–2. pH range of indicators. (Diem, K. (ed.): Documenta Geigy Scientific Tables. Basle, Switzerland, 1962. (With acknowledgments to Distillation Products Industries, Rochester, N.Y.)

intake of foods, salts, and water, there must be flexible but precise and selective reabsorption of water and other substances from the glomerular filtrate by the tubular cells in order to maintain constancy of composition of the extracellular fluid, a condition of life. For this reason, the solid content of urine varies, in health, in both directions from the solid content of plasma (excluding protein); that is, it may be more or less concentrated, both situations requiring work by the renal tubular epithelial cells.

Concentration of solids in urine, the best index of the concentrating ability of the kidneys, can be measured in a number of ways in the clinical microscopy laboratory:

1. Weighing aliquots of urine on an analytical balance
2. Determination of specific gravity (usually with a hydrometer)
3. Determining light refraction (light refraction in a TS meter)
4. Determining osmolality (usually by measurement of depression of the freezing point, or the vapor pressure)
5. Determining surface tension

All of these measurements have inherent problems or difficulties when applied as clinical methods. They are interrelated, but no two are identical.[10]

Highly accurate and precise measurements of specific gravity can be performed by weighing aliquots of known volumes of urine on an analytical balance, and comparing these weights with known weights of distilled water at the same temperature. This procedure is not sufficiently practical to be a routine method but may be useful for a patient with sudden onset of severe oliguria if no other method is available for the amount of urine sent to the laboratory.

"Osmolality" may be defined as "the number of active particles (osmoles) of solute present per kg of solvent (water, in this case).[10] The number of osmoles is equal to "θn mols," where θ is the osmotic coefficient and n the number of particles or ions formed upon dissociation of the solute in solution, and M is molality.

$$\text{Osmolality} = \theta n M$$

For example, the θ for NaCl is 0.93; then 1 kg water containing 1 mole of NaCl will contain $2 \times 0.93 \times 1$ mole $= 1.86$ osmoles of NaCl. The osmotic coefficient (θ) for nonelectrolytes such as glucose and urea is one.

As Joseph Holmes has pointed out, specific clinical applications of the urine osmolality determination include:[10]

1. Calculation of free water clearance
2. Study of the ratio of plasma to urinary osmolality in the differential diagnosis of diabetes inspidus and compulsive water-drinking

3. More precise evaluation of concentration-dilution tests
4. To differentiate, when used with the specific gravity measurement, an increase in urinary excretion of small molecular metabolites as compared with those of large molecular size
5. For evaluating renal solute excretion in patients with kidney disease

The urine or serum osmolality determination has been used diagnostically:

1. To evaluate hyper- and hyponatremia
2. To determine the extent of solute retention in acute renal failure
3. As a substitute for multiple electrolyte determinations
4. For evaluation of various metabolic disturbances within the body when chemical procedures for measuring solutes concerned are not available

According to Joseph Holmes, the last application is useful in patients with liver disease. Holmes reports an average normal value of 290 mOsm/kg (currently designated as mmol/Kg) of serum for males and 285 mmol/Kg of serum for females, based on determinations on medical and nursing students and hospital personnel in the age range of 20 to 40 years.

Otto Beckmann devised the first relatively sensitive apparatus for determining the freezing point of a solution in 1888.[11] Numerous instruments suitable for routine clinical use are now available commercially in the United States (see yearly Scientific Instruments Guide, published as a special issue of Science for the American Association for Advancement of Science).

In dilute solution, reduction in freezing temperature is proportional to the total number of particles of solute per unit volume of solvent. The freezing point itself is defined as that temperature at which an infinitesimal amount of solid phase will exist in equilibrium with the liquid phase at standard pressure. In practice, for determining osmolality, the solution is super-cooled. Crystallization is then induced by agitation, producing heat of fusion, resulting in plateauing of the temperature curve at a point slightly below the freezing point. This point, however, is used for calculations, and by comparing unknowns to standards, no correction is needed. (The temperature of the solution never does rise to the freezing point of the original solution because the concentration is decreased after the beginning of crystallization.)

If a single molecular species is present in solution, such as sodium chloride, a close correlation exists between the number of osmotically active particles (osmolality) and the density of the particles (specific gravity) (Fig. 1–3). For a solution such as urine, with variable and complex composition, this correlation is not as close. Nevertheless, there is a correlation between urine osmolality and specific gravity.

Osmolality may be calculated from the freezing point depression, since 1 g molecular weight of any substance will release Avogadro's number (6.023×10^{23}) of particles and will depress the freezing point by 1.86° C. A specific gravity of 1.025 is roughly equivalent to an osmolality of 800 mmol/Kg.[13] Correlation is poorer in subjects on special diets. Patients with sodium-restricted diets, for example, have specific gravities decreased proportionately more than osmolality.

The hydrometer method is probably still widely used for measuring specific gravity, unfortunately. In most clinical microscopy laboratories, this method involves use of a urinometer (a hydrometer calibrated at 16° C for this measurement). Although the method is inaccurate, poorly reproducible, and subject to many variabilities, including interinstrument as well as intertechnologist bias, the method is still capable of generating useful clinical information. Specific gravity may be defined as the mass of a unit volume divided by the mass of a similar volume of distilled water under standard conditions.

Most urinometers are manufactured to read 1.000 in distilled water at 16° C. Since temperature affects the specific gravity, a correction

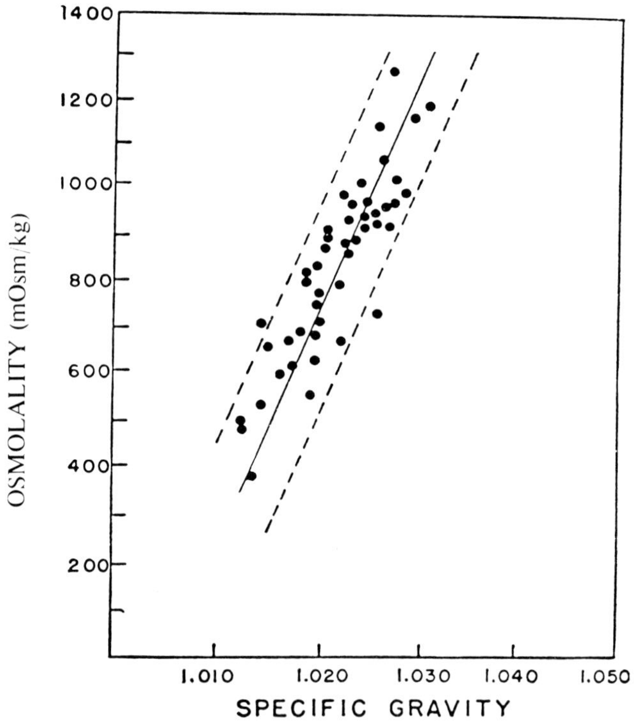

Fig. 1–3. Specific gravity vs osmolality. There is a somewhat linear relationship between specific gravity and osmolality, although the two techniques measure different parameters. (Dusten, H., and Corcoran, A. Courtesy of Med. Clin. N. Am.)

must be made by adding or subtracting 0.001 for every 3° C above or below 16° C. There are difficulties with use of urinometers: the scales on some instruments are not accurate, and are sometimes difficult to read; turbidity of the urine may make it difficult to read the scale; the plummet may adhere to the sides of the vessel; the urinometer may be calibrated inaccurately during manufacture. Since glass is theoretically a supercooled liquid and not a solid, the plummet may change shape and size, and therefore, require recalibration. Urinometers should be calibrated with standard solutions of sodium chloride or glucose. They should be cleaned as specified in National Bureau of Standards Circular 555 (on hydrometers). Formulas for standard calibrating solutions can be found in CRC Laboratory Handbook of Chemistry and Physics.

Table 1–3 compares specific gravities obtained by a carefully calibrated Squibb urinometer, a NaCl solution-standardized Spee-Grav temperature-compensated instrument, a factory-calibrated American Optical TS meter, and a Fiske osmometer. In general, the TS meter read low in most instances as compared to the urinometer and Spee-Grav instrument. For calibration purposes, 20 readings should be made with each solution, and the standard deviation should be calculated. The

TABLE 1–3. Comparison of Urine Specific Gravities and Osmolality Determined by Osmometer, Speegrav Temperature-Compensated Photoelectric Hydrometer, TS Meter, and Carefully Calibrated Squibb Urinometer.

Specimen Number	Osmolality (mmol/Kg)	Specific Gravity		
		SPEE-GRAV	URINOMETER	TS METER
1	300	1.008	1.007	1.005
2	462	1.011	1.010	1.010
3	626	1.018	1.015	1.013
4	791	1.022	1.025	1.021
5	758	1.021	1.019	1.018
6	851	1.024	1.022	1.021
7	892	1.025	1.025	1.022
8	754	1.022	1.020	1.022
9	660	1.016	1.018	1.017
10	421	1.010	1.011	1.007
11	536	1.014	1.015	1.015
12	393	1.012	1.011	1.009
13	547	1.015	1.015	1.014
14	503	1.011	1.012	1.010
15	873	1.018	1.021	1.021
16	769	1.017	1.020	1.018
17	308	1.006	1.009	1.007
18	725	1.018	1.021	1.016
19	461	1.010	1.012	1.010
20	295	1.006	1.006	1.004

(Prepared by the authors in the laboratories of the Ochsner Clinic, New Orleans, La., 1965.)

departure of the readings from the known specific gravities should not be more than 0.002 specific gravity units, or the urinometer should be discarded and a new one calibrated. Furthermore, different measurements by different individuals on different solutions show variability (1 SD) of about 0.003 specific gravity units. We suggest, for greater accuracy, that routine measurements be performed in duplicate and the results averaged. Photoelectrically temperature-compensated hydrometers available on the market today have a reproducibility of ±0.0005 specific gravity unit. They are, however, expensive, costing about $350; large numbers of specimens would have to be measured to justify this expense.

Since specific gravity and refractive index measurements are related, both reflecting the quantity of dissolved solid, the TS meter or other refractometers can also be used to calculate specific gravity. The value of the TS meter lies in its rapidity, its simplicity, and the extremely small volume (1 drop) of urine necessary; all of which compensate for the cost of over $500 for the instrument. (For most hydrometers, by contrast, approximately 15 ml of urine are required, although some operate effectively on less.) George Leonard and Myrton Beeler, in an unpublished study at Ochsner Clinic, found that readings with a TS meter purchased through regular commercial sources on 100 haphazardly selected urine specimens averaged lower by 0.002 specific gravity unit than average values obtained with a carefully calibrated Squibb urinometer. This suggests the necessity for checking calibration of TS meters. At Earl K. Long Memorial Hospital, we have found similar discrepancies. We make corrections by adding 0.002 specific gravity unit to the readings in urine with patients in renal failure or when critical measurements are necessary. Calculation, incidentally, cannot be done with sugar or salt solutions as for hydrometers, because the TS meter is especially adjusted for the usual comparison of urine.

For the 1965 National Comprehensive Laboratory Survey by the Subcommittee on Surveys of the Standards Committee of American Society of Clinical Pathologists, 70% of participants used urinometers for determining specific gravity, 25.5% used refractometers, and 4.5% used other unspecified methods.[14] A graphic representation of the data is shown in Figure 1–4. Results are very similar to those obtained in the 1964 Comprehensive Survey. Sixty-seven per cent of the participants obtained acceptable results using a urinometer, whereas 92% of the participants using a refractometer obtained acceptable results, as defined by the Committee (mean ± 2 SD of peer group). The difference between the two methods seemed remarkable in the published results of the survey; however, the material was "ersatz" urine, for which the TS meter is not properly calibrated.

Of the series just referred to, numbering more than 500 specimens measured by both methods, differences greater than .006 specific gravity

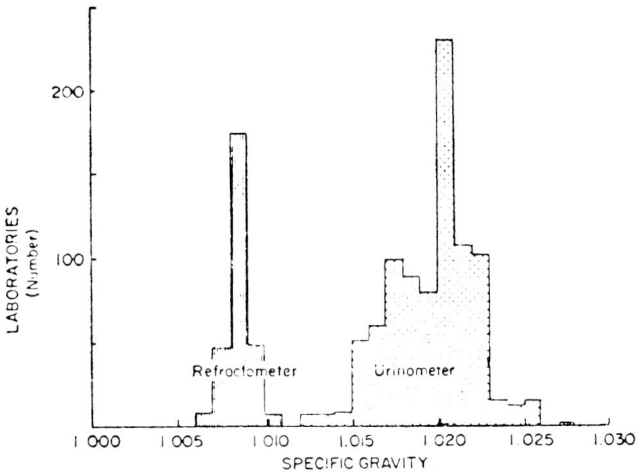

Fig. 1–4. Report of the Standards Committee, College of American Pathologists, 1965 National Comprehensive Laboratory Survey (a part of which was specific gravity determinations done on a sodium sulfide solution). Reference laboratory values obtained on this specimen were as follows: urinometer (calibrated against distilled water at 25° C), 1.018 ± 0.004; specific gravity by weight, 1.019 ± 0.002; refractometer, 1.008 ± 0.001; osmolality, 349 mOsm/kg. The results are very similar to those obtained on the 1964 comprehensive survey. More than 500 laboratories throughout the United States were surveyed. The differences between the two methods should be evaluated in light of the "ersatz" urine used in the survey. The TS meter is not calibrated to yield correct results for solutions other than urine.

unit were found in most instances. In the study, specific gravity was measured on uncentrifuged urine. Centrifugation did not change the results by the urinometer method. It is of interest that all of the specimens in which there were significant differences between methods contained considerable numbers of bacteria as well as epithelial cells and white cells in the urine sediment. The refractometer readings were almost invariably lower than the urinometer results, in part because of the use of "ersatz" urine.[14]

Probably the greatest usefulness of the measurement of specific gravity of random urine specimens lies in interpreting other findings in the urine analysis. Red cells and casts are not stable in dilute alkaline urine, and abnormal quantities of protein are diluted to nearer normal concentration.

Though urea, sodium, and chloride normally comprise the bulk of dissolved solids in urine, glucose and protein content also affect specific gravity. For every 1 g of glucose/100 ml of urine, 0.004 must be subtracted from the value of the specific gravity; and, for every 0.4 g of protein/100 ml of urine, 0.001 must be subtracted.

If the specific gravity of a random urine specimen is 1.025 or more or if the osmolality is 800 mmol/Kg or higher, it is usually not necessary to perform more sophisticated tests for renal concentrating ability.[12]

The average 70-kg man excretes about 60 g of solids in the urine/24 hours. After age 45, this becomes less; and by age 75, it is approximately 30 g of solids/24 hours, assuming average intake of fluids in each age group. Total solids of urine can be estimated from the specific gravity by multiplying the last two figures of the specific gravity of a 24-hour urine by 2.6 (Long's coefficient), giving amount of total solids (g) per L of urine. Under conditions of stress involving water deprivation, concentrating ability of the kidneys can be estimated from measurement of specific gravity or osmolality of the urine (Table 1–4). Tests of concentrating ability are unreliable in edematous patients, especially if they are undergoing diuresis. Otherwise, loss of concentrating ability is an indication, as a rule, of kidney disease, including, especially, pyelonephritis. It may also be seen in patients with renal calcinosis associated with hypercalcemia, and in those with sickle cell disease. Transient losses of concentrating ability may result from low potassium nephropathy, and there may be rapid loss in acute tubular necrosis.

When there is sudden onset of oliguria, precise and accurate measurements of specific gravity or osmolality are of greater value than is examination of urinary sediment in differentiating prerenal causes of oliguria, such as salt depletion and dehydration, from acute tubular necrosis. Concentrated urine is found in the latter states. The differentiation is particularly important because of the need to restrict fluids in patients with acute tubular necrosis and to give fluids and electrolytes to patients who are salt-depleted or who are dehydrated.

The most sensitive test for renal damage early in this condition is the free water clearance test, which is equal to volume of urine excreted per unit of time minus the volume of plasma osmotically cleared per the same unit of time (VP or osmotic clearance). The latter,

$$\mathrm{Vp} = \frac{\mathrm{Cu} \times \mathrm{Vu}}{\mathrm{Cp}}$$

where C = osmolality, V = volume, p = plasma and u = urine. True water clearance is normally negative when it becomes zero or positive following, for example, shock or surgery. It provides early warning of impending acute renal failure.

Many different concentration tests have been devised, and of these, Fishberg's is perhaps the most widely used. This test requires restriction of fluid intake for approximately 12 hours; three subsequent urine collections, 1 hour apart; and measurement of specific gravity of each specimen. When determining renal concentrating ability, it is good practice to place the patient on a diet high in protein for 3 days prior to the test, requesting that he eat a dry supper at 6 P.M. the evening before the test is to be done. He should void and discard the specimen

TABLE 1–4. Serum and Urine Osmolalities in Various Disorders, and the Mechanism of Their Deviation from Normal.

Pathologic condition	Serum osmolality	Urine osmolality	Mechanism
Post surgery	Decreased	Increased	Increased adrenal stimulation, decreased ADH secretion
Hepatic cirrhosis	Decreased	Increased	Decreased GFR, 2° hyperaldosteronism
Congestive heart failure	Decreased	Increased	Decreased GFR, 2° hyperaldosteronism
1° Aldosteronism	Normal to increased	Normal to decreased	Retention of Na, diuresis of water
Addison's Disease	Decreased	Normal to increased	Increased Na excretion
Diabetes insipidus	Increased	Decreased	Decreased ADH
Nephrogenic diabetes inspidus	Increased	Decreased	Decreased response of distal tubules to ADH
Hypokalemia and Hypercalcemia	Increased	Decreased	Increased water loss
Compulsive water drinking	Decreased	Decreased	Dilution
Iatrogenic water loading	Decreased	Decreased	Dilution (5% D/W)
Iatrogenic sodium loading	Increased	Increased	Normal saline (155 meq/L Na^+ and Cl^-)
High-protein diet	Increased	Markedly increased	Tube feeding with high-protein mixture
Inappropriate ADH secretion	Decreased	Increased	Water retention

(Holmes, J.: Workshop on Urine Analysis and Renal Function Studies, Pre-Workshop Manual. Commission on Continuing Education. Courtesy of American Society of Clinical Pathologists, 1962.)

at bedtime. Allow no fluid following this until the test has been completed. He is to collect a urine specimen at 8 A.M. the next day. Normal subjects are able to concentrate sufficiently for one of these urines to reach a specific gravity greater than 1.029. However, one specific gravity of at least 1.025 or greater (equivalent to an osmolality of 800 mmol/Kg or higher) indicates normal concentrating ability. According to Andrew Haraway and E. Lovell Becker, the normal patient will concentrate to over 800 mmol/Kg.[11] Values between 600 and 800 mmol/Kg indicate minimal impairment; 400 to 600 mmol/Kg, moderate impairment; and less than 400 mmol/Kg, severe impairment of renal concentrating ability. One can determine this more accurately by determining the ratio of urine to serum osmolality which is normally greater than three. Measurement of urine concentration only, however, provides an adequate test of renal concentrating ability in most patients.[15] In prolonged concentration testing, one frequently finds that the later specimens have lower specific gravity than the first specimens. On most occasions (approximately 90%) the first morning specimen is the most concentrated, and, therefore, indicative of the patient's ability to concentrate urine. While the urine concentration test is very sensitive and shows changes early in chronic renal disease, it is useless and may even be dangerous when, as in diabetes insipidus, the patient may be seriously dehydrated by withholding water from the diet. Decreased renal function may be discerned with this test before either phenolsulfonphthalein excretion or serum urea nitrogen is abnormal. Usually by the time the specific gravity is fixed at 1.010 or 1.008, phenolsulfonphthalein tests and others also reflect deficits in renal plasma flow and tubular excretory functions. Abnormal elevations of the serum urea concentration begin to appear when the specific gravity will no longer exceed approximately 1.015. Maximal concentration of urine can be achieved only when antidiuretic hormone (ADH) secretion is fully stimulated by adequate dehydration and the kidney is excreting a minimal amount of water. If the tubules cannot respond to ADH, or if ADH is lacking, water will not be conserved, and therefore, the urine will be relatively dilute despite need to conserve water. Failure to concentrate urine to a specific gravity greater than 1.008 occurs in very severe renal tubular disease; in the case of defective formation or release of ADH; and in certain reversible states such as severe anemia and hypokalemia. Pyelonephritis, hypokalemia, hypercalcemia, and sickle cell disease may cause the tubular dysfunction, as previously mentioned. Failure to concentrate urine may be as much a defect in tubular function or renal blood flow as a defect in ADH secretion. The phenolsulfonphthalein test, developed by Lawrence Roundtree and J.P. Gehardy in 1910, although crude, is still clinically useful in measuring tubular excretory function.

PROTEIN

Glomerular filtrate normally contains 10 to 25 mg protein/dl. Therefore, about 18 to 45 g of protein are normally presented to the tubules during each 24-hour period, and this amount is almost completely resorbed by the tubular epithelial cells. The resultant urine protein concentration is too low to be detected in random samples subjected to the heat and acetic acid test, sulfosalicylic acid test, or tests based on the protein error of indicator dyes. About 150 mg/24 hours, or about 20 mg/dl generally are regarded as the upper limit of normal. Proteins with molecular weights less than 40,000 daltons comprise a significant fraction of the total as do those between 40,000 daltons and 90,000 daltons, especially albumin. Proteinuria refers to protein in the urine in sufficient quantities to be detected by most clinical tests, thus implying abnormally high excretion of protein.[21] It is a very sensitive indicator for diffuse renal disease. The commonest pathologic cause of proteinuria is probably increased leakage through a damaged glomerular basement membrane rather than diminished reabsorptive capacity of the tubules. As proteinuria increases, proteins of increasingly high molecular weight escape into the urine, including not only albumin, but also more of the higher molecular weight globulins; although, even in normal urine, significant amounts of IgA and IgG are present. Albumin, because of its relatively small molecular weight (about 60,000 daltons) is more readily filtered than are the globulins, and is therefore usually abundant in pathologic conditions. This is why the term "albuminuria" has been used synonymously with "proteinuria," although the latter is more accurate. In pathologic states, the level of proteinuria, while continuous, is rarely constant, and not every sample of urine will be abnormal in patients with advanced nephritis. Different but characteristic electrophoretic patterns have been demonstrated for tubular and glomerular proteinuria. In the latter, selective proteinuria suggests a better prognosis than nonselective proteinuria. (Manuel, Y., Revillard, J., and Betuel, H.: Proteins in Normal and Pathologic Urine. Baltimore, University Park Press, 1970.)

Benign albuminuria, which is not dependent upon organic disease, can occur following violent exercise, severe emotional stress, prolonged exposure to cold (for instance, cold baths), ingestion of excessive amounts of protein (such as egg albumin), in pregnancy, and during the premenstrual state. However, in these conditions the proteinuria is generally mild and transitory.

Concentration of urinary proteins can increase from a normal 0.02 mg/ml at rest to as much as 5 mg/ml during exercise. However, since the urinary flow during exercise is reduced, the excretion of protein usually will not exceed 2 mg/minute under such circumstances. Most often, especially with strenuous exercise, the urinary protein content of urine will rise to its highest point within 30 minutes of the recuperative phase.

Immunodiffusion studies reveal regular occurrence in urine, during exercise, of albumin, prealbumin, α-1-acid-glycoprotein, α-1-antitrypsin, α-2-HS-glycoprotein, Zn-α-2-glycoprotein, α-2-Gc-globulin, ceruloplasmin, haptoglobin type 1-1 and 2-1, transferrin, hemopexin, β-1-microglobulin, β-1A-globulin, β-2-glycoprotein 1, 3S-α-1-globulin, α-A-globulin, α-G-globulin subunits, and α-G-globulins.[23] This excretion represents a quantitative increase in the patterns of proteins seen in normal urine, when the patient is at rest.[23]

Transitory proteinuria can also occur following injections of epinephrine or norepinephrine, in dehydration, following hemorrhage, in salt depletion, and in fevers. In addition, there is a benign condition, orthostatic albuminuria, in which morning urines collected before the patient arises tend to be negative; those collected while the patient has been in the erect position are positive. Orthostatic proteinuria can be induced in the majority of young adults by prolonged standing in an erect lordotic position, probably as a result of renal circulatory changes.

It is usually well below 1.5 g/24-hour volume. It is not usually clinically significant, although a small percentage of these individuals may have underlying renal disease indicated by minimal glomerular basement membrane changes. Normally, transglomerular diffusion of proteins is less during recumbency, since blood flow rate through the glomerulus is then higher and opportunity for resorption in the tubules is greater. A urine sample collected immediately after standing for 30 minutes in a lordotic position may contain as much as 1 to 3 g protein/L, and some (but usually less) protein is present following normal daytime activities.

Organically-caused albuminuria (albuminuria that results from disease) is commonly found in patients with cardiac disease, ascites, abdominal tumors, febrile states, convulsive disorders, hyperthyroidism, intestinal obstruction, hepatic disease with jaundice, hematologic disorders (leukemia, anemia, purpura), poison ingestion (turpentine, phosphorus, mercury, sulfosalicylic acid, phenol, lead, opiates, sulfonamides, barbiturates), and drug therapy (Table 1–5 and Fig. 1–5).

Proteinuria occurs not only in renal diseases affecting primarily the glomeruli, but also in all cases of severe tubular disease, such as acute tubular necrosis secondary to hypoxia, chronic interstitial pyelonephritis, primary renal tubular acidosis (Butler-Albright syndrome), multiple aminoaciduria syndromes (Fanconi's syndrome), chronic hypokalemia with hyperkaluria (Bartter's syndrome, or potassium-losing nephropathy), nephrogenic diabetes insipidus, and others.[23]

The dipstick tests for protein suffer from poor reproducibility for values of protein near normal; therefore, color changes that are slight ("trace") most often are an inaccurate observation. They may not detect abnormal protein, such as Bence-Jones light chains.

Proteinuria may occur during pregnancy without any demonstrable pathologic condition; with toxemia, with urinary infection, or following delivery (disappearing immediately postpartum). There is a close relationship between the severity of the toxemia and the degree of proteinuria. Proteinuria in patients with urinary tract infections may originate in part from degenerating leukocytes and renal tubular epithelial cells. In patients with active pyelonephritis (whether pregnant or not), proteinuria may be marked ($>$3 g/24 hours). Bacterial counts and culture of the urine are suggested in the event that active pyelonephritis is suspected (even in the absence of increased white blood cells, glitter cells, or pus casts). Many workers consider proteinuria of pregnancy to result primarily from a renal vascular change, rather than from an organic renal disorder.[23]

A trace or 1+ reaction for protein with Albustix, Labstix, or Multistix, or conventional screening test indicates significant proteinuria and implies significant renal disease. Reliability of Albustix compared with other protein tests is greater with lower than with higher concentrations of protein. Albustix estimations agreed with immunoassay results in

TABLE 1–5. Protein Excretion Rates in Various Renal Disorders.

	Protein Excretion Rate*			
Disease State	0.05–0.1 2/24 hrs.	0.1–1 2/24 hrs	1–3 2/24 hrs.	Over 3 2/24 hrs.
Exercise proteinuria	+			
Febrile proteinuria	+			
Postural proteinuria	+	+		
Arteriosclerotic renal vascular disease	+	+		
Hypertension, arterial	+	+	+ (rare)	
Congestive heart failure		+	+	+
Pyelonephritis	+	+	+ (rare)	
Polycystic renal disease	+	+		
Acute glomerulonephritis (Ellis Type I)	+	+	+	+
Membranous glomerulonephritis (Ellis Type II)		+	+	+
Drug-induced nephrotoxic agents (Mg, CCl_4, etc.)	+	+		
Nephrotic syndrome			+	+
Kimmelstiel-Wilson syndrome			+	+
Systemic lupus erythematosus	+	+	+	+
Polyarteritis nodosa	+	+	+ (rare)	
Multiple myeloma†	+	+	+	+
Systemic sclerosis	+	+		

*Approximate ranges of daily protein excretion in some common diseases of the kidney; divisions should be taken as a guide, rather than absolute range of excretion in these diseases.
†Does not refer to Bence Jones proteinuria but to more general proteinuria frequently seen in multiple myeloma.
(Harvey, A., et al. (eds.): The Principles and Practice of Medicine. 17th Ed. Courtesy of Appleton-Century-Crofts, 1968.)

74% of 250 samples, with sulfosalicylic acid methods in 71%, and with both methods in 65% of the cases in one series.

The finding of abnormal proteins in the urine is rare.[24] Under certain conditions, however, proteins may appear that are not normally found in serum, the most prominent of these being Bence Jones protein, the presence of which is highly suggestive (but not absolutely diagnostic) of multiple myeloma. Bence Jones proteins are light-chain (lambda-type) globulins (having a Svedberg constant of 3.5 to 4, and a molecular weight between 25,000 and 40,000 daltons). These proteins are seen in up to 85 percent of patients with multiple myeloma. "M-bands" may also be seen with protein electrophoresis. These are sharp peaks, lying between the β- and α-globulins, and may be seen in the presence or absence of Bence Jones protein.

The uncontrolled growth of a clone of plasma cells in multiple myeloma is slow and may be asymptomatic; however, it may be manifest

Quantitative protein excretion in various renal disorders

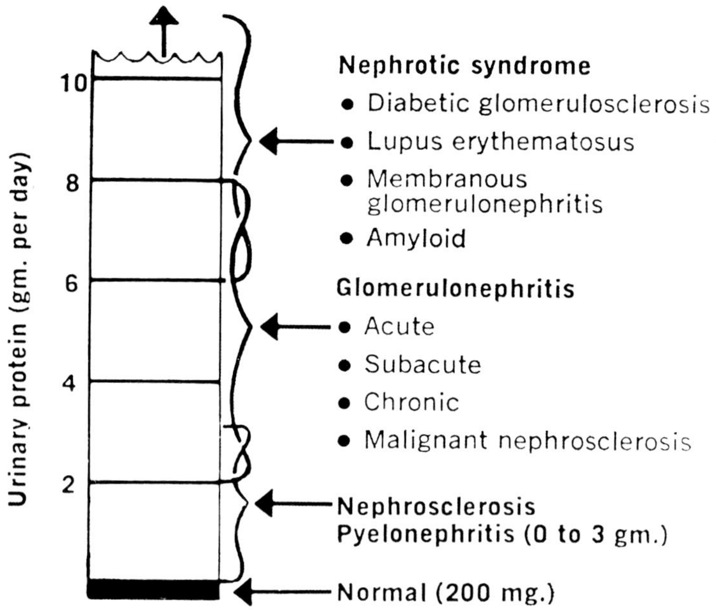

Fig. 1–5. Quantitative protein excretion in various renal disorders. (Garrett, J. Courtesy of Missouri Med.)

by demonstration of a monoclonal spike in serum protein electrophoresis, by demonstration of an abnormal light chain or immunoglobulin in urinary protein electrophoresis. There is a direct relationship between the size of the tumor mass and the quantity of protein present. Death of the patient may occur when the plasma cell tumor mass reaches 5×10^{12} myeloma cells, and only three doubling times may occur between diagnosis and death. In IgG myeloma, the doubling time had been estimated at 3 months, which closely relates to the mean survival of 7 months in untreated patients. Early diagnosis by demonstration with the above mentioned techniques can permit an earlier treatment and a more favorable prognosis according to Robert Mass (Brief review: Diagnosing and managing plasma cell (multiple) myeloma. Geriatrics, 33:53, 1978).

Monoclonal abnormal proteins in urine and in serum can be found in myeloma and also in other diseases, as follows:

Diagnosis	*Percentage of Cases*
Plasma cell myeloma (multiple myeloma)	60–65
Localized plasmacytoma	3–5
Waldenstrom's macroglobulinemia	5–8
Chronic lymphocytic leukemia and lymphocytic lymphoma	5–6
Benign monoclonal gammopathy	20–25
Hodgkin's disease and others	<1

Not all protein immunoglobulin abnormalities can be demonstrated by concentration of urine proteins and subsequent electrophoresis. When demonstrated, however, the relative frequency of protein abnormalities is as follows:

Immunoglobulin	*Percentage of Cases*
IgG	61
Light chain (lambda-type) globulins	19.5
IgA	17
IgD	1.5
IgE	<1
IgM (usually occurs in Waldenstrom's macroglobulinemia or benign monoclonal gammopathy)	—

GLUCOSE

Under stress, normal kidneys are capable of reabsorbing 250 to 350 mg of glucose/minute from the glomerular filtrate. If one assumes an average filtration rate of 125 ml/minute and a maximal arterial blood sugar concentration of 200 mg/dl after glucose ingestion, it may be seen that the quantity of glucose delivered to the tubules seldom exceeds 250 mg/minute in normal subjects. The maximal rate of reabsorption of glucose by the tubules is called the "maximal tubular reabsorption capacity (Tm_G)."

The term "mellituria" is used to designate abnormally increased amounts of sugar in the urine; whereas the terms "glycosuria" and "glucosuria" usually signify the presence of abnormally increased amounts of glucose in the urine.[16] Glucosuria may result from diabetes mellitus, phlorizin intoxication, intravenous glucose infusions, lowered renal threshold, brain injury, excitement, myocardial infarction, hyperthyroidism, and pregnancy. The renal threshold level for glucose (about 160 to 180 mg/dl blood, depending upon the method used to quantitate the glucose) may exhibit rather wide variations among healthy individuals. Since, in mild diabetes, the fasting blood sugar may stay below the threshold, glucosuria may occur only intermittently in such patients, usually following ingestion of carbohydrate-rich meals. Then, too, the threshold may be increased in longstanding diabetes. By combining semiquantitative measurements of urinary glucose (on a trace to 4^+ scale) with serial serum glucose determinations, an estimation of the renal threshold can be made.[17] Knowledge of the renal threshold level of glucose excretion in any individual patient will aid the physician in controlling the patient's blood sugar. For instance, if the urine is sugar-free, the physician cannot tell whether the patient's blood sugar is 140 mg/dl or 40 mg/dl, the latter value being near the hypoglycemic shock level in most patients. However, if the patient's urine is known to exhibit 1^+ glycosuria at a blood sugar level of 180 mg/dl, regulating the patient to spill a trace to 1^+ glucose test level will prevent hypo-

TABLE 1–6. Comparison of Urinary Sugar Screening Test, Glucose Oxidase Test, and Chromatographic Analysis of Sugars Found in Urine in Various Disorders.

Sugar Disorders	Screening Reducing Tests	Specific Test for Glucose (Glucose Oxidase Test)	Sugar Found by Chromatography
Primary pentosuria	positive	negative	Xylulose
Alimentary pentosuria	positive	negative	Arabinose
Essential fructosuria	positive	negative	Fructose*
Hereditary fructosuria	positive	negative	Fructose*
Galactosemia	positive	negative	Galactose†
Galactose-fructose intolerance	positive	negative	Glucose, galactose
Diabetes mellitus	positive	negative	Glucose
Glucose-galactose malabsorption	positive	positive	Glucose
Alimentary glycosuria	positive	positive	Glucose
Renal glycosuria	positive	positive	Glucose
Lactulosemia	positive	negative	Lactulose
Disaccharide intolerance‡	positive	negative	Lactose, galactose, (±) sucrose
Monosaccharide malabsorption	positive or negative	positive or negative	Glucose, galactose

*Tolerance tests must be done to confirm diagnosis.
†Red blood cell galactose-1-phosphate-uridyl transferase deficiency must be demonstrated.
‡The screening tests are highly unreliable for the detection of the disaccharide intolerances, inasmuch as these sugars are not absorbed in patients with monosaccharide and disaccharide intolerances. (Fecal sugars may be more helpful in these disorders.)
(Kodak CHROMAT/O/SCREEN Analysis Kit for Sugars, publication JJ-173, Eastman-Kodak Company, Rochester, p. 5, 1971; compiled partially from Stanbury, J., Wyngaarden, J., and Fredrickson, D. (eds.): The Metabolic Basis of Inherited Disease. 2nd Ed. Courtesy of McGraw-Hill, 1966.)

glycemic shock; while at the same time the blood sugar level will be under reasonable control. Recently, determination of glycosylated hemoglobin in the blood has been found to correlate very well with recent control of diabetes; but patients cannot, of course, perform the test themselves.

Diabetes, a disease of insulin deficiency characterized by glucosuria and hyperglycemia, is the most common disorder of carbohydrate metabolism. It has been estimated to occur in up to 4 to 8% of the population over age 40, so there are over 5 million diabetic patients in the United States, at least half of whom are undetected as patients. Tests for glycosuria should be included routinely in the performance of any urinalysis, since diabetes mellitus is a serious and common disease, and this is a simple (though relatively insensitive) screening method.

The Clinistix test is usually more sensitive than the Benedict's reaction for detection of glucose in the urine, the latter reacting to a level of 0.25 g/dl or higher; whereas the former may detect lower levels than this. Furthermore, the old screening tests (Benedict's test and Clinitest tablets) are not specific for glucose, but measure a variety of reducing agents. This may be an advantage when screening children for other metabolic disorders. Whenever the nonspecific screening tests are positive, a more specific test, such as provided by the Labstix, Multistix, Tes-tape test strips (glucose oxidase determination), Chemstrips, and other "dipstick tests," should be applied.[7] There is little need for use of the cumbersome Benedict's qualitative test, since the introduction of Clinitest tablets, which are simple to use and do not require a boiling water bath (as does Benedict's test).

Whenever the Clinitest result is positive and the Clinistix or Labstix examination is negative, investigations for conditions other than diabetes mellitus should be instituted, by such techniques as paper chromatography. The following is a list of the range and type of sugars that may be found in normal human urine:

Sugar	*mg/dl*
Sucrose	0–15
Lactose	0–10
Fructose	0–5
Galactose	0
Xylose	0–3
Glucose	0–12
Ribose	0
Xylulose	0

Unfortunately, the urine sugar test is not a very sensitive screening procedure for detecting diabetes mellitus. The diagnostic sensitivity and specificity achieved depend in part on the interval between the last meal and the urine specimen collection, as illustrated in the following chart:

Hours Post-Prandial	*Sensitivity (% diabetics +)*	*Specificity (% + diabetics)*	*Predictive Value (% true positives ÷ all positives for the general population)*
Fasting	34.4	88.3	15
1 hour	37.7	83.5	13
2 hours	54.1	80.6	16

(Note that this definition of specificity differs from that used earlier.) After 2 hours, sensitivity decreases and specificity increases again. (See discussion of diabetes mellitus under "Amino Acids and Metabolites of Disorders of Metabolism.") Predictive value can be dramatically increased by screening only adults who are prone or who have a family history of diabetes mellitus.

REDUCING SUBSTANCES AND SUGARS OTHER THAN GLUCOSE

Fructose, lactose, galactose, pentose, and sucrose may each be encountered in urine. All except sucrose are reducing agents and may react to the nonspecific tests for glucosuria, based on reducing capacity. Identification of sugars can be made readily by thin-layer or paper chromatographic techniques (see technique section).[18,19]

Normal human urine rarely contains more than five or six sugars, and then only in very low concentrations. Most abnormal urine specimens show only one or two sugars, but in much higher concentrations. The same is true of fecal extracts. Therefore, separation and identification of such mixtures are possible with one-dimensional chromatography.

Galactosuria, a hereditary metabolic disorder, occurs in 1:30,000 live births and is inherited as an autosomal recessive trait. It is caused by low activity of galactose-1-phosphate-uridyl-transferase which converts galactose-1-phosphate to glucose-1-phosphate. Galactosuria occurs a few days after ingestion of lactose. Unless detected early and treated by elimination of lactose and galactose from the diet, it may lead to development of cataracts, mental retardation, cirrhosis of the liver, and renal tubular dysfunction causing aminoaciduria. The diagnosis should be confirmed by demonstrating the enzyme deficiency in red blood cells. Galactosuria also may occur in advanced liver disease.

Pentosuria may occur in patients as a rare metabolic disorder and has also been reported to occur in morphine addicts. It is inherited as an autosomal recessive trait.

Lactosuria may occur during pregnancy and lactation.

Fructosuria is a rare metabolic abnormality inherited as an autosomal recessive trait with an incidence of 1:130,000. It causes no symptoms. Excretion of fructose is said to be stopped when fructose or sucrose is withdrawn from the diet. Hereditary fructose intolerance is also a rare condition, but not benign, in which fructosuria, proteinuria, and aminoacidurias occur. Clinically, symptoms include anorexia, emesis, hypoglycemic fits, and hepatosplenomegaly. Since recovery is possible when fructose is completely removed from the diet, early detection is important.

Sucrosuria may be accompanied by diabetic-like symptoms of thirst, loss of weight, and susceptibility to infection. It has been reported on occasion to be associated with mental retardation. Some patients excrete sucrose after only minimal intake. Ingestion of 100 g of sucrose results in pronounced sucrosemia. Levels as high as 35 to 45 mg of sucrose/dl of blood may be reached between 1 and 2 hours after ingestion. Normal individuals excrete sucrose only after a dose of 2 to 3 g/

TABLE 1–7. Sugars Found in Urine Due to Various Disorders.

Disorder	Glucose	Galactose	Fructose	Xylose	Ribose	Sucrose	Lactose
Renal Glycosuria	+						
Diabetes Mellitus	+						
Galactosuria		+					
Essential Fructosuria			+			+	
Hereditary Fructose Intolerances			+				
Familial Galactose and Fructose Intolerance		+	+				
Essential Pentosuria				+			
Ribosuria					+		
Endogenous Lactosuria							+
Congenital Lactose Malabsorption							+
Gastrointestinal Disorders						+	+
Congenital Lactosuria							+
Galactosemia		+					
Alimentary Glycosuria	+						

(Kodak CHROMAT/O/SCREEN Analysis Kit for Sugars, publication JJ-173, Eastman-Kodak Company, Rochester, 1971.)

kg of body weight. Unfortunately, sucrose is not a reducing sugar and therefore is not detected by the usual laboratory tests. If chromatography is used, the color developer must not rely on reducing ability if sucrose is to be detected.

Other reducing substances that may cause false positive "sugar" tests include preservatives (chloroform, formaldehyde), ascorbic acid, creatinine, homogentisic acid, glucuronic acid, and some antibiotics (penicillin and streptomycin). Sodium hypochlorite (household bleach) and vitamin C can cause false positive strip tests for glucose in urine. The glucose strip tests (Multistix and Chemstrip 8) should not be used to quantitate glucose in urine, because trained observers get inconsistent results with values less than 2.5 g/L of urine.[22]

Thin-layer chromatographic techniques are rather simple when compared to other chemical analyses. An experienced worker will be able to identify most sugars by their position (Rf value) and color after visualization. Rf value is defined in the following equation:

$$Rf = \frac{\text{Distance the sugar travels}}{\text{Distance the solvent front travels}} \times 100$$

Such proficiency can be gained only by testing many specimens of urine and plasma. When specific identification of the sugars present in urine is required, chromatography is indispensable (Table 1–7). Spot-test techniques based only on the reducing properties of sugars lack the specificity of thin-layer chromatographic techniques. Standards and normal urine samples should be run simultaneously.

KETONE BODIES

The ketone bodies include acetone, acetoacetic (diacetic) acid, and beta-hydroxybutyric acid, although the latter is not a ketone (Fig. 1–6). Acetone is a decomposition product of diacetic acid and is probably not produced as such within the body, although it is invariably found in the urine when the other two compounds are present. Normally, beta-hydroxybutyric acid constitutes about 40 to 70% of the ketone bodies. (There are no clinical tests for it, but when it is present, diacetic acid is also invariably present, and this can be detected.)

Ketone bodies are formed in the liver as intermediates in the metabolism of fatty acids, and in health they are almost completely further metabolized, so that only negligible amounts appear in the urine (up to 20 mg [expressed as acetone] /24-hour urine volume). Under conditions of abnormal carbohydrate metabolism such as occur in diabetes mellitus, they accumulate in the blood (ketonemia) and are excreted into the urine (ketonuria), a general condition known as ketosis. Ketosis is characterized by excessive formation and accumulation of these ketone bodies.[20,21] The accumulation of ketone bodies is often the cause of acidosis and coma in diabetics. Ketone bodies may occur in increased concentration in patients with other situations in which there is altered carbohydrate and fat metabolism, such as following exposure to cold, after violent exercise, in starvation, cachexia, eclampsia, pernicious vomiting of pregnancy, severe diarrhea, following administration of anesthesia, in von Gierke's (Cori type I) disease, and in patients on a high-fat, low-carbohydrate (ketogenic) diet. Severe ketosis almost invariably causes acidosis, except in patients in whom there is concomitant loss of hydrogen ions from constant gastric lavage or persistent vomiting.

Routine determination of urinary (and plasma) ketones should be performed for any patient showing greater than normal excretion of sugar or reducing substances. It is useful for following effects of treatment and in judging severity of the acidosis. Urine content may be surprisingly labile! Diabetic children who awaken following a day of

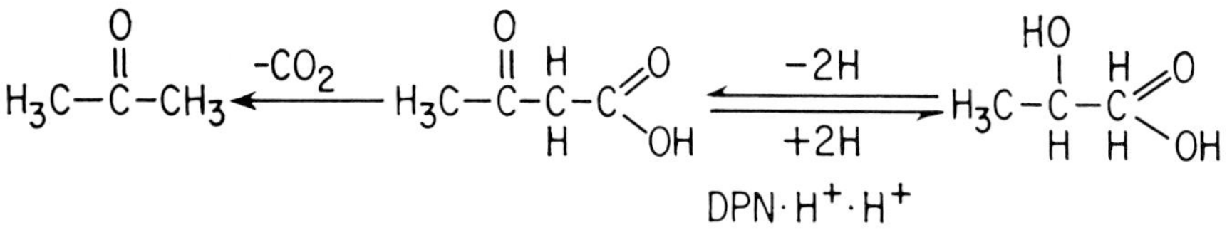

Acetone — Acetoacetic acid — β-hydroxybutyric acid

Fig. 1–6. Metabolic breakdown of acetoacetic (diacetic) acid and beta-hydroxybutyric acid.

inactivity with headache, malaise, and 4+ ketones in their urine may have a negative urine within an hour or so of strenuous exercise, such as running around a track. Since the development of the Acetest tables and Ketostix by the Ames Company, the Gerhardt test has been largely supplanted for screening of urinary ketones. There is no simple test for beta-hydroxybutyric acid, as has been mentioned. The substance can be oxidized to diacetic acid and estimated by the Hart's test, although there is no good reason for doing so.

To follow therapy, measurement of blood ketone levels frequently provides a more reliable estimate of the severity of acidosis than does measurement of ketones in the urine, sugar in the urine, sugar in the blood, or carbon dioxide content of the blood. The blood level of ketones (normally about 0.3 to 2 mg/dl) may exceed 50 mg/dl in diabetic acidosis. In other metabolic acidoses, the level rarely reaches 20 mg/dl.

PHENOLIC ACID AND CATECHOLAMINE METABOLITES (ESPECIALLY VANILMANDELIC ACID)[25–27]

It is alleged that one of every 200 hypertensive patients that are refractory to therapy with nonganglionic blocking agents, may have a phenolic acid or catecholamine secreting tumor. Judged by the Mayo Clinic series, the patients are as likely to have sustained as paroxysmal hypertension. (Those with persistent hypertension are 4 times more likely to have a malignant tumor, and about half the patients with sustained hypertension also have severe diabetes and evidence of hypermetabolism.) Since catecholamine and phenolic acid-secreting tumors are surgically curable, it is desirable to screen all hypertensive patients for elevations of catecholamines and other phenolic acids and their metabolites.

The adrenal medulla secretes two hormones: epinephrine (adrenaline, the major stored hormone) and norepinephrine (noradrenaline), the former being a methylated derivative of the latter. These compounds contain a catechol nucleus and an amine group; hence they are referred to as catecholamines (Fig. 1–7).

Hydroxylation of a benzene ring yields phenol (a weak acid). Meta-

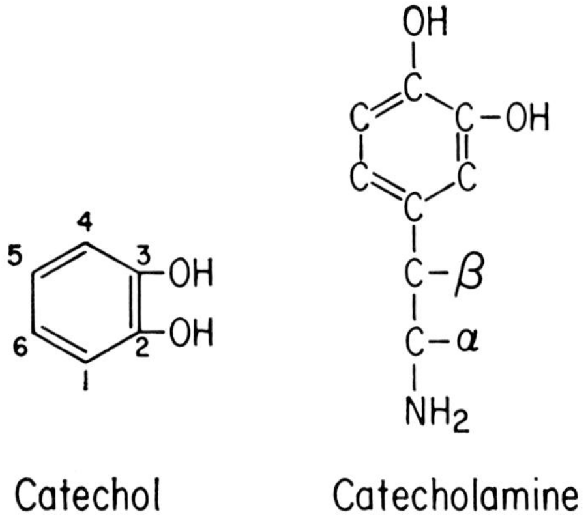

Fig. 1–7. Catechol and catecholamine nuclei. The ring carbons of the catechol nucleus are numbered counterclockwise. The side chains are identified by Greek letters starting with the carbon adjacent to the nitrogen. (Modified from Wortman, R. Courtesy of N. Engl. J. Med.)

bolic derivatives of the phenol ring, therefore, are collectively termed phenolic acids. Catecholamines are phenolic acids in which an additional hydroxyl group is present. There are some 50 or more phenolic acids that have been identified in human urine (Table 1–8).[26]

Epinephrine and norepinephrine are also synthesized in brain, chromaffin cells other than those of the adrenal medulla, and in postganglionic sympathetic neurons (the major source of the neurotransmitter norepinephrine), especially of the heart. Only a fraction of the catecholamines secreted by the arenal medulla is epinephrine. However, most of the epinephrine entering the blood stream comes from this source. Both epinephrine and norepinephrine are synthesized from the amino acids tyrosine and phenylalanine, and both are highly active pressor substances (Fig. 1–8). Norepinephrine elevates systolic and diastolic pressure by causing peripheral arterial constriction, while epinephrine causes a rise only in systolic pressure by its direct effect on the heart. Small amounts of epinephrine and norepinephrine are excreted in urine, partly as such, and partly as glucuronide and sulfate conjugates. The major portions of the hormones are transformed by enzymatic activity into a variety of deaminated metabolites, the principal one being 3-methoxy, 4-hydroxymandelic acid (vanilmandelic acid; VMA) (Fig. 1–9).

Biosynthesis and Metabolism of Catecholamines

Normally, 10 to 15 mg/L tyrosine are present in the blood stream. By an active transport mechanism it is removed from the circulatory system and concentrated in brain and other tissues. Within the chromaffin cells, it migrates from cytoplasm to mitochondria, back to cytoplasm, and finally to the chromaffin granules (which are specialized subcel-

TABLE 1–8. Major Phenolic Acids in Human Urine and Their Relative Rf Values in Two Different Solvents (Ipn-Ntlz Isopropyl Alcohol-Aqueous Ammonia-H_2O 8:1:1; Bz-Prop Acid Propionic Acid-Benzene-H_2O 3:3:1).

Compound No.	Description	RF Ipr-NH_3	RF Bz-Prop Acid
1	*p*-Hydroxyphenylacetic acid	0.42	0.49
2	Dark yellow (DzSA); light purple (DzPNA)	0.43	0.16
3	*m*-Hydroxyhippuric acid	0.33	0.09
4	*p*-Hydroxyhippuric acid	0.20 (0.15)	0.07
5	5-Hydroxyindoleacetic acid	0.28	0.16
6	Salicyluric acid	0.25	0.38
7	Homovanillic acid	0.37	0.68
8	Dark red (DzSA); gray (DzPNA)	0.06	0.21
9	*p*-Hydroxymandelic acid	0.34	0.07
10	Orange → red (DzSA); blue (DzPNA)	0.31	0.14
11	*m*-Hydroxyphenylacetic acid	0.45	0.49
12	*p*-Hydroxybenzoic acid	0.29 (0.23)	0.55
13	*o*-Hydroxyphenylacetic acid	0.75	0.58
14	*p*-Hydroxyphenyllactic acid	0.44	0.13
15	*m*-Hydroxybenzoic acid	0.45 (0.39)	0.47
16	Feruloylglycine	0.18	0.17
17	Vanilloylglycine	0.16	0.16
18	Orange-red (DzSA); blue-gray (DzPNA)	0.34	0.25
19	Vanillic acid	0.25	0.78
20	Dihydroferulic acid	0.45	0.74
21	*m*-Hydroxyphenylpropionic acid	0.56	0.61
22	*p*-Hydroxyphenylpropionic acid	0.53	0.59
23	αResorcylic acid	0.22	0.09
24	Dark yellow (DzSA); red (DzPNA)	0.35	0.37
25	Dark yellow (DzSA); reddish purple (DzPNA)	0.62	0.55
26	Reddish orange (DzSA); light purple (DzPNA)	0.63	0.33
27	Salicylic acid	0.78	0.88
28	Red (DzSA); blue (DzPNA)	0.37	0.93
29	Orange → gray (DzSA); light brown (DzPNA) (pregnancy urine)	0.44	0.03
30	Dark brown (DzSA); purple-brown (DzPNA)	0.16	0.02
31	Ferulic acid	0.29	0.78
32	Dark yellow (DzSA); light brown (DzPNA)	0.10	0.02
33	*p*-Hydroxycinnamic acid	0.33	0.60
34	Purple (DzSA); blue-purple (DzPNA)	0.06	0.07
35	*p*-Hydroxycinnamoylglycine	0.27	0.10
36	Orange (DzSA); yellow (DzPNA)	0.34	0.07
37	Reddish purple (fades) (DzSA); gray (DzPNA)	0.27	0.04
38	Purple (DzSA); blue-purple (DzPNA)	0.46	0.18
39	Maroon (DzSA); purple (DzPNA)	0.13	0.03
40	Gray (DzSA); blue-gray (DzPNA)	0.33	0.03
41	Light orange red (DzSA); purple (DzPNA)	0.21	0.04
42	Purple (DzSA); purple (DzPNA)	0.50	0.14
43	Brown (DzSA); gray (DzPNA)	0.07	0.00

(Armstrong, M., Shaw, K., and Wall, P. Courtesy of J. Biol. Chem.)

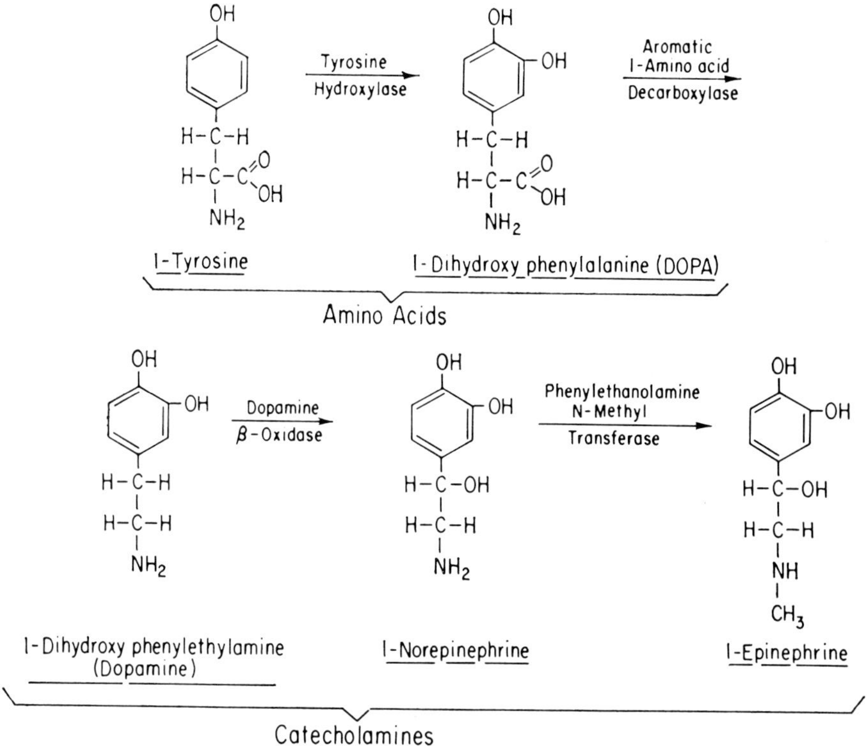

Fig. 1–8. Biosynthesis of catecholamines. Both epinephrine and norepinephrine are synthesized from phenylalanine and tyrosine. Phenylalanine hydroxylase converts phenylalanine to tyrosine. Dopamine, norepinephrine, and epinephrine are collectively termed catecholamines.

lular vesicles). At each site, an enzymatic reaction occurs, resulting in the final production of norepinephrine (Fig. 1–10). These enzymes are tyrosine hydroxylase, aromatic 1-amino acid decarboxylase, dopamine beta-oxidase, and phenylethanolamine N methyl transferase (the latter is found only in adrenal medulla, heart, and midbrain). In those chromaffin cells containing the enzyme for production of epinephrine, there is an added migration from chromaffin granules to the cytoplasm for n-methylation, then back to the granules for storage. In the rabbit there is an additional pathway for formation of epinephrine from tyramine.

Small amounts of epinephrine and norepinephrine are released continuously, and they are also released in spurts in response to sympathetic nerve impulses, hypoglycemia, and other physiologic stimuli. It has been suggested that tyrosine hydroxylation can control the rate of norepinephrine synthesis, secondary to stimulation by sympathetic nerve impulses from the central nervous system. Those organs with extensive sympathetic innervation take up the circulating catecholamines and store most of them in their original form. Receptor organs

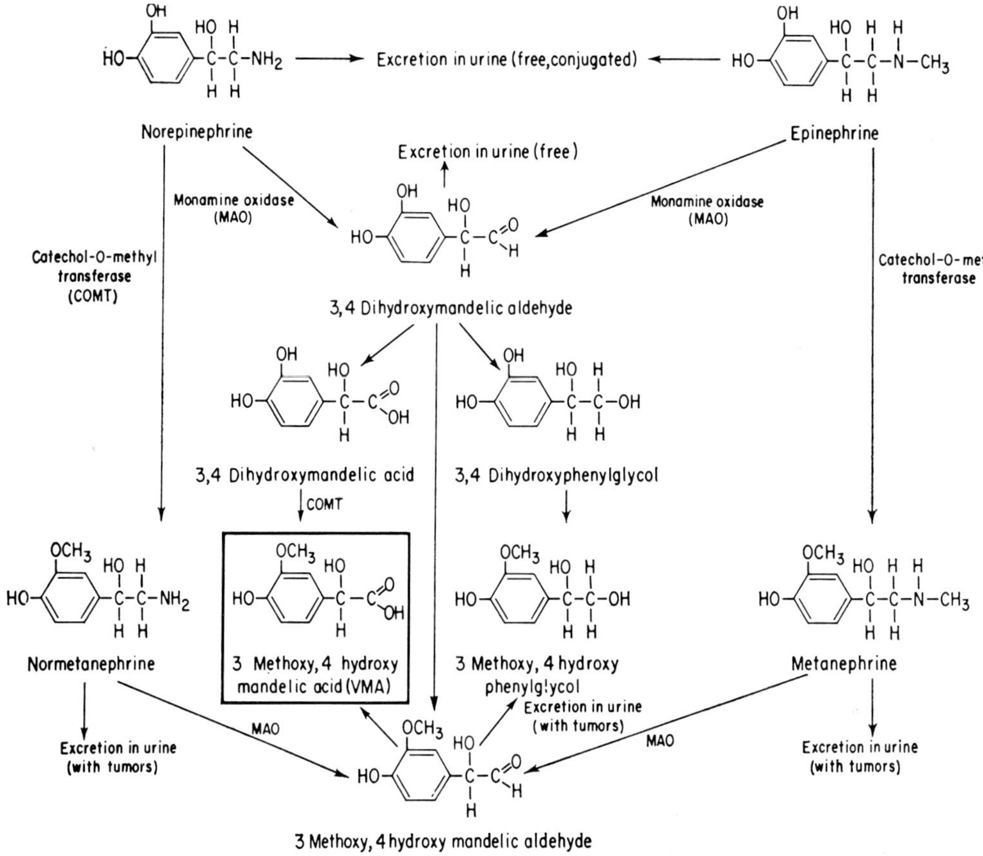

Fig. 1–9. Metabolism of epinephrine and norepinephrine with formation of vanilmandelic acid (VMA).

take most of them up within the first minute after delivery into the blood stream. Receptor sites responsible for smooth-muscle contraction have been labeled alpha receptors, and those responsible for relaxation, beta.

Catecholamines are metabolized by two routes, differing in that the initial deactivation is either by the enzyme catechol-O-methyltransferase (COMT), yielding metanephrine or normetanephrine, or by monoamine oxidase (MAO), yielding 3,4-dihydroxymandelic acid (DHMA). Epinephrine and norepinephrine taken up by organs which harbor high concentrations of the enzyme catechol-O-methyltransferase are transformed to their orthomethylated products, metanephrine and normetanephrine, respectively. This enzyme is largely responsible for the destruction of circulating catecholamines and is found in almost all tissues,

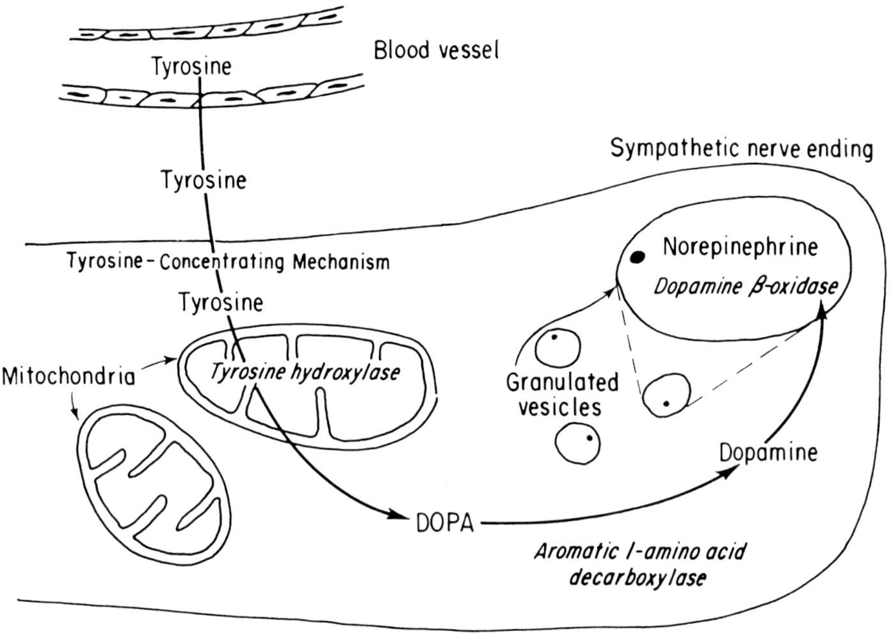

Fig. 1–10. Anatomical relationships of biochemical activity and biosynthesis of epinephrine in sympathetic nerve endings. (Wortman, R. Courtesy of N. Engl. J. Med.)

but is especially highly concentrated in liver and kidney, which receive a large share of the cardiac output.

Newly formed metanephrine and normetanephrine undergo further biochemical transformation (unless excreted in the urine as such) by the enzyme monoamine oxidase into 3-methoxy, 4-hydroxymandelic acid (VMA), and are excreted as such or as the glucuronide and sulfate conjugates.

A second pathway of catecholamine metabolism resulting in production of vanilmandelic acid is by direct action of the enzyme, monamine oxidase, on catecholamines within the nerve endings to yield 3-4 dihydroxymandelic acid. Small amounts of "free" material are released by the nerve endings, some of which interact with receptor sites, while the remainder is deprived of biologic activity by o-methylation. Catechol-O-methyltransferase action on 3-4 dihydroxymandelic acid, probably released independently of nerve impulses, yields 3-methoxy, 4-hydroxymandelic acid, and is the source of most of the VMA found in urine (Fig. 1–9).

The laboratory techniques most commonly applied to detection of catecholamine-secreting tumors in the past have been biologic or chemical assays of catecholamines. The most popular are modifications of the method of Lund, and involve adsorption on alumina, elution with acid, oxidation to adrenochrome and noradrenochrome, and tautomerization in alkali to form the fluorescent trihydroxyindoles. These assay procedures are not simple, especially because of difficulties inherent in use of fluorometric techniques. Partly for this reason, pharmacologic tests have been fairly widely employed. These tests depend on blood pressure response to such substances as histamine, phentolamine, and tyramine. They are unreliable and some are dangerous.

F. William Sunderman, Jr., devised a quantitative extraction technique in 1964 that has received widespread use throughout the United States.[28] After acidification of urine and removal of pigments and other interfering constituents by adsorption upon activated magnesium silicate, vanilmandelic acid is extracted with ethyl acetate from which it is re-extracted with carbonate. It is then oxidized to vanillin with potassium ferricyanide at an acid pH in the presence of zinc; the vanillin is extracted from the oxidation mixture with toluene, then re-extracted and reacted with indole phosphoric acid reagent to produce a salmon-colored complex that is measured photometrically at 495 nm. A simpler technique involving extraction and then diazotization with para-nitroanaline has been developed by the Hycel Corporation. This technique has also been widely used throughout the United States. Quantitative-recovery experiments by the authors have averaged about 85% for both these techniques.

Pheochromocytoma is a relatively rare tumor, usually benign, that may arise at any site of occurrence of chromaffin tissue, most commonly in the adrenal medulla. There is no race or sex predilection for occurrence of the tumor. There is, however, a familial tendency, and the tumor frequently coexists with van Recklinghausen's disease. Over 1,000 cases of pheochromocytoma have been reported since Albert Fraenckel recorded the first one in 1886. We have seen and diagnosed 13 such tumors during the past 10 years since being at the Earl K. Long Memorial Hospital. The right gland is affected more commonly than the left. Extra adrenal tumors have been recorded in about 7% of cases. Pheochromocytomas produce symptoms by secretion of large amounts of 1-epinephrine and 1-norepinephrine; and symptoms and signs include increased basal metabolic rate, hyperglycemia, sweating, trembling, and widened pulse pressure. The chief effect of norepinephrine secretion is increased total peripheral vascular resistance, giving rise to manifestations closely simulating those of essential hypertension (Fig. 1–11). The hypertension is purely paroxysmal in about 20% of cases and sustained in about 50%. The most useful diagnostic methods depend upon the demonstration of increased urinary excretion of 3-methoxy, 4-hydroxymandelic acid, or of epinephrine and norepinephrine, and their methoxy derivates.[27] VMA or metanephrine determinations are probably the most reliable.

Neuroblastomas and ganglioneuromas are rarer than pheochromo-

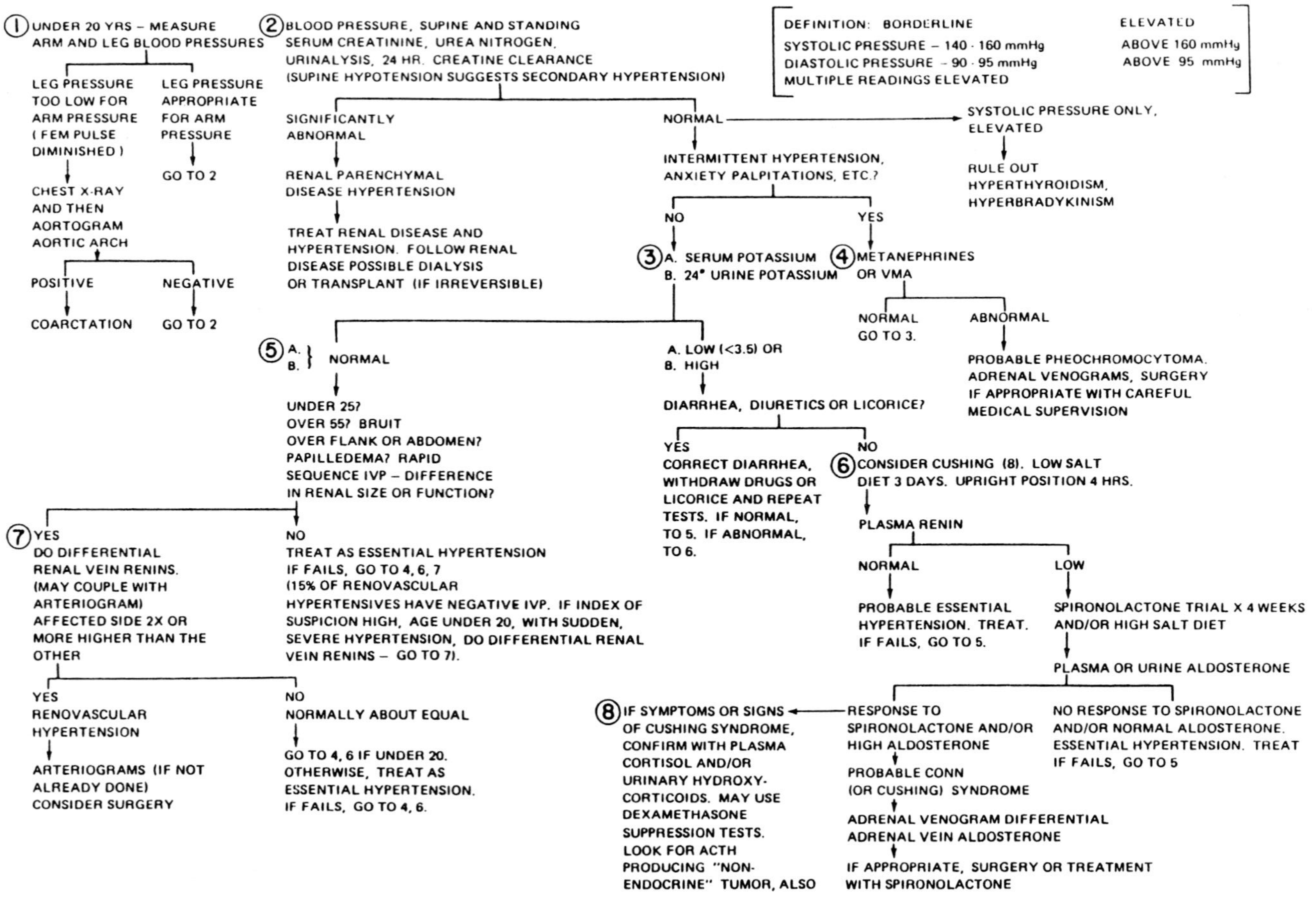

Fig. 1–11. An algorithm for the diagnosis of hypertension (if any Rx for essential hypertension fails after 6 months, consider missed etiology or lack of compliance). (From Beeler, M.: Interpretations in Clinical Chemistry. Chicago, American Society of Clinical Pathologists, 1978.)

cytomas. The former are highly malignant. Symptoms produced by such tumors may commonly be only mechanical. Neuroblastomas and ganglioneuromas secrete a wide variety of catecholamine metabolites; and not all tumors produce elevated urinary vanilmandelic acid. Homovanillic acid excretion is frequently elevated in patients with neuroblastomas but is usually normal in patients with pheochromocytomas. Therefore, measurement of urinary homovanillic acid and VMA may help in the differential diagnosis of neuroblastoma and pheochromocytoma (Table 1–9).

Carcinoid syndrome is characterized, biochemically, by presence of increased urinary serotonin metabolite—5-hydroxy-indoleacetic acid (5-HIAA). Levels of 5-HIAA in urine of normal subjects are not more than 15 mg/day, while the urine of patients with extensive carcinoid rarely contains less than 50 mg/day. (See discussion of chromagens.)

Phenylketonuria (PKU; see discussion of aminoacidurias)

Before the diagnosis of phenylketonuria can be made and dietary treatment instituted, the three criteria on page 46 must be met.

TABLE 1–9. Catecholamines and Other Phenolic Acids Detectable in Urine in Various Disorders.

Disorders	Compounds Sometimes Found in Increased Quantities in the Urine
Pheochromocytoma	(Vanilmandelic acid) 4-hydroxy-3-methoxymandelic acid, Metanephrine, Normetanephrine, (Homovanillic acid) 4-hydroxy-3-methoxyphenylacetic acid
Ganglioneuroma	Normetanephrine, (Vanilmandelic acid) 4-hydroxy-3-methoxymandelic acid, (Homovanillic acid) 4-hydroxy-3-methoxyphenylacetic acid, Vanillic acid
Neuroblastoma	Norepinephrine, Dopamine, (Vanilmandelic acid) 4-hydroxy-3-methoxymandelic acid, Normetanephrine, (Homovanillic acid) 4-hydroxy-3-methoxyphenylacetic acid, Dihydroxyphenylalanine, Vanillic acid
Wilms' tumor	p-hydroxyphenylacetic acid
Malignant melanoma	p-hydroxyphenylacetic acid
Ascorbic acid deficiency and tyrosinosis of the newborn	p-hydroxyphenylacetic acid, p-hydroxyphenyllactic acid, p-hydroxyphenylpyruvic acid, Tyrosine
Chemodectoma	(Vanilmandelic acid) 4-hydroxy-3-methoxymandelic acid
Ganglioneuroblastoma	(Vanilmandelic acid) 4-hydroxy-3-methoxymandelic acid, Normetanephrine, Dopamine, Norepinephrine
Imidazoiuria	Imidazolelactic acid, Histidine
Carcinoid syndrome	5-hydroxyindoleacetic acid
Histidinemia	Imidazolelactic acid, Histidine
Phenylketonuria	o-hydroxyphenylacetic acid

(Kodak CHROMAT/O/SCREEN Analysis Kit, publication JJ-174, Eastman-Kodak Company, Rochester, 1971.)

1. Serum phenylalanine levels are 20 mg/dl or higher on at least two occasions.
2. Serum tyrosine levels are "normal" (below 5 mg/dl in blood samples drawn at the same time as those for phenylalanine determination).
3. The classical phenylalanine metabolites such as o-hydroxyphenylacetic acid are present in high concentration in the urine (Table 1–14).

METABOLITES OF DISORDERS OF METABOLISM AND AMINOACIDURIAS[23,29]

As is now so well known, Archibald Garrod, over a half-century ago, described four diseases (pentosuria, albinism, alkaptonuria, and cystinuria) as "inborn errors of metabolism." He considered them to be the result of inherited abnormalities of certain enzymes, resulting in disordered intermediary metabolism. Since his time, our understanding of biochemical genetics has expanded enormously. It is now known that the sequence of purine and pyrimidine bases in deoxyribonucleic acid (DNA) of the chromosomes provides the code for the amino acid sequence of polypeptides synthesized by the cells. The structural gene or cistron is the part of the chromosome responsible for each such polypeptide. The codon is the subunit of the cistron responsible for the placement of a single amino acid. There are, in addition to operator genes, regulator genes, which determine how much of a particular polypeptide will be synthesized. Messenger ribonucleic acid (mRNA) transfers the code from the nucleus to the cytoplasm, where protein is formed in the ribosomes. Mutation is caused by a change in base sequence of DNA; and the results may be decreased synthesis of a protein (operator or regulator gene mutation), complete failure of synthesis, or synthesis of an abnormal protein with an altered amino acid sequence (cistron or codon mutation). The mutation may result in disease and death. Probably most mutations are lethal to the fetus. If the protein affected is an enzyme, the subsequent disease may result from absence of an important metabolite, as in albinism; accumulation of metabolites prior to the reaction catalyzed by the defective or absent enzyme, as in phenylketonuria; or from increased amounts of metabolites normally present only in small quantities, as in phenylketonuria also.

Diseases may also be produced less directly by alterations of the renal tubular transport mechanisms, as well as other transport systems, such as those of the liver and gut.

Because of the association of such disorders with mental retardation, attempts at early detection of carriers and diseased individuals, with hope of early institution of control measures designed to lessen or prevent damage or to give parental guidance, have received great emphasis in recent years. Schemata have been developed for screening urine, blood, and other materials in the laboratory; and one of the most recent and comprehensive of these is that described by J.P. Berry and associates.

In addition to the classical "inborn errors of metabolism," there are, of course, numerous other metabolic disorders, most of them hereditary and presumably the result of altered genes; although because the specific abnormality may result in a complex phenotype, they are not yet fully understood. Some of these, such as diabetes mellitus and disorders of pigment metabolism, are briefly considered elsewhere in this book. Others, including altered sensitivity to pharmacologic agents, coagulation disorders, and disorders of lipid metabolism, are not discussed in this book.

The disorders classified as "aminoacidurias" may result from a classic inborn error of metabolism (overflow type).[28] The overflow type of aminoacidurias may also result from severe liver disease, and so need not result from a metabolic disorder. Also, aminoacidurias secondary to tubular transport mechanisms may be the result of a hereditary disorder that primarily, or only secondarily, affects the tubules (such as galactosuria) (Tables 1–10 to 1–14).

In the most sophisticated laboratories, urinary metabolites are now being studied by gas-liquid chromatography followed by mass spectrometry.

Phenylpyruvic Oligophrenia

"Male, aged 5, idiot, urine contains phenylpyruvic acid; unable to walk, talk, or stand; he can now crawl a little, but hardly uses his legs at all, and sits tailorwise; wet and dirty in habits; brachycephalic; . . . fits started when he was a few months old; they consisted of twitching associated with apparent loss of consciousness. They have continued ever since and often occur several times in one day."

Lionel Penrose described this patient in 1935, a year following the original description of the syndrome by Asbjorn Folling in Sweden. The patient's 19-year-old brother was similarly afflicted, but five other siblings were healthy. The epileptic seizures were felt to be unusual. Skin pigmentation and spasticity were characteristic findings. The gene for the disease is not completely recessive, according to Penrose, but predisposes heterozygotes to mental breakdown.

George Jervis, in 1947, demonstrated that feeding phenylalanine to fasting normal patients results in an increase of substances in the blood reacting positively with the Millon reagent for tyrosine. Patients with this disorder, however, failed to show such increases, although both patients and normals showed an increase following feeding of tyrosine. This was interpreted to demonstrate an inability of the patient to hydroxylate phenylalanine to tyrosine. Jervis later reported that crude liver extract from patients with phenylketonuria failed to form tyrosine

TABLE 1–10. Primary Renal Transport Aminoacidurias.

Aminoacid Transport Groups	Disease Caused by Inherited Transport or Overflow of One Amino Acid with Competitive Inhibition of Transport of other Members of the Group	Clinical Features
1. Dibasic amino acids (ornithine, lysine, arginine, cystine)	CYSTINURIA *Type I* Homozygotes have defective intestinal and renal transport of dibasic amino acids and cystine. Heterozygotes have normal amino acid excretion. *Type II* Homozygotes have defective intestinal transport of lysine, but normal absorption of cystine. Heterozygotes have cystine-lysinuria. *Type III* Homozygotes have normal intestinal transport of dibasic amino acids and cystine. Heterozygotes have cystine-lysinuria.	Renal Calculi
2. Monocarboxylic, monoaminoacids	HARTNUP DISEASE Transport defect present in kidney and intestine. Intestinal flora produce abnormal indoles from tryptophan.	
3. Proline, hydroxyproline and glycine	MILD PROLINURIA Slight to moderate increased excretion of proline, hydroxyproline and glycine. Heterozygotes may excrete only glycine in excess. SEVERE PROLINURIA (Joseph's syndrome) May excrete up to 3 gm per day proline, 300 mg. per day hydroxyproline, and 600 mg. per day glycine. HYPERPROLINEMIA Prolinuria due to overflow. Hydroxyprolinuria and glycinuria are renal.	
4. Methionine	METHIONINE MALABSORPTION SYNDROME Methionine prominent in urine and stools with lesser increase of branched-chain amino acids, tyrosine, phenylalanine, and tryptophan. Possibly specific absorption defect in methionine with consequent competitive inhibition by increased methionine in another transport system. Intestinal bacteria make alpha-hydroxybutyric acid from methionine.	Mental retardation, excretion of alpha-hydroxybutyric acid with offensive odor, white hair, edema.
5. Beta-alanine, beta-amino*iso*-butyric acid, taurine	HYPERBETA-ALANINEMIA Beta-alanine and gamma aminobutyric acid overflow into urine. Normal plasma concentrations, suggesting possible competitive inhibition of transport due to excess β-alanine. Gamma-aminobutyric acid elevated in CSF and urine. (GABA is poorly transported.)	Somnolence, fits, early death in only reported patient.

(Kodak CHROMAT/O/SCREEN Analysis Kit for Aminoacids, publication JJ-172, Eastman-Kodak Company, Rochester, 1971.)

TABLE 1–11. Secondary Inherited Renal Aminoacidurias.

Disease State	Type of Aminoaciduria	Other Biochemical Abnormalities	Clinical Features	Inherited Abnormality
Galactosemia	Generalized renal. (Like plasma.)	Galactosuria; glucosuria if severe	Mental retardation; liver disease; cataract	Galactose-1-phosphate-uridyl transferase deficiency
Cystinosis	Generalized renal. (Like plasma.)	Glucosuria; phosphaturia; potassium loss; water loss; bicarbonate loss	Renal rickets; cystine deposits; death from dehydration, acidosis or uremia	Unknown. Possible defect in efflux of amino acids from cells.
Wilson's disease	Generalized renal. (Like plasma.) Terminally may also show picture of hepatic insufficiency with methionine, cystine, ethanolamine	Ceruloplasmin usually low in plasma; increased free copper in liver	Hepatic cirrhosis; basal ganglia disease; gray-brown corneal ring (Kayser-Fleischer ring)	Unknown. Ceruloplasmin deficiency may be primary defect.
Lowe's syndrome	Generalized renal.	Glucosuria; phosphaturia	Mental retardation; cataract; glaucoma; renal rickets; pronounced hypotonia	Unknown. Appears to be X-linked.
Adult Fanconi syndrome	Generalized renal.	Glucosuria; phosphaturia	Renal osteomalacia	Unknown. Most are inherited as dominant.
Tyrosinosis	Generalized renal with addition of overflow of tyrosine.	Glucosuria; phosphaturia	Hepatic cirrhosis; renal rickets	*p*-hydroxyphenylpyruvic acid oxidase deficiency
Phosphate-losing rickets	Glycine	Few families have glucosuria.	Renal rickets	Unknown. Usually X-linked. Recessive inheritance.

(Kodak CHROMAT/O/SCREEN Analysis Kit for Aminoacids, publication JJ-172, Eastman-Kodak Company, Rochester, 1971.)

from phenylalanine although controls were positive. He concluded that the specific enzyme responsible was absent.

More recently, Marvin Armstrong and associates investigated the presence of other substances in the urine of these patients, using the techniques of paper chromatography, and they proposed a more complete scheme of the metabolism of patients with this defect. With the normal pathway of metabolism of phenylalanine blocked, alternate pathways assume greater importance, and many substances other than phenylpyruvic acid are present in increased amounts. Phenylketonuria,

TABLE 1–12. Secondary Acquired Renal Aminoacidurias.

Clinical Disease	Type of Aminoaciduria and Biochemical Features
Heavy Metal Poisoning	Renal, generalized but certain characteristic features may be present.
Lead	Beta-amino*iso*butyric acid and alanine prominent.
Mercury	Glycine prominent.
Uranium	Alanine prominent.
Cadmium	Serine and threonine prominent.
Acute tubular necrosis	Renal, generalized. Varies from case to case.
Burns	Renal, generalized. Varies from case to case. Peptides prominent.
Multiple myeloma	Renal, generalized. May produce adult Fanconi syndrome.
Muscular dystrophies	Taurine prominent. May be generalized.
Leukemia and other tumors	Generalized. Beta-amino*iso*butyric acid may be prominent, reflecting increased tyrosine degradation. Thymine.
Neuroblastoma	May be generalized. May excrete cystathionine. A few excrete homocystine.
Bone disease, growth, uterine involution	Increased peptide-bound hydroxyproline reflecting increased turnover.
March hemoglobinuria	Cystine and beta-amino*iso*butyric acid may be present in morning urine.
Vitamin D deficiency	Renal, generalized.
Scurvy	Taurine, tyrosine, and phenylalanine may be prominent.
Liver disease	Overflow cystine, taurine, beta-amino*iso*butyric acid, and ethanolamine present. Blood methionine may be elevated disproportionate to other amino acids.
Nephrotic syndrome	Renal, generalized.
Kwashiorkor	Taurine, beta-amino*iso*butyric acid, and ethanolamine prominent. May have generalized renal aminoaciduria.

(Kodak CHROMAT/O/SCREEN Analysis Kit for Aminoacids, publication JJ-172, Eastman-Kodak Company, Rochester, 1971.)

tyrosinosis, and alkaptonuria all occur as results of blocks in phenylalanine metabolism (Table 1–14 and Fig. 1–12).

Presumably there is a critical period, between 4 months and 2 years of age, during which subsequently irreversible damage may be done to the central nervous system unless the diet is modified to include little or no phenylalanine. Because of this assumption, in the State of Louisiana (and elsewhere), laboratory testing of all newborns has become mandatory by law.

The screening test most widely used is Robert Guthrie's bacterial inhibition test. A filter paper disc is impregnated with capillary blood from an infant, no sooner than 1 day following beginning ingestion of milk. (Unfortunately it is customary to administer dextrose-in-water to newborns the first 24 to 48 hours of life, because, in case of a tracheoesophageal fistula, the dextrose-in-water would be diverted into the lung and would be absorbed; whereas milk, being fatty, would not be absorbed and would produce an irresolvable lipoid pneumonia. Therefore, blood for the test can rarely be collected before the third day of life, and many hospitals discharge the infant by that time!) A special

TABLE 1–13. Primary (No Threshold) Aminoacidurias.

Disease	Amino Acid in Great Excess in Urine	Amino Acid Pattern of Blood	Clinical Features	Deficient Enzyme
Homocystinuria	Homocystine (30–300 mg/day)	Homocystine about 4 mg/dl. Methionine may be markedly elevated. Plasma cystine subnormal	Mental retardation; dislocated lenses; Marfan-like syndrome; vascular accidents; osteoporosis	Cystathionine synthetase
Cystathioninuria	Cystathionine (may be over 1 g/day)	Cystathionine slightly elevated	Mental retardation; congenital acidosis; thrombocytopenia; pituitary-gland abnormalities	Cystathioninase
Argininosuccinicaciduria	Argininosuccinic acid (2.5–9 g/day)	Argininosuccinic acid about 4 mg/dl	Mental retardation; ataxia, trichorrhexis nodosa; early refusal to eat protein; ammonia intoxication	Argininosuccinase
Hypophosphatasia	Phosphoethanolamine (up to 150 mg/day)	Phosphoethanolamine slightly elevated, about 0.4 mg/ml	Bone disease	Alkaline phosphatase
Carnosinuria	Carnosine (20–100 mg/day)	Not available	Some have had convulsions, mental retardation, retinitis pigmentosa	?

(Kodak CHROMAT/O/SCREEN Analysis Kit for Aminoacids, publication JJ-172, Eastman-Kodak Company, Rochester, 1971.)

medium is prepared without phenylalanine, and a microorganism requiring phenylalanine for growth is inoculated onto the medium. A number of impregnated discs are placed on the surface. The organisms will grow only around discs impregnated with blood containing increased amounts of phenylalanine.

If newborns are discharged before the test can be performed, urine is usually tested for phenylpyruvic acid before the end of the fourth week of life, either with the Phenistix dip test or with ferric chloride reagent. Both depend on similar reactions, development of a green color, when increased amounts of phenylpyruvic acid are present. The Phenistix test will detect 75 to 80% of cases with urine concentration of phenylketones of 8 mg/dl or higher. However, blood levels of phenylpyruvic acid have to reach 10 to 20 mg/dl to produce these urine levels. Since blood levels greater than 3 mg/dl in the first 2 to 3 days of life are considered suggestive of phenylketonuria, the test is obviously helpful only in those cases with high levels of phenylketones. The Phenistix

TABLE 1–14. Primary Overflow Aminoacidurias.

Disease	Amino Acids Increased in Blood	Abnormal Enzyme	Tissue in which Enzyme Abnormality has been Demonstrated	Clinical Features	Abnormalities in Urine in Addition to Overflow Aminoaciduria	Other Abnormalities
Phenylketonuria	Phenylalanine	Phenylalanine hydroxylase	Liver	Mental retardation Fits Eczema Fair hair	*o*-hydroxyphenylacetic acid, phenyl pyruvic, acetic, and lactic acids	Blood tyrosine does not rise, and may drop after phenylalanine load
Tyrosinosis	Tyrosine (methionine may be markedly elevated)	*p*-hydroxyphenylpyruvic acid oxidase	Liver	Hepatic cirrhosis Fanconi syndrome	*p*-hydroxyphenylpyruvic, acetic, and lactic acids. Methionine may be prominent	Generalized aminoaciduria, renal glycosuria, renal rickets
Histidinemia	Histidine (alanine may also be increased)	Histidase	Skin	Mild or severe mental retardation (speech defect)	Alanine may be increased. Imidazole pyruvic, acetic, and lactic acids	Urocanic acid absent in sweat and in urine after oral histidine load
Maple Syrup urine disease	Valine Leucine Isoleucine Alloisoleucine	Branched-chain keto-acid decarboxylase		Vomiting, hypertonicity, severe mental retardation, early death	Branched-chain keto-acids in great excess	Urine has odor of maple syrup
Severe infantile		Enzyme deficiency nearly complete	Leukocytes			
Intermittent	Same but activity of enzyme 10–20% of normal		Leukocytes	Same but occur only with infections or trauma. May die during attack	Keto-aciduria only during attacks	Urine odor present only during attacks
Hypervalinemia	Valine	Valine-alpha keto *isovaleric* acid transaminase	Leukocytes	Mental retardation		
Hyperglycinemia	Glycine	Not known (one patient had carbamylphosphate synthetase deficiency)	?	Periodic vomiting, lethargy, ketosis, neutropenia and thrombocytopenia, osteoporosis		
Severe infantile		Glycine oxidase (?)	Liver		Acetone	May have ammonia intoxication
With hypooxaluria	Glycine			Mental retardation	Decreased oxalate excretion	
Citrulinemia	Citruline	Argininosuccinic acid synthetase	Liver	Mental retardation Liver disease		Ammonia intoxication. May have low blood urea nitrogen

Congenital lysine intolerance	Lysine, Arginine	Lysine dehydrogenase	Liver	Mental retardation		Ammonia intoxication
Hyperlysinemia	Lysine	Not known		Mental retardation Fits Muscular asthenia (may be normal)	Ornithine. Gamma-aminobutyric acid and ethanolamine in excess	Delayed conversion of injected lysine to CO_2
Hyperprolinemia: Type I	Proline	Proline oxidase	Liver	Mental retardation Fits	Hydroxyprolinemia, glycinuria	May have hereditary nephritis and deafness
Type II	Proline	Δ′-pyroline-5-carboxylate dehydrogenase	Liver	Mental retardation Fits	Δ′-pyroline-5-carboxylate, hydroxyprolinemia, glycinuria	
Hydroxyprolinemia	Hydroxyproline	Hydroxyproline oxidase		Mental retardation (?)		No excretion of Δ′-pyroline-3-hydroxy-5-carboxylate or gamma hydroxyglutamic acid after hydroxyproline feeding
Hyper-beta-alaninemia	Beta-alanine	Beta-alanine-alpha keto glutarate transaminase (?)		Somnolence Fits	Beta aminobutyric acid, gamma aminobutyric acid and taurine in excess	GABA and Beta-alanine increased in CSF
Sarcosinemia	Sarcosine Ethanolamine	Sarcosine dehydrogenase (?)		Mental retardation Difficulty swallowing (?)		
Homocystinuria	Methionine Homocystine	Cystathionine Synthetase	Liver	Mental retardation Dislocated lenses Vascular accidents Marfan-like syndrome Osteoporosis	Homocystine in great excess in urine	Plasma cystine may be low
Ornithinemia	Ornithine	? Ornithine Transcarbamylase		Mental retardation Fits Refusal of protein foods	Ornithine may be in normal concentrations in urine	Ammonia intoxication
Tryptophanemia	Tryptophan	? Tryptophan Pyrrolase or Formylase		Mental retardation Short stature Photo-sensitivity Ataxia	Decreased excretion of kynurenine after tryptophan load	

(Kodak CHROMATO/O/SCREEN Analysis Kit for Aminoacids, publication JJ-172, Eastman-Kodak Company, Rochester, 1971.)

test is almost twice as sensitive as the ferric chloride test. Positive test results should be confirmed by quantitative determination of serum phenylalanine levels by the fluorescent technique. It is calculated that 1 in 7,000 persons in the general population of the United States may develop phenylketonuria. Premature newborn infants (less than 5 pounds) without the genetic defect may have elevated phenylalanine and tyrosine levels, probably as a result of delayed development of appropriate enzyme activity. These premature patients will have a positive Guthrie bacterial inhibition test, but usually not a positive ferric chloride or Phenistix test. They also excrete phenylacetic acid, which gives the urine and sweat a "musty" or "athlete's" odor.

Treatment, of course, is purely dietary, and may avert the usual consequences of the disease. Frankly, we see little reason to single this disease out for mandatory legal testing to the exclusion of the others.

Alcaptonuria

"The patient is a child of 4 years. . . . The mother consulted me because she thought there was blood on the diaper. When the diaper stood in water, the water looked exactly as if it contained blood. When the diapers were boiled with soap, they stained black. This child's skin was stained black where soiled by the urine. This could not be washed off by ordinary means, but gradually wore off." This patient reported by Elmer Bagnall, in 1929, had alcaptonuria. The disease, a hereditary one, transmitted probably by a single autosomal recessive gene, is characterized by inability to oxidize homogentisic acid, a normal intermediary metabolite in phenylalanine and tyrosine metabolism. There is as yet no proof that the disease is not caused by presence of enzyme inhibitors, but it seems more likely to result from a defective enzyme system (Fig. 1–12).

As a result of the metabolic disability, increased quantities of homogentisic acid are excreted in the urine.[28] Emil Aberholden is stated by Elmer Bagnall to have found homogentisic acid in normal urine after 50 g of phenylalanine were taken. The output in alcaptonuria varies considerably. In Neuberger's case, the patient's output on a basal diet ranged from 3.57 to 5.23 g. The blood levels are low, however, and the renal clearance values are said to be 400 to 500 ml. The urine may look normal when freshly voided. When exposed to air, it becomes pink, then black. No other aromatic substances are excreted in abnormal quantities in this condition, according to Neuberger.

The alcaptonuric is likely to be asymptomatic until middle life, then, over a period of years, to develop deposition of a melanin-like pigment, particularly in the cartilages, and not infrequently, to develop arthritic symptoms, a syndrome known as ochronosis.

Laboratory diagnosis depends on observation of blackening of the urine by addition of sodium hydroxide; on application of the ferric

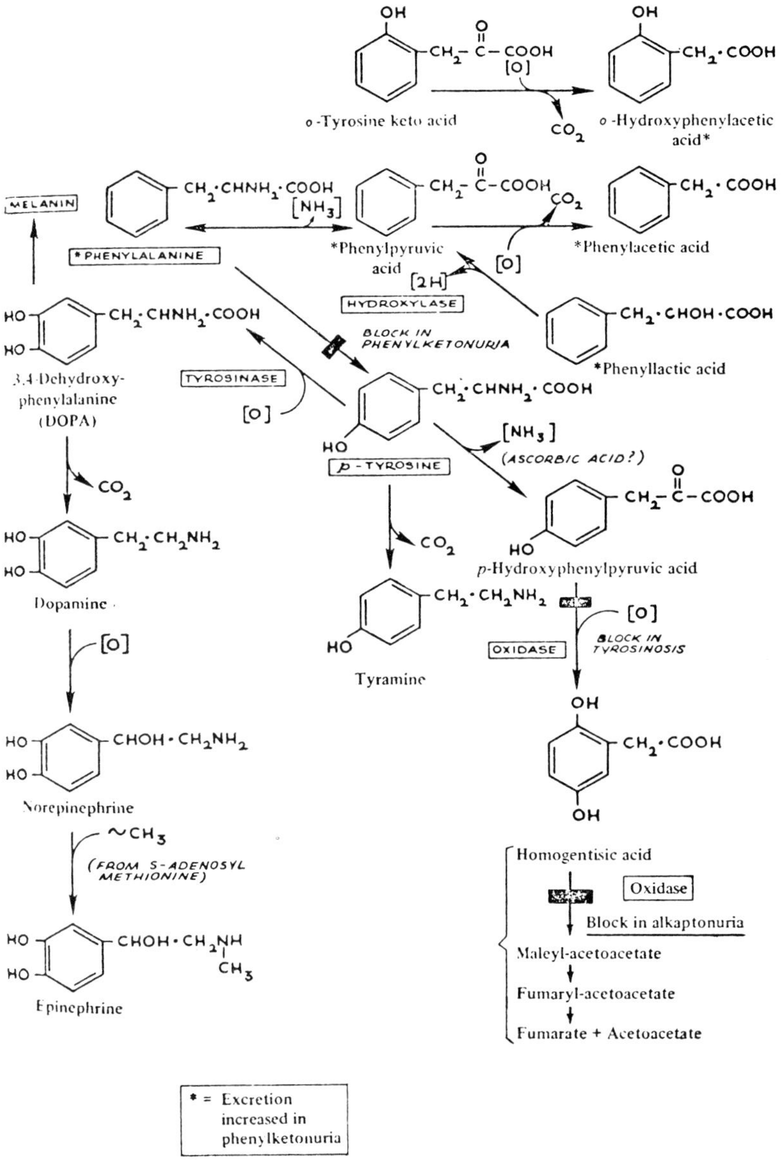

Fig. 1–12. Metabolism of phenylalanine and tyrosine with inherited metabolic defects producing phenylketonuria, tyrosinosis, alcaptonuria. (Harper, A.: Review of Physiologic Chemistry. 12th Ed. Courtesy of Lange Medical Publications.)

chloride test to urine, which, as in the case of phenylpyruvic oligophrenia, develops a transitory green color (followed by development of a black precipitate, however); or, on ability of alkalinized urine to turn photographic paper, exposed to light, black. More definitive tests include two-dimensional paper chromatography.

Cystinosis

This is a disease usually associated with hypophosphatemic rickets, dwarfism, glycosuria, aminoaciduria, and deposits of cystine crystals throughout the reticuloendothelial system in children. The disease is probably inherited as a Mendelian recessive, and the prognosis is poor; death often occurs before puberty. A similar disease occurs in adults, with osteomalacia rather than rickets. Probable synonyms include the de Toni Fanconi syndrome, Debré and Lignac's disease, and Milkman's syndrome.[28]

The fundamental defect appears to be inability to reabsorb glucose, amino acids, and in some cases phosphates in the proximal convoluted renal tubules, which have been demonstrated to lack alkaline phosphatases. Some patients appear to lack ability to reabsorb bicarbonate, uric acid, and potassium properly, as well (Table 1–11). The diagnosis may be complicated by secondary kidney disease which may ultimately result in a raised serum phosphorus. Laboratory diagnostic aids include depression of serum phosphorus, elevated serum alkaline phosphatase, glucosuria, and aminoaciduria. Cystine crystals may be demonstrable in the bone marrow, but may not appear in urine.

Cystinuria

Normally 30 to 100 mg cystine are excreted daily in the urine. There is a group of people who excrete approximately 1 g daily, along with increased amounts of lysine, arginine, often ornithine, and perhaps cadaverine and putrescine. These are cystinurics. Cystine is the least soluble of these substances, and the urine of the patients is frequently saturated with it. Renal calculi composed of cystine often result. Eight of 15 patients reported by Charles Dent were so afflicted. The plasma levels of cystine normally average 10 mg/dl. Two patients of Dent, an English physician who popularized the technique of two-dimensional paper chromatography, had plasma levels of 15 and 18 g/dl, respectively. For this reason it is thought that the primary fault is with the resorption mechanism of the kidney tubule, rather than with the metabolism of cystine.

Cystine is present normally in urine, but only in small quantities. When present in excessive amounts, part of it is usually in crystalline form, and can be detected microscopically. Spot tests are also available, as well as the nitroprusside test for its detection. About 30 to 100 mg of cystine are excreted daily into the urine. Laboratory diagnosis of cystinuria depends on demonstrating increased renal excretion of cystine in the absence of other demonstrable causes for this. The cystine crystals are typically hexagonal and moderately birefringent, and so are readily recognizable when present in urinary sediment. Two-dimensional paper chromatographic demonstration of increased cystine, as well as other amino acids, is more definitive.

Gout

Gout is a familial disease characterized by a greatly increased body pool of uric acid, often accompanied by hyperuricemia and by intermittent attacks of acute colchicine-responsive arthritis, usually affecting the lower extremities. The former may be caused by overproduction of uric acid, the result of a shunt that permits an abnormally rapid conversion of glycine to uric acid.[29,30]

Uric acid is liable to sudden precipitation in serum at a level of 6.5 mg/dl. Since kidney tubules normally reabsorb a large proportion of the uric acid present in the glomerular filtrate, and since the normal serum uric acid level is at least 5 mg/dl serum ± 2 mg/dl (± 2 standard deviations), it may be seen that the gouty individual stands in jeopardy of sudden precipitation of urates in all of his tissues. This may explain the acute arthritic attacks and the gradual development of *tophi* (tumor-like accumulations of sodium urate), as a result of hydrogen-binding of uric acid and lysosomal membranes, with subsequent membrane rupture and cell autolysis.[30]

The predilection of the acute arthritic attacks for the first metatarsal-phalangeal joint and the precipitating mechanisms are not easily explained. Most arthritic attacks follow some kind of stress. It has been noted that gouty individuals have a one-third lower than normal 17-ketosteroid excretion with clinical evidence of normal androgen activity. Also, excessive excretion of water and sodium chloride precedes the attack. These facts suggest the possibility that relative adrenal cortical insufficiency plays a role.

Neither is the efficiency of colchicine in relieving the acute attacks explainable, since unlike salicylates and probenecid, it does not increase excretion of uric acid. The latter drugs, however, while lowering the body pool of uric acid, will not abort an acute attack.

Laboratory diagnosis depends on demonstration of an elevated serum uric acid in a person with characteristic symptoms, demonstration of urate crystals in cells of arthritic joint fluid, or identification of a tophus histologically. In research laboratories, the miscible pool of body uric acid may be measured with ^{15}N-labeled uric acid. In normal individuals it averages about 1 g. Patients with gout may have 20 or 30 times this amount.

Hemochromatosis and Hemosiderosis[28]

These two diseases of excess iron storage may result from different fundamental mechanisms. Normally, iron in the ferric state is absorbed from the duodenum and caecum, but crosses the cell membrane in the ferrous state. In the mucosal cell, it combines with a protein, apoferritin, to form ferritin. At the opposite pole of the cell, the iron crosses the membranes and is reconverted to the ferric state and released into the blood stream, where it combines with a globulin, siderophilin (transferrin), for transport in the blood stream.

In primary hemochromatosis, excess iron in the form of hemosiderin appears in the parenchymal and reticuloendothelial cells of many organs, including, at times, just about every organ of the body. Another noniron-containing pigment, hemofuschin, also accumulates intracellularly. There is little doubt that the patients have increased iron absorption. Whether the cause is an inborn error of metabolism, however, is in doubt. The clinical diagnosis is based on the triad of pigment (hemosiderin) cirrhosis, bronze or slate gray (melanin) discoloration of skin, and diabetes.

Hemosiderosis may be associated with anemias or malnutrition. A common type follows exogenous administration of iron in the form of blood transfusions over a period of years. As the excretion of iron other than through blood loss is limited to approximately 1 mg/day normally, primarily by cellular desquamation, the body cannot dispose of the excess iron, so hemosiderin deposition occurs. The body contains about 4 to 5 g of iron. Patients with hemochromatosis may have 30 g or more; those with hemosiderosis have intermediate amounts.

Hemochromatosis is invariably characterized by finely granular cirrhosis of the liver. This is usually absent in hemosiderosis. Other points of differentiation include pancreatic fibrosis, diabetes mellitus, skin pigmentation, and testicular atrophy, all common in hemochromatosis, but absent in hemosiderosis. Finally, pigment deposition in organs other than the liver, spleen, lymph nodes, and bone marrow is much less in hemosiderosis than in hemochromatosis. There is not a sharp line of demarcation between the amount of liver iron seen by special staining of biopsy or autopsy material from patients with Laennec's cirrhosis and those with hemochromatosis; all gradations of quantities of iron being seen. This has suggested to some that hemochromatosis may not be an entirely separate and distinct disease, but rather a form of portal cirrhosis in subjects whose intake of iron is increased.

Laboratory diagnosis depends largely on serum iron, iron-binding capacity, and transferrin determinations. Normal serum iron may be taken to be about 100 mcg/dl $\pm$ 60 for males and $\pm$ 70 for females. The serum iron is elevated in both hemochromatosis and hemosiderosis. Total serum iron-binding capacity averages about 300 mcg/dl.

Serum iron-binding protein is normally about 30 to 40% saturated with iron, while that from patients with hemochromatosis is often 90% saturated. Patients with hemosiderosis show lesser degrees of saturation. Deposition of iron-containing ferritin occurs within renal tubular epithelial cells, and as the cells slough into the urinary stream, iron can be detected in urine sediment by the Prussian blue stain. Stainable iron is demonstrable in longstanding hemolytic states, such as sickle cell hemoglobinopathy, also.

Normally, approximately 10% of an oral dose of radioactive iron is absorbed. In patients with hemochromatosis, 60% may be absorbed; in patients with hemosiderosis, however, absorption is normal. Patients with hemochromatosis may exhibit glycosuria and a diabetic-type glucose tolerance test. Liver function tests may be abnormal also. Morphologic study of a liver biopsy specimen is a helpful procedure.

Hepatolenticular Degeneration (Wilson's Disease)

This progressive, familial disease was first described by Samuel A.K. Wilson in 1912 (Table 1–11). Characteristic findings are liver disease; neurologic symptoms, usually appearing before the age of 30, and including muscular rigidity, tremor, a mask-like face, a fixed smile, and emotional disturbance; a low plasma ceruloplasmin level; a variable, but usually decreased plasma copper level; increased urinary excretion of copper; and aminoaciduria. Some patients have brown or yellow-green pigment deposited in Descemet's membrane at the limbus of the cornea, the Kayser-Fleischer rings. The liver, at autopsy, exhibits morphologic alterations resembling portal cirrhosis; the lenticular nucleus is degenerated and cystic. Both contain increased amounts of copper. The liver, brain, and perhaps, kidney disease is presumably related to the increased copper content. It has been suggested that the disease is primarily a congenital defect of a specific plasma protein, ceruloplasmin (copper oxidase), into which copper is normally incorporated. The disease usually runs a fatal course in months to years.

Laboratory diagnosis generally involves determination of copper oxidase activity by its ability to decolorize a buffered substrate of p-phenylene-diamine or by radial immunodiffusion techniques, and demonstration of increased urinary excretion of copper.

Hypophosphatasia

Hypophosphatasia is a rare inborn error of metabolism characterized by abnormal mineralization of bone, somewhat resembling rickets; diminished alkaline phosphatase activity in the serum in the presence of normal phosphorus; normal or elevated serum calcium; and increased urinary phosphorylethanolamine (Table 1–13).

Diabetes Mellitus

Diabetes mellitus is a disease characterized by inappropriate elevation of the blood sugar caused by a relative or absolute lack of insulin. It is associated with atherosclerosis, probably because of deranged fat metabolism; and also with a pathologic condition of the basement membrane of small blood vessels, producing microaneurysms that may or may not be secondary to the metabolic disturbance.

Two types of hereditary diabetes are recognized: the juvenile type, with onset in childhood, relatively severe as a rule; and the adult type, with onset during adult life, usually relatively mild. Obesity is often the precipitating factor for the second type, which is usually controllable by diet alone or diet and oral antidiabetic agents; whereas, patients with the juvenile type generally require insulin for control.

Insulin presumably acts to facilitate transport of glucose across the cell membrane, except in the case of parenchymal liver cells, upon which its action appears to enhance phosphorylation of glucose, presumably by stimulation of hexokinase enzymes. The result of these actions of insulin is increased utilization of glucose via all of its pathways of metabolism; while an absolute or relative lack of insulin results in decreased utilization via all of its pathways, causing, among other things, high blood sugar concentration. As the hexosemonophosphate shunt, one of the pathways of glucose metabolism, normally generates triphosphopyridine nucleotide (TPN) necessary for synthesis of fatty acids, this pathway of fat metabolism is also blocked. As pyruvate is not supplied from the Embden-Myerhof pathway, acetyl-Co-A, a product of fat metabolism, cannot be metabolized via the Krebs cycle either. The two remaining pathways for metabolism of acetyl-Co-A not requiring adequate carbohydrate metabolism are cholesterol synthesis and ketone body production. This explains ketosis and associated acidosis as well as high levels of serum cholesterol in patients with uncontrolled diabetes mellitus.

Diagnosis of diabetes is not based primarily on insulin assay, although radioimmunoassay techniques are available. It is measurement of carbohydrate tolerance that forms the basis of laboratory diagnosis (see discussion of glucose under "Routine Urinalysis"). Insulin is formed by the beta cells of the islets of Langerhans in the pancreas. Strangely enough, in 33% of autopsies of patients with diabetes, the islet cells appear normal by light microscopy. One can make a presumptive diagnosis of diabetes mellitus from the cellular alterations observable by light microscopy at autopsy in only one-half to two-thirds of cases.

Various pathologic alterations of the islet cells may be seen, the most common of which is hyaline degeneration, consisting of pink amorphous deposits in intercellular locations in and about the capillaries of the islet. Other changes include hydropic degeneration, glycogenation, fibrosis, lymphocytic infiltration, hypertrophy, and even adenoma. The kidneys in patients with diabetes mellitus are often the site of disease. Pyelonephritis is common, hence, urinary abnormalities are detectable and measurable. In addition, alterations of the blood vessels, including hyaline degeneration of the small arteries, are almost universally present in patients with diabetes mellitus, as previously mentioned.

ACID MUCOPOLYSACCHARIDES

Acid mucopolysaccharides are polymers of repeating disaccharide units that contain hexosamines, uronic acid, and sulfates. Within body tissues, the polysaccharides are thought to be linked to protein through galactose and serine residues. Polymers of the polysaccharides are present in the ground substance of connective tissue. Their physiologic roles involve the concentration of electrolytes and water in extracellular fluid, calcification, wound healing, resistance to infection, lubrication of joints, blood coagulation, and maintenance of intraocular environmental stability.

Acid mucopolysaccharides are excreted in the urine of patients with Hurler's syndrome in amounts ranging from 10 to 100 times normal.[28] In normal persons, the principal isomers of mucopolysaccharides found in urine are chondroitin sulfates A and C. In urine from patients with typical Hurler's syndrome, chondroitin sulfate B and heparitin monosulfate may be excreted in abnormal quantities. L-Iduronidase deficiency has been identified as one of the various lysosomal defects in mucopolysaccharide degradation in patients with Hurler's syndrome (type I).

Other disorders in which abnormal urinary acid mucopolysaccharides have been reported include Morquio-Ullrich disease (keratosulfate excretion), Marfan's syndrome (hyaluronic acid, chondroitin sulfates A and B excretion), and hereditary arthro-osteoonychodysplasia (hyaluronic acid excretion). Increased excretion of acid mucopolysaccharides in amounts 1.5 to 2 times normal also have been reported in patients with some inflammatory conditions, rheumatic disease, diabetes, arterial hypertension, and disseminated lupus erythematosus.

One quantitative determination of urinary acid mucopolysaccharide is based on precipitation with cetyl trimethyl ammonium bromide, subsequent measurement of the uronic acid production by the Dische carbazole reaction. With this technique, excretion of acid mucopolysaccharides range from 5 to 15 mg/day (expressed as mg of carbazole uronic acid), varying primarily as a result of the nature of the polysaccharides. Variations due to age and sex have been reported, but the data are not uniform (Manley, G., and Hawksworth, H.: Arch. Dis. Child., *41*:91, 1966, and Dische, A.: J. Biol. Chem., *167*:189, 1927). Clear distinction between the quantities of mucopolysaccharide excreted by pa-

TABLE 1–15. Distinguishing Features of the Mucopolysaccharidoses.

MPS	Somatic and Skeletal Changes	Mental Retardation	Cardio-pulmonary	Hepato-spleno-megaly	Corneal Clouding	Hearing Loss	Inheritance	Predominant Urinary MPS
I (Hurler syndrome)	Marked	Severe after first year	Valvular and coronary disease, impaired ventilation	Marked	Progressive	Present	Autosomal recessive	Dermatan sulfate; heparan sulfate
II (Hunter syndrome)	Moderate to marked	Severe but gradual in onset	Valvular disease; pulmonary hypertension; impaired ventilation	Marked	Rare	Present, early onset	X-linked recessive	Dermatan sulfate; heparan sulfate
III (Sanfilippo syndrome)	Mild	Severe	Not described	Moderate	Absent	Present	Autosomal recessive	Heparan sulfate
IV (Morquio syndrome)	Marked	Absent or slight	Aortic regurgitation	Slight	Present, late onset	Present, not severe	Autosomal recessive	Keratan sulfate
V (Scheie syndrome)	Mild	Essentially absent	Aortic valvular disease	Variable	Marked	Variable	Autosomal recessive	Dermatan sulfate
VI (Maroteaux-Lamy syndrome	Marked	Absent	Cardiac murmurs	Moderate	Present	Variable	Autosomal recessive	Dermatan sulfate

tients with Hurler's syndrome and by normal individuals can be made even with screening tests.

A simplified screening test involves "eyeballing" of the metachromasia produced when urine is dried on filter paper and stained with toluidine blue (MPS test, Ames Company, Elkhart, Ind.). The screening test is capable of detection of mucopolysaccharides in urine above the level of 0.2 mg/ml. Specimens from patients with Hurler's syndrome are stained purple, whereas negative tests are stained pale blue. Another screening test consists of adding 5 volumes of acidified bovine serum to 1 volume of urine; a positive test is indicated by the development of dense white turbidity as a result of protein precipitation (Berenson, G., and Sena, M.: Fed. Proc., *18*:190, 1959).

CHROMOGENS

Innumerable substances excreted in the urine (many of which are exogenous) can produce abnormally colored urine (see discussion under "Color"). Some of them result from hereditary abnormalities of metabolism (see "Metabolites of Disorders of Metabolism and Aminoacidurias"). Others do not lend themselves to any convenient categorization.

The following chromogens will be discussed in this section:

1. Porphyrins (and porphyrias)
2. Hemoglobin and myoglobin
3. Bile pigments and urobilinogen
4. Melanogens
5. Indican

Porphyrins (and Porphyrias)

Porphyrins are substances intermediate in the formation of hemoglobins, cytochromes, catalases, oxidases, and peroxidases. They function in oxygen transport and electron transfer. The basic structure of all porphyrins is the pyrrole ring, four of which, when bound cyclically, form the porphin ring (Fig. 1–13 and Table 1–16). Porphyria refers to hereditary disorders of porphyrin metabolism. Normally, 100 to 250 mg of coproporphyrin and about 20 mg of uroporphyrin are excreted daily in the urine. In addition, 200 to 500 mg of coproporphyrin are excreted daily in the feces. Porphyrins are excreted in both the urine and the feces in the oxidized form (porphyrin) and in the reduced form (porphyrinogen); but evidence indicates that most are probably excreted in reduced form—uroporphyrinogen and coproporphyrinogen—and later oxidized to coproporphyrin and uroporphyrin. The reduced porphyrins do not fluoresce, but the oxidized porphyrins do fluoresce. Fluorescence forms the basis for their qualitative detection in the laboratory. The oxidation process occurs quickly during contact with air,

TABLE 1–16. Summary of the Primary Porphyrias and Their Clinical Aspects.

Type	Synonyms	Clinical Manifestations	Laboratory Findings	Inheritance
Congenital (erythropoietic porphyria)	Congenital photosensitive; Gunther's disease	Photosensitivity; hemolytic anemia with splenomegaly	Large amounts of uroporphyrin I and coproporphyrin I in bone marrow, erythrocytes, and urine	Homozygous for abnormal gene
	"Hydroa estivale" Erythropoietic protoporphyria	Solar urticaria or solar eczema	Increased protoporphyrin in bone marrow, erythrocytes, plasma and feces	Heterozygous for abnormal gene; latent cases frequent
Intermittent acute porphyria	Acute porphyria; porphyria hepatica; pyrroporphyria; Swedish type	Abdominal colics, hypertension, nervous system involvement; acute attacks frequent; photosensitivity absent	ALA and PBG in liver and urine	Heterozygous for abnormal gene; latent cases frequent
Photosensitive hepatic porphyria	Porphyria cutanea tarda hereditaria; mixed hepatic porphyria; South African genetic porphyria Variegate porphyria	Cutaneous abdominal, and neurologic. Acute attacks occur, usually precipitated by drugs	Copro- and protoporphyrin in liver and feces; during attacks, ALA, PBG, and porphyrins in urine	Heterozygous for abnormal gene; latent cases frequent

with dilute iodine solution, and with other oxidizing agents. Porphobilinogen and delta-aminolevulinic acid may normally be present in urine in extremely small amounts (usually undetectable by routine qualitative clinical methods), but not in feces. Uroporphyrins and coproporphyrins each have four possible isomers (I, II, III, IV, depending on side group combinations of methyl, vinyl, ethyl, and proprionic acid), but only uroporphyrin types I and III and coproporphyrin types I and III exist in nature. Protoporphyrin is formed from coproporphyrinogen III. When the former is combined with iron, it forms heme, the functional group of hemoglobin, myoglobin, catalase, cytochrome, and peroxidase.

Erythropoietic protoporphyria (congenital porphyria) results from a Mendelian recessive hereditary defect of hemoglobin synthesis. Clinical manifestations, which appear in early childhood (about 1–2 years of age), include excretion of burgundy-colored urine containing increased amounts of type I uroporphyrin and coproporphyrin and, rarely,

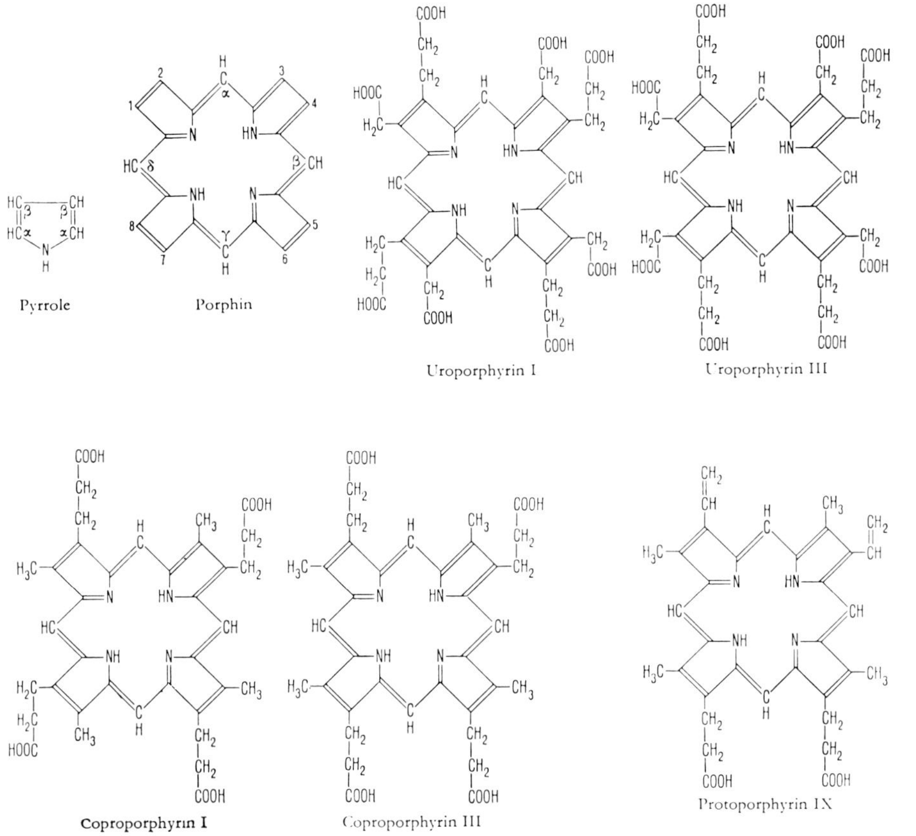

Fig. 1–13. Pyrolle nucleus and porphyrin ring. Carbons of the pyrolle nucleus closest to the nitrogen are labeled with the Greek letter alpha, and those farthest with the Greek letter beta. The parent compound of the porphyrin is a cyclic tetrapyrolle in which the four pyrolle rings are linked together through their alpha-carbon atoms by means of methene (=C—) bridges. The porphyrin molecule thus forms a closed ring of carbon and nitrogen atoms lying in one plane and containing a central 16-numbered ring of 12 —C— and 4 —N— atoms. The simplest of the porphyrins is etioporphyrin, which has four methyl and four ethyl groups in positions one and eight of the porphyrin ring. Depending upon the arrangement of the attached groups, four isomeric forms of etioporphyrin are possible. The isomers, known as types I to IV porphyrins, provide the basic classification of porphyrins. All porphyrins in the human body are derived from porphobilinogen and are related structurally to uroporphyrin I and uroporphyrin III compounds in which the eight beta hydrogen atoms of the porphyrin are replaced by four acetic acid and four propionic acid groups. Decarboxylation of the four acetic acid groups gives rise to coproporphyrin which contains four methyl and four proprionic acid groups. Only uroporphyrin I and uroporphyrin III and coproporphyrin I and coproporphyrin III are of clinical significance in humans. (Reproduced from Documenta Geigy Scientific Tables, 6th and 7th editions, by permission of the publishers, CIBA-GEIGY Limited, Basle, Switzerland.)

type III coproporphyrin (Table 1–16). Patients characteristically have reddish discoloration of teeth and bones, and skin photosensitivity, lesions identical to those seen in hydroa vacciniforme developing after exposure to sunlight and healing with scarring. They may also have hemolytic anemia with splenomegaly, and some patients have hirsutism. It is only sometimes possible to control hemolysis by splenectomy; if so, and if the patient can avoid ultraviolet light, he may lead a relatively normal existence. Patients also develop hyperpigmentation of skin, secondary to increased melanin deposition. Red blood cells with increased protoporphyrins will fluoresce in ultraviolet light.

Paroxysmal hepatic porphyria (intermittent acute porphyria) may be chemically induced or may result from a Mendelian dominant inherited defect of hepatic porphyrin metabolism, possibly because of increased manufacture of delta-aminolevulinic acid synthetase in liver mitochondria. Clinical manifestations tend to occur in young adulthood and include attacks of abdominal pain and vomiting; neurologic disturbances resembling Landry's paralysis (secondary to nerve demyelization); mental symptoms; red urine during the acute attacks, containing increased amounts of uroporphyrin I and III and increased coproporphyrin III, as well as porphobilinogen and its precursor, delta-aminolevulinic acid (the latter two compounds being absent in the previous type). Skin photosensitivity is lacking. Barbiturates, arsenic, chloroquine, and griseofulvin may precipitate attacks. The mortality rate is high.

Photosensitive hepatic porphyria (chronic porphyria or porphyria cutanea tarda) differs from the foregoing chiefly in the presence of skin photosensitivity, blisters forming after exposure to sunlight or mild trauma and often resulting in scarring. This type often is associated with alcoholism, syphilis, or diabetes. Porphobilinogen is usually absent and the urine may contain uroporphyrin I and III, coproporphyrin I and III, or both (Table 1–16).

Other types may occur with findings intermediate between those of paroxysmal hepatic porphyria.

Although there may be increased urinary excretion of coproporphyrin and delta-aminolevulinic acid in urine of patients with myocardial infarction, the observation has no known clinical significance. It has also been observed that coproporphyrin excretion is increased in patients who are alcoholics. Coproporphyrins alone may be excreted in abnormally large amounts in patients with toxicity from lead, arsenic, mercury, sedatives, sulfonamides, ethyl alcohol, carbon tetrachloride, and chloroform, as well as with hypervitaminosis, hepatic disease, hematologic disease, and "hypermetabolism." Such conditions are frequently termed secondary porphyrias or porphyrinurias.[31]

Delta-aminolevulinic acid and porphobilinogen, being nonfluorescent porphyrin precursors, are assayed photometrically, the latter with

Ehrlich's aldehyde reagents. Semiquantitative tests for porphyrinurias have been designed by Cecil Watson and Samuel Schwartz, and are sufficiently quantitative to permit routine use in the clinical microscopy laboratory. Uro- and coproporphyrins fluoresce bright red when excited with long wavelength "black light" (wavelength 3600 to 3800 Angstroms); hence, the Wood's lamp (Robert Wood, physicist, Johns Hopkins University, 1903) is often used as the exciting energy source for the qualitative detection of these compounds. Protoporphyrins will also fluoresce (red) and can be visualized with ultraviolet microscopy of red blood cell precursors of bone marrow in patients with erythropoietic protoporphyuria.

A rapid screening test for urinary porphyrins involves preliminary adsorption by anion exchange resin (Dowex), subsequent elution of the porphyrins from the resin with hydrochloric acid, and observation of fluorescence using the Wood's light. The test is considered positive when reddish-pink fluorescence is present.[32]

Hemoglobin and Myoglobin

Plasma normally contains about 5 mg/dl of free hemoglobin, the remainder being bound to an alpha-2-globulin—haptoglobin.[33] Because haptoglobin specifically binds hemoglobin, when there is intravascular hemolysis there is a direct relationship between the hemoglobin-binding capacity of serum and the appearance of hemoglobin in the urine. There is normally sufficient haptoglobin present to bind only up to approximately 135 mg hemoglobin/dl. Thereafter, hemoglobin may be found free in the urine. Haptoglobin may combine with nonhuman hemoglobin, but does not combine with heme or with myoglobin pigments. The hemoglobin-haptoglobin complex is not excreted in the urine but is fairly rapidly removed from circulation. Low haptoglobin levels, therefore, are characteristic of acute as well as chronic hemolytic processes. In mild hemolytic disorders with plasma hemoglobin levels below 135 mg/dl, heme pigments present in the blood stream may unite with albumin to form methemalbumin (Fairley's pigment). This can be detected with Schumm's test, in which plasma is treated with ammonium sulfide ether, following which an ammonium chromagen is formed with an intense spectral absorption band at 558 nm.[33] The presence of methemalbumin in the blood, therefore, is an indication that significant amounts of free hemoglobin were at one time present. If the plasma hemoglobin concentration is greater than 135 mg/dl, renal clearance of hemoglobin from the blood begins, and free hemoglobin appears in the urine—hemoglobinuria. In the course of excretion, some hemoglobin is taken up by the tubular cells of the kidneys and metabolized to hemosiderin. When sloughed into the urine, these cells can be detected by iron stains (Prussian blue reaction). Disintegration of the renal tubular cells may liberate hemosiderin granules into the urine that can also be identified by staining for iron. The term hemosiderinuria is used when stainable iron can be found within the urine. (Following massive intravascular hemolysis, hemoglobin casts can also be found in the urine.)

Screening sticks for urinalysis may incorporate tests for red cells whose significance is discussed later under "microscopic examination." Tests are based on hemolysis of cells and the usual tests for hemoglobin (using its ability to act as a peroxidase and visualize colorless substrates, such as toluidine, when changed to a blue color). The sticks may include tests for urobilinogen—a product of the breakdown of hemoglobin.

The following is a list of the types and causes of hemoglobinuria:

1. Paroxysmal nocturnal hemoglobinuria: Hemosiderinuria is present.
2. "March" hemoglobinuria: Unaccustomed excessive exercise and low renal threshold.
3. Glucose-6-phosphate dehydrogenase deficiency: (a) Ingestion of fava beans; (b) Drug ingestion, primaquin and probably phenothiazine, nitrofurantoin, and others.
4. Cold hemoglobinuria: Donath-Landsteiner antibody.
5. Autoimmune hemolytic anemia: (a) Cold antibody with lupus, lymphomas, and viral pneumonias; (b) warm antibody (rare) with lupus erythematosus.
6. Incompatible blood transfusion: Severe intravascular hemolysis.
7. Infections: (a) Plasmodium falciparum, especially on quinine therapy (blackwater fever); (b) Clostridial infections.
8. Drugs: Sulfonamides, phenacetin, quinine, arsenic.
9. Trauma: Muscle-crush injury, electrocution, convulsions.

Myoglobin is not normally detectable in urine. Myoglobinuria occurs as a result of crush injuries to muscles (crush syndrome). In many patients with muscle damage, there is also red cell destruction, and hemoglobinuria occurs along with myoglobinuria. Idiopathic recurrent myoglobinuria is a syndrome characterized by severe muscle pain and spasms followed by pseudoparalysis and the appearance of myoglobin in the urine. Haff disease, described in German and Swedish patients, may result from poisonous fish and eel resins causing muscle destruction, followed by myoglobinuria. Myoglobinuria in McArdle's disease has been associated with mild phosphorylase deficiency in some but not all cases.

The types and causes of myoglobinuria are as follows:

1. Paroxysmal myoglobinuria: Muscle cramps with myoglobinuria for 72 hours after attack.

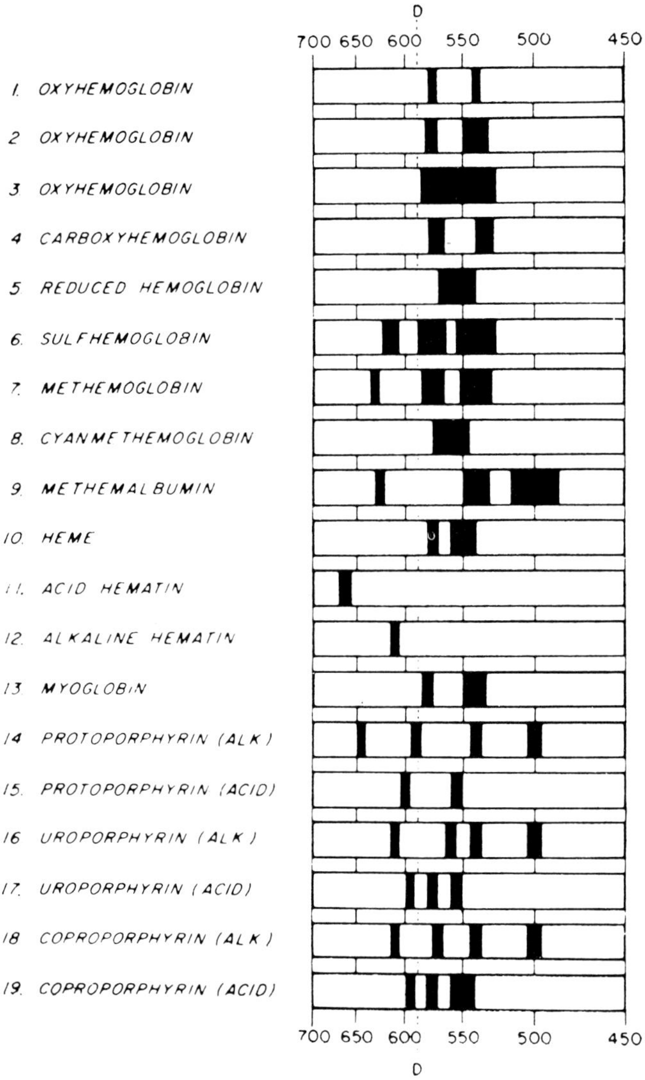

Fig. 1–14. Comparison of characteristic absorption spectra of hemoglobin, its derivatives, and myoglobin. (Miale, J.: Laboratory Medicine—Hematology. 3rd ed. Courtesy of C.V. Mosby.)

2. "March" myoglobinuria: Excessive unaccustomed exercise, anterior tibial syndrome.
3. Trauma: Beating, bullet, crush injury, electrocution, following convulsions.
4. Primary muscle disease: Muscular dystrophy, dermatomyositis, polymyositis.
5. Toxin: Fish poisoning (Haff disease), sea snake bite.
6. Carbon monoxide poisoning.
7. Arterial occlusion to muscle: diabetic atherosclerosis, thromboembolization.

Urinary screening tests for hemoglobin or myoglobin depend upon their peroxidase activity, releasing oxygen from hydrogen peroxide, which oxidizes a substrate (usually benzidine, orthotolidine, or gum guaiacum) from colorless to blue (Fig. 1–15).[35]

The benzidine test is the most sensitive of these and can detect about 1 part of blood in 64,000 parts of urine. (Caution should be employed in handling benzidine, which has been shown to be carcinogenic in animals.) The orthotolidine (Hemastix, Labstix, Multistix) tests are half this sensitive to about as sensitive (corresponding to 20–25 RBC's/HPF and 10–15 RBC's/HPF, respectively). Microscopic examination, however, is unsurpassed in sensitivity for detection of a few red cells (less than 10/HPF) in the urine.

Because plants and certain bacterial components produce peroxidase activity, benzidine and orthotolidine tests may be positive in their presence in the absence of hemoglobin. The Hemastix test is more reactive in urine containing free hemoglobin than in urine containing intact red cells, inasmuch as hemoglobin directly catalyzes oxidation, whereas red cells must first be lysed.

Myoglobin has peroxidase activity and, therefore, gives positive results with the orthotolidine and guaiac tests.

If the hemoglobin normally present in 20 ml of whole blood (3 g hemoglobin) or more is rapidly released by hemolysis, the hemoglobin-binding capacity of circulating haptoglobin will be saturated and free hemoglobin will appear in the plasma and the urine. With hemoglobinuria, urine may not be red at all times depending on concentration. Also, the hemoglobin can be reduced to methemoglobin (dark brown color) in the urinary bladder as a result of the acid pH of the urine. Hemoglobinuria can be distinguished from hematuria by the absence of intact red blood cells, and it may have a distinctly different clinical significance (the latter indicating abnormal permeability of the glomerulus or leakage of red cells from some parts of the urinary tract). In order to distinguish hematuria from hemoglobinuria, microscopic examination should be performed on sediment from a fresh centrifuged urine specimen. Markedly hypotonic urine (specific gravity less than

1.010 or osmolality less than 400 mmol/kg) may cause lysis of red blood cells and produce positive tests for hemoglobin, but yield a negative microscopic examination for red blood cells. Therefore, both urinary pH and concentration of solids in urine should be considered in the differentiation of hematuria versus hemoglobinuria.

Presence of myoglobin can be differentiated from hemoglobin by ammonium sulfate saturation, inasmuch as 80% (w/v) ammonium sulfate will not precipitate myoglobin, but will precipitate hemoglobin (and other proteins).[36] Myoglobinuria can be distinguished more definitively from hemoglobinuria by spectroscopic or electrophoretic methods, but ammonium sulfate saturation may be good enough for screening purposes. (Urines that contain porphyrins, homogentisic acid, drugs, dyes [pyridium] will color the urine red, but will not yield a precipitate with 3% [w/v] sulfosalicylic acid, and urine should be tested with this reagent prior to proceeding further with ammonium sulfate saturation tests for detection of myoglobin.) A schema for the spectroscopic differentiation of hemoglobin and myoglobin is presented in Figure 1–14. Spectroscopically, however, the bands for carboxyhemoglobin and myoglobin usually cannot be distinguished from those of oxyhemoglobin, unless a mercury arc lamp is used. This makes the method more difficult to interpret inasmuch as there are frequently mixtures of abnormal pigments when any is present in urine.

Verdoglobin, a product of hemoglobin degradation in the reticuloendothelial system, can occur in the urine in burned patients who have pseudomonas infections.[34] It has been theorized that pseudomonas toxins hinder further degradation of verdoglobin, which is, therefore, excreted in the urine. There is some uptake of verdoglobin by the liver, with subsequent excretion in bile; however, most plasma verdoglobin is excreted in the urine. Pseudomonas organisms cause hemolysis, thus making available more hemoglobin for metabolism in the reticuloendothelial system. A fairly accurate screening method for detecting ver-

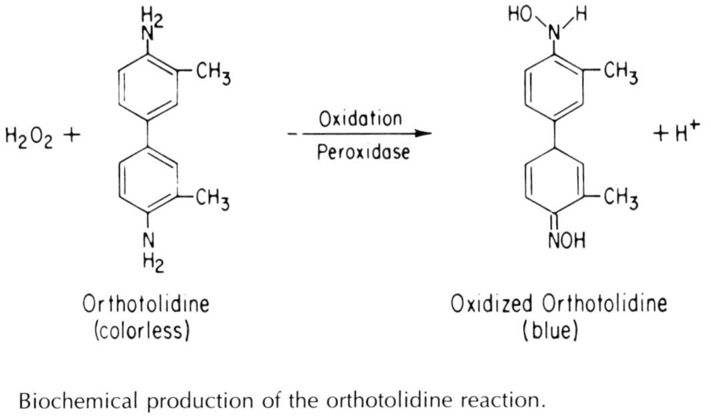

Fig. 1–15. Biochemical production of the orthotolidine reaction.

doglobin in the urine is based on its ability to fluoresce when excited with ultraviolet light (380 nm). Pseudomonas organisms themselves produce a fluorescent pigment that can be distinguished from verdoglobin by its ability to fluoresce in acid, neutral, and alkaline solutions—verdoglobin being demonstrable in all three, and the pseudomonas pigments being demonstrable only in neutral or alkaline media.

Bile Pigments and Urobilinogen

Degradation of red blood cells and hemoglobin occurs primarily in the reticuloendothelial system of the liver and spleen.[37] During reticuloendothelial phagocytosis, the protoporphyrin IX nucleus of hemoglobin is opened by oxidation of the methene bridges between rings I and II (with retention of globin and iron). The resulting pigment is called biliverdin or verdoglobin. The iron and globin are then removed, the former entering the ferritin pool, and the latter being metabolized to amino acid. The remaining green pigment formed is termed bilirubin (Fig. 1–16). This is transported in the blood as an albumin or globulin complex to the liver where it is esterified within the parenchymal cells either with glucuronic acid (approximately 76%), sulfate (14%), or unknown acids (10%). After passing into the gallbladder, bilirubin may be reoxidized to biliverdin, thus giving rise to the green color of gallbladder bile.[37–39]

The bilirubin pigments generally are represented as linear tetrapyrrole chains with terminal hydroxyl groups. However, their structure probably should be represented by a tetrapyrrole ring closed by a hydrogen bond between the oxygen atoms (Fig. 1–17).[37] (The blue and green eggshells of certain birds and the scales of some fish, as well as integument of some insects and secretion of gastropods, owe their color to protein conjugated bile pigments.)

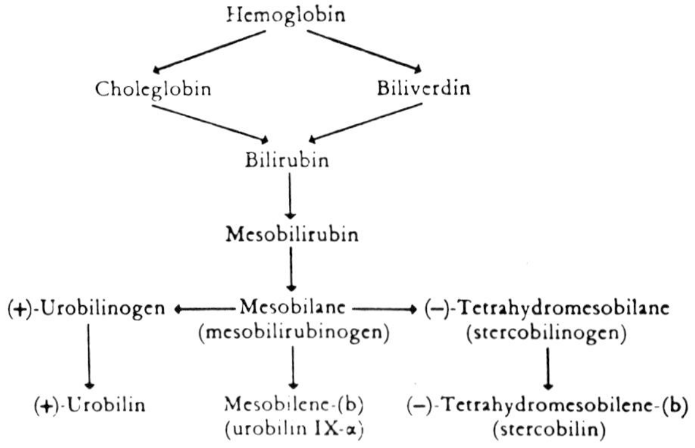

Fig. 1–16. Formation of bilirubin.

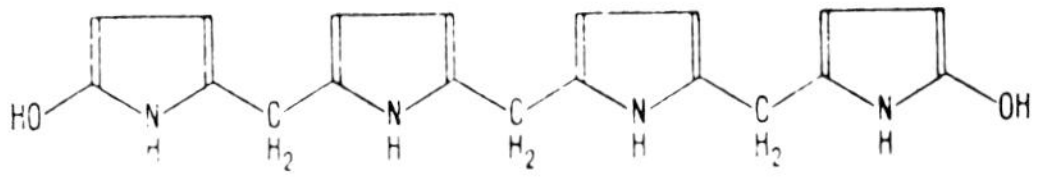

(a) Linear tetrapyrrolic structure of bile pigments

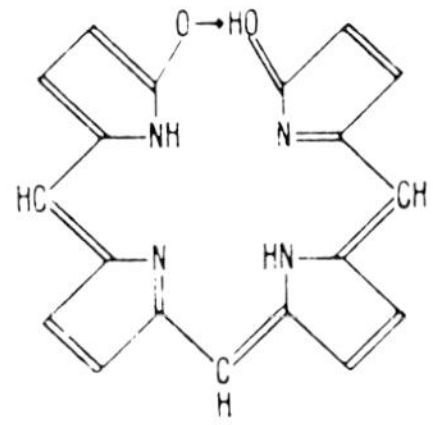

(b) 'Ring' structure of bile pigments

Fig. 1–17. Structure of bile pigments. Although bile pigments are frequently represented as linear tetrapyrolles (a), chemically it is structurally more correct to represent them as "ring" structures (b).

Bilirubin is catabolized to mesobilirubinogen, then to stercobilinogen and urobilinogen in the intestinal tract. Some urobilinogen is normally absorbed and returned to the liver, which reoxidizes it to bilirubin. Stercobilinogen, upon standing, is further oxidized to brown stercobilin, giving rise, in part, to the color of human feces. Some urobilinogen escapes the liver and is secreted by the kidney. (Urobilin is not normally formed in vivo, but when urobilinogen is exposed to the air it is oxidized to urobilin, or further to d-urobilin.) One to 2 mg/day of metabolized bile pigments are excreted in human, while fecal excretion level is from 50 to 250 mg/day (Fig. 1–18).

Obstruction to the flow of bile into the intestine deprives the stool of bile pigments resulting in clay-colored acholic stool. This also, of course, results in decreased urine urobilinogen, which is characteristic of obstructive jaundice.

Bilirubin esterified with glucuronic acid and sulfate is water-soluble, so it yields a direct reaction with Ehrlich's aldehyde reagent, conjugated bilirubin; therefore, it is called direct reacting bilirubin. Unconjugated bilirubin is usually referred to as indirect bilirubin. Because conjugated bilirubin is water-soluble, it is filtered at the glomerulus and appears in the urine, whereas bilirubin itself (unconjugated), while soluble in lipids, is insoluble in water. Unconjugated bilirubin circulates attached to protein and does not filter through the glomerulus.

The liver excretes approximately 500 to 1000 ml bile/day (about 6 g bilirubin/day), and serum level of total bilirubin usually does not normally exceed 1.1 mg/dl. Presence of increased amounts of bilirubin in

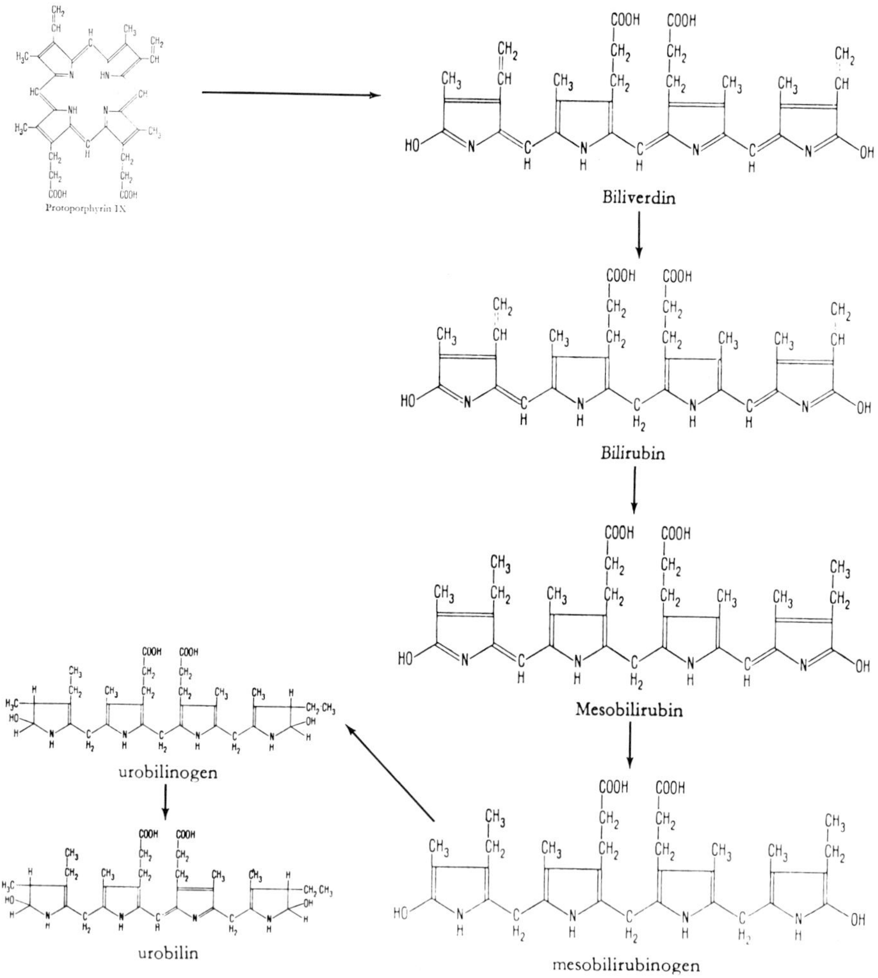

Fig. 1–18. Formation of the various bile pigments from protoporphyrin IX nucleus of hemoglobin with probable structure of urobilinogen and its oxidation product, urobilin. The actual formulas for urobilinogen and urobilin are uncertain. (Diem, K. (ed): Documenta Geigy. 7th ed. Courtesy of Geigy.)

the blood produces a condition called jaundice (icterus), in which bilirubin and its related pigments are deposited in body tissues (Fig. 1–19), including the skin, causing them to appear yellow. The solubility difference explains some of the physiologic behavior of the two types of pigments and accounts for the fact that bile pigments are excreted in the urine in patients with obstructive jaundice and various types of hepatitis with an obstructive component but not in those with pure hemolytic jaundice. (In the latter case, indirect or unconjugated bilirubin is present in the blood in increased amounts.) Because lipid-

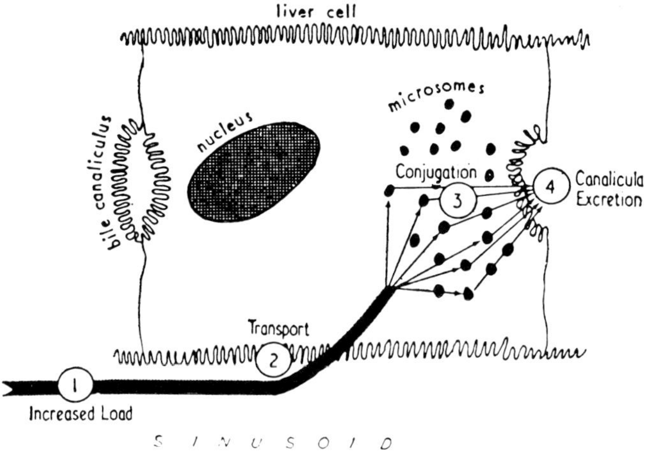

Fig. 1–19. Mechanisms of production of jaundice within hepatic parenchymal cells. Jaundice could theoretically result from (1) increased load of bilirubin presented to the cell, (2) defective uptake and transport within the cell, (3) defective conjugation within hepatic microsomes, or (4) defective canalicular excretion or mechanical block in the bile duct system. (Sherlock, S. Courtesy of Br. Med. J.)

soluble substances have an affinity for central nervous system tissues, a great excess of indirect-reacting bilirubin in the blood may result in deposition of bilirubin pigment in and damage to basal ganglia of the brains (kernicterus) of newborns with severe hemolytic disease of the newborn (erythroblastosis fetalis).

The simplest test for bile pigments involves acidic oxidation of bilirubin into a rainbow of colors resulting from formation of biliverdin (green), bilicyanin (blue), choletelin (yellow), and others, a reaction named after Gmelin in the mid-19th century. This reaction is also the basis of the Harrison spot test. At their normal concentration in urine (about 0.5 mg/dl), bile pigments are not detected by screening methods. Alfred Free's Ictotest, introduced by the Ames Company, involves coupling bilirubin with paranitrobenzene diazonium paratoluene sulfonate (bilazo) to produce a blue to purple reaction. Because the tablets are inexpensive, the reaction rapid, the test simple, they have been widely used for detection of increased amounts of bile pigment in urine. They are said reliably to detect more than 0.1 mg bilirubin/dl urine. Quantitative and semiquantitative tests for bile pigments and urobilinogen are based on formation of colored substances by reaction with various reagents. The most common tests include Watson's and Wallace-Diamond's, which involve use of Ehrlich's aldehyde reagent to produce a red reaction product. Ehrlich's aldehyde reagent will also react with porphobilinogen, melanogens, and many other nonurobilinogen substances. We prefer Watson's test for measurement of urobilinogen since

Richard Henry has shown that the color produced in the Wallace-Diamond test is not caused primarily by urobilinogen. Richard Henry's modification of the Watson test involves use of phenolsulfonphthalein (PSP) as a secondary standard to replace the old pontacyl dye secondary standards, because the spectral absorbance of the PSP dye and urobilinogen is about the same at 560 nm and curves are reproducible from lot to lot, which is not the case with the pontacyl dyes.[40] (There are no pure urobilinogen standards!)

Presence of urobilin in urine has the same diagnostic significance as presence of urobilinogen. If the urobilinogen test is negative, the urine should be checked for urobilin, since the former is oxidized to the latter upon standing.[41] Urobilin can be detected by formation of green fluorescent zinc-urobilin when reacted with alcoholic zinc acetate in the presence of iodine (Schlesinger's test) (Fig. 1–20). The zinc-urobilin complex has spectral absorption maxima at 637, 601, 551, and 521 nm. The screening test is 22.5 times more sensitive for detection of urobilinogen than is spectroscopic analysis.

Because some authorities have found diurnal variation in urobilinogen output (maxima occurring in the afternoon between 12:00 noon and 4:00 P.M.), it is usual to collect urine for urobilinogen determination over a 2-hour period in mid-afternoon during these hours. Also, urobilinogen clearance varies widely with urinary pH—from a rate of 2 ml/minute at a pH of 5, to a rate of 5 ml/minute at a pH of 8. More reproducible results can be obtained by inducing an alkaline urine in the patient, which can be accomplished before the test sample is collected by oral administration of sodium bicarbonate. Inasmuch as sunlight and air speed oxidation of urobilinogen to urobilin, specimens should be collected in dark bottles and tests performed as soon as possible after collection of urine.

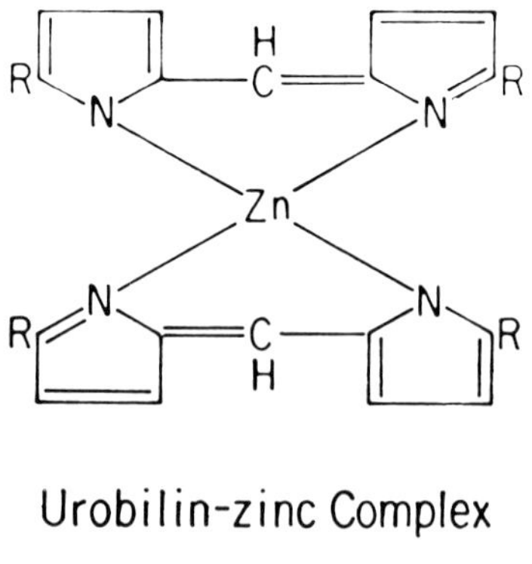

Fig. 1–20. The urobilin-zinc complex that fluoresces green color in visual light.

Melanogens

Presence of *melanin*, or its colorless precursors, melanogens, in urine in sufficient quantities to detect by simple tests is abnormal. The condition occurs in about 20% of the patients with malignant melanoma—those who have widespread metastases.[42]

The simple Thormählen test (utilizing nitroprusside reagent in a strongly alkaline solution) produces a blue to black color, when melanogens are present, immediately after acidifying with glacial acetic acid.

The ferric chloride test can also detect melanogens, but it is neither specific nor sensitive. The Ehrlich test is more sensitive, but it is also nonspecific. A more definitive test depends on extraction of urine with ethyl acetate, two-dimensional paper chromatography, and development of color with paranitrobromoanaline (see discussion of phenolic acids). The levels of several urinary phenolic acids, including homovanillic acid, are consistently elevated in patients with pigmented melanomas. The latter acid is also excreted in large amounts in patients with neuroblastoma, as previously noted.

5-Hydroxyindoleacetic Acid (5-HIAA)

The liver metabolizes serotonin (itself produced from the essential amino acid tryptophan) to the principal urinary metabolite 5-hydroxyindoleacetic acid (5-HIAA), which is normally excreted in urine in amounts ranging from 2 to 8 mg/24 hours (Fig. 1–21). In patients with argentaffinomas (Kulchitsky cell or carcinoid cell tumors), excretion of 5-HIAA may be greater than 25 mg/day, although excretion is variable.[43] Two-thirds of carcinoid tumors occur in the appendix; the ileum is the next most common site. Most carcinoids of the appendix are small and do not metastasize; ileal carcinoids metastasize and produce obstruction. In general, however, metastases are very slow to develop, and 15 to 25 years may elapse between the time of diagnosis and detection of metastasis. Excessive serotonin excretion from carcinoids, especially

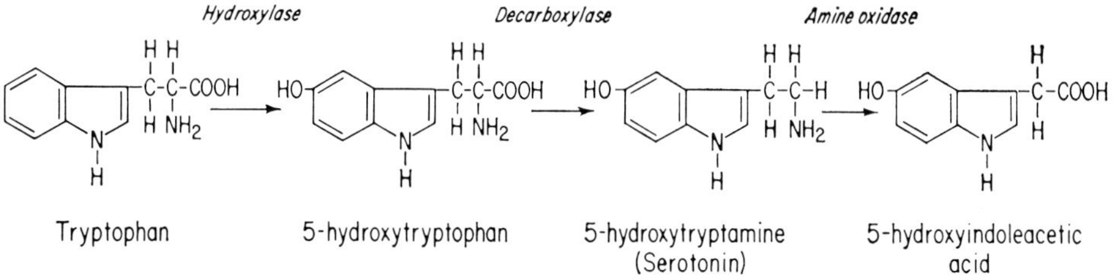

Fig. 1–21. The formation of serotonin and its metabolic product, 5-hydroxyindoleacetic acid (5-HIAA), from tryptophan.

when there are liver metastases, produces the carcinoid syndrome—skin flushing, patchy cyanosis, hypertension, valvular (tricuspid) right heart disease, congestive heart failure, "asthma," and watery diarrhea. We have seen 5 carcinoid tumors but never a carcinoid syndrome.

In the clinical laboratory, 5-HIAA, when present in the urine in amounts greater than 8 mg/L, can be detected by the Sjoerdsma screening test. This test is diagnostically useful, but patients should be followed after surgery with quantitative determinations of serotonin and 5-HIAA.

Indican

Indole, skatol, cresol, and phenol arise from action of intestinal bacteria, especially from the action of Escherichia coli, on tyrosine and tryptophan, or from ingestion of benzene, or other phenolic compounds. Some are normally absorbed, detoxified in the liver, and excreted in the urine. Higher levels of indole are produced when there is increased intestinal putrefaction. In patients with intestinal infarction, they are absorbed in increased amounts into the blood stream. In the liver, indole is converted to indoxyl conjugated with sulfate and excreted in the urine as indoxyl blue or indican (potassium indoxyl phosphate).[44] Indican is normally present in the urine in concentrations ranging from 2 to 4 mg/24 hours.

A modification of the ferric chloride test, known as the Obermayer test, can detect increased levels and point the finger of suspicion to increased intestinal putrefaction or increased absorption in the presence of gangrene or infarction. Lesser increases are said to be seen in patients with constipation.

IONS

Determination of concentration of some ions present in urine has some clinical significance, especially when balance studies are called for. These include sodium, potassium, hydrogen, calcium, magnesium, iron, chloride, and bicarbonate. Most of these procedures are carried out quantitatively in the clinical chemistry laboratory. In the past, chloride has been assayed by the Fantus procedure, now outmoded because of the ease of performance of quantitative tests for chlorides. Furthermore, since the advent of atomic absorption spectrophotometry, fewer calcium determinations by the Sulkowitch method are requested of our clinical microscopy laboratory. Nevertheless, the usefulness of calcium determinations by the patient at home for regulating his own intake of vitamin D as therapy for hypoparathyroidism justifies its continued use.

Calcium

Although 9 g of calcium are filtered daily through the kidneys, 99% is reabsorbed in the tubules, leaving calcium excretion rather constant at a level of about 100 to 150 mg/day. At the normal concentration of calcium in serum (9 to 11 mg/dl), the average patient is just above his renal threshold (7.5 to 9.0 mg/dl of serum). Above a serum level of 11.5 mg/dl of serum, calcium is excreted in the urine in increasing amounts, and there is the potential for development of nephrolithiasis or nephrocalcinosis. At a serum level of 16 mg/dl, there is danger of sudden death from hypercalcemia. Lower-than-normal serum levels are usually associated with hypoparathyroidism caused either by disease of the glands or by accidental removal of them during thyroidectomy. Below the renal threshold, no calcium is excreted in the urine. Therefore, qualitative evaluation of calcium in the urine by semiquantitative or qualitative techniques gives an estimate of the serum calcium level. The test is simple enough to be carried out by a patient in his own home to regulate his own medication for hypoparathyroidism.[50]

Hypercalciuria is usually defined as excretion of more than 200 mg calcium/day.[51] Hypercalcemia caused by hyperparathyroidism usually results in constant 3+ to 4+ urinary calcium as judged by the Sulkowitch test. Conversely, hypocalcemia associated with hypoparathyroidism is usually associated with a negative reaction. A large dietary intake of calcium (as in excessive milk intake) may produce 3+ or 4+ reactions. Increased urinary calcium also may be seen in patients with primary carcinomas (of breast and lung); primary or metastatic bone tumors, including multiple myeloma; the milk-alkali syndrome; hypervitaminosis D; sarcoidosis; hyperthyroidism; Cushing's syndrome; and renal tubular acidosis. Decreased urinary calcium may be seen in patients with vitamin D deficiency, either primary or secondary to malabsorption syndromes (such as sprue and celiac disease); nephrosis; and decreased calcium intake. As calcium intake is decreased, there is a proportionate increase in excretion of phosphorus, whose renal threshold is about 2 mg/dl of plasma.

Iron

Urine contains so little iron that it is undetectable by routine examination of urine from an adult on a balanced diet (0.045 mg/24 hours). Consequently, demonstration of presence of iron in the urine is abnormal. Most iron in the urine is found in the form of hemosiderin (an aggregate of ferritin molecules).

It may be found in patients with hemolytic anemias and transfusion reactions. It is quite common to find patients with sickle cell anemia (who frequently have aplastic crises and sometimes hemolytic crises). In general, hemosiderin found in the urine of these patients is within tubular cells. However, as cells degenerate, hemosiderin becomes incorporated into casts; the casts degenerate, especially in alkaline urine upon standing, to liberate iron. In patients with hemochromatosis and hemosiderosis, there is deposition of iron within epithelium throughout the urogenital tract.

In the urine, ferrous iron can be demonstrated with Turnbull's blue stain, while ferric iron can be stained with Prussian blue stain. Alternatively, ferrous iron can be oxidized to ferric iron by ferricyanide in an acid environment (the Prussian blue reaction). With low concentrations of iron, a pH less than 3 to 4 is essential to produce the blue color. Otherwise, a green conjugate will develop.

LIPIDS

Neutral Fats, Fatty Acids, and Lipoids

Stainable fat rarely appears in the urine except within cells. Chylomicrons are less dense than urine, so they are not found in centrifuged sediment. Also, lipemia is not usually accompanied by lipuria, inasmuch as fats will not traverse the glomerulus into the urinary filtrate.[45] Chyluria is caused by rupture of dilated lymphatics in renal tubules secondary to obstruction of abdominal lymphatics and the thoracic duct. As noted above, these chylomicrons float to the surface of urine, of course.

Stains for fats depend on the partition coefficient between solvent and lipid—that is, greater solubility of the dye in lipids than in other solvents, thus "staining" the lipids. Sudan III or IV provides good stains for most lipids including neutral fats (triglycerides), but not for lipids and lipoids of high melting point, such as cholesterol, carotenoids, and paraffins.

Embolism of bone marrow fat from fracture sites may, however, cause lipuria, but only when there is glomerular infarction. Fats occur most often in the urine of patients with degenerative tubular disease (with fat within the renal tubular epithelial cells), in the form of oval fat bodies and fatty casts. Unclean collection containers, oiled catheters, and soaps may contaminate urine, thus mimicking stainable fats or lipoids.

Under the microscope, unstained droplets of fat appear as round, highly refractile areas. They may appear black and sometimes only slightly refractile under low-power examination with subdued light. Some lipids seen in urine of patients with the nephrotic syndrome exhibit anisotropism; that is, they rotate a beam of polarized light, appearing as shining "Maltese crosses" against a dark field. Waxy casts may also exhibit anisotropism. Cholesterol esters are anisotropic, so it has been assumed that Maltese crosses are cholesterol esters. Neutral fats (triglycerides) and fatty acids do not exhibit anisotropism.

Metachromatic Granules (Sulphatides)

Cerebroside sulfuric acid esters (sulphatides) are formed by demyelination of the central nervous system and by alterations of epithelium (renal, biliary, and otherwise). These esters may be seen as granules in urine that stain brown with toluidine blue O. The reaction has yet to be fully characterized.

The stain test is only a screening procedure, but when it is properly interpreted and the results of the test are positive, indicative of (but not diagnostic of) hereditary metachromatic leukodystrophy.[52] Confirmation of excess sulphatide excretion should be made by chemical determination of arylsulfatase-A activity. The granules under polarized light are doubly refractile ("Maltese-cross" effect); they migrate electrophoretically toward the anode at pH 12. Metachromatic granules can be stained with para-aminosalicylic acid, aniline, methylene blue (red color), thionine, and other dyes, but Toluidine Blue I has been used more widely. The granules will not stain with Sudan IV or Turnbull blue neutral fat stains. Recently, the validity of the relationship between metachromatic granules and metachromatic leukodystrophy has been questioned.[53] A rapid screening test for deficiency of arylsulfatase-A activity in the urine of patients with diffuse cerebral sclerosis (metachromatic leukodystrophy) has been advocated for evaluation and confirmation of suspected cases (Austin et al., Arch. Neurol., *14*:529, 1966).

Polarization microscopy affords a ready means of identifying numerous lipids in urinary sediment.[54]

MICROSCOPIC EXAMINATION OF URINARY SEDIMENT

Not only do various diseases manifest themselves in the urine by the formation of certain sediment elements (urinary sediment), but the courses of many diseases affecting the urinary tract may be followed by accurate sediment examination. Finally, in an attempt to predict the prognosis of a patient with certain varieties of intrinsic renal diseases, the urinary sediment provides discriminating data that cannot be as easily obtained through any other investigative method.[55]

QUALITY ASSURANCE IN MICROSCOPIC URINALYSIS

Prior to the actual microscopic examination of the sediment, the laboratory worker must ensure that quality-assurance procedures are followed. The concept of quality-assurance procedures in urinalysis is relatively new, but, as is to be expected in the chemistry laboratory, the procedures ensure that each urinalysis specimen sampled will be treated similarly enough to provide results that are accurate, precise, consistent, and dependable. Standardization of a procedure in microscopic urine analysis have been shown to provide results that are more

TABLE 1–17. Characteristic Urinary Findings and Correlated Clinical Features in Renal Lesions and Disorders of the Kidney and Genitourinary Tract.

Disease State	Urinary Findings	Clinical Features
Exercise	Microscopic hematuria, mild proteinuria, cylindruria	History of vigorous exercise immediately preceding the examination
Trauma	Hematuria varying from microscopic to gross	History of trauma to region of kidney
Cystitis	White blood cells especially in clumps Proteinuria (mild) Bacteriuria No casts	Urgency, frequency, dysuria
Renal calculi	No casts or protein unless pyelonephritis or other renal disease present	Flank pain varying from dull ache to severe renal colic. Occasionally gross hematuria
Genitourinary tumors	Hematuria of variable severity	Local symptoms depending upon the location of the tumor
Hereditable disorders Hemoglobinopathies Osler-Weber-Rendu disease Polycystic disease	Hematuria usually grossly visible No casts	Usually no symptoms Occasionally mild flank pain Rarely severe flank pain
Thrombocytopenic purpura	Only red blood cells in urine, no casts	No symptoms
Glomerulonephritis		
Acute	Red blood cell casts, white blood cells, proteinuria, granular casts	Smoky urine Occasionally clinical features of uremia only, or heart failure and/or hypertension
Chronic	Red blood cell casts, white blood cells, proteinuria, granular casts and cellular casts	Few symptoms until malignant hypertension or uremia supervene

Systemic lupus erythematosus }	May resemble those of acute glomerulonephritis	Fever and joint pain are most prominent features but many systems may be involved
Polyarteritis }	Telescoped urine sediment with all types of casts plus red blood cells and white blood cells	May present as acute glomerulonephritis with uremia but no hypertension; fever, anemia and nervous system involvement also common
Lung Purpura with Nephritis (Goodpasture's syndrome)	Red blood cell casts, gran. casts, proteinuria	Severe recurrent hemoptyses which precede onset of symptoms or uremia
Allergic Nephropathies		
Henoch-Schoenlein Purpura	Urinary findings of acute glomerulonephritis with gross hematuria	Gastrointestinal and joint manifestations and purpura
Thrombotic Thrombocytopenic Purpura	Proteinuria and red blood cell casts	Fever Neurologic manifestations Hemolytic anemia, jaundice
Focal Embolic Glomerulitis	Red blood cell casts Mild proteinuria	Subacute bacterial endocarditis usually present; mild renal insufficiency
Malignant Hypertension	Rarely gross hematuria	Headache, decreasing vision, and other manifestations of severe hypertension
Chemical or Drug Induced		
Carbon Tetrachloride	Red blood cell casts, protein	Progressive uremia, jaundice, hepatomegaly
Sulfonamides	Crystals in urine	Occasionally progressive renal insufficiency
Dicoumarol	None	Other manifestations of bleeding diathesis

(Harvey, A. (ed.): Principles and Practice of Medicine. 17th ed. Courtesy of Appleton-Century-Crofts.)

reproducible. Commercially available systems (such as Kova) offer a microscopic slide in which a standard volume of urine is observed (see Fig. 1–44).

Once the urine has been received in the laboratory, the time of receipt should be recorded and the specimen promptly examined. Strict criteria for specimen acceptability—that is, whether or not to perform a microscopic examination on the sediment—need to be established in each laboratory and understood by the clinical staff. These criteria include collection of a midstream sample in an appropriate clean container, sufficient urine to analyze, accurate patient identification, and no visible signs of contamination.

The urinalysis sediment specimen must be properly identified prior to and during the examination.

Any results obtained, whether they be positive or negative, should be correlated with the clinical history and symptomatology (Table 1–17). This is especially true when an asymptomatic patient presents with obviously abnormal urinary findings. Procedures should be followed that ensure that the urine sediment has not remained at room temperature for longer than a few hours. The sooner the urinalysis specimen is examined, the better. Sediment elements, especially casts and cells, tend to disappear on standing. This is due to the fact that urine contains enzymes that cause protein disruption. In addition, routine urinalysis specimens are often contaminated with microorganisms whose metabolic products alter or destroy sediment elements and change the urine pH towards the alkaline side, a factor that also produces sediment disruption.

CENTRIFUGED VERSUS UNCENTRIFUGED URINE

There is continuing argument as to whether it is best to centrifuge and examine sediment or to examine uncentrifuged urine for formed elements. The finding of 2 to 5 WBC/HPF during microscopic examination of sediment from a centrifuged specimen may have no clinical significance, whereas, the same finding in an uncentrifuged urine specimen may indicate presence of urinary tract infection. Likewise, the presence of bacteria in a fresh, uncentrifuged urine sample may have great clinical importance; in centrifuged specimen sediment, however, this finding could be insignificant. An incidental finding of an occasional red blood cell in an uncentrifuged sample of urine from an ostensibly normal person would not warrant much attention; when it is a consistent finding, however, minor hematuria is an indication that the patient needs further workup for a possibly severe problem.

Most authorities in the United States agree that concentration enables the microscopist to recognize and identify most of the elements present with greater accuracy and precision than if centrifugation were not performed.

Most pediatricians who obtain urine samples by suprapubic taps, with catheterizations, and in bags fixed over the genitalia prefer centrifugation of all specimens to obtain maximum information about patients with potential disease processes. In the laboratories of Earl K. Long Memorial Hospital, *we centrifuge all specimens,* because we feel that abnormal findings, even if they do not necessarily indicate disease, can easily be followed up to rule out this possibility. This is especially true of specimens from patients with urinary tract infections resulting from Escherichia coli, for example, who may have, microscopically, large numbers of bacteria but very few pus cells. Such a finding in urine sediment should be followed with a bacteriologic culture of the urine.[56]

As in all other sections of the laboratory, a centrifuge with a fixed speed should be utilized for urine-sediment concentration. The spin time should be constant and the volume of urine centrifuged should be the same for each sample studied. A recommended time for centrifugation is 5 minutes at 400 RCF (relative centrifugal force) using a volume of urine of 12 ml. The volume used is not critical and varies in different laboratories (usually 10–12 ml); however, it should be consistent from specimen to specimen. If any given sample of urine does not contain the required volume for quality assurance, a normal saline solution should be added to reach this volume. Obviously, if such a dilution of the sample is made, an appropriate calculation should be performed when quantitating any elements present.

Once the urine sample is centrifuged, the supernatant should be poured off, and the remaining 1 ml concentrated specimen at the bottom of the centrifuge tube should be thoroughly mixed. After an aliquot is taken, the sample should be placed on a microscopic slide for examination. As stated previously, the beginning volume of urine undergoing centrifugation may vary from laboratory to laboratory. The concentrated volume of urine containing the sediment elements (1 ml, 1/2 ml, etc.) should be representative of the sample handled. Plastic microscopic slides that have built in chambers that receive a standard amount of urine to ensure reproducible results, such as Kova, are commercially available.

The microscope utilized to observe the sediment should be a modern standard binocular microscope that provides Koehler illumination (see Chapter 9, "The Microscope and Microscopy"). Since many sediment elements have a low refractive index, it is imperative that the observer be familiar with the workings of the microscope and be able to provide himself with a field of high contrast. This is ordinarily done by lowering the condenser and stopping down the iris diaphragm. If more than one microscope is used in a laboratory to examine urine sediments, the microscopes should have similar eyepieces and objectives so that the area of view will be the same and the number of cells or other elements present in a given field will be comparable.

Having followed quality-assurance procedures in the preparation of the centrifuged urine specimen for microscopic analysis, the observer can be certain that microscopic findings will reflect accurately the patient's health. It is imperative that the observer be experienced, conscientious, and able to identify correctly any and all elements present. Perhaps the microscopist's most important task is differentiating the normal sediment from the abnormal. In many instances, this differentiation is simply a matter of degree—that is, the presence of white blood cells in the urine does not necessarily reflect disease of the urinary tract, because this finding may be normal if the cells are present in small numbers. On the other hand, certain elements always reflect an abnormal state (red blood cell casts, for example).

ROUTINE MICROSCOPIC EXAMINATION OF SEDIMENT

Conventionally, the routine urinalysis has included examination of the microscopic sediment; unfortunately, this portion of the examination has often been relegated to relatively poorly trained individuals.

G. Berry Schumann and Associates reported in 1977, at a meeting of the American Society of Clinical Pathologists in Las Vegas, that "In a random screening such as for insurance physicals, hospital admission examinations, and so on, much time and expense could be saved by omitting the microscopic examination of those urine specimens that are yellow, clear, and have a negative reagent strip chemical reaction. . . ." They calculated their false negative results not to exceed 1.0%. We vehemently disagree with this thesis, especially in samples from patients who are admitted to hospitals.[55]

NORMAL URINARY SEDIMENT

It is rare that a microscopic examination of the sediment will fail to reveal any solid components even in patients without known diseases of the genitourinary tract. Table 1–18 lists the sediment elements that may be present in a given normal urinalysis specimen. Basically, these elements originate from the blood stream, from epithelium lining the renal tubules or urinary tract, from products of metabolism (that is, crystals), or from contaminants (microorganisms or spermatozoa, especially in the female).

Traditionally, the routine microscopic examination includes examination for the following:

1. Red blood cells
2. White blood cells
3. Casts
4. Mucus
5. Epithelial cells
6. Microorganisms
7. Spermatozoa
8. Crystals

To enhance the observation and diagnosis of all sediment elements, but especially casts, the experienced urinoscopist often uses phase contrast and/or interference contrast microscopy.[55,56–60] In both instances, these techniques have capitalized on relatively small differences in refractive index in an attempt to enhance the viewing of the sediment elements present. Although adding to the cost of the equipment necessary for urine observation, cells, casts, and crystals are seen more readily when phase or interference contrast microscopy is utilized. A variety of commercially available stains can aid in the recognition of any elements that may be present. The most commonly used stain is a gentian violet/safranin mixture (the Sternheimer-Malbin stain).[48]

Red Blood Cells[56–60]

Red blood cells in the urine most commonly appear as biconcave discs, just as they do in stained smears of the peripheral blood. Due to the high osmolar concentrations commonly found in urine (over 800 mmol/Kg), however, these cells are frequently crenated; less frequently, the cells may imbibe water, whereupon they assume spherical shapes. In either instance, rupture of the red cell membrane may occur, leading to a positive hemoglobin test. In such cases, further investigation of the patient, including retesting a freshly collected urine sample, is indicated. The color of the cells is usually pale reddish-tan, since they

TABLE 1–18. Sediment in Normal Urine.

Sediment	Quantity
Blood cells:	
Red blood cells	0–2/hpf
White blood cells	3–5/hpf
Casts:	
Hyaline	0–2/lpf*
Granular	o–1/lpf*
Mucus	variable
Epithelial cells:	
Renal	0–1/hpf
Transitional	0–2/hpf
Squamous	variable/hpf
Crystals in acid, neutral, or basic urine	variable
Microorganisms:	+
Bacteria	
Fungi (yeasts)	
Spermatozoa	+ present in both men and women

*May be greatly increased in number when exercise/stress occurred within 24 hours prior to sediment examination.

contain hemoglobin and do not exhibit birefringence under polarized light (a feature that can distinguish them from oval fat bodies and certain crystals). In normal concentrated urine, red blood cells are present in small numbers, and an increase is usually pathologic. The physiologic increase of red blood cells can occur following violent exercise or fever without indicating significant urinary disease. Increase in red blood cells is clinically termed hematuria.

White Blood Cells

White blood cells of normal urinary sediment are most often *polymorphonuclear leukocytes (polys)*. Other mononuclear cells, usually lymphocytes, are rarely found; monocytes or macrophages are found much less frequently. Increased numbers of polys in the urine are indicative of a pathologic condition and are most frequently associated with inflammatory conditions involving the kidneys or lower urinary tract. Polys are recognized by their cytoplasmic granularity, multilobed nuclei, and size (usually about 12 to 15 μ diameter).

Casts

Casts are often present in the normal urinary sediment.[61,62] Although this fact was not commonly recognized until recently, both hyaline and granular casts in the urine accompany stress and strenuous physical exercise in the normal patient.[72] In such instances, they may be seen in rather large numbers in the sediment (sometimes as many as 50 per low-power microscopic field). In the patient who has not undergone extensive physical exercise within the preceding 24-hour period, occasional hyaline or granular casts in the sediment are a frequent occurrence.

Casts are produced in the distal renal tubules or collecting ducts. Cast formation is poorly understood and thought to consist of an agglutination or gelation of certain concentrated protein components of the urine present in the nephron.[62] Appropriate conditions of pH, ionic concentration, and solubility are necessary for this gelation process to occur. They commonly occur in the distal tubes, where the pH is acidic and water reabsorption occurs. Casts, by definition, are cylindrically shaped, semisolid protein molds of the renal tubules. Even in the normal urine, casts vary greatly in size, especially in length, and are usually seen as relatively narrow, elongated cylindrical structures; their ends are curved (cigar-shaped), their sides smooth and molded and, in the urine of a normal patient, do not contain cellular inclusions. Some casts have a long, tapered end that looks like a tail; these are called "cylindroids" and have absolutely no clinical significance. Both hyaline and granular casts have a low refractive index and for that reason are often very difficult to visualize without appropriate microscopic conditions.

A basic protein structure has been detected in casts by using scanning electron microscopic technology. Chemical analysis of casts has shown that they consist, at least in part, of a peculiar protein derived from the kidney (Tamm-Horsfall protein).[63] It has also been shown that this special protein forms fibrils under appropriate conditions (especially a relatively low pH) in the laboratory. Since similar environmental conditions also prevail in the renal tubules during concentration and dilution of urine, one may assume that this is indeed a partial mechanism of cast formation. In addition, numerous other serum proteins are present in the varieties of urinary casts, including normal urinary proteins. These proteins include albumin and various types of globulins.

Granular casts are also present in normal urinary sediments and may be defined as basically hyaline casts containing granules. The exact origin or composition of the granular matter in these casts in normal urinary sediment is unknown, although the granules are suspected to be products of epithelial cells lining the nephron such as lysosomes. Few experimental data have been offered to confirm this hypothesis, and until more are available, it may be premature to say that these granules originate from cells. Gerald Rutecki and Associates (Characterization of proteins in urinary casts. N. Engl. J. Med., *284*:1049, 1971), however, identified Tamm-Horsfall mucoproteins in all casts and other serum proteins only in granules, suggesting that granular casts may be made up of aggregates of serum protein, and therefore, may not be evolutionary.

Scanning electron microscopy has been very helpful in elucidating the features of normal granular casts.[65] Basically, they are composed of a hyaline cast matrix in and on which granular matter has been incorporated. The granules appear to be derived from the cytoplasmic granules or lysosomes of renal tubular epithelial cells.

Although the experienced microscopist is able to evaluate most details of the formed elements in urinary sediment in an unstained preparation with proper microscopic illumination, some elements, especially casts, can be more easily recognized after differential staining with crystal violet and safranin dyes, a technique introduced by Richard Sternheimer and Barney Malbin in 1951.[48] With the Sternheimer-Malbin stain (in acid or neutral urine), the red blood cells will remain colorless or stain slightly purple. In alkaline urine, the red cells are usually lysed and alkaline hematin forms, which stains dark purple. The nuclei of ordinary leukocytes usually stain dark orange-purple, and significant granularity is discernible in the cytoplasm. Some cells may be intermediate between light and dark forms. Granular motility cells ("glitter cells"), large polymorphonuclear leukocytes that have imbibed water, generally have light blue to almost colorless cytoplasm, while other leukocytes have dark blue cytoplasm. The nuclear staining makes differentiating epithelial cells from white blood cells somewhat less difficult than it is in unstained sediment. Much of the value of differential urinary-sediment staining lies in the ease with which casts can be recognized.[61,62] Hyaline casts appear pink to light purple and homogeneous. When other elements, such as red blood cells, white blood cells, and renal cells, are encased within the protein coagulum of the cases, they also are readily identified. Hemoglobin casts are deep purple, red blood cells and fibrin producing granularity in them at times. Hemoglobin casts, however, are best identified in unstained sediment because they are difficult to differentiate from clumped material with the Sternheimer-Malbin stain. Granular casts appear purple and, as stated, granular. The highly refractile globules of fat in fatty casts will remain unstained within the pink hyaline matrix.

Mucus

Mucus is present in the urinary sediment in variable amounts. It has no clinical importance except for the fact that the inexperienced observer may confuse mucus with hyaline casts. To differentiate the two, phase and/or interference microscopy is helpful. Mucus does not ordinarily stain with the usual urine sediment stains or stains very lightly. Mucus may assume a wide variety of shapes and forms but it does not have a clear margin, does not appear as a solid element, and is not ordinarily cylindrical in shape. It can best be described as a fibrillar protein product of certain epithelial cells lining the nephron, lower urinary tract, or vagina. It is present in variable amounts in both men and women.

Epithelial Cells[66–68]

Three varieties of *epithelial cells* may be present in both normal and abnormal urinary sediment; for the most part, they have little clinical significance and are observed frequently.[66] The most easily recognized of these epithelial cells is the squamous cell. This cell derives from the lower urinary tract and is not present in the normal kidney; it lines the distal one-third of both the male and female urethra and the entire vagina. It may be present in variable numbers and is recognized as a large flat cell (20–50 μ in diameter) with a small central spherical nucleus. The nucleus itself measures approximately the size of a leukocyte (8–12 μ). The cytoplasm of squamous cells may be finely wrinkled (an indication of drying of the specimen) and often contains granules.

Cells deriving their origin from transitional epithelium lining the renal pelvis, ureters, urinary bladder, and proximal two-thirds of both the male and female urethra are also seen in the normal urine. They may occur in clumps. Using light microscopic techniques, they are difficult to distinguish from epithelial cells that line the nephron, because both cell types are polyhedral in shape. Transitional epithelial cells, however, have a peculiar characteristic that, when present, distinguishes them from other epithelial cells. This feature is the tendency of the cell to accept water, which induces a marked swelling of the cell itself so that it becomes bloated or spherical. Transitional cell nuclei are central and approximately the size of a white blood cell (12–14 μ in diameter). If the transitional cell accepts sufficient amounts of water, its diameter may be greatly increased and reach as much as 20–25 μ.

The renal epithelial cell is perhaps the most difficult of all epithelial cells to recognize and distinguish.[49] It is approximately the same size as the transitional epithelial cells, polyhedral in shape, and often contains cytoplasmic vacuoles. The nucleus cannot be distinguished readily from the nucleus of the transitional epithelial cell. The nucleus is single-lobed and differential staining reveals a nucleolus. The cell ordinarily measures approximately 15 to 20 μ in diameter and does not have a tendency to imbibe water; therefore, it does not appear swollen in the sediment. Differential and histochemical staining enables one to identify the exact origin of this epithelial cell—that is, whether it be from the proximal or distal tubule. Sometimes these cells in the sediment have a microvillus border along one margin; these microvilli permit ready differentiation of them from transitional epithelial cells.[61]

Ordinarily, small numbers of renal epithelial cells have little or no pathologic significance. They may appear in markedly increased numbers in the sediment, however, and may point to a disease affecting the renal tubule. When present in abnormal numbers and in certain disease states, renal epithelial cells may contain visible fat droplets in their cytoplasm. In these instances, they are called oval fat bodies. This feature will be discussed later.[49,72]

Certain other epithelial cell types may, on occasion, be seen in the urine. They derive from the various glands lining the genitourinary tract, including the prostate gland in males, are columnar, and may be mucus-secreting. Using ordinary microscopic methods, it is exceedingly difficult to identify these cells accurately and to distinguish them from renal epithelial cells, even with staining. Histochemical techniques, as well as cytocentrifugation methodology, may provide assistance, however.[49] These forms of epithelial cells have little, if any, clinical significance.

Microorganisms

Bacteria are commonly present in sediments from normal patients. This is due to the fact that, in routine analysis, nonsterile collection techniques are utilized. Since urine is a fluid that is abundant in products that promote and enhance bacterial growth, bacteria thrive and multiply.

The bacteria usually seen in urine are gram-negative bacilli (Enterobacteriaceae), but coccal forms are also common (Enterococci).[67] The presence of large numbers of bacteria in fresh urine is distinctly abnormal; however, some may normally appear in fresh urine, especially in centrifuged sediments. Usually fewer than 1,000 bacteria per ml of uncentrifuged urine are present. They are not usually seen in wet mounts unless 10,000/ml or more are present, a number suggesting the presence of infection. Proper patient preparation can make the difference between a diagnostically significant or useless specimen. For most accurate results, the periurethral area must be washed thoroughly with surgical disinfectant. The specimen should be clean catch and examined within 1 hour of collection (2 hours if refrigerated). If 0.02 ml of uncentrifuged urine is placed on a microscopic slide and stained with Gram's iodine, presence of bacteria in ten consecutive oil immersion fields is considered significant bacteriuria (defined more accurately as 100,000 bacteria/ml or more). As many as 40% of pregnant women have significant bacteriuria and may develop acute pyelonephritis during pregnancy. Bacteriuria is frequently accompanied by pyuria (white blood cells in urine) in infections caused by most organisms. This is not always true in infections with Escherichia coli, in which the inflammatory response may be minimal, but it is, nevertheless, a clinically significant infection. Therefore, cultures are indicated for all urine specimens in which significant numbers of bacteria appear, whether or not pyuria is present.

Fungi (usually simple yeasts) are also found in the sediment in normal urine, but less frequently than bacteria; if the urine is allowed to stand for a sufficient length of time. When hyphae are seen, however, they usually indicate a pathologic condition. In normal urine, the presence of bacteria and yeast organisms in the sediment is not accompanied by an increase in the number of white blood cells.

Yeast forms of candida are common in urine of patients with diabetes mellitus. They appear as ovoid and spherical forms that can easily be confused with red blood cells. Look for budding forms and resistance to acid for differentiation from red blood cells (red cells lyse!). In female diabetics, chronic candida vaginitis can contribute yeast to urine sediment and be misinterpreted as urinary tract infection. It may be necessary to obtain catheterized specimens for clear differentiation. In such cases, however, the mycelial form of the organisms, as well as the yeast form, can frequently be found in wet preparations of vaginal fluid.

Spermatozoa

Spermatozoa are commonly found in the urinary sediment of both men and women. They have no clinical significance unless the pathologist is investigating rape cases, and their presence or absence is not a feature that is universally noted by laboratory technologists. Spermatozoa may or may not be motile.

Parasites

The flagellated protozoa, Trichomonas vaginalis, is slightly larger than a leukocyte, but the flagellum can seldom be seen in wet mounts of urine. They are readily demonstrable, however, in dry preparations stained with OG-6 (eosin) and EA-65 (light green, eosin, and Bismark brown) of the Papanicolaou stain.

Crystals

Crystalluria, or the presence of crystals in the urine, is a common finding that often provokes considerable thought and speculation. Normal urine may contain a wide variety of crystals. These precipitate frequently (especially if the urine is refrigerated) and are dependent for their formation on several factors, mainly urinary acidity and solute concentration.

The most commonly observed crystals in acid urine are the crystals of uric acid. These may assume a multiplicity of shapes and sizes and vary from an amorphous, nondescript granular shape to that of rhombic plates. Uric acid crystals are usually yellowish brown in color, but they may be colorless. They may also assume a six-sided configuration and must not be confused with cystine crystals. Urate crystals have little, if any, clinical significance, although they may be present in large numbers in patients with leukemia or lymphoma, due to the high cell-turnover rate. During cell destruction that occurs in chemotherapy of these disorders, the excretion of uric acid into urine may be increased. Sodium urate crystals appear as pale yellow or colorless, thin, elongate prisms that regularly occur in fan-shaped clusters.

Calcium oxalate crystals also assume pleomorphic shapes and forms and are most commonly associated with either acid or neutral urine pH. These crystals most frequently assume a dumbbell or octahedral shape and are usually colorless. Calcium oxalate crystals will be seen in large amounts in the urine of patients who have recently consumed certain foods rich in oxalic acid, such as rhubarb, asparagus, tomatoes, and certain berries; they are ordinarily of no pathologic significance. They are often present in the urine of infants and children after milk ingestion. However, they are present in large numbers in the urine of patients who have ingested ethylene glycol, a major component of automobile antifreeze.

The main crystals seen in alkaline urine are crystals of the salts of calcium. These include calcium phosphate and triple phosphate crystals (ammonium-magnesium phosphate) as well as amorphous phosphates. In addition, ammonium biurate crystals, which are yellow and assume peculiar, tortuous, starfish, or thorn-apple shapes, are commonly observed. Amorphous phosphates are colorless or pale gray granules that may precipitate out of the urine in large quantities upon refrigeration. Triple phosphate crystals usually occur in the form of a prism and assume a coffin-lid appearance. They may also take on a feathery or leaf-like shape and are colorless. Calcium phosphate crystals (dicalcium phosphate), in addition to being most commonly found in alkaline urine, may also appear in neutral or slightly acid urine. These crystals most frequently assume a large, thin, plate-like, ice-sheet appearance and frequently contain granules. They have no clinical significance. Calcium carbonate crystals are small, colorless, dumbbell-shaped crystals that often appear in masses and may simulate casts (pseudocast).

Many abnormal crystals, which will be discussed later in this chapter, assume shapes and other characteristics that may simulate these normal crystals. Abnormal crystals predominately occur in acid urine, whereas normal crystals appear in urine with acid, neutral, or alkaline pH. Therefore, in instances in which an abnormal crystal is suspected, the observer should obtain a fresh specimen and promptly do a pH determination.

The following is a review of crystals found in normal urine (see also Chapter 4, Urinary Stone Analysis):

1. Acid urines
   Uric acid: often rhombic-shaped and reddish-brown (a distinguishing feature); the most pleomorphic of all crystals
   Sodium urate: needle- and fan-shaped clusters; amorphous brown clumps
   Calcium oxalate: envelope-shaped
2. Alkaline urines
   Ammonium urate: thorn-apple–shaped
   Ammonium magnesium phosphate (triple phosphate): coffin-lid–shaped
   Calcium carbonate: dumbbell-shaped
   Calcium phosphate: amorphous or wedge-shaped

There is no constant relationship between the presence of crystals in urine and predisposition to stone formation or any particular disease state.

ABNORMAL URINARY SEDIMENT

In many instances, the abnormal sediment is simply defined by an increase in the number of sediment elements, especially blood cells; therefore, a semiquantitative analysis of the constituents of the urinary sediment is essential. In addition, this semiquantitation will enable the physician to follow the course of a given patient with renal disease and assist in predicting the prognosis. In this section, particular emphasis will be given to certain sediment elements present in the abnormal urine that essentially are never associated with the normal sediment.

Blood Cells

Finding small numbers of both red and white blood cells in the sediment has already been described as normal. Finding increased numbers of these cells, however, is definitely abnormal and suggests that a disease of the urinary tact is present. Only further investigation and careful observation of the entire urinary sediment, as well as a thorough macroscopic and chemical analysis, will enable the physician to accurately diagnose the specific disease present.

Red Blood Cells

The microscopic examination of sediment is the most sensitive method for detecting hematuria. Neoplasms of the kidneys or urinary bladder often cause hematuria. Red blood cells are also found in certain medical diseases of the kidney, such as hypertension and glomerulonephritis, which are usually accompanied by some degree of cylindruria and proteinuria. In any case, the finding of increased numbers of red blood cells in the sediment suggests to the physician that further workup of the patient is necessary, even mandatory. Athletic pseudonephritis is a term that has been coined to denote the abnormality of increased red blood cells and hemoglobin in the urine in the absence of an intrinsic renal disease. This finding has been noted in individuals undergoing severe physical exercise, such as long-distance running and playing football. This phenomenon is not associated with the presence of red blood cell casts, but it may be associated with increased numbers of hyaline and granular casts. In addition, when proteinuria is present in these patients, it is mild and reverts to normal within 24 to 48 hours after the physical stress ceases. In the abnormal patient with hematuria, proteinuria is ordinarily persistent.

White Blood Cells

An increased number of polys in the urinary sediment is an exceedingly common finding and is associated with many diseases. Inflammatory conditions of the genitourinary tract, such as urethritis, cystitis, and pyelonephritis, produce increased numbers of leukocytes in the urine. The distinction between an upper versus a lower urinary tract infection is important clinically, since both treatment and prognosis differ. To assist the clinician in making this differentiation, several ancillary tests are currently in use—among them, the so-called antibody-coated bacteria test (ACB test). The urinoscopist often will be able to make this distinction on the basis of the microscopic sediment examination, since renal infections are frequently accompanied by proteinuria and cylindruria, whereas lower urinary tract infections are not.

The presence of increased numbers of white blood cells in the urine is termed "pyuria." Acute pyelonephritis is usually characterized by pyuria, but chronic pyelonephritis is not. Granular motility cells (glitter cells), which are often found in the urine of patients with pyelonephritis, are polys showing Brownian movement of granules. The nuclei of ordinary leukocytes are stained orange-purple with the Sternheimer-Malbin stain, and the nuclei of the large, inflammatory glitter cells are colorless or stain lightly. Active granular motility ceases if urine osmolality exceeds 600 mmol/Kg; hence, glitter cells may disappear in concentrated urine.

White blood cells may be increased in the urine in certain medical diseases of the kidney besides those of an infectious nature. This fact should not be overlooked and should not trap the observer into making a diagnosis of pyelonephritis when, in fact, the patient may have a noninfectious condition in which white cells are but a part of the overall picture. Lupus erythematosus, as well as other collagen diseases of the kidney, often show increased numbers of polys in the urine. These conditions are ordinarily accompanied by other urinary features, usually hematuria and cylindruria.

Epithelial Cells

Epithelial cells may be seen in normal sediment as well as in abnormal sediment; they may be squamous, transitional, or renal. Squamous cells have little, if any, clinical significance. Normally, transitional epithelial cells are constantly being sloughed into the urine, but they may be increased in number in inflammatory conditions affecting the urinary tract, especially the bladder. If large numbers of these cells are present in the urine, the observer should attempt to ascertain whether or not there are any nuclear abnormalities, in which case a fresh specimen should be sent to the cytology section of the laboratory for Papanicolaou stains and cytological interpretation.

Renal epithelial cells, when present in the sediment in large numbers, have clinical significance. These cells are sloughed into the urine in the event of an injury to the tubular portion of the nephron. They are prominent in the sediment in generalized viral diseases, such as hepatitis and cytomegalic inclusion disease, and are also seen in various toxic conditions, such as heavy metal poisoning (lead, mercury), and after the ingestion of ethylene glycol (antifreeze). Some of these cells may become incorporated into casts (epithelial casts).

The sloughed renal epithelial cells often will show marked signs of degeneration. These features include nuclear and cytoplasmic disruption, breakdown of cell membranes, and the appearance of lipid globules in the cytoplasm. These lipid globules, when present, are easily seen as spheres in the cytoplasm with a pale yellow or tan color. When present, the particular cell is called an *oval fat body*. Intracellular lipids may be further identified by means of polarizing prisms, since the lipid has the physical property of birefringence and displays a "Maltese-cross" pattern with polarized light.

Acellular Casts

In the preceding section, it was pointed out that certain casts (predominantly hyaline and granular casts) occur frequently in normal persons who have been stressed. These casts are also found in the abnormal sediment in patients having intrinsic renal disease. Several other varieties of urinary casts are seen in the abnormal patient that are peculiar to disease states and not associated with the normal. Each of these casts will be discussed in some detail.

HYALINE CASTS

Hyaline casts are the prototype of all urinary casts. They have a low refractive index and are difficult to see when using ordinary light microscopy, but they may easily be diagnosed when phase or interference contrast microscopy is used. Their appearance is similar in both normal and abnormal urinary sediments. In disease states, accompanying proteinuria is usually present and persistent—that is, it does not disappear after 48 hours. In patients with abnormal numbers of hyaline casts in the urine, a follow-up urinalysis is warranted in order to distinguish whether or not the finding is stress produced.

GRANULAR CASTS

Granular casts are a frequent finding in the urinary sediment of abnormal patients. In such instances, the granules are often larger than in the normal (coarsely granular casts) and are thought to be derived from the breakdown of cells that become entrapped in or adherent to the cast matrix. The specific origin of many other granular casts is not known, but it is suspected that some granular casts arise from the cytoplasmic products (lysosomes) of renal tubular epithelial cells.

Granular casts have a considerably higher refractive index than do hyaline casts. They may have tortuous shapes, but are most often cigar-shaped, sometimes with one end tapered to a point (cylindroid). Certain granular casts evolve into waxy casts. Granular casts also may be broad or narrow. Broad casts, in general, indicate a more severe form of renal disease, and when present in large numbers, a poorer prognosis.

One specialized form of granular cast is the so-called "hemoglobin cast." This cast is basically a degenerated red blood cell cast that maintains its hemoglobin pigmentation and appears granular to the microscopist. For the sake of completeness, it is discussed here but will also be considered with red blood cell casts.

Commonly mistaken for granular casts and recently correctly identified, is the so-called "bacterial cast." This cast is associated with patients who have acute pyelonephritis; it is basically a hyaline cast in and upon which bacteria have collected. Many microscopists, unaware of the fact that bacterial casts exist and are essentially pathognomonic for pyelonephritis, commonly mistake these casts as granular casts. Only with special stains, such as the Gram stain, or with the use of phase or interference contrast, will bacterial shapes be observed in the cast itself. Many bacterial casts have associated polys in their matrix. These may also be misdiagnosed as white blood cell casts and the bacterial component totally missed unless the specialized microscopic techniques mentioned previously are utilized.[68]

WAXY CASTS

Many waxy casts evolve from pre-existent granular casts. They are of extremely high refractive index and appear to be thick and brittle when using ordinary bright field light microscopic techniques. They have parallel margins, are often broad and have ends that are squared or broken-off. Their margins are often notched and sometimes show cracks or fissures, a feature that has been called "serrated." The presence of many broad waxy casts in the urine indicates an extremely poor prognosis and severe degeneration of the nephron.

BILE CASTS

Bile is often found in the urine of patients with severe jaundice resulting from a variety of causes. This metabolic product of hemoglobin breakdown may be absorbed into a pre-existent hyaline cast, thereby forming a *bile cast*. These casts are easily seen in the urine because of their deep brownish-green pigmentation and may be present in large numbers in patients having viral hepatitis, various hemolytic diseases, and obstructive jaundice.

FATTY CASTS

Casts that contain significant numbers of yellowish-tan fat globules and differently sized spherical bodies of lipid (cholesterol) are called fatty casts. They may be present in urine of patients with many types of renal disease, but especially in patients having the nephrotic syndrome. Fatty casts are easily diagnosed, but the inexperienced observer may often confuse them with red blood cell casts. Urinary lipid globules may be easily differentiated from red blood cells simply by polarizing the microscopic field.

Fats will exhibit birefringence when polarizing prisms are used, manifesting a "Maltese-cross" pattern.[69] One must be careful, however, not to mistakenly diagnose certain crystals or starch granules as fat, since these substances also show birefringence with polarized light.

Fatty casts are acellular and should not be confused with oval fat body (OFB) casts, which will be considered later under cellular casts. Both of these casts contain lipids and display the "Maltese-cross" pattern with polarized light. The oval fat body, however, is actually a renal tubular epithelial cell, and the lipid is present within this cell; whereas, in a fatty cast, the lipid has no cellular association. Fatty casts and oval fat body casts often are seen together in the same patient. This is due to the fact that the nephrotic syndrome is a common denominator of many diseases affecting the kidney.

Cellular Casts

Several kinds of cells may become incorporated into urinary casts. These include cells derived from the blood stream, as well as epithelial cells that have their origin in the kidney itself. Cellular casts, therefore, are classified on the basis of the predominant type of cell contained. Cellular casts are not found in normal urinary sediment, so when present, they are pathologic. The primary disease process within the kidney may be indicated by these types of casts. These casts should be scrutinized carefully to determine the specific cell type therein.

All cells in the urine show some degree of degenerative changes characteristic of cellular death. This is especially true of cells incorporated within cellular casts. For this reason, degenerative signs, including both cytoplasmic and nuclear degeneration and subsequent autolysis are often seen in the cells within casts. Special microscopic techniques enhance the recognition of these particular cell types, especially interference contrast microscopy.[56] When the cells degenerate, the remnants and granular material thus produced can often be discerned in the casts that subsequently are formed. These granular casts may provide valuable clues about the precursor cell of origin and may even contain products of the cell (that is, hemoglobin from a pre-existent red blood cell cast).

WHITE BLOOD CELL CASTS

White blood cell casts frequently appear in the urine in a wide variety of disease states. However, they are most consistently observed in infections of the kidney such as acute pyelonephritis. They are present in various other inflammatory conditions affecting the kidneys, such as lupus erythematosus, polyarteritis nodosa, and poststreptococcal glomerulonephritis. White blood cell casts, therefore, are not pathognomonic for any given disease state, and their relative number becomes an important differential point in attempting to make a specific clinical diagnosis.

White blood cell casts are basically formed by the incorporation and adherence of polymorphonuclear leukocytes (polys) to a hyaline cast matrix. Scanning electron microscopic studies have shown these leukocytes are closely applied to the cast surface by delicate proteinaceous fibrils. In cases of acute pyelonephritis due to bacteria, the microorganisms may often be found on the cast surface as well.[68]

Leukocytic casts are relatively easy to recognize when the white blood cells remain intact. The polys have multilobed nuclei, are about 15 μ in diameter, and have granular cytoplasm. When staining techniques are used (Sternheimer-Malbin stain), the casts are observed with great facility and the multilobate structure of the nuclei is perceived with ease. White blood cells, however, are relatively fragile and tend to degenerate easily as the casts transit the tubular portions of the nephron. In such instances, lobes of the nuclei may be extremely difficult to recognize, and the granularity of the cytoplasm becomes prominent. In addition, the cell walls may become discontinuous, and the granules may leak into the surrounding cast matrix.

White blood cell casts are usually accompanied in the urine by white blood cells and protein. A major factor in differentiating upper from lower urinary tract infections is that these casts are ordinarily present in infections of the kidney, whereas they are absent in inflammatory diseases of the lower genitourinary tract.

RED BLOOD CELL CASTS

Red blood cell casts are extremely important diagnostic indicators when found in the urinary sediment. They are ordinarily seen in conjunction with diseases that induce damage to the glomerulus, especially the glomerular basement membrane, thereby causing leakage of red blood corpuscles from the blood stream into the urine. Many diseases disturb the integrity of the glomerulus, but among the most common are acute glomerulonephritis, lupus erythematosus, and immune complex disorders. Hematuria is a common accompaniment of renal cell carcinoma, but red blood cell casts are not usually found in this condition. Red blood cells may also enter the urinary flow by diapedesis across the basement membrane of the renal tubule. This mechanism is often associated with vascular diseases of the kidney, such as renal infarction, nephrosclerosis, and hypertension.

Red blood cell casts are relatively easy to identify in the urinary sediment. They have a high refractive index and, if the red blood cells are intact, appear on the cast surface as biconcave corpuscles, often closely packed together, with their typical brownish-red hemoglobin pigmentation. The red cells within the cast often show signs of crenation. In the urine of patients with red blood cell casts, red cells are usually present in the surrounding urine. Proteinuria is also a common accompaniment.

Red blood cells in the casts commonly show degenerative signs with loss of cell walls and leakage of hemoglobin into the surrounding matrix. In such instances, in which red blood cells are not intact within the cast, the cast is called a *blood cast*. In many such casts, special stains for fibrin and hemoglobin will be positive.

EPITHELIAL CASTS

Renal epithelial cells are damaged and then sloughed into the urinary flow in various diseases affecting the kidney, especially in generalized viral diseases, and when toxins are introduced into the body. These epithelial cells may become incorporated into a hyaline cast matrix and are bound to its surface by thin, proteinaceous fibrils, thereby creating an epithelial cast. Renal epithelial cells are derived from the tubular epithelium, and epithelial casts are usually formed in the distal or collecting tubules of the nephron. Specific disease prototypes that often induce the formation of epithelial casts are lead intoxication, diethylene glycol poisoning, and cytomegalic inclusion disease. Large numbers of bile-pigmented epithelial cells are commonly sloughed into the urinary flow in viral hepatitis, in which case epithelial casts may form and are seen in the urine early in the acute phase.

The sloughed renal tubular epithelial cells show marked signs of degeneration. These features include nuclear and cytoplasmic disruption and may include the appearance of fat globules within the cytoplasm. When these globules are present, the cell is called an oval fat body. These cells may be seen singly within the cast or dissociated from it, in the urine. When several of the oval fat bodies are present in the cast itself, it is called an oval fat body cast.

BACTERIAL CASTS

In studying a series of patients with acute pyelonephritis using the technique of scanning electron microscopy, it was shown that many of the white cell casts in these patients also contained bacteria on their surfaces. Retrospectively, when these WBC casts were studied with phase or interference microscopy or when the sediment was stained with the Gram stain, bacterial forms could also be distinguished in the cast. We have not seen this variety of cast in any other disease state, and it is therefore incumbent on the urinoscopist to examine carefully the sediments of patients suspected of having pyelonephritis for the presence of this variety of cast. If these casts are present, a specific clinical diagnosis of pyelonephritis may be made. Bacterial casts may also appear in a "pure" form; they do not contain white cells. In such instances, these casts appear as granular casts on light microscopy, and it is also necessary, for accurate diagnosis, to apply the aforementioned microscopic techniques.[68,72] Rarely, casts containing fungi, usually yeasts, have been seen in patients with severe fungal infections of the kidneys.

Abnormal Crystals

Many crystals found in the abnormal urinary sediment are also present in the normal sediment. These normal crystals were previously described and will not be considered further.

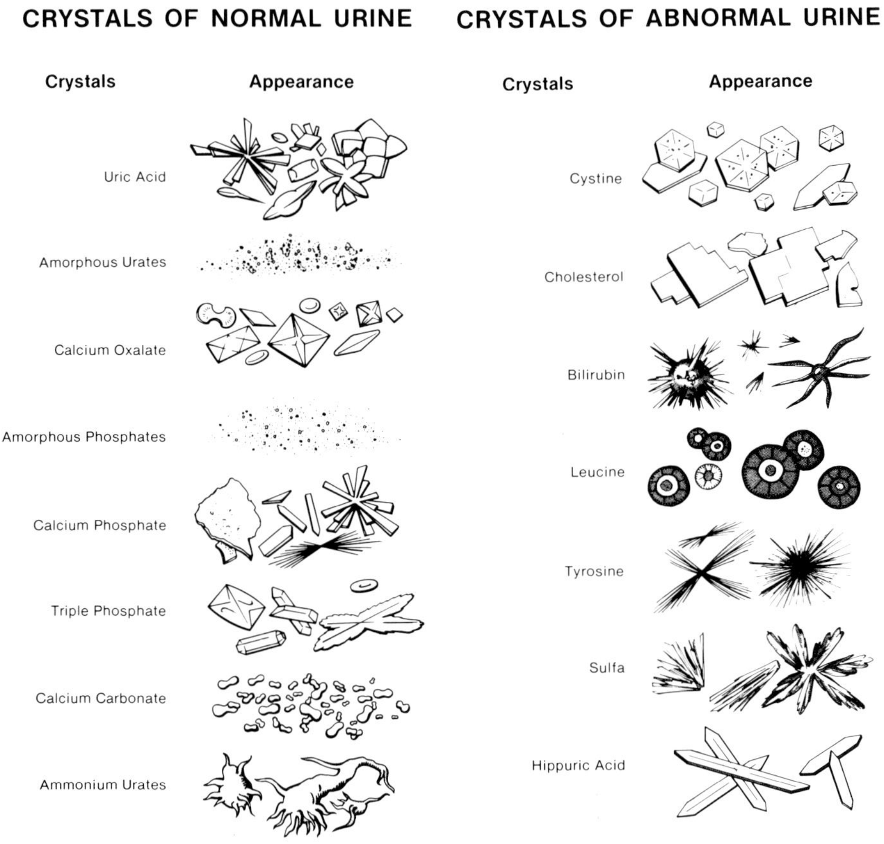

Fig. 1–22. Schematic representation of various forms of crystals in urine. (Haber, M.: *A Primer of Microscopic Urinalysis*. Fountain Valley, Calif., ICL Press, 1978.)

Abnormal crystals are ordinarily found in acid urine (and sometimes neutral urine) (Fig. 1–22). They are highly pleomorphic in their appearance and shall be considered individually. Most are metabolic byproducts of various disease states. In recent years, however, and with the intervention of a wide variety of pharmaceutical agents in the treatment of disease, many of these drugs or their byproducts may be found in the urine. A month rarely passes when a new crystal is described in a current medical journal as being present in the urine from a new medication. No attempt will be made to discuss every one of these crystals.

Uric acid crystals are commonly found in acid urine. They are extremely pleomorphic, often rhombic, and can assume practically any form. A distinguishing feature of uric acid crystals is their usual reddish-brown tint. When in the form of sodium urate, the crystals appear as needle- or fan-shaped clusters and can be mistaken for sulfanilamide derivatives. Uric acid stones can form even in the absence of increased uric acid excretion by the kidneys, depending on the acidity of urine, although urine can easily become supersaturated with uric acid at pH 5. Increased uric acid excretion, as well as formation of uric acid stones, is associated with gout, polycythemia, leukemia, lymphoma, liver diseases, theophylline and thiazide therapy, acid isohyduria, and rapid catabolic breakdown of cells (such as destruction of white cells in peripheral blood, as may occur in childhood leukemias under therapy). There is a lack of correlation between serum uric acid levels, concentration of uric acid in urine, and attacks of gouty arthritis.

A note of caution regarding crystals: the stained sediment will infrequently contain crystals that look abnormal. The observer should recognize that the stain may crystallize in the urine and appear abnormal. The usual urinary sediment stain (Sternheimer-Malbin), a mixture of crystal violet and safranin dye, appears as delicate, needle-like, purple fans that may simulate the appearance of various abnormal crystals, especially tyrosine. Whenever an abnormal crystal is found in the urine, a correlation should be made with the patient's clinical diagnosis and any therapeutic measures utilized. More often than not, this correlation will prove to be valuable and will enable the urinoscopist to specifically identify the characteristic crystal. Therapeutic and diagnostic agents often precipitate in the urine (Renograffin, an agent used in genitourinary tract radiography, for example). Finally, patients undergoing heavy doses of chemotherapeutic agents for the treatment of cancer commonly show abnormal crystals in urine. Formation of these crystals is induced by agents that act in destroying malignant cells in the body, the metabolic byproducts of which are found in the urine.

It has been said all too often that crystals in the urine are unimportant. Proper and accurate identification in certain instances is of more than academic interest, because the information can assist the clinician in accurately diagnosing the disease of his patient, as noted above, or in predicting the prognosis.

BILIRUBIN CRYSTALS

Bilirubin crystals are seen in the urine, in only few patients with jaundice. They are pleomorphic, often granular, and yellowish-brown. They may also be present as rhombic plates or in needle-like clusters and are most frequently seen in patients with intrinsic liver disease; serum direct bilirubin is usually elevated, and the urine is invariably acid.

LEUCINE CRYSTALS

Leucine crystals are birefringent, highly refractile, and easily recognized in the urine. They are pale yellow to brownish-yellow in color and ordinarily spherical. Close observation reveals intrinsic concentric striations often with radiating spokes from a central nidus. (They can be mistaken for sulfanilamide crystals.) When polarized, they do not reveal the typical "Maltese-cross" pattern as would be seen with urinary lipid. This difference in birefringent pattern is helpful in their differentiation.

TYROSINE CRYSTALS

Tyrosine crystals are among the most unique of all the abnormal urinary crystals, because they are colorless or pale yellow and appear as sheaves of fine, silky needles, although they may be single as well. If stained with the Sternheimer-Malbin technique, they characteristically appear pale purple. This crystal frequently occurs in patients with liver disease and in patients with bilirubinuria.

CYSTINE CRYSTALS

Cystine crystals are seen in the urine as flat, thin, hexagonal plates. They are colorless and highly refractile. They may occur singly or in clumps. They should not be confused with urate crystals, which are also often six-sided, and this differentiation can be made on the birefringent patterns that are multiple and complex with urates. Cystine crystals are readily identifiable as hexagonal flakes of varying size, up to 100 μ in diameter. Legal's nitroprusside test (for acetone) has been used for many years for the detection of cystine in urine. In any case, significant cystinuria is accompanied by presence of cystine crystals in the urine that can be identified microscopically. Chemical screening tests for cystine (Brand test, Legal test, and others), therefore, do not have great clinical usefulness. Secondary cystinuria may be present in patients with a transient acute phase of chronic renal disease (such as pyelonephritis), with heavy metal nephrotoxicity, aminoaciduria (including Wilson's disease), and renal tubular acidosis (see discussion of aminoacidurias). They are also characteristically present in patients with cystine stones.

CHOLESTEROL CRYSTALS

Cholesterol crystals, which are also present in acid urine, are thin, broad, large, flat plates, with an irregularity of one or more of the corners. This feature has been called a "stair-step" appearance. They are colorless or pale greenish-yellow, birefringent, and are often present in large numbers in the urine of patients with nephrotic syndrome.

HIPPURIC ACID

Hippuric acid crystals may be found in the urine of normal and abnormal patients and are perhaps the only crystals considered to be abnormal that are found in alkaline urine. They appear as colorless or pale-yellow prisms or as needles of relatively high refractive index (in contrast to tyrosine), usually with triangular or "pointed-finger" ends.

SULFA CRYSTALS

Sulfa crystals are not commonly seen in the urine of present-day patients, since the sulfa drugs used to treat urinary tract infections are more soluble than those drugs manufactured in prior years, and the new sulfa compounds do not tend to crystalize in the urine. When present, however, they are usually pale yellow or colorless and show birefringence with polarized light. They often appear in clumps or sheaves, and present as highly refractile irregular spicules or fans. Each form of sulfa crystal appears differently in the urine; their characteristic individual shapes may be correlated with the specific type of sulfa drug the patient is receiving. Sulfanilamide and drugs related to it, alone or in combination with other drugs (such as tolbutamide, chlorothiazide, and other thiazide diuretics), may precipitate in renal tubular lumina in acid urine, especially when proteinuria is present, and hence, may block the renal tubules. Many of these crystals may be tentatively identified by microscopic examination, inasmuch as they have characteristic shapes. Confirmation of the identity of sulfanilamide and related drugs may be obtained by reacting the arylamine group of the compound with cellulose (such as that in paper towels, matchsticks, for example) to form a colored complex (a yellow to orange complex); this is called the Lignin test. Polarization microscopy offers a fast and simple method to locate crystals for identification. When examining urine for sulfa crystals, however, a fresh urine specimen is needed, since crystals may dissolve with progressive alkalinization of urine upon standing. Furthermore, patients who are receiving alkalinizing agents (Mandelamine and other drugs) can have significant damage from precipitation of sulfanilamide crystals within the kidney tubules, but without accompanying crystaluria in alkaline urine.

CALCIUM CRYSTALS

Mild acidity to near neutrality of urine (pH 5.5 to 6) favors calcium oxalate precipitation. Many patients with calcium oxalate stones have oxalate and normal concentrations of urine calcium. Except in patients with oxalosis, there seems to be no correlation between magnitude of urinary oxalate excretion and appearance of calcium oxalate stones. Calcium oxalate crystals are common in urine of children or patients with a high milk intake, in patients with oxaluria, diabetes mellitus, or conditions causing excess glycogen breakdown, or in patients receiving carbonic anydrate inhibitors (acetazolamide). These crystals are also common in urine of patients who are immobilized because of bone fractures or central nervous system injuries.

Contamination

Urine specimens may become contaminated with feces, vaginal secretions, or menstrual blood, and thus, are not ordinarily suitable for examination. In the case of fecal contamination, various forms of undigested plant and animal cells may be present and should not be confused with abnormal sediment elements. Examination of contaminated specimens is not cost effective, may waste the time of the technologist and provide the physician with the wrong information.

MICROORGANISMS

Bacteria and fungi are commonly found in the urinary sediment of man. These microorganisms often infect the upper and/or lower urinary tract and are manifested in the abnormal urine by their presence, usually accompanied by inflammatory cells, especially polys. Specific diagnosis is made using appropriate cultures. Since urine is not ordinarily collected using sterile techniques, the specific identification of various pathogenic microorganisms depends on collecting the specimen under aseptic conditions.

Bacteria are most often Gram-negative bacilli (Enterobacteriaceae). Gram-positive cocci (Enterococci), however, are also found frequently. Essentially, any microorganism can produce urinary tract infection. Bacteriuria occurs frequently in pregnancy, and it is thought that as many as 40% of women in their third trimester will experience some degree of significant bacteriuria or urinary tract infection (significant bacteriuria is defined as over 100,000 bacteria/ml urine).

Candida is the most common yeast form present in the urine. Patients afflicted with diabetes mellitus often experience candida infections of the urinary tract. Budding yeast forms (which must be differentiated from red blood cells) are frequently found in the urine and are accompanied by polys. In many of these patients, mycelial forms of the organisms may be found in the sediment.

Parasites are rarely found in the urine of patients living in the United States; Trichomonas vaginalis is the exception to this statement, but this organism presents no difficulty in diagnosis as it is a pear-shaped, motile protozoan with an undulating membrane centrally located along the midline of its body. The flagellae are difficult to see in wet mounts, but the organisms are easily demonstrable in dry preparations using various staining techniques, especially the Papanicolaou stain.

Schistosoma haematobium, with its characteristic terminal spine, is frequently seen in other parts of the world. This organism usually involves the lower urinary tract of man. It is not found in this country, since its natural host (a peculiar type of snail) does not reside in the United States. Certain forms of lice and mites often drop into the urine during voiding and are identifiable when found.[72]

ARTIFACTS

Various plant and animal cells, fibers (both natural and manmade), scratches on slide-cover slips, pollen grains, and a variety of other materials, may be found in the urinary sediment. The observer must learn to recognize such contaminant or artifactual materials and to not diagnose them as pathologic. The only way to do this is with experience and appropriate training. There is no easy way to obtain either training or experience, except by multiple examinations of a wide variety and large number of urinary sediments under appropriate conditions, using good equipment in a suitable, well-equipped laboratory. Under optimum conditions, the experienced and well-trained observer will rarely misdiagnose sediment elements; therefore, the observer will be able to provide appropriate and timely information leading to a high level of patient care.

ADDIS COUNT

Standardization of quantitative examination of urinary sediment was introduced by Thomas Addis and subsequently popularized in his book,

TABLE 1–19. Typical Results of Addis Counts.

	Casts/ 24 hours	WBC and epith. cells/ 24 hours	RBC/ 24 hours	Protein/ 24 hours
Normal children	0–29,000	9,000–2,000,000	0–800,000	3–90 mg
Normal adult	0–9,000	32,000–3,000,000	0–1,500,000	0–35 mg
Glomerulonephritis (active)	100,000–700,000	up to 300,000,000	50,000 gross hematuria	1.0–3.0 g
Glomerulonephritis (chronic) or nephrosis	50,000–19,000,000	3,500,000–300,000,000	0–190,000,000	1.0–17 g
Lipoid nephrosis	5,000–20,000,000	300,000–58,000,000	0–2,500,000	0.3–18 g
Pyelonephritis (active)	0–450,000	59,000,000–1,000,000,000	0–8.5 billion	0.3–3 g
Pyelonephritis (inactive)	0–70,000	600,000–102,000,000	100,000–4,000,000	0.4–2 g
Lobar pneumonia	0–9,700,000	0–420,000,000	0–11,000,000	0–11 g
Rheumatic fever	0–1,000,000	500,000–140,000,000	860,000–4,000,000	Trace to 0.5 g
"Collagenoses"/ angiitis*	100,000–5,000,000	3,000,000–500,000,000	1,000,000–3.5 billion	0.07–2.2 g

*Includes periarteritis nodosa, lupus erythematosus, etc.

(Modified from Henry, J. Manual of Principles and Techniques for Clinical Microscopy Laboratory. State University of New York, Upstate Medical Center, Syracuse.)

Glomerular Nephritis, in 1948.[47] Elements that are too few in number to be observed or counted in routine specimens may be observed in significant numbers in concentrated sediment from a specimen collected over a longer period of time; estimates of progress or regression of disease prognosis may be made more precisely (Table 1–19). Since the test is based on rate of excretion of specific elements, the urine collection must be timed. It is convenient and conventional to collect urine for a 12-hour period. In advanced renal disease, the urinary output may be decreased to the point that only a few milliliters are excreted per hour. For this reason, too, the 12-hour collection period from midnight to noon has become favored.

REFERENCES

1. Smith, H.: DeUrina. Kaiser Foundation Med. Bull., *6*:1, 1958.
2. Wallnöfer, H., and von Rottauscher, A.: Chinese Folk Medicine. New York, Crown, 1965, p. 71.
3. Wells, C.: Bones, Bodies and Disease. New York, Praeger, 1964, p. 83.
4. Kiefer, J.: Uroscopy: The clinical laboratory of the past. Trans. Am. Assoc. Genitourin. Surg., *50*:161, 1958.
5. Kingsbury, F.: Progress in quantitative laboratory methods. Association of Life Insurance Medical Directors of America, *14*:383, 1928.
6. Needham, R.: Biochemical Values in Clinical Medicine. 3rd Ed. Bristol, John Wright & Sons, 1967.
7. Kark, R., et al.: A Primer of Urinalysis. 2nd Ed. New York, Hoeber Medical Division, Harper & Row, 1963, pp. 13 and 38.
8. Freeman, J. and Beeler, M.: Kidney stone analysis. Postgrad. Med. J., *46*:51, 1969.
9. Oser, B. (ed): Hawk's Physiological Chemistry. 14th Ed. New York, McGraw-Hill Book Co., 1965, p. 43.
10. Holmes, J.: Workshop on Urinalysis and Renal Function Studies, Pre-Workshop Manual. Chicago, Commission on Continuing Education, American Society of Clinical Pathologists, 1962.
11. Haraway, A. and Becker, E.: Clinical application of cryoscopy. J.A.M.A., *205*:506, 1968.
12. Dustan, H. and Corcoran, A.: Functional interpretation of renal tests. Med. Clin. N. Am., *39*:947, 1955.
13. Wolf, A. and Pillay, V.: Renal concentration tests (editorial). Am. J. Med., *46*:837, 1969.
14. Report of Standards Committee, College of American Pathologists, 1965 National Comprehensive Laboratory Survey: Hematology, Blood Banking, Clinical Microscopy, 1965, p. 17.
15. Warhol, R., Eichenholz, A., and Mulhausen, R.: Osmolality. Arch. Int. Med., *116*:743, 1965.
16. Cahill, G. (ed.): Diabetes. New York, Medom, Inc., USV Pharmaceutical Corp., 1970.
17. Wilkerson, H.: Oral glucose tolerance tests, in Diabetes Mellitus: Diagnosis and Treatment. Edited by Danowski. New York, American Diabetes Association, 1964.
18. Smith, I. (ed.): Chromatographic and Electrophoretic Techniques. 2nd Ed. Bath, Pitman Press, 1968.
19. Stabe, E.: Thin Layer Chromatography. New York, Academic Press, 1965.
20. Nash, J., Lister, J., and Vobes, D.: Clinical tests for ketonuria. Lancet, *1*:801, 1954.
21. Gerhardt, C.: Diabetes mellitus and acetone. Wein. Med. Pr., *6*:672, 1865.
22. James, G., and Bee, D.: Glycosuria: Accuracy and precision of laboratory diagnosis by dipstick analysis. Clin. Chem., *25*:996, 1979.
23. James, G.P., Bee, D.E., and Fuller, J.: Proteinuria: Accuracy and precision of laboratory diagnosis by dipstick analysis. Clin. Chem., *24*:1934, 1978.

24. Garrett, J.: The interpretation and significance of proteinuria. Missouri Med., *64*:111, 1967.
25. Rennie, I., and Keen, H.: Evaluation of clinical methods for detecting proteinuria. Lancet, *2*:489, 1967.
26. Beeler, M., Freeman, J., and Morgan, L.: Vanilmandelic Acid and Catecholamines. 2nd Ed. Chicago, Commission on Continuing Education, American Society of Clinical Pathologists, 1974.
27. Armstrong, M., Shaw, K., and Wall, P.: The phenolic acids of human urine. J. Biol. Chem., *218*:293, 1956.
28. Sunderman, F.: Measurements of vanilmandelic acid for the diagnosis of pheochromocytoma and neuroblastoma. Am. J. Clin. Path., *42*:481, 1964.
29. Stanbury, J., Wyngaarden, J., and Fredrickson, D. (eds.): The Metabolic Bases of Inherited Disease. 4th Ed. New York, McGraw-Hill, 1978.
30. Talbot, J.: Gout. 2nd Ed. New York, Grune & Stratton, 1964.
31. Weissmann, G.: Molecular basis of gout. Hospital Practice, *6*:43, 1971.
32. Patterson, J., Catanzaro, C., and Dede, D.: Manual for Workshop on the Porphyrins and Porphyrias. Chicago, Commission on Continuing Education, American Society of Clinical Pathologists, 1966.
33. Castrow, F., Mullins, J., Flowers, R., and Mills, G.: Anion exchange resin screening test for urinary porphyrins. Arch. Derm., *96*:204, 1967.
34. Miale, J.: Laboratory Medicine—Hematology. 3rd Ed. St. Louis, C.V. Mosby, 1967, pp. 533 and 697.
35. Stone, H., Martin, J., and Graber, C.: Verdoglobinuria: An ominous sign of pseudomonas septicemia in burns. Ann. Surg., *159*:991, 1964.
36. Derman, H., and Pauker, J.: Detection of occult blood in feces and urine. *In* Hemoglobin, Its Precursors and Metabolites. Edited by F. Sunderman and F. Sunderman, Jr. Philadelphia, J.B. Lippincott Co., 1964, p. 70.
37. Blondheim, S., Margoliash, E., and Shafir, E.: A simple test for myohemoglobinuria (myoglobinuria). J.A.M.A., *167*:453, 1958.
38. Bouchier, I. and Billing, B.: Bilirubin Metabolism. Philadelphia, F.A. Davis, 1967.
39. Harris, J.: The Red Cell. Cambridge, Harvard University Press, 1965, p. 233.
40. Zimmerman, H.: Tests of hepatic function. *In* Clinical Diagnosis by Laboratory Methods. 14th Ed. Edited by I. Davidsohn and J. Henry. Philadelphia, W.B. Saunders, 1969, p. 673.
41. Henry, R.: Clinical Chemistry, Principles and Techniques. New York, Hoeber Medical Division, Harper & Row, 1964.
42. Schwartz, C., Sborov, B., and Watson, C.: Studies on urobilinogen I-V (series of articles on urobilinogen). Am. J. Clin. Path., *14*:605, 1944.
43. Beeler, M., and Henry, J.: Melanogenuria—evaluation of several commonly used laboratory procedures. J.A.M.A., *176*:136,1961.
44. Sjoerdsma, A.: Serotonin. N. Engl. J. Med., *261*:181, 231, 1951.
45. Everett, M.: Medical Biochemistry. 2nd Ed. New York, Hoeber Medical Division, Harper & Row, 1946, p. 430.
46. Lippman, R.: Urine and the Urinary Sediment. 2nd Ed. Springfield, Charles C Thomas, 1957.
47. Addis, T.: Glomerular Nephritis. New York, Macmillan Publishing Co., 1948.
48. Sternheimer, R. and Malbin, B.: Clinical recognition of pyelonephritis with new stain for urinary sediments. Am. J. Med., *11*:212, 1951.
49. Kern, W.: Epithelial cells in urine sediments. Am. J. Clin. Path., *56*:67, 1971.
50. Haber, M.: Interference contrast microscopy provides 3-D images of urinary sediment. Lab. Med., *2*:9, 1971.
51. Barney, J. and Sulkowitch, H.: Progress in the management of urinary calculi. J. Urol., *37*:746, 1937.
52. Latner, A.: Cantarow and Trumper Clinical Biochemistry. 7th Ed. Philadelphia, W.B. Saunders, 1975, p. 239.
53. Austin, J.: Metachromatic form of diffuse cerebral sclerosis. Diagnosis during life by urine sediment examination. Neurol., *7*:415, 1957.
54. Helfaut, M., Borgeson, M., and Hellstrom, B.: The value of urinary sediment examination as a screening method in suspected cases of metachromatic leukodystrophy. Acta Paediat., *51*:49, 1962.

55. Lancaster, R., Cannon, D., Freeman, J., and Lehman, R.: Urinary Sediment: Formed Elements and Casts. Chicago, Commission on Continuing Education, American Society of Clinical Pathologists, 1970.
56. Haber, M.: Interference contrast microscopy for identification of urinary sediment. Am. J. Clin. Path., *57*:316, 1972.
57. Thomas, T.: A rapid slide method for urine cell counts. Med. Lab. Tech., *28*:38, 1971.
58. Brady, L., Webster, M., and Kark, R.: Identification of elements of urinary sediment with phase contrast microscopy. J.A.M.A., *206*:1777, 1979.
59. Free, A., and Free, H.: Urinalysis in Clinical Laboratory Practice. Cleveland, CRC Press, 1975.
60. Lindquist, B., and Wahlin, A.: Differential count of urinary leukocytes and renal epithelial cells by phase content microscopy. Acta Med. Scand., *198*:505, 1975.
61. Schumann, G., Harris, S., and Henry, J.: An improved technique for examining urinary casts and review of their significance. Am. J. Clin. Path., *69*:18, 1978.
62. Haber, M.: Urine Casts. Their Microscopy and Clinical Significance. 2nd Ed. Chicago, Am. Soc. Clin. Path., 1976.
63. McQueen, E.: Composition of urinary casts. Lancet, *1*:397, 1966.
64. Tamm, I., and Horsfall, F.: A mucoprotein derived from human urine which reacts with influenza, mumps, and newcastle disease viruses. J. Exp. Med., *95*:71, 1952.
65. Haber, M., and Lindner, L.: The surface ultrastructure of urinary casts. Am. J. Clin. Path., *68*:547, 1977.
66. Kern, W.: Epithelial cells in urine sediments. Am. J. Clin. Path., *56*:67, 1971.
67. Riedasch, R.: Antibody coating of urinary tract bacteria. N. Engl. J. Med., *299*:606, 1978.
68. Lindner, L., Jones, R., and Haber, M.: A specific urinary cast in acute pyelonephritis. Am. J. Clin. Path., *74*:809, 1980.
69. Hudson, J., Dennis, A., Gerhardt, R.: Urinary lipid and the maltese cross. N. Engl. J. Med., *299*:586, 1978.
70. Behrman, R.: Urinary findings before and after a marathon race. N. Engl. J. Med., *225*:801, 1939.
71. Bolande, R.: Inclusion bearing cells in the urine in certain viral infections. Pediatr., *24*:7, 1959.
72. Haber, M.: *The Urinary Sediment. A Textbook Atlas*. Chicago, American Society of Clinical Pathologists, 1981.

HYDROGEN ION CONCENTRATION (pH)

METHOD. pHydrion, Nitrazine, Labstix, Chemstrip, or Multistix tests.

PRINCIPLE. Paper impregnated with mixed indicators or nitrazine (sodium dinitrophenolazo-naphthol disulfonate) with the pH range 4.5 to 7.5 on paper reacts with H^+ ions to produce different colors, depending upon H^+ activity. The color is compared with a reference color chart.

PROCEDURE

1. Dip nitrazine, pHydrion paper, or Labstix into urine and gently shake off excess fluid.
2. Compare color immediately with reference chart.

INTERPRETATION, DISCUSSION, AND CLINICAL SIGNIFICANCE. pH of normal urine ranges from 4.5 to 8.0, with an average of 6.0 for 24-hour samples. Normally, the pH is chiefly a reflection of the NaH_2PO_4: Na_2HPO_4 ratio.

At pH 4.8, ratio is 50 to 1.
At pH 6.0, ratio is 9 to 0.
(The blood ratio at pH 7.4 is 4 to 1.)

Control samples should be run periodically to determine reliability of the pH paper.

MATERIALS AND REAGENTS

1. Nitrazine (E.R. Squibb & Sons, New York, N.Y. 10022)
2. pHydrion (Micro Essential Laboratory, Brooklyn, N.Y. 11200)
3. Labstix (Ames Company, Elkhart, Ind. 46514)
4. Chemstrip (Bio-Dynamics/BMC, Indianapolis, Ind., 46250)

REFERENCES

1. Kark, R., et al.: A Primer of Urinalysis. 2nd Ed. New York, Hoeber Medical Division, Harper & Row, 1963, p. 13.
2. Page, L., and Culver, P.: Syllabus of Laboratory Examinations in Clinical Diagnosis. Cambridge, Harvard University Press, 1961, p. 294.

SPECIFIC GRAVITY

METHOD. Hydrometer method.

PRINCIPLE. Markedly diminished concentrating ability of the kidneys results in presence of lesser numbers of solute molecules per unit volume of urine. Specific gravity is defined as the mass of a unit volume of fluid under standard conditions of temperature and pressure, divided by the mass of a similar volume of distilled water under similar conditions. Since specific gravity of urine varies with the number and weight of urine solute molecules, it normally reflects concentrating ability of the kidneys unless altered by glycosuria, heavy protein content, or presence of foreign substances such as x-ray contrast media. The specific gravity is measured by the buoyancy of a hydrometer plummet calibrated in specific gravity units.

We do not recommend use of the hydrometer.

PROCEDURE

CALIBRATION OF URINOMETER. Clinically employed urinometers yield results that are both inaccurate and imprecise (Yamblas, J., et al. N. Engl. J. Med., *270*:506, 1964). Therefore, it is mandatory to calibrate urinometer scales with distilled water and standard solutions of known specific gravities—NaCl or glucose solutions, using at least two different solutions, one around 1.010, one around 1.020 (consult CRC Handbook of Chemistry and Physics).

1. Clean urinometer by washing it with soap and rinse thoroughly with tap water. It may be desirable to clean urinometer by soaking it in acid cleaning solution before initial use and intermittently thereafter. They may be cleansed as specified in National Bureau of Standards Circular 555 (on hydrometers).

2. It is a good rule to rinse the urinometer vessel with a small amount (ca. 2 ml) of the solution to be measured prior to the measurement.
3. Determine the temperature of the solution with a calibrated centigrade thermometer. (Reference immersion thermometers certifiable by the National Bureau of Standards are available from the Arthur H. Thomas Co. of Philadelphia.)
4. Pour aliquot of solution to be measured into vessel.
5. Float urinometer in fluid and gently spin it (to prevent adherence to the walls of the vessel).
6. Read fluid level at bottom of meniscus with the meniscus at eye level and urinometer in a vertical position.
7. Perform each determination 20 times on the same sample, merely removing and replacing the urinometer each time if you do this conscientiously, attempting to avoid bias, you will find variability in measurements.
8. Record each specific gravity value.
9. Determine the mean reading, temperature of sample and standard deviation of measurements.
10. Compare your results with the true values for specific gravity of the solutions. Some urinometers are calibrated at 16° C (Squibb, for example), which means that they will read correctly, relative to water at 4° C (as 1.000), if the solution is at 16° C. Since room temperature (and, therefore, urine temperature) is often higher than this, readings must be temperature corrected. The usual correction is to subtract 0.001 S.G. Units for each 2° C above the specified calibration temperature, although Mansfield Clark quotes a figure of .001 S.G. Unit for each 5° C difference.
11. If you calculate the departure from accuracy of your urinometer to be greater than ±0.002 specific gravity units from the known value, you should exchange the urinometer for a new one and recheck the new one in similar fashion.
12. Calculations:

    1. Mean

    $$\bar{x} = \frac{\Sigma x}{n}$$

    2. Standard deviation

    $$SD = \sqrt{\frac{\Sigma(x-\bar{x})^2}{n-1}}$$

Where Σ = sum of
$\bar{x}$ = mean (average)
x = individual readings
Σx = sum of individual readings
n = number of readings (20, in this case)
$\Sigma(x-\bar{x})^2$ = sum of squared difference from mean
$\sqrt{\ }$ = square root of
SD = estimate of standard deviation

13. Calculations:

	Urinometer #1			Urinometer #2			Urinometer #3			Urinometer #4		
	Value	Diff. mean	Sq. Diff. mean	Value	Diff. mean	Sq. Diff. mean	Value	Diff. mean	Sq. Diff. mean	Value	Diff. mean	Sq. Diff. mean
1.												
2.												
3.												
4.												
5.												
6.												
7.												
8.												
9.												
10.												
11.												
12.												
13.												
14.												
15.												
16.												
17.												
18.												
19.												
20.												
Sum of values												
Sum of squared differences from mean												
	#1			#2			#3			#4		

Mean = $\frac{\text{sum of values}}{\text{number of values}}$

$$\bar{x} = \frac{\Sigma x}{n}$$

$$\bar{x} = \frac{\Sigma x}{20}$$

Standard deviation = $\sqrt{\frac{\text{sum sq. diff. from mean}}{\text{no. values} - 1}}$

$$S.D. = \sqrt{\frac{\Sigma (x-\bar{x})^2}{n - 1}}$$

$$S.D. = \sqrt{\frac{\Sigma (x-\bar{x})^2}{19}}$$

RESULTS

	#1	#2	#3	#4
Mean				
S.D.				

DETERMINATION OF SPECIFIC GRAVITY OF URINE

1. Pour a sufficient aliquot of urine into a clear urinometer vessel.
2. Float urinometer in fluid and gently spin it to prevent adherence to the wall of the vessel.
3. Read fluid level at bottom of meniscus with meniscus at eye level and urinometer in a vertical position.
4. Correct for temperature, protein, and glucose (see "Discussion and Clinical Significance").

INTERPRETATION. Specific gravity of the first morning urine specimen usually ranges from 1.007 to 1.030. Under extreme stress, specific gravity may range from 1.001 to 1.040.

DISCUSSION AND CLINICAL SIGNIFICANCE. Specific gravity, refractive index, and osmolality are related to one another, because they reflect the quantity of dissolved solids in the urine; however, they are not identical. Solids in urine are a heterogeneous group that may affect each measurement differently.

As mentioned, urinometers are manufactured to read 1.000 in distilled water at a specific temperature, recorded on them, such as 16° C. Correction for temperatures other than this has already been discussed.

Although urea, sodium, and chloride are normally the solids present in greatest concentration in urine, glucose and protein may also be present and will alter the specific gravity significantly. So that the measurement better reflects the concentrating capability of the kidney, correct for presence of glucose and protein as follows:

For every 0.4 g of protein/dl subtract 0.001 from specific gravity; and for every 1.0 g of glucose/dl, subtract 0.004 from specific gravity. Specific gravities higher than 1.040 suggest presence of abnormal substances, such as glucose and radiopaque dyes. In severe renal disease, specific gravity tends to be fixed near specific gravity of protein-free blood plasma (ca. 1.007). In isosthenuria, specific gravity is fixed at 1.007, and with hyposthenuria, specific gravity is less than 1.007. The term "hypersthenuria" is not used.

The urinometer reading is repeatable to ±0.002 unit with multiple determinations by one person on one specimen.

Proper design and use of hydrometers are described in National Bureau of Standards Circular 555.

About 12 years ago, an unpublished experiment was conducted under the direction of Bradley Copeland at the New England Baptist Hospital involving testing of 46 urinometers representing 27 different types from 10 different suppliers, ordered and obtained in the usual manner. Throughout the experiment, suggestions in Circular 555 were met. Each urinometer was tested in replicate, independently, by eight different observers, by immersing in distilled water and in 5.4% (w/v) dextrose solution (S.G. 1.020) at the temperature for which the urinometer was calibrated.

Reproducibility, including instrument-to-instrument and observer-to-observer error, was such that, in the case of about 40% of the urinometers, ±2 standard deviations was greater than ±0.004 at the 1.000 level; and on 80%, ±2 standard deviations was greater than ±.004 at the 1.020 level. The average of the measurements indicated an inaccuracy greater than .002 units for 30% of the urinometers.

Comments by different observers included statements that many were hard to read; some did not float perpendicularly; many had no mark at the 1.000 level. In addition, the urinometers varied considerably in the degree of adherence to National Bureau of Standards recommendations regarding materials and form. Similar findings have been reported by others.

For these reasons, we do not recommend use of manual specific gravity measurements.

MATERIALS AND REAGENTS

1. Urinometer float and vessel.

2. Thermometer.
3. NaCl or glucose standards (prepared from CRC Handbook of Chemistry and Physics).

REFERENCES

1. Copeland, B., Sherman, M., and Beeler, M.: Unpublished observations.
2. Kark, R., et al.: A Primer of Urinalysis. 2nd Ed. New York, Hoeber Medical Division, Harper & Row, 1963, p. 9.
3. Page, L., and Culver, P.: A Syllabus of Laboratory Examinations in Clinical Diagnosis. Cambridge, Harvard University Press, 1961, p. 295.
4. Yalambas, J., Hernden, E., and Reynolds, G.: Specific gravity determinations fact and fancy. N. Eng. J. Med., *270*:506, 1964.

SPECIFIC GRAVITY

METHOD. Speegrav (photoelectric hydrometer) method.

PRINCIPLE. Same as hydrometer; however, the Speegrav is automatically temperature compensated and semiautomatic. (Calibration of the instrument with at least two standard NaCl solutions, one of low and one of high specific gravity, should be performed every morning before the instrument is used.)

PROCEDURE

STANDARDIZATION OF INSTRUMENT

1. Place instrument on level table. Connect aspirator to cold water faucet. Turn on moderate stream of water.
2. Pour lower range specific gravity standard into sample chamber (without introducing air bubbles). If sucking noise develops, increase flow of water from faucet slightly!
3. Turn "LOW SCALE ADJUST" and "FULL SCALE ADJUST" knobs fully to right. (Do not turn switch until knobs are adjusted!) Then turn switch "ON."
4. Place index finger lightly over finger stop and aspirate solution from sample chamber. Prefill with standard.
5. Set "LOW SCALE ADJUST" knob (to left), so that meter reads specific gravity of low standard.
6. Aspirate solution.
7. Flush chamber with high-range standard, then fill with this standard.
8. Set "FULL SCALE ADJUST" knob, so that meter reads specific gravity of high standard.
9. Repeat procedure again with low standard, using "LOW SCALE ADJUST" knob to set reading; and with high standard, using "FULL SCALE ADJUST" knob.
10. Turn switch "OFF" when finished at the end of the day.

UNKNOWN DETERMINATIONS

1. Flush sample chamber with urine. Then fill chamber with specimen.

2. Read immediately.
3. Aspirate by placing finger over stopper.
4. Repeat with next sample.

INTERPRETATION. Same as with hydrometer procedure.

DISCUSSION AND CLINICAL SIGNIFICANCE. The instrument is a photoelectric temperature-compensated hydrometer and is subject to the same variations as is the hydrometer. However, repeatability is better than with the hydrometer, one standard deviation being in the range of ± 0.0005 unit for replicate determinations on one sample by one person.

Standards can be obtained from the manufacturer, which consist of solutions of known concentration of NaCl, stabilized by "colloid." They can also be prepared in the same manner as for calibration of the manual urinometer. We prefer the latter procedure. Although the instrument is temperature-compensated, we prepared the NaCl solutions at 20° C, and initially standardize the instrument with the solutions at 20° C. Subsequently, we use the NaCl solutions at room temperature.

Because the instrument is expensive and requires a volume of urine greater than 5 ml and because the refractometer (TS meter) is readily available, we do not recommend the use of the Speegrav.

MATERIALS AND REAGENTS

1. Speegrav instrument model 101 (Biological Research, St. Louis, Missouri)
2. NaCl standards

REFERENCE

Clinical Speegrav Instruction Manual (model 101), 1965.

SPECIFIC GRAVITY AND TOTAL SOLIDS

METHOD. Goldberg refractometer (TS meter).

PRINCIPLE. The refractive index of urine varies with the nature and concentration of dissolved solid. It can be determined rapidly with 1 drop of urine by means of the TS meter, which is calibrated to read in specific gravity units.

PROCEDURE

1. Clean surface of the cover and prism of the TS meter with a dry, soft, nonabrasive cloth or lens paper, and close the cover.
2. Apply a drop of urine at the notched (bottom) closed portion of the cover so that it flows over the prism surface by capillary action.
3. Point the instrument toward a fluorescent light source, rotate the eyepiece until the scale is in focus, and read, on the specific gravity scale, the dividing line between the light and dark contrast.

INTERPRETATION. See interpretation with hydrometer procedure.

DISCUSSION AND CLINICAL SIGNIFICANCE. Specific gravity, refractive index, and osmolality are related as has been previously mentioned in that they each vary with the quantity of dissolved solids in the urine; however, they are not identical, as the same often influences each of these measurements to a different degree.

The specific gravity scale of the Goldberg refractometer "acquires" an increasing error with greater amounts of solids; but the measurement is precise enough for clinical purposes over the essential range encountered. The instrument cannot be calibrated by use of a standard binary solution, such as salt, because urine is a mixture of components, in which urea, for example, has a specific gravity increment of 0.0028 per g/dl and sodium chloride, a specific gravity increment of .0071 per g/dl. With a standard sodium chloride solution of concentration 20.2 g/L, in the TS meter, the refraction $(n - M_o) \times 10^4$ is 35. A refraction of 35 (which is what the instrument really "sees") corresponds to a $D^{20}{}_{-20}$ of about 1.009. This was pointed out to us in a communication from A.V. Wolf, Ph.D., in which he stated that TS meters need no calibration other than the zero point, which should be set at a temperature preferably close to 20° C. According to Dr. Wolf, it will then yield accurate refractions, total solids for serum and urine, and specific gravities of human urine to ±.001 units. (An interesting side note: The composition of cat urine is sufficiently different from that of human urine that a single scale will not do for both.)

Because of its simplicity of use, relatively good reproducibility and accuracy, and because of the small size of the sample required, we recommend the routine use of the TS meter. (Refer to earlier discussion of error under "Concentration of Solids in Urine.")

The TS meter is temperature-compensated between 60° and 100° F. It will be changed by heat above 150° F, or by immersion of the eyepiece and focusing ring into water.

The refractometer (A.O. model 10400) can also be used to measure total serum protein. For this purpose, it has few advantages over conventional ones, but it is rapid.

George Leonard and Myrton Beeler at Ochsner Clinic, as mentioned earlier, found that with a TS meter purchased through commercial sources, specimens of 100 haphazardly selected urines averaged lower (by 0.002 specific gravity unit) than results obtained with carefully calibrated Squibb urinometers. This suggests the necessity for checking calibrations.

The relationships between specific gravity and total solids are related in Table 1–20.

MATERIALS

1. TS meter (catalog no.10400, American Optical Co., Buffalo, N.Y. 14215).
2. Dropping pipettes.

TABLE 1–20. Relationships Between Specific Gravity and Total Solids.

Specific Gravity	Total Solids (g/dl)	Specific Gravity	Total Solids (g/dl)	Specific Gravity	Total Solids (g/dl)	Specific Gravity	Total Solids (g/dl)
1.000	.0	1.010	2.5	1.020	5.0	1.030	7.5
1.001	.3	1.011	2.7	1.021	5.2	1.031	7.7
1.002	.5	1.012	3.0	1.022	5.5	1.032	8.0
1.003	.7	1.013	3.2	1.023	5.7	1.033	8.2
1.004	1.0	1.014	3.5	1.024	6.0	1.034	8.5
1.005	1.2	1.015	3.7	1.025	6.2	1.035	8.7
1.006	1.5	1.016	4.0	1.026	6.5	1.036	9.0
1.007	1.7	1.017	4.2	1.027	6.7	1.037	9.2
1.008	2.0	1.018	4.5	1.028	7.0	1.038	9.5
1.009	2.2	1.019	4.7	1.029	7.2		

REFERENCES

1. Leonard, G., and Beeler, M.: Unpublished observations, 1964.
2. Rubini, M. and Wolfe, A.: Refractometric determination of total solids in water of serum and urine. J. Biol. Chem., *225*:869, 1957.
3. TS meter Manual, Buffalo, American Optical Co.
4. Wolf, A.V.: Personal communication, 1966.
5. Wolf, A.V., and Pillay, V.: Renal concentration tests (editorial). Am. J. Med., *46*:837, 1969.
6. Wolf, A.V.: Urinary concentrative properties. Am. J. Med., *32*:329, 1962.
7. Wolf, A.V., Fuller, J., Goldman, E., and Mahony, E.: New refractive methods for the determination of total proteins in serum and in urine. Clin. Chem., *8*:158, 1962.

RENAL CONCENTRATION TEST

METHOD. Fishberg concentration, modified by Haraway and Becker.

PRINCIPLE. Measurement of renal concentrating ability is more valuable for the purpose of assessing the ability of the kidney to perform work (by concentrating against a gradient), than is determination of solids in a random sample of urine.

PROCEDURE. (The patient should be on a high-protein diet for at least 3 days prior to the test.)

1. At 6:00 P.M. the evening before the test, instruct the patient to take a usual meal, but do not permit consumption of free fluids.
2. Instruct patient to fast until test is completed.
3. Instruct patient to void at bedtime and discard urine.
4. Instruct patient to void and discard urine at 6:00 A.M., then return to bed and collect a specimen in a clean container at 8:00 A.M. that is labeled with patient's name, time, and date of collection, and send to the laboratory.
5. Measure temperature of each urine specimen.
6. Determine osmolality or specific gravity of each specimen. Check for protein and glucose.

INTERPRETATION. Normal subjects are able to concentrate urine to a specific gravity of 1.029 to 1.032. If the specific gravity is 1.025 or higher (corresponding to an osmolality of about 800 mmol/Kg), it is considered to be a normal test result. Values between 600 and 800 indicate minimal impairment; 400 to 600 moderate impairment; and less than 400 severe impairment of renal concentrating ability.

One can evaluate this more accurately by determining the ratio of urine to serum osmolality (normally greater than 3); but, according to Haraway and Becker, measurement of urine concentration alone is adequate for most patients.

DISCUSSION AND CLINICAL SIGNIFICANCE. This test is one of the most valuable of the renal function tests, and is capable of detecting renal (tubular) functional defects early in the course of renal disease, even when functional impairment is well compensated. It is one of the earliest tests to exhibit impairment in asymptomatic chronic pyelonephritis. Impairment may also occur early in the course of diabetes mellitus and essential hypertension. Lowering of renal functional capacity may be discernible with this test before either phenolsulfonphthalein excretion or blood urea nitrogen are abnormal. Maximal concentration of urine can be achieved only when antidiuretic hormone (ADH) is fully stimulated by adequate dehydration, and when the kidney is excreting a minimum amount of water. If the tubules cannot respond to ADH or ADH is lacking, water will not be conserved; therefore, the urine will be relatively dilute despite the need to conserve water. Failure to concentrate urine above a specific gravity of 1.008 or to 400 mmol/Kg occurs in severe renal tubular disease, in the case of defective formation or release of ADH, and in reversible states, such as severe anemia and hypokalemia.

Although urea, sodium, and chloride are normally the most important of the dissolved substances measured in urine by these techniques, glucose and protein also alter specific gravity significantly. Therefore, correct for these as previously described. Each of the following substances in the quantities listed is capable of increasing the measured specific gravity (at 16° C) by .001 unit:

Urea	3.595 g
Glucose	2.700 g
Sodium chloride	1.473 g
Albumin	3.892 g
Sodium phosphate	3.792 g
Disodium phosphate	0.979 g
Sodium sulfate	1.405 g

MATERIALS. Urinometer, Speegrav instrument, TS meter (refractometer), or osmometer.

REFERENCES

1. Fishberg, A.: Hypertension and Nephritis. 5th Ed. Philadelphia, Lea & Febiger, 1954, p. 96.

2. Haraway, A.W., and Becker, E.L.: Clinical application of cryoscopy. J.A.M.A., *205*:506, 1968.
3. Lashmet, F., and Newburgh, I.: An improved concentration test of renal function. J.A.M.A., *99*:1883, 1930.
4. Wolf, A.V., and Pillay, V.: Renal concentration tests (editorial). Am. J. Med., *46*:837, 1969.

RENAL TUBULAR EXCRETION TEST

METHOD. Phenolsulfonphthalein Excretion.

PRINCIPLE. Phenolsulfonphthalein (PSP), when injected intravenously, is excreted by the kidney tubules. The appearance of the dye in the urine over a fixed time is an empirical measure of renal blood flow and tubular excretory function. The pink dye color of PSP can be quantitated spectrophotometrically or semiquantitated visually by comparison with standards.

SAMPLE

1. No preparation is necessary until the morning of the test.
2. Ask patient not to void before test begins.
3. To start test, have patient drink at least 600 ml of water ($2\frac{1}{2}$ glasses, 8 oz each).
4. 30 minutes after patient ingests water, inject intravenously 6 mg (1 ml) sterile PSP dye.
5. In separate, clean containers, collect all urine voided at 15 minutes, and again at 60 minutes after injections of dye.

PROCEDURE

1. Record volumes of each sample of urine.
2. Transfer each urine specimen to a 1,000-ml dilution container.
3. Add drops of sodium hydroxide (enough for alkalinization) for maximum PSP color development.
4. Dilute each specimen to 1,000 ml with tap water.
5. Pour into colorimeter tube and read absorbance at 540 nm to 565 nm (or semiquantitative visual measurement can be made in a Dunning colorimeter).
6. Calculation: Read percentage of dye in sample from prepared chart relating absorbance to percentage of dye (for spectrophotometric quantitation).

INTERPRETATION. Normal range of PSP excretion (percentage excretion).

	Minimum (%)	*Maximum* (%)	*Mean* (%)
15 minutes after injection	28	51	35
1 hour	9	17	12
2 hours	3	10	6
Total: 2 hours	63	84	70

DISCUSSION AND CLINICAL SIGNIFICANCE. About 85% of PSP dye injected intravenously is bound to albumin, transported to the kidney, and excreted by the renal tubules. (Since this PSP is albumin-bound, it is not filtered at the glomerulus.) The rate of excretion depends on renal blood flow and tubular cell integrity; hence, PSP excretion is an empirical measure of renal blood flow and tubular excretory function.

Normally 10 to 15% of the injected PSP dye will be excreted by the liver. In severe liver disease, this fraction may be transported to and excreted by the kidney, thus giving spuriously high results. The PSP excretion is 10 to 15% lower when the patient is in the erect position than when he is in the recumbent position; this is also true of the other renal-clearance tests. This postural difference is aggravated in patients with glomerulonephritis and nephrosclerosis. Inaccurate timing of urine sample will cause spurious results. This is commonly the fault when excretion of PSP is calculated to be greater in subsequent samples than in the 15-minute sample.

Note: There is more than 1 ml PSP dye in the injection ampule; therefore, the amount of dye injected into the patient should be properly measured in the syringe.

Substances that will color urine (pyridium, beets, Ex-Lax, bile, blood, bromsulfonphthalein dye, abnormal urinary pigments) or deep amber-colored urine specimens will yield inaccurate results because of color interference.

If the patient is unable to void, catheterization may be necessary (this should be done by a nurse, not a medical technologist). Because of the possibility of infection, however, this should be avoided whenever possible. Large residual urine volumes cause unacceptable errors. If the red color developing after the addition of alkali is pale, urine may be diluted to 500 ml rather than 1,000 ml; however, appropriate correction must be made in results by dividing the percentage by 2.

MATERIALS AND REAGENTS

1. Phenolsulfonphthalein dye (1 ml = 6 mg) sterile vial
2. Sodium hydroxide, 10% (w/v)
3. Spectrophotometer (or Dunning colorimeter)
4. 1000 ml dilution containers
5. Dropping pipettes
6. A 2 ml sterile syringe and a 24 to 25 gauge needle
7. Water glass

REFERENCES

1. Chapman, E.: Further experience with the fractional phthalein test. N. Engl. J. Med., *214*:16, 1936.
2. Page, L., and Culver, P.: Syllabus of Laboratory Examination in Clinical Diagnosis. Cambridge, Harvard University Press, 1962, p. 351.
3. Rowntree, L, and Gerhardy, T.: An experimental and clinical study of the functional activity of the kidneys by means of phenolsulfonphthalein. J. Pharmacol. Exp. Ther., *1*:579, 1910.

GLUCOSE

METHOD. Clinistix, Combistix, Labstix, Multistix, Chemstrip, and TesTape tests.

PRINCIPLE. These "strip tests" contain glucose oxidase, peroxidase, and orthotolidine. Glucose oxidase reacts with glucose, if present in the urine, removing two hydrogens, to form gluconolactone; which is, in turn, promptly hydrated to gluconic acid. The freed hydrogen ions then combine with atmospheric oxygen to form hydrogen peroxide, which, in the presence of peroxidase, oxidizes the orthotolidine to form a blue color. The principle of the TesTape reaction is similar, differing only in the accessory chemicals.

PROCEDURE

1. Rapidly dip the test end of the strip in urine or briefly pass through urine stream.
2. Compare dip test area with the color reference guide after 10 seconds.
3. Positive and negative controls should be examined simultaneously.

INTERPRETATION. The tests are specific for glucose, but the enzyme may be inhibited by various substances, including high concentrations of ascorbic acid. Absence of color change indicates an absence of glucose, while a change to blue on the red glucose area of the stick indicates a positive test result. Generally, a light color corresponds to a smaller amount of glucose and a dark color to a larger amount, but accurate quantitation is not possible. (Test results should probably be interpreted as indicating presence or absence of more than 0.1 g of glucose/dl of urine.)

DISCUSSION AND CLINICAL SIGNIFICANCE. The test reliably detects 0.1 g glucose/dl or more in urine and is more sensitive than Benedict's test or Clinitest tablets. Because of this sensitivity, the test may be positive in the presence of a negative Clinitest and Benedict's test. The dipstick method is not routinely used for therapeutic control of diabetics in whom it is not desired to maintain the urine sugar-free. It is often not used for screening children's urines, either, as the less specific tests can detect a wider variety of disease.

MATERIALS. Clinistix, Combistix, and Labstix (Ames Company, Elkhart, Ind. 46514), and TesTape (Eli Lilly Co., Indianapolis, Ind. 46206), Chemstrip (Bio-Dynamics/BMC, Indianapolis, Ind. 46250).

REFERENCES

1. Ames Company and Eli Lilly Co. brochures on tests.
2. Bio-Dynamics Co. brochure on test.
3. Kark, R., et al.: A Primer of Urinalysis. 2nd Ed. New York, Hoeber Medical Division, Harper & Row, 1963, p. 38.

REDUCING SUBSTANCES (QUALITATIVE)

METHOD. Clinitest method.

PRINCIPLE. Cupric sulfate, in the presence of heat and alkali (sodium carbonate), will oxidize reducing agents (sugars), and in return be reduced to cuprous oxide. Sodium carbonate and citric acid act as effervescents to facilitate rapid solution of the tablet. Sodium carbonate also provides the alkaline pH necessary for the reaction; the heat required is generated both by solution of alkali and by heat of solution of citric acid. Result of reduction of copper is a color change from blue through green to orange, depending on the amount of reducing substance present.

PROCEDURE

1. Place 5 drops of urine in a test tube.
2. With a separate dropper, place 10 drops of water into the same test tube.
3. Place 1 Clinitest tablet into the test tube. (Do not shake while reaction is occurring!)
4. Wait 15 seconds after boiling stops, then shake the tube gently and compare the color of the solution with the colors of the reference chart.
5. Controls should be tested.

INTERPRETATION. Color changes occurring later than 15-second waiting period should be disregarded.

Negative	Blue (none)
Trace	Dark green ($\leq$0.25 g/dl)
1+	Light green (0.50 g/dl)
2+	Green-yellow (0.75 g/dl)
3+	Orange-yellow to orange-tan (1.00 g/dl)
4+	Orange to red ($\geq$2.00 g/dl)

DISCUSSION AND CLINICAL SIGNIFICANCE. Clinitest tablets, like Benedict's reagent, react with glucose, fructose, lactose, galactose, and pentose. Unlike Benedict's solution, however, they do not react with creatine, homogentisic acid, uric acid, salicylates, penicillin, chloral hydrate, streptomycin, isoniazid, or PAS. Large quantities of ascorbic acid (vitamin C) may cause a false positive, as with the Benedict's test.

Glycosuria can occur following ingestion of sucrose or glucose, especially in patients who have undergone gastrectomy (alimentary glycosuria), in individuals with decreased maximal renal tubular reabsorption capacity (renal glycosuria), in patients with various intestinal metabolic disorders (galactosuria, pentosuria), and in patients under severe stress, or in those with relative or absolute insulin deficiency (diabetes mellitus, Cushing's syndrome, phlorizin poisoning).

MATERIALS AND REAGENTS

1. Clinitest tablets (Ames Company, Elkhart, Ind. 46514)
2. Test tubes, 13 × 100 mm

REFERENCES

1. Ames Company brochure on test.
2. Free, A., and Free, H.: Urine Analysis in Clinical Laboratory Practice. Cleveland, CRC Press, 1975, p. 39.
3. Kark, R., et al.: A Primer of Urinalysis. 2nd Ed. New York, Hoeber Division, Harper & Row, 1963, p. 38.

GLUCOSE AND KETONES

METHOD. Diastix and Keto-Diastix methods.

PRINCIPLE. Glucose in urine, in contact with atmospheric oxygen, is converted to glucuronic acid and hydrogen peroxide when exposed to reagent strips impregnated with glucose oxidase. Then the peroxide, in the presence of peroxidase in the strips, oxidizes a potassium-iodide dye combination to variable degrees from green through a series of orange-brown colors in a fashion similar to the Benedict's test. Glucose concentration is determined by comparison of the color to a reference chart.

Another portion of the strip is impregnated with sodium nitroprusside and glycine, which will form a purple ferropentacyanide compound with isonitroamine derivatives of ketones. Estimation of concentration of ketones is made by comparison of color to a reference chart.

TABLE 1–21. Rf and Color of Urine Sugars by Paper Chromatography.

Source	Rf	Color
Xylulose	155	gray-brown
Ribose	137	gray-brown
Xylose	130	gray-brown
Arabinose	112	gray-brown
Fructose	105	brown
Mannose	105	gray-blue
Glucose	100	blue
Galactose	80	blue
Sucrose	80	brown
Maltose	47	blue
Inositol	35	
Lactose	32	blue
Glucuronic acid	20	brown

PROCEDURE

1. Dip reagent strip into urine for 2 seconds, then remove.
2. Compare reagent strip to chart.
   KETONES—Read the ketone test exactly 15 seconds after dipping.
   GLUCOSE—Read the glucose test 30 seconds after dipping.
   (Ketone levels of 2+ or greater may suppress color development of glucose test area.)

INTERPRETATION. Presence or absence of glucose and ketones can be semiquantitated by a series of color changes as follows:

Glucose	
Blue	negative
Light green	trace (≤0.1 g/dl)
Green	1+(0.25 g/dl)
Greenish-brown	2+(0.5 g/dl)
Orange-brown	3+(1 g/dl)
Red-brown	4+(≥2 g/dl)
Ketones	
Tan	negative
Light purple	1+ (≤0/1 g/dl)
Moderately purple	2+
Deep purple	3+

DISCUSSION AND CLINICAL SIGNIFICANCE. The significance of finding glucose and ketones in the urine has already been noted. Varying temperatures, pH, and osmolality do not affect the test significantly; the accurate timing of the test, however, is essential for optimum importance.

The test is more sensitive to urinary glucose than the Clinitest, but slightly less sensitive than TesTape. Concentration of glucose as low as 0.1 g/100 ml of urine can be detected with Clinistix and TesTape, 0.25 g/100 ml of urine with Clinitest. A 3+ or 4+ reaction with Clinitest or Clinistix has the same significance as a 3+ or 4+ result with Keto-Diastix; not so, however, with 1+ or 2+ reactions.

The Keto-Diastix, therefore, may give positive results with degrees of glycosuria that may not be clinically significant. Another disadvantage is that the strips may show a speckled color rather than a solid color.

If ketones exceed 2+, the urine should be retested with another reagent, such as Clinitest, to get a more accurate estimation of the glycosuria, because high ketone levels may suppress some color development of the glucose reaction.

The sticks are useful for diabetic patients who test their own urine at home, especially because they are simple to use and inexpensive.

MATERIALS AND REAGENTS. Diastix and Keto-Diastix (Ames Company, Elkhart, Ind. 46514).

REFERENCE

1. Levine, R. (ed.): Proceedings of the Keto-Diastix Clinical Conference. Elkhart, Ind., 1970.

SUGARS

METHOD. One-dimensional ascending paper chromatography.

PRINCIPLE. Urine aliquots and standards are spotted on duplicate sheets of filter paper. These are sewed into cylindrical form, placed in a jar, and the chromatogen is allowed to develop overnight in isopropanol-water. The paper is removed, dried, cut in half, and sprayed with citric acid-aniline solution and glucostat reagent (one on one half, the other on the other half), heated appropriately, then interpreted. Spots indicate presence of sugars.

SPECIMEN. Use a first morning urine, or a 24-hour specimen as for amino acids.

PROCEDURE

1. Test for reducing substances to determine if present (use Clinitest method).
2. Pour solvent into glass jar, cover, and allow to equilibrate for 30 minutes.
3. Place 8″ square sheet of Whatman no. 3 filter paper on clean towel on hard surface.
4. Draw pencil line across paper 2 cm from bottom. Make 15 tiny cross marks, along the line, 1 cm apart.
5. On each side make similar marks 4″ from bottom.
6. Spot 5 unknowns on points 1 through 6 2 to 3 μL at a time, then repeat the same specimens on points 8 through 15, drying with portable hair dryer to keep the spreading to a minimum. Spot standards at positions 7 and 14. If results with the preliminary tests were found to be positive, spot a total of 20 μL of the specimens; if negative, spot 40 μL. Spot 2 to 4 μL of the standard solution.
7. Sew or staple edges of paper together, aligning marks, to form a cylinder.
8. Place in jar containing water-isopropanol, replace the lid, and let develop overnight (17 hours).
9. Remove paper from jar, unfasten and unroll, and dry in air.
10. Cut paper into two similar halves. Spray one-half with glucostat reagents and incubate for 10 minutes at 60° C. Spray the other half with citric acid-aniline solution, and dry at 120° C for 5 minutes.

INTERPRETATION. A spot developing with both reagents is glucose. Identify sugar by its Rf:

$$\text{Rf} = \frac{\text{DISTANCE TRAVELED BY SUGAR}}{\text{DISTANCE TRAVELED BY SOLVENT FRONT}}$$

and by comparison with the movement of the standards. If glucose is present and interferes with other sugars, it can be destroyed prior to spotting by incubation with glucose oxidase. The sugars can also be identified by their Rf value:

$$\text{Rf} = \frac{\text{DISTANCE TRAVELED BY SUGAR}}{\text{DISTANCE TRAVELED BY GLUCOSE}} \times 100$$

MATERIALS AND REAGENTS

1. Solvent. 160 ml isopropanol plus 40 ml distilled water, citric acid (0.2 M). In a volumetric flask, place 4.2 g citric acid and dilute to volume with distilled water. Mix.
2. Alcoholic aniline, 25% (v/v). Add 25 ml redistilled aniline to 75 ml absolute ethanol.
3. Citric acid-aniline solution. Mix equal volumes of 0.2 M citric acid and alcoholic aniline-glucostat reagent. (Washington Biochemical Corp., N.J.) Prepare as directed.
4. 1 gallon glass tank with lid
5. Whatman filter paper no. 3, 8″ × 8″
6. Hair dryer
7. Atomizer

REFERENCES

1. Cawley, L., and Goodwin, W.: Workship on paper chromatographic analysis of amino acids and sugars in blood and urine. New Orleans, Louisiana Pathology Society Meeting, Feb. 12–14, 1965.
2. Henry, J. (ed.): Clinical Diagnosis and Management by Laboratory Methods. 16th Ed. Vol. 1. Philadelphia, W.B. Saunders, 1979, p. 587.
3. Smith, J.: Chromatographic and Electrophoretic Techniques. Vol. 1. New York, Interscience Publishers, 1961, p. 246.

SUGARS

METHOD. Thin-layer silica gel chromatography.

PRINCIPLE. Urine is diluted with isopropyl alcohol, and an aliquot is spotted on a silica gel chromatogram sheet, upon which standard solutions are also spotted. The chromatogram is developed in ethyl acetate-isopropanol-water and visualized by spraying with naphthoresorcinol. Identification of sugars is made by comparison of Rf's of unknowns with those of standards.

PROCEDURE

1. Place 1 ml aliquot of patient's first morning specimen of urine in a test tube; add 1 ml of isopropyl alcohol; mix well by inversion.
2. Spot 6 μL sample of diluted urine in 2 μL aliquots about 2 cm from lower edge of paper. (A Hamilton syringe is convenient for this purpose.) Dry with warm air after each application.
3. Spot standard solution (mixture of sugars) similarly, lateral to unknown.
4. Place in developing chamber and allow to migrate for about 10 cm distance (about 40 minutes).
5. Dry with warm air.
6. Spray with visualizing agent.

7. Place in 110° C oven for no more than 3 minutes.
8. Spray with acrylic for preservation.

INTERPRETATION. Sugars will appear as blue to blue-gray to violet spots. Rf value of each sugar can be calculated as follows:

$$Rf = \frac{\text{DISTANCE SUGAR TRAVELS}}{\text{DISTANCE SOLVENT TRAVELS}}$$

DISCUSSION AND CLINICAL SIGNIFICANCE. This method is more rapid than paper chromatography and, therefore, may be more convenient for screening.

MATERIALS AND REAGENTS

1. Standard: 0.5 g/dl isopropyl alcohol: lactose, sucrose, D (+) galactose, D (+) fructose, L (+) arabinose, D (+) xylose, D (−) ribose, D glucuronic acid.
2. Developing reagent: Ethyl açetate-isopropanol-water, 55:36:12.
3. Visualizing agent: Phosphoric acid, 85% (w/v), 10 ml in dl of 0.2% (w/v) naphthoresorcinol in ethyl alcohol. (Methyl alcohol should be a suitable alternate.)
4. Krylon acrylic spray coating (Krylon, Inc., Norristown, Pa. 19401)
5. Chromatography medium: Eastman Silica Gel G chromatography sheet—type K301-RO
6. Developing apparatus: Eastman chromatography developing apparatus

REFERENCES

1. Becker, S., and May, P.: Chromatography of urine sugars. Am. J. Clin. Path., 49:436, 1968.
2. Henry, J. (ed.): Clinical Diagnosis and Management by Laboratory Methods. 16th ed. Vol. 1. Philadelphia, W.B. Saunders, 1979, p. 587.

TABLE 1–22. Rf and Color of Urine Sugars by Silica Gel Chromatography.

Sugar	Color	Rf
Lactose	blue	0.09
Sucrose	violet-black	0.21
Galactose	blue	0.25
Glucose	blue	0.28
Fructose	violet-black	0.34
Arabinose	blue-gray	0.39
Xylose	blue-gray	0.49
Ribose	blue-gray	0.51
Glucuronic Acid	blue-violet	0.87

SUGARS

METHOD. Kodak Chromat/O/Screen (Thin Layer Chromatographic Analysis).

PRINCIPLE. Urinary sugars are preserved with Merthiolate or thymol, then spotted on chromatographic strips and allowed to migrate in one dimension with butanol:pyridine:hydrochloric acid gel, along with known standards of sugars. The gel contains analine hydrogen phthalate that stains most monosaccharides and disaccharides (lactose, galactose, etc.) varying colors from red-brown through green-brown. Rf values can also be calculated.

SPECIMEN COLLECTION AND PRESERVATION

1. Urine should be preserved with 1 drop of 10% (w/v) Merthiolate or a small crystal of thymol. Samples should be stored at 4° C (39° F) until ready for analysis. Specimens contaminated with feces are not suitable for chromatography.
2. Feces—Estimation of fecal sugar derivatives provides an important contribution to the diagnosis of sugar malabsorption. In practice, immediate estimation of fecal pH must be done along with Clinitest and Clinistix tests. Feces must be frozen immediately on powdered dry ice to prevent continuing bacterial degradation of sugar compounds. For chromatography, feces should be homogenized immediately with an equal amount of acetone (w/v). Centrifuge and discard any fat that appears above the acetone layer. Use 10 μL samples of the acetone phase for chromatography.
3. Blood should be preserved in a vacutainer tube (fluoride additive) until ready for analysis.

   An advantage of the CHROMAT/O/SCREEN Analysis Kit is that no additional sample preparation is necessary. Urine requires no desalting, and plasma requires no deproteinization.

PROCEDURE

SAMPLE APPLICATION

1. Remove chromatographic sheet from package. Chromatographic sheets are wrapped in a shrink package and stacked with the coated sides facing in one direction. The top sheet is a blank, protective piece of Mylar film. Use a sharp instrument to cut open the plastic shrink package on either the top or bottom. Remove a chromatographic sheet, being careful not to scratch or touch the coated side with the bare fingers. Always use the forceps provided for handling the sheets. Place the sheet on a clean horizontal surface.
2. Apply the sample using the pipette. Put a 1 μL pipette into the pipette holder. With the pipette in as nearly a horizontal position as possible, fill it completely by touching it to the surface of the liquid sample (plasma, urine, standard, etc.) The liquid can be seen moving up the pipette as it fills the tube by capillary action. The liquid will stop when the pipette is full.

   To apply the sample, hold the pipette in a perpendicular position so that the tip just touches the chromatographic sheet between two of the cut-out circles. Do not scratch or break the coating by pressing the pipette on the sheet. Squeeze the holder and apply its entire volume in one application. The sample should spread to the edges of the circles. Preliminary examination can be attempted with 1 μL of urine, plasma, or feces extract. If the chromatogram reveals no sugars, or too high a concentration, the volume should be adjusted for further chromatograms. In some cases, applications of as much as 10 μL may be required. This is best done by applying 1 μL at a time, and completely drying the spot between applications with gentle heat from a hair dryer.

3. Apply the standard solution. A vial containing a standard solution of three sugars is included with the kit. Composition and concentration of this standard are shown in the following table:

Sugar	*Glucose*	*Lactose*	*Ribose*
Concentration g/dl	0.5	2.0	1.0

Apply 1 μL of the standard to the chromatogram between two other circles, in the same manner as the sample. To minimize the chances of error, always apply spots to the chromatogram in the same order, *i.e.*, left to right or right to left, with the standard in the same position. After chromatography, visual comparison of the sample with the standard will simplify the location and identification of sugars present in the urine.

4. Identify the specimen. Write the patient's name or identification on the back of the developing chamber. The top of the chromatographic sheet can also be numbered with a sharp pencil.
5. Dry the sheet completely before proceeding. It may be air dried, but use of a hair dryer will speed the operation.

METHOD OF DEVELOPMENT

1. Fill the chamber trough with gel. Remove the cap and puncture the top of the tube of KODAK CHROMAT/O/SCREEN Gel. CAUTION: Care should be taken if the tube has been warmed, because a ribbon of the gel several centimeters long may be expelled upon opening. After using the gel, replace the cap tightly to prevent any leakage or evaporation. Completely fill the trough of the development chamber by squeezing the tube of gel into the trough until a peak projects just above the developing chamber floor. Use the special scraper to mold and remove excess gel. Otherwise, the solvent will migrate in an uneven front causing Rf values to change.
2. Insert the spotted sheet and close the chamber. Place the opened developing chamber on a table or other horizontal surface with the trough toward your left and the door to your right.

   Insert the spotted, dried chromatographic sheet, coated side up, on the chamber door, with the spots toward you. With the door on the table, close the trough side over the door. Keep the chamber on the flat surface.

Close the chamber tightly by pressing the edges with your thumb. For proper contact between the chromatographic sheet and the gel surface, gently tap the closed chamber, trough-side up, once or twice against a table edge. During development, the chamber may be left in a horizontal or vertical position (ascending or descending chromatography), or it may be transported, with no change in results.

3. Develop the chromatogram. The advance of the solvent front can be seen by holding the chamber up to the light. It should reach the top in approximately 20 to 30 minutes. This will vary slightly, depending upon temperature and humidity. If migration takes more than 45 minutes, it means that the gel has become dry. Good results can still be achieved, but care should be taken in interpretation since Rf values may change.

   Better resolution of the sugars is possible if the chromatogram is allowed to develop for several minutes after the solvent front reaches the top of the sheet. Total developing time can be increased to as much as 60 minutes. For comparison, it is essential to run a standard mixture beside the unknown. Glucose can be used as a reference point with this modification. Glucose is substituted in the usual calculation for Rf value determination, so that the other sugars are related to the position of glucose, and expressed as Rg values. As explained above,

$$\text{Rg} = \frac{\text{Distance sugar travels}}{\text{Distance glucose travels}} \times 100$$

4. Dry the chromatogram. After development, remove the sheet from the chamber with the forceps. Allow the solvents to evaporate from the sheet in air for 5 to 10 minutes. The solvents must be completely evaporated before proceeding to the visualization step.

METHOD OF VISUALIZATION. The gel contains aniline hydrogen phthalate, a reagent that stains most mono- and disaccharides. To visualize the separated zones, it is only necessary to heat the chromatogram in an oven at 100° C (212° F) for 3 minutes. Do not overheat. Overheating will increase the intensity of the background color, which covers the lower $^3/_4$ of the chromatogram. The sugars can be identified by comparison with the standard and by referring to the chart below, which lists colors and both Rf and Rg values.

Comparison with reference chromatograms illustrating the separation of normal and abnormal specimens will also be helpful. The specimen

TABLE 1–23. Identification of Sugars after Thin-Layer Chromatography.

Sugar	Color with Analine Hydrogen Phthalate	Rg Values	Rf Values	Detection Limit (μg)
Ribose	red-brown	160	72	10
Xylose	red-brown	160	72	2
Fructose	yellow-brown	115	52	20
Sucrose	light brown	107	48	50 (after 30′ at 100° C)
Glucose	green-brown	100	45	5
Galactose	green-brown	100	45	2
Lactose	gray-brown	56	25	1
Glucuronic acid	red-brown	40	18	5

may be analyzed further by two-dimensional thin-layer chromatography or electrophoresis.

The background color will vary from light yellow to tan, depending upon temperature and other variables. This will influence the colors of the sugars, so it is always best to compare the chromatogram to a standard chromatogram run at the same time.

Note: Rf values may vary under the influence of factors such as laboratory temperature and humidity, and quantity of sugar present. Variations in Rf values are observed with different runs. Therefore, a statement of Rf values is only a guide and is of value to the analyst only after comparison with values observed in his laboratories on many known samples tested under controlled conditions.

The relative position of the separated sugars is not likely to change using the KODAK CHROMAT/O/SCREEN Gel and the chromatographic sheets supplied with the kit. Chromatography of a number of known samples will establish these positions.

DISCUSSION AND CLINICAL SIGNIFICANCE

1. Glycosuria. Glucose is normally present in the urine in concentrations not exceeding 100 mg/24 hours or 15 mg/dl. "Alimentary glycosurias" are the result of a postprandial rise in plasma glucose sufficient to exceed the renal glucose theshold. This can occur in some hyperthyroid or post-gastrectomy patients, in those with advanced liver disease, or even in otherwise normal persons.

   Renal glycosuria is caused by glucose leakage from the kidney. It can occur at normal plasma levels and may be congenital. Some forms of the congenital type usually also involve problems with urine acidification, ammonia production, and transport of water, phosphates, and amino acids. Such tubular defects occur in patients with the Fanconi syndrome and cystinosis. Glucose-galactose malabsorption usually results in defective renal transport of glucose. Acquired renal glycosuria is found in patients with the nephrotic syndrome and with renal tubular damage, resulting from mercury, uranium, or Lysol disinfectant poisoning, in patients with Wilson's disease, and with myelomatosis. Mild temporary renal glycosuria may be found in patients with acute glomerulonephritis and during pregnancy.

In diabetics, plasma glucose levels may exceed the renal threshold. This can also occur in patients with Cushing's syndrome, acromegaly, pheochromocytoma, and certain intracranial lesions.

2. Galactosuria occurs in paients with advanced liver disease and with galactosemia. The latter, which occurs in 1 in 30,000 live births, is inherited as an autosomal recessive trait. Here, the defect results from low activity of the enzyme galactose-1-phosphate-uridyl-transferase, which converts galactose-1-phosphate to glucose-1-phosphate. The disease is characterized by galactosuria in the first days following ingestion of lactose. It usually is manifest in the first weeks of life by vomiting, diarrhea, hepatomegaly, and jaundice. Within several months, patients may exhibit cataracts, mental deficiency, and cirrhosis, and may progress to early death. Diagnosis should be confirmed by demonstrating the enzyme deficiency in a red cell preparation. Prompt withdrawal of lactose from the diet is desirable; otherwise, the prognosis is poor. Therefore, early detection is vital.
3. Fructosuria may result from severe liver disease or from essential fructosuria. The latter is inherited as an autosomal recessive trait with an incidence of 1 in 130,000. It is benign and diagnosed by appearance of frustosuria or sucrosuria after ingestion of these sugars. It results from lack of hepatic fructokinase.
4. Hereditary fructose intolerance is also a rare inherited condition. It is not benign and is characterized by a fructosuria with proteinuria and aminoaciduria. Clinically, its symptoms are hypoglycemic fits, anorexia, vomiting, and frequently, hepatosplenomegaly with jaundice. Since recovery is possible when fructose is completely removed from the diet, early detection is very important. It results from absence of the fructose-phosphorate-splitting liver aldolase.
5. Familial galactose and fructose intolerance is characterized by alimentary galactosuria and fructosuria. The ingestion of either of the sugars produces hypoglycemia.
6. Essential pentosuria is another rare, autosomal recessive trait that is completely benign. L-Xylulose and occasionally, L-arabital may be found in the urine. It probably results from a defect in glucosuriac acid metabolism.
7. Ribosuria occurs in patients suffering from certain types of muscular disease. It is presumably due to catabolized muscle nucleoprotein resulting in excretion of the ribose.
8. Disacchariduria has been described in several forms, and the ex-

cretion of lactose and sucrose following ingestion of these sugars has been associated with many gastrointestinal disorders. It may accompany the congenital deficiencies of intestinal disaccharidosis, discussed subsequently, as well as sprue, celiac disease, hiatal hernia, infantile gastroenteritis, intestinal scleroderma, cystic fibrosis, regional enteritis, acrodermatitis enteropathica, intestinal lymphangiectasia, ulcerative colitis, giardiasis, and after gastric and intestinal surgery. The detection of disaccharides in the urine is of practical value, since it coincides with the symptoms of intestinal sugar intolerance such as abdominal distension, cramps, and fermentative diarrhea, which improve when the offending sugars are removed from the diet. Thus, early detection is very important.

A good example of the unreliability of the common reducing sugar tests to detect meliturias is the diagnosis of the disaccharidurias. Case mortality is high in the disaccharide intolerance of infancy partly because the diagnosis is sometimes missed because of reliance solely on the usual reduction tests for sugars. Furthermore, reducing sugars are found in stools of these patients, presumably because of bacterial hydrolysis of disaccharides. The disaccharides can, however, be detected by chromatography. Gross aminoaciduria very often occurs with disaccharidurias.

9. Endogenous lactosuria occurs during late pregnancy and lactation. Lactose appears in the urine and increases greatly at the onset of lactation, after which it gradually decreases even though lactation continues.
10. Congenital lactose malabsorption is characterized by diarrhea and a constant failure of the infant to thrive after first being given lactose-containing foods. Vomiting may or may not accompany these symptoms. Lactose is found in the stool and in the urine after oral ingestion of the sugar. The presence of lactosuria after a lactose load does not differentiate congenital from acquired lactose malabsorption. The estimation of disaccharidase activities from jejunal or duodenal mucosal biopsies is necessary for final diagnosis. Lactose intolerance may be secondary to other causes of diarrhea such as gastroenteritis, celiac disease, or trauma to the small intestine, as mentioned above.

MATERIALS AND REAGENTS

1. KODAK CHROMAT/O/SCREEN Gel (Butanol:pyridine: hydrochloric acid. Aniline hydrogen phthalate added for visualization.)
2. Chromatographic sheets, 30 two-channel sheets
3. Pipette, 1 μL
4. Pipette holder
5. Developing chambers, 30 chambers
6. Instruction booklet

7. Forceps
8. Standard
9. Scraper

TABLE 1–24. Trouble Shooting.

Problem	Probable Cause	Remedy
Uneven advance of solvent front	1. Gel not leveled in trough 2. Chamber not tightly closed	1. Level gel with scraper 2. Tightly close chamber
Plasma chromatogram has vertical smudge	Presence of protein in sample	Spot sample completely across the narrow neck between holes on the chromatographic sheet
Broad bands of separated sugars or long tails on either side (difficult to determine Rf values)	1. Sample has spread out too far on application 2. Too high a concentration of sugars	1. Spot several smaller applications 2. Use smaller sample
Long running time	Dried solvent gel	No effect on results if a standard is run along with unknowns
Smudged chromatograms, or specimens which do not run	Excess gel in trough is squeezed past sample when chamber is closed. Sample dissolves in gel	Level gel in trough
Final, visualized chromatogram has dark background	Chromatogram heated too long or at too high a temperature	Warm chromatogram 100° C for 3 minutes
Poorly resolved sugars	Migration time too short	Increase migration time to one hour

REFERENCES

1. Carson, A., and Neely, R.: Disaccharide intolerance in infancy. Arch. Dis. Child., *38*:574, 1963.
2. Dormandy, T., and Porter, R.: Familial fructose and galactose intolerance. Lancet, *1*:1189, 1961.
3. Flynn, F.: Essential pentosuria. Br. Med. J., *1*:391, 1955.
4. Levin, B., et al.: Congenital lactose malabsorption. Arch. Dis. Child., *45*:173, 1970.
5. Levin, B., et al.: Fructosuria. Arch. Dis. Child., *38*:220, 1963.
6. Long, C.: Biochemists Handbook. Princeton, D. Van Nostrand, 1961, p. 923.
7. Moncrieff, A., and Wilkinson, R.: Sucrosuria with mental defects and hiatus hernia. Acta Scand., *43*:(Suppl. 100) 495, 1954.
8. Smith, I.: Chromatographic and Electrophoretic Techniques. Vol. 1. New York, Interscience Publishers, 1969.
9. Stanbury, J., Wyngaarden, J., and Fredrickson, D. (eds.): The Metabolic Basis of Inherited Diseases. 3rd Ed. New York, McGraw-Hill, 1972, p. 83.
10. Tocci, P.: The biochemical diagnosis of metabolic disorders by urinalysis and paper chromatography. *In* Amino Acid Metabolism and Genetic Variation. Edited by W. Nyhan. New York, McGraw-Hill, 1967, p. 461.
11. Walton, J., and Latner, A.: Ribosuria in muscular dystrophy. Arch. Neurol. Psych., *72*:362, 1954.

12. Young, D., and Jackson, A.: Thin-layer chromatography of urinary carbohydrates. A comparative evaluation of procedures. Clin. Chem., *16*:954, 1970.

GALACTOSE

METHOD. Dipstick test.

PRINCIPLE. Galactostix involves the formation of galacto hexodialdose and hydrogen peroxide from the oxidation of galactose by galactose oxidase on the plastic stick. A second enzyme, peroxidase, catalyzes the reaction of hydrogen peroxide to react with orthotolidine, incorporated on the stick, to form the oxidized orthotolidine, which is blue.

PROCEDURE

1. Immerse reagent strip into fresh urine specimen and allow it to become thoroughly wet for approximately 2 seconds.
2. Remove excess urine by blotting edge of strip against urine container or on filter paper.
3. Compare test area with color chart in 60 seconds.

INTERPRETATION. Only concentrations of 0.1% or over can be detected; if detected, the test is considered *positive.* Normal concentrations of galactose cannot be measured with this test.

DISCUSSION AND CLINICAL SIGNIFICANCE. The test is most useful for screening of children for a hereditary metabolic disorder, galactosuria. Galactose can also be demonstrated in the urine of lactating or pregnant women and may occur in patients with advanced liver disease.

The reaction of the galactose stick is inhibited by a high concentration of ascorbic acid, tetracycline antibiotics, and other strong reducing agents. It is advisable to dilute concentrated urine prior to testing, because the strength of color of the strip decreases as specific gravity of the urine (especially a specific gravity over 1.010) increases. The test is more sensitive than the copper reduction test or Clinitest reagent tablets for reducing substances. The reagent area of the strip does not react with lactose, glucose, or fructose, but it is quite specific for galactose.

The reagent strips are fastidious and will deteriorate with oxygenation; therefore, the bottle should be tightly capped. The strips should be protected from light and heat.

A positive control may be prepared by adding a measured amount of lactose to dilute urine (specific gravity less than 1.010) and by permitting the urine to stand for 1 hour (to permit mutarotation to occur) before testing.

MATERIAL AND REAGENTS

1. Urine container
2. Galactostix (Ames Company, Elkhart, Ind. 46514)

REFERENCES

1. Ames Company brochure on the test, 1975.
2. Roth, H., Segal, S., and Bertoli, D.: The quantitative determination of galactose—an enzyme using galactose oxidase with applications to blood and other biological fluids. Anal. Biochem., *10*:32, 1965.
3. Stanbury, J., Wyngaarden, J., and Frederickson, D.: The Metabolic Basis of Inherited Disease. 4th Ed. New York, McGraw-Hill, 1978, p. 174.

GALACTOSE AND LACTOSE

METHOD. Mucic acid test.

PRINCIPLE. A fine, white precipitate of mucic acid ($C_6O_4H_6(OH)_4$) crystals will be formed in urine upon the oxidation of lactose or galactose by nitric acid and heat with the presence of these sugars.

PROCEDURE

1. Pour 50 ml of urine into a beaker.
2. Carefully add 10 ml of concentrated nitric acid.
3. Boil until volume is reduced to about 10 ml.
4. Add 10 ml of water and let it stand overnight.

INTERPRETATION. A normal amount of galactose or lactose in urine will not be detected by this test. If galactose or lactose is present in an increased amount, a fine, white precipitate will form.

DISCUSSION AND CLINICAL SIGNIFICANCE. In hereditary galactosuria, in which there is a decrease or absence of galactose-1-phosphate-uridyl-transferase, the sugar will be found in the urine only a few days after the ingestion of lactose. Unless detected in the first few days of life and treated by a diet free of lactose and galactose, cataracts, mental retardation, cirrhosis of the liver, and renal tubular aminoaciduria will occur.

Galactosuria and lactosuria occur most commonly during pregnancy and lactation.

MATERIALS AND REAGENTS

1. HNO_3, concentrated
2. Beaker, 100 ml
3. Serologic pipettes, 10 ml
4. Test tube, 16 × 100 mm

REFERENCE

1. White, W., Erickson, M., and Stevens, S.: Chemistry for Medical Technologists. St. Louis, C.V. Mosby, 1970, p. 381.

GALACTOSE AND PENTOSES

METHOD. Tollen's phloroglucin test.

PRINCIPLE. Pentoses and galactose, if heated with mineral acids, yield furfurol which produces a purple colored compound when combined with the sweet crystalline phenol phloroglucin, $C_6H_3(OH)_3$.

nitroprusside in an acid environment, despite the buffering capacity of the tablet. Also, creatinine may interfere.

The tablets are stable if protected from light, and they can tolerate temperatures to 120° F. Tablets that turn yellow or orange are no longer usable. If the urine is not absorbed within 30 seconds after being dropped on the tablet, the tablet is not good, already having absorbed too much moisture.

MATERIALS AND REAGENTS

1. Acetest tablets (Ames Company, Elkhart, Ind 46514)
2. Acetone (Baker Analyzed Reagents; J. T. Baker Chemical Company, Phillipsburg, N.J. 08865)
3. Dropping pipette

REFERENCES

1. Ames Company brochure on test.
2. Brand, E., Harris, M., and Biloon, S.: Cystinuria. The excretion of a cystine complex which decomposes in the urine with the liberation of free cystine. J. Biol. Chem., 86:315–331, 1930.
3. Kark, R., et al.: A Primer of Urinalysis. 2nd Ed. New York, Hoeber Medical Division, Harper & Row, 1963, p. 42.

KETONE BODIES

METHOD. Ketostix, Multistix tests.

PRINCIPLE. Reagent strips contain similar reagents to those in Acetest tablets and react in similar fashion.

PROCEDURE

1. Dip test strip in urine or briefly pass through urine stream.
2. Compare color with chart after 15 seconds.

INTERPRETATION AND CLINICAL SIGNIFICANCE. Interpretation is the same as with the Acetest tablets. Ketostix will demonstrate reliably as little as 10 mg of diacetic acid/dl serum, plasma, or urine. Do not use a Ketostix that has a brown discoloration. Moisture content will decrease sensitivity, so sticks should be stored in a tightly closed bottle.

MATERIALS AND REAGENTS. Ketostix, Multistix (Ames Company, Elkhart, Ind. 46514).

REFERENCES

1. Ames Company brochure on test.
2. Kark, R., et al.: A Primer of Urinalysis. 2nd Ed. New York, Hoeber Medical Division, Harper & Row, 1963, p. 44.

PROTEIN

METHOD. Heat and acetic acid test.

PRINCIPLE. Urinary protein is coagulated by heat, and the degree of turbidity produced is proportional to the quantity of protein present.

Phosphates and mucins, which may also produce turbidity, are dissolved by the acetic acid.

PROCEDURE

1. Fill a 5 ml test tube to within 1 inch of the top with urine.
2. Heat the upper portion of the tube with a small flame until it just begins to boil.
3. Add 5 drops acetic acid.
4. Reheat to boiling in similar manner and observe for clouding at the top of the tube.

INTERPRETATION. Read results against a dark background and record as follows:

Negative	Clear at the top of tube
Trace	Faint, barely visible clouding (5–15 mg/dl)
1+	Distinct but nongranular cloud (25–50 mg/dl)
2+	More dense granular cloud (about 100 mg/dl)
3+	Dense cloud with heavy flocculation (about 200–300 mg/dl)
4+	Heavy precipitate or solid flocculant (≥500 mg/dl)

DISCUSSION AND CLINICAL SIGNIFICANCE. Normal urine contains too little protein (up to 100 mg/24-hour volume) to be detected by this test. False positive test results may be caused by x-ray contrast media, tolbutamide (Orinase), penicillin in massive doses, and para-aminosalicylic acid (PAS). False negatives may occur in highly buffered alkaline urine or in presence of severe urinary tract infections by urea-splitting organisms. If the urine is turbid before the test, it should be centrifuged to clear it.

Proteinuria can occur as a result of fever, lower urinary tract disease, following severe exercise, exposure to cold, or in a benign condition known as "orthostatic proteinuria," in which proteinuria occurs only when the subject is in an upright position. Because of its almost universal presence in patients with organic renal disease, however, a renal biopsy should be considered to establish a diagnosis if these other conditions can be ruled out.

MATERIALS AND REAGENTS

1. Acetic acid, 5% (w/v)
2. Test tubes, 13 × 100 mm
3. Bunsen burner

REFERENCES

1. Air Force Manual, Laboratory Procedures in Clinical Chemistry and Urinalysis. Gunter AFB, Alabama, Section 18–9, March 15, 1962.
2. Kark, R., et al.: A Primer of Urinalysis. 2nd Ed. New York, Hoeber Medical Division, Harper & Row, 1963, p. 26.

PROTEIN

METHOD. Sulfosalicylic acid.

PRINCIPLE. Most, if not all, proteins (albumin, globulins, Bence Jones protein, hemoglobin, for example) are coagulated by dilute sulfosalicylic acid (or by most other weak acids, for that matter), and the amount of turbidity produced can be estimated visually.

PROCEDURE

1. Filter or centrifuge urine specimen to obtain 5 ml of clear supernate.
2. Check urine acidity with nitrazine or pHydrion paper.
3. If urine is alkaline or neutral, add acetic acid drop by drop until pH is just slightly below 7.
4. Add 2 ml of sulfosalicylic acid, mix, and observe for white precipitates.
5. Controls should also be run.

INTERPRETATION. A white precipitate forms when protein is present. Report as follows.

Negative	Urine remains clear (no protein)
Trace	Faintly turbid (<10 mg/dl)
1+	Definite turbidity (10–50 g/dl)
2+	Heavy turbidity but no flocculate (50–200 mg/dl)
3+	Heavy cloud with flocculation (200–500 mg/dl)
4+	Heavy cloud with heavy flocculation (>500 mg/dl)

DISCUSSION AND CLINICAL SIGNIFICANCE. False-positive tests may occur in the presence of mucin, high concentrations of uric acid, tolbutamide (Orinase) metabolites, high concentrations of penicillin, para-amino-salicylic acid, and some x-ray contrast media. False-negative test results could occur in highly buffered alkaline urine, if they were not first acidified.

This method has been modified in some laboratories, using a much smaller aliquot of urine and more dilute acid, yielding a light precipitate that can be quantitated photometrically or densitometrically.

MATERIALS AND REAGENTS

1. Acetic acid, 10% (v/v)
2. Sulfosalicylic acid, 3% (w/v)

Sulfosalicylic acid ($C_7H_6O_6S \cdot SH_2O$)	3 g
Distilled water q.s. to	100 ml

3. Test tubes, 13 × 100 mm
4. Filter paper and funnel
5. Volumetric pipette, 2 ml

REFERENCES

1. Air Force Manual, Laboratory Procedure in Clinical Chemistry and Urinalysis. Gunter AFB, Alabama, Section 18–10, March 15, 1962.

2. Naumann, H.: A system of testing for Bence Jones protein. South. Med. J., 59:157, 1966.

PROTEIN

METHOD. Albustix, Combistix, Multistix, Chemstrip, or Labstix tests.

PRINCIPLE. The test is based on the "protein error" of hydrogen ion indicators: that is, at the same pH, certain indicators have one color in the presence of protein and another color in the absence of protein. The stick contains citrate buffer which provides a hydrogen ion concentration corresponding to pH 3. At this pH, tetrabromphenol blue indicator dye has a yellow color when no protein is present. At the same pH, the indicator dye will change to a yellow-green, green and blue with increasing amounts of protein. Therefore, the color of the stick provides a method for rough quantitation of the amount of protein present.

PROCEDURE

1. Dip stick in urine according to directions on container.
2. Remove from urine and compare color with reference chart.

INTERPRETATION

Negative	No protein or < 10 mg/dl
Trace	< 30 mg/dl
1+	30 mg/dl
2+	100 mg/dl
3+	300 mg/dl
4+	≥ 1 mg/dl

DISCUSSION AND CLINICAL SIGNIFICANCE. Test positive and negative control material in addition to unknown. False positive dipstick tests for protein may occur with highly buffered alkaline urine, but do not occur with drugs and contrast media that do produce false positives with the heat and acetic acid test. Numerous medications interfere with the reaction and can produce unusual colors or unusual results.

MATERIALS AND REAGENTS. Albustix, Combistix, Multistix, or Labstix (Ames Company, Elkhart, Ind. 46514).

REFERENCES

1. Bio-Dynamics Co. brochure on test.
2. Kark, R., et al.: A Primer of Urinalysis. 2nd Ed. New York, Hoeber Medical Division, Harper & Row, 1963, pp. 18 and 24.
3. Latner, A.: Cantarow and Trumper Clinical Biochemistry. 7th Ed. Philadelphia, W.B. Saunders, 1975.

PROTEIN (QUANTITATIVE)

METHOD. Shevky-Stafford method (slightly modified).

PRINCIPLE. All proteins are coagulated by phosphotungstic acid, and the amount of settled precipitate is measured in standardized volumetric tubes precalibrated and marked by manufacturer according to Marian Shevky's original technique.

PROCEDURE

1. Dip Albustix, Combistix, Multistix, or Labstix strip into urine and compare color with reference chart upon removal from urine.
2. Dilute urine specimen as follows depending on the qualitative result of urine.

Trace	No dilution of urine
1+	Dilute urine 1 in 2
2+	Dilute urine 1 in 4
3+	Dilute urine 1 in 8
4+	Dilute urine 1 in 16 and 1 in 32

3. Tranfer urine into Shevky-Stafford tube to 4.0 (ml) mark.
4. Add Tsuchiya's reagent to 6.5 (ml) mark.
5. Mix by inverting slowly 3 times.
6. Allow to stand 10 minutes; again mix by inversion. Centrifuge at 1600 rpm (or at an acceleration sufficient to supply an RCF of 420) for 5 minutes at room temperature.
7. Read volume of column of precipitate from tube.
8. Calculation:
   ml ppt. × 7.2 × dilution factor = g protein/L (Shevky used 13 ml tube, so then 1.0 ml ppt. is equivalent to 3.6 g protein/L; the newer tubes call for a final value of 6.5 ml. So 1.0 ml ppt. is equivalent to 7.2 g protein/L; hence, the reason for the factor 7.2.)
9. Controls should also be run.

INTERPRETATION. The test is very sensitive and can detect a wide spectrum of proteins, including albumin, globulin, Bence Jones protein, abnormal uroglobulins, hemoglobin, and so on (even when the amount of protein is too small to be detected by Labstix or similar test strips). Results vary with temperature, the same volume of precipitate signifying less protein at lower temperatures than at higher.

DISCUSSION AND CLINICAL SIGNIFICANCE. The method should give results within about 6.5% of the true value of the amount of protein (as determined by Kjeldahl nitrogen determination). The specific gravity of the urine does not affect results. However, careful standardization of centrifugation is necessary. The method is slightly more accurate than Esbach's method (according to Shevky and Stafford's original studies).

MATERIALS AND REAGENTS

1. Tsuchiya's reagent:

Phosphotungstic acid	1.5 g
Conc. HCl	5 ml
95% (v/v) ethanol q.s. to	100 ml

2. Shevky-Stafford (or McNaught protein) tube (Arthur H. Thomas Co., [no. 2998-G55], Vine St., at Third, Philadelphia, Pa. 19105)

3. Labstix (Ames Company, Elkhart, Ind. 46514)
4. Serologic pipettes, 5 ml and 1 ml
5. Clinical centrifuge
6. Test tubes, 13 × 100 mm

REFERENCES

1. Lipmann, R.: Urine and the Urinary Sediment. Springfield, Charles C Thomas, 1967, p. 106.
2. Shevky, M., and Stafford, D.: A clinical method for the estimation of protein in urine and other body fluids. Arch. Int. Med., 32:222, 1923.
3. Simmons, J., and Gentzow, C.: Medical and Public Health Laboratory Methods. Philadelphia, Lea & Febiger, 1955, p. 280.

PROTEIN (QUANTITATIVE)

METHOD. Esbach's method.

PRINCIPLE. Protein is precipitated from urine with picric acid, and the volume of precipitate is measured in standardized precalibrated volumetric tubes.

SAMPLE. Collect an accurately timed 24-hour urine specimen and record the volume.

PROCEDURE

1. Fill an Esbach tube with urine to the "U" mark (10 ml mark).
2. Add Esbach's reagent to the "R" mark (20 ml mark).
3. Place cork stopper on tube and mix by inversion.
4. Read the level of the volume corresponding to precipitate after allowing precipitate to settle for 30 minutes at room temperature.
5. Calculations:
   Reading on tube = g/1,000 ml urine

OR

$$\frac{\text{Reading on tube} \times \text{24-hour vol. (ml)}}{1{,}000} = \text{g/24-hour urine}$$

INTERPRETATION. The reading on the tube indicates the number of g protein/L of urine as stated above. If the urine is diluted, multiply final result by reciprocal of dilution.

DISCUSSION AND CLINICAL SIGNIFICANCE. Normally healthy adults excrete less than 100 mg protein/24 hours, an amount too small to be detectable by usual tests for proteinuria. Most organic proteinuria results from abnormal glomerular filtration, as has been stated previously. The test is accurate and simple. However, we prefer the Shevky-Stafford method.

MATERIALS

1. Esbach's reagent (stable with shelf storage in a brown bottle)

Picric acid	1g
Citric acid	2g
Distilled water	100 ml

2. Esbach tube
3. Cork and stopper

REFERENCES

1. CRC Practical Manual for Clinical Laboratory Procedures. Cleveland, Chemical Rubber Co., 1965, p. U-26.
2. Esbach, G.: Dosage clinique de l'albumine (modification du procede de 1874). Bull. de Therap. (Fr.) 98:497, 1880.

PROTEIN (QUANTITATIVE)

METHOD. Sulfosalicylic acid turbidity.

PRINCIPLE. Sulfosalicylic acid precipitates protein in urine with a turbidity that is approximately proportional to the concentration of protein in a solution. The turbidity is measured with a spectrophotometer. Each acidified urine is used as its own blank to offset the effects of urinary pigments. Most proteins (albumin, globulin, hemoglobin, myoglobin, Bence Jones immunoprotein) can be coagulated.

SAMPLE. For collection of the 24-hour sample, the patient is provided with written instructions. The patient is instructed to void first thing in the morning. From that time, all urine passed during the day and night is collected in the clean bottle provided. Final collection is made the next morning at the same hour that collection was started. After collection is completed, the urine should be refrigerated, if necessary, for it to stand for longer than 1 to 2 hours before analysis. No added preservative is necessary.

PROCEDURE

1. Measure total volume of the sample and record in ml.
2. Centrifuge an aliquot of the urine and use the supernatant for analysis.
3. Pipette into cuvettes:

Unknown	*Blank (for Each Patient)*
1 ml urine	1 ml urine
4 ml sulfosalicylic acid	4 ml HCl

4. Mix tubes by inversion; let stand for 5 minutes before reading.
5. Read in spectrophotometer at 500 nm using the blank set to zero Absorbance. Read results in Absorbance units.
6. Read the values from the standard curve. If greater than 140 mg/dl, repeat with 1:10 dilution with normal saline.
7. Results are reported in two fashions: mg/dl or mg/24 hours. To obtain mg/24 hours, multiply mg/dl by urine volume in ml and divide result by 100. Report result as 14 mg/dl or 210 mg/24 hours.

PREPARATION OF STANDARD CURVE. Determine the total protein concentration of a pooled serum with a normal protein distribution. Do not include lipemic or hemolyzed specimens in the pool. Run this sample on an automated chemistry analyzer. The protein concentration of the standard will be:

$$\text{protein (mg/dl)} = \frac{\text{TP} \times 1{,}000}{200} = \text{TP} \times 5$$

where TP is total protein concentration in the serum in g/dl. For example, if the pooled serum has a total protein concentration of 7.0 g/dl, the dilute standard has a protein concentration of 35 mg/dl. Prepare an appropriate number of dilutions to obtain a standard curve. Use the 100-ml volumetric flasks for making dilutions. Using saline as a blank, read the Absorbance of each dilution, and plot the results on log paper. You can use the guidelines provided in Table 1–25 to establish a standard curve.

INTERPRETATION. Two to 8 mg/dl or up to 150 mg/24 hrs. Values greater than 4,000 mg/dl in adults or greater than 2,000 mg/dl in children should be reported to the physician. If the results obtained are "zero," report as "undetectable."

DISCUSSION AND CLINICAL SIGNIFICANCE. Normal urine contains a small amount of protein, because the normal glomerulus prevents passage of albumin and larger proteins from plasma to the glomerular filtrate. Detection of protein in urine is usually considered evidence of renal (especially glomerular) disease. The degree of proteinuria varies with the type of disease and with the severity of the disease process. Measuring the amount of protein excreted is helpful in diagnosis and in following the course of disease. Proteinuria may be absent in phases of acute pyelonephritis, in chronic pyelonephritis, and in cases of obstructive nephropathy, kidney stones, kidney tumors, and congenital malformations.

Measurement of urine protein by turbidimetric methods is much more precise and accurate than the original Esbach method. Sulfosalicylic acid or trichloracetic acid are commonly used as precipitants. Sulfosalicylic acid precipitates albumin, globulin, polypeptides, proteoses, and Bence Jones proteins. More precise measurements that are suitable for small amounts of protein are available, but in routine clinical practice, quantitative measurement by the turbidimetric procedure with sulfosalicylic acid is satisfactory. Screening tests for proteinuria should not be too sensitive, because they are required to differentiate normal protein excretion from abnormal. Quantitative measurement by this method is satisfactory for clinical use.

Acid precipitation tests will give false positive results when organic iodine x-ray media are present. Urinary excretion may persist for 3 days after administration of the dye. An excretion product of the oral hypoglycemic agent, tolbutamide, will also cause turbidity with acidification of the urine. Some false positive and false negative reactions include:

Agent	*Problem*
Urine turbidity	May confuse reading
X-ray contrast media	May cause false positive
Tolbutamide and its metabolites	May cause false positive
Penicillin (large doses)	May cause false positive
Aminosalicylic acid in urine containing preservatives	May cause false positive
Highly buffered alkaline urine	May cause false negative
Quaternary ammonium compounds	No effect
Nitrofurantoins	Pink color
Dilute specimen (sp. gr. < 1.010)	False low-protein value

MATERIALS AND REAGENTS

1. Sulfosalicylic acid, 3% (w/v) in distilled water
2. Hydrochloric acid, 1.25% (w/v)
3. Test tubes, 15 × 100 mm
4. Spectrophotometer at 500 nm
5. Volumetric pipettes, 5 ml

TABLE 1–25. Guidelines for Establishing a Standard Curve.

Amount of Pooled Serum	Conversion of g/dl to mg/dl		Value in mg/dl
0.1	$\frac{TP \times 1000}{1000}$	$\frac{.1}{100}$	TP × 1
0.25	$\frac{TP \times 1000}{400}$	$\frac{.25}{100}$	TP × 2.5
0.5	$\frac{TP \times 1000}{200}$	$\frac{.5}{100}$	TP × 5
0.75	$\frac{TP \times 1000}{133.3}$	$\frac{.75}{100}$	TP × 7.5
1.0	$\frac{TP \times 1000}{100}$	$\frac{1.0}{100}$	TP × 10
1.25	$\frac{TP \times 1000}{80}$	$\frac{1.25}{100}$	TP × 12.5
1.5	$\frac{TP \times 1000}{66.7}$	$\frac{1.5}{100}$	TP × 15

REFERENCES

1. Annino, J.S.: Clinical Chemistry: Principles and Procedures. 4th Ed. New York, Little, Brown, 1976.
2. Henry, J. (ed.): Clinical Diagnosis and Management by Laboratory Methods. 16th Ed. Philadelphia, W.B. Saunders, 1979, p. 604.

BENCE JONES PROTEIN

METHOD. Sulfosalicylic acid test and sulfosalicylic acid-heat method.

PRINCIPLE. Bence Jones protein (light polypeptide chains produced in excess by plasma cells in certain pathologic conditions) will precipitate at about 60° C, will redissolve as the temperature is raised to 100° C, and will reappear with cooling of urine to 60° C; whereas, other proteins will usually not appear at 60° C, and will precipitate with boiling at 100° C. However, since Bence Jones proteins are often accompanied by other proteins, sophisticated modifications of this basic procedure are necessary for some specific identification and quantitation.

SAMPLE. Urine should be free from bacteria and should be centrifuged until clear.

PROCEDURE

SULFOSALICYLIC ACID TEST

1. Use protein-containing urine as a control.
2. Place 5 ml patient's urine in a 15 ml test tube; in a separate tube, place 5 ml of control urine.
3. Add 2 ml sulfosalicylic acid and observe for precipitate.
4. If a precipitate does not form, the test is negative and can be discontinued here.

SULFOSALICYLIC ACID-HEAT METHOD

1. Use protein-containing urine as a control.
2. Place 4 ml control urine in a 15 ml test tube. In a separate test tube, place 4 ml patient's urine.
3. Add 1 ml acetate buffer to each tube.
4. Place thermometer in tube with urine-buffer mixture.
5. Heat buffered urines for 15 minutes in a 56° C water bath. Observe for formation of precipitate.
6. Transfer to boiling water bath and heat until temperature reaches 100° C. Observe while in the boiling water bath for dissolution of precipitate. (This can be observed in the presence of albumin and globulin, which will precipitate here. Pseudo-Bence Jones protein will fail to dissolve.)
7. Filter urine while it is still close to boiling temperature. (Use care, or Bence Jones protein may precipitate prematurely and be lost on the filter paper.) Allow to cool and observe for re-formation of precipitate. If the precipitate does not re-form, the test is negative.

8. If protein is present, reheat filtrate as in steps 5 and 6 and observe for precipitate to appear, disappear, then reappear again after placing tubes in cold water bath.
9. If precipitation does re-form, this is either Bence Jones protein or uric acid. Add 1 ml of sulfosalicylic acid and mix. Uric acid dissolves. Bence Jones protein precipitate intensifies.

INTERPRETATION. Mobility of Bence Jones protein varies from that of the slow gamma globulins to those of the faster-moving alpha globulins, varying from patient to patient (but characteristically appearing as a narrow, sharply-defined band). In the presence of large amounts of globulin, the pattern may be difficult to interpret.

DISCUSSION AND CLINICAL SIGNIFICANCE. It has become customary to refer to proteins with typical thermal solubility properties as Bence Jones proteins, while those that are typical or atypical in this regard but that react only with specific antisera for light chains of gamma globulins are called "light chains." There are two types of light chains: kappa and lambda. Polymerized forms and pigments may also be present. Large amounts may be found in the sera of patients with myeloma, but seldom in the absence of urinary Bence Jones proteins. They may also be present in the urine of patients with macroglobulinemia. They originate in the plasma cells in bone marrow.

Franklin's disease is characterized by a lymphoproliferative malignancy without bone, but with liver and spleen, involvement. These patients may have Bence Jones proteinuria. Rarely, Bence Jones proteinuria may be encountered in patients with benign hyperglobulinemia, or in patients with serum monoclonal gammopathies of unknown origin. These probably eventuate in myelomas, in most cases.

MATERIALS AND REAGENTS

1. Sodium chloride, 0.9% (w/v)
2. Sulfosalicylic acid, 20% (w/v)
3. Test tubes, 15 ml conical
4. Serologic pipettes, 5 ml
5. Filter paper (Whatman no. 4) and filter funnel
6. Water bath capable of boiling (100° C), and cool water bath
7. Thermometer capable of 100° C

REFERENCES

1. Bence Jones, J.: On a new substance occurring in the urine of a patient with mollities ossium. Philos. Trans. R. Soc. Lond., *138*:55, 1848.
2. Manuel, Y., Revillard, J.P., and Betuel, H.: Proteins in normal and pathologic urine. Baltimore, University Park Press, 1970.
3. Naumann, H.: A system of testing for Bence Jones protein. South. Med. J., *59*:157, 1966.
4. Osserman, E., and Lawlor, D.: Abnormal serum and urine proteins in 35 cases of multiple myeloma as studied by filter paper electrophoresis. Am. J. Med., *28*:462, 1955.

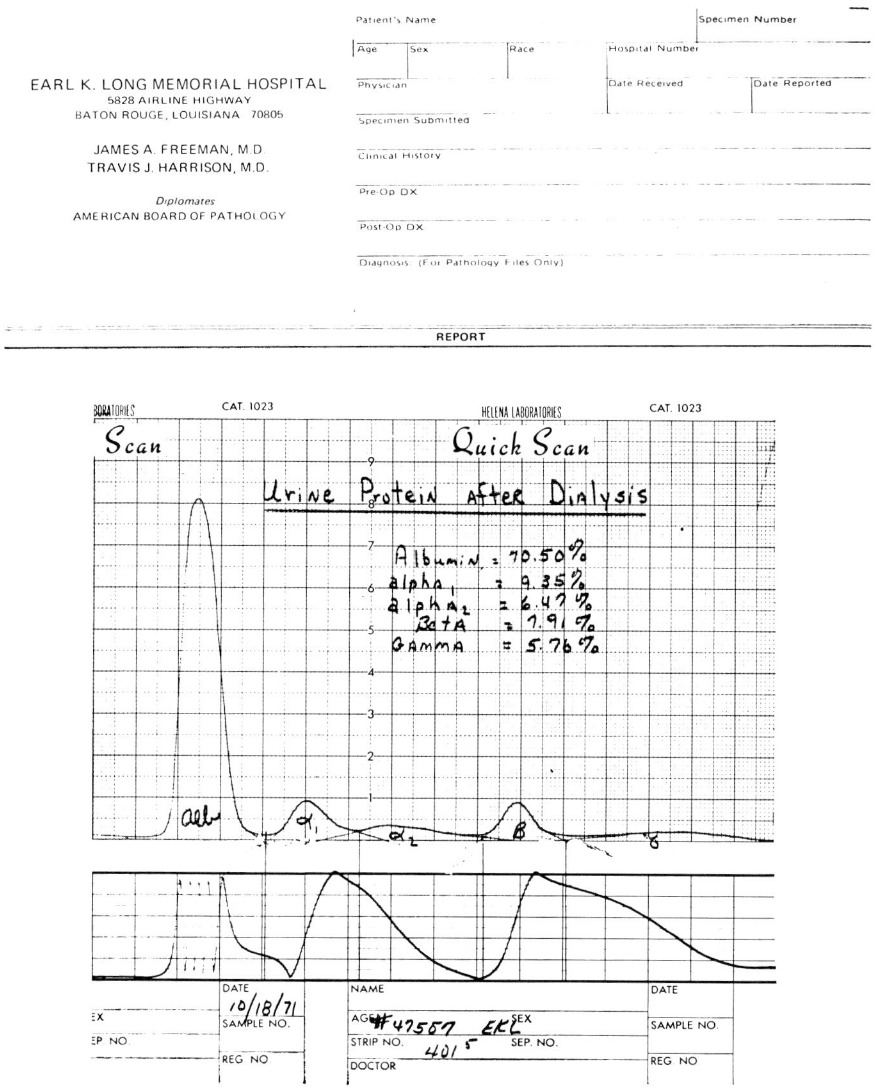

Fig. 1–23. Densitometric tracing of electrophoretic strip of urine protein after dialysis.

5. Putnam, F., et al.: The heat precipitation of Bence Jones proteins. I. Optimum conditions. Arch. Biochem., *83*:115, 1959.

PROTEIN CONCENTRATION

METHOD. Minicon disposable dialysis ultramicrofilter.

PRINCIPLE. A chamber with semipermeable membrane and a solvent in a well is used to dialyze and concentrate body cavity fluids, especially urine. Different types of semipermeable membranes are used depending upon the molecular weight of proteins to be dialyzed. The capacity of the absorbant is about 3 times the total sample volume; the chamber is graduated at levels 5X through 100X, indicating concentration ratio. It takes approximately 3 hours to concentrate a sample 100 times.

SAMPLE

1. Urine: Concentration of urine requires Minicon-A25, a filter with a molecular weight cut-off at 25,000 or an A75 filter with molecular weight cut-off at 75,000.
2. Spinal fluid: Concentration requires B15 filter with a molecular weight cut-off at 15,000.

PROCEDURE. A small aliquot sample can be tested with a couple drops of salicylic acid to determine whether protein is present. Sulfosalicylic acid will precipitate all proteins, including immunoglobulins, Bence Jones, hemoglobin, myoglobin. It is fruitless to try a concentration in the event that no protein is present.

1. Determine the required concentration level with protein dipstick tests (Multistix, Labstix, Chemstrips). The percentage of recoverable macrosolute decreases with the degree of concentration.

   Example 1: A dipstick determination of 100 mg/dl is found as the protein content of an abnormal urine sample. Analysis by electrophoresis or immunoelectrophoresis requires that macrosolute content be at least 2.5 g/L. Concentration by dialysis to 50% (v/v) assures the required degree of enrichment for analysis.

   Example 2: To achieve concentrations above 100X, fill chambers 1 to 5 with 5 ml of sample and allow concentration of 25X in each chamber. This reduces the volume in each chamber 0.2 ml. Pool the concentrated samples (1 ml) and transfer to chamber 6. Allow to concentrate an additional 10% (v/v) and withdraw. The final concentrate is 250X.
2. Prefilter urine through Whatman paper no. 1 or equivalent.
3. Insert sample to level no higher than the "fill" line using a Pasteur pipette or syringe. Care should be taken to avoid scratching the membrane surface. Mark chamber numbers on sample identity record.
4. Sample volume will decrease to approximately 100X. Volume at each graduation line is shown below. For samples smaller than 5 ml, graduations are determined proportionally.
5. To recover sample, insert pipette or syringe to base of chamber and withdraw. Mixing the sample by drawing in and out of the pipette or syringe several times improves recovery.

INTERPRETATION. Protein concentrated in the chamber can be aspirated and thereafter, spotted for electrophoresis or chromatographic techniques.

DISCUSSION AND CLINICAL SIGNIFICANCE. Retention of pro-

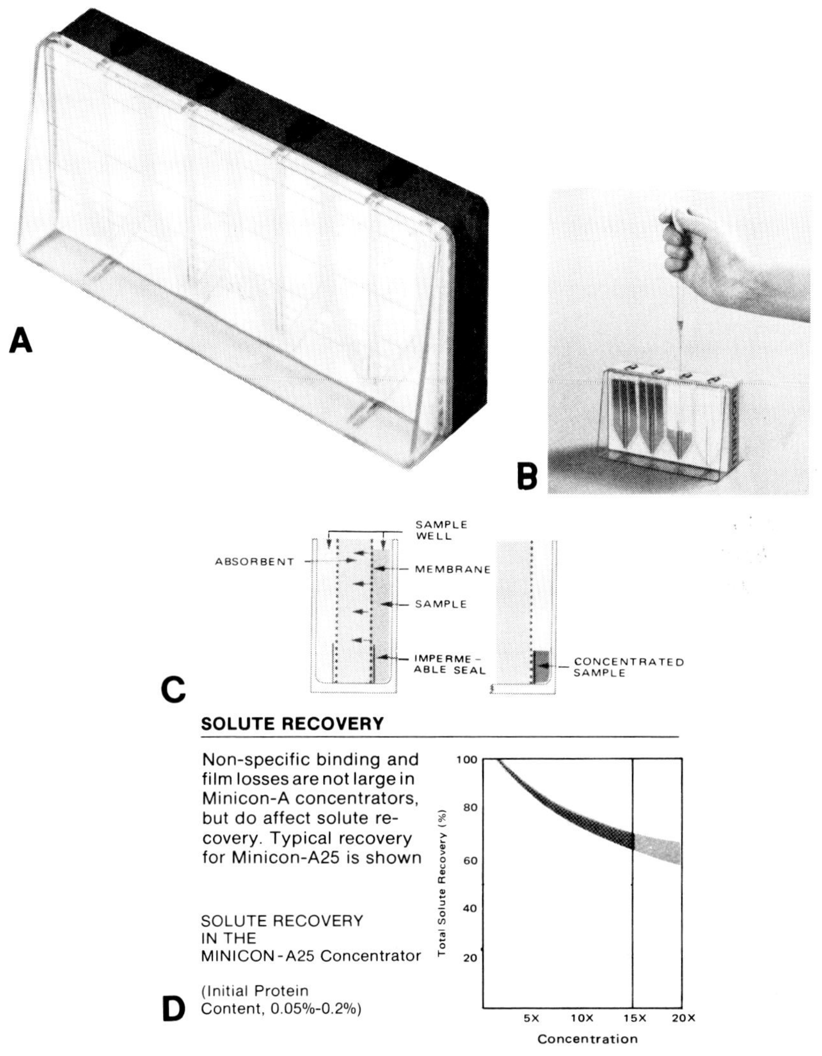

Fig. 1–24. Protein concentration. **A,** Minicon concentration cell. **B,** Pipetting of urine (or other body fluid) into cell. **C,** Cross-section of cell wall. **D,** Graphic analysis of solute recovery (concentration).

tein in the Minicon-B concentrator is closely related to molecular size and shape, but molecular weight is a more convenient parameter. Protein whose molecular weights are close to the membrane cut-off are partially retained. A typical concentration of urine and spinal fluids with the Minicon-B15 unit is noted. Since there is some nonspecific binding of solute on the membrane as well as nonrecoverable loss through the wetting of the chamber, Minicon-B15 filter is not recommended when analytic results are required for exacting research. It is, however, suitable for qualitative or semiquantitative evaluations, such as subsequent electrophoretic or chromatographic migrations.

MATERIALS AND REAGENTS

1. Minicon filter systems (Amicon Corporation, 21 Hartwell Ave., Lexington, Mass. 02173)
2. Pasteur pipettes and bulbs (Fisher no. 13-687-5B or equivalent)
3. Sulfosalicylic acid, 20% (v/v)
4. Dipsticks (Albustix, Combistix, Labstix, Chemstrips)

The content of permeating solute in the final concentrate may be computed by:

$$Cf = \left(\frac{1^n}{R}\right) \times Co$$

where Cf = final solute content; Co = starting solute content; R = reduction of dilution factor; and n = number of reduction-dilutions. For example, reducing the volume to 10X and rediluting, followed by a second 10X reduction, redilution:

$$Cf = \left(\frac{1}{10}\right)^2 \times Co$$

$$Cf = 0.01 \times Co$$

reduces the final content to 1% of the initial content or 99% washout. The same relationship holds for exchange of salts. At higher MW, permeating solutes are increasingly retained, and this simple formula no longer applies. For example, inulin (5,000 MW), which has about a 40% retention in the Minicon-A25, requires two 10X concentrations and redilutions for a 90% (v/v) washout.

TABLE 1–26. Minicon-A Concentration* Time in Minutes (Sample Volume: 0.75 ml)

	A25				A75
Concentration Factor	Albumin 0.05%	Albumin 0.2%†	*Serum Protein* 0.05%	*Serum Protein* 0.02%	7S Globulin 0.05%
5X	27	33	26	27	62
10X	34	43	34	38	79
15X	40	51	41	49	89

*Ambient temperature—concentration times increase slightly with reduced temperatures
†Initial protein content

REFERENCES

1. Amicon Corporation brochure on test.
2. Blatt, W.: Products for concentrating dilute samples. Clin. Lab. Products, April, 1974.

PROTEIN ELECTROPHORESIS

METHOD. Cellulose acetate electrophoresis and densitometric scanning.

PRINCIPLE. A sample of urinary protein, concentrated by Amicon ultrafiltration, is electrophoresed on cellulose acetate strip previously soaked in an alkaline buffer. The strip is then stained in ponceau S dye, in acid, dehydrated in methanol, cleared in acid, and quantitated by densitometric scanning.

SAMPLE. Urinary sedimented protein, concentrated 100 times.

PROCEDURE

1. Pour 50 ml of buffer in each of the outer compartments of the electrophoresis chamber.
2. Wet two disposable paper wicks in the buffer, then drape one over each support bridge making sure it makes buffer contact.
3. Chamber is now ready for electrophoresis, but should be kept covered while not in use.
4. Wet the required number of Titan III cellulose acetate plates (each plate holds 8 samples) by slowly (10 seconds) and uniformly lowering strips into buffer.
5. Soak strips approximately 20 minutes prior to use. Prior to wetting a strip, code by marking on the glossy, hard (Mylar) side with a Helena marker (the mark should be placed in the upper left corner so that it can later be used to help distinguish the multiple samples).
6. Using the Microdispenser, fill each well in the sample well plate with 3 μL of sample (for economy and convenience, do not change the bore with each new sample; merely wash out in water).
7. Load the applicator by depressing the tips into the sample wells 3 or 4 times. The first loading should be applied to a blotter. This primes the applicator and the second loading is much more uniform. Once the applicator is loaded, it must be used within 15 seconds. (Move quickly through the next two steps!)
8. Remove the wetted cellulose acetate plate from the buffer with finger tips and blot firmly once.
9. Quickly place the strip in the aligning base, cellulose side up. One end of the strip should align with the black line marked "center application." The mark made by the Helena marker should be on the left side. From this point on, sample no. 1 will always be on the same side as the mark, while sample no. 8 will be on the opposite side.

10. Depress the applicator tips once more into the sample wells to insure maximum pick-up.
11. Now promptly transfer the applicator to the aligning base. Press the button quickly and hold the button down for 5 seconds.
12. Quickly place the strip—cellulose acetate side down—in the chamber.
13. Place a weight (coin or glass slide, for example) on the strip.
14. Cover the chamber, turn timber to 15 minutes and adjust voltage to 180 volts.
15. Power must be applied within 15 minutes after a strip has been placed in the chamber. (Power is automatically cut off at the end of the time period.)
16. Stain for 6 minutes in ponceau S dye. If only one strip is run, it is easiest to carry out the staining protocol in a single staining dish. Approximately 40 to 50 ml of each reagent will be needed. The ponceau S dye may be reused, but the other solutions should be discarded after use. When staining two or more strips, carry out the protocol with the strips in a rack.
17. Destain in 3 successive washes of acetic acid for 2 minutes each or until the background is white. The strips may be dried and stored as a permanent record at this point. If a transparent background is desired (that is, for densitometry), proceed to the next step.
18. Dehydrate the acetate by transferring to methanol for 2 minutes. (Some clearing problems can be solved by passing through 2 methanol washes.)
19. After removal from both the acetic acid rinse and the methanol rinse, allow the racks and plates to drain for 5 to 10 seconds before placing in the next solution.
20. Place the strips into a clearing solution that is 30 parts acetic acid, 70 parts methanol, and 6 parts Clear Aid. Leave the strips in the solution for 5 minutes.
21. Place the plates—acetate side up—onto a blotter and dry for 3 to 4 minutes under the microevaporation hood.
22. Scan strips in densitometer using a 525-nm filter.

INTERPRETATION. Densitometric tracing is interpreted by the pathologist, and a written report is submitted with graphic tracing.

DISCUSSION AND CLINICAL SIGNIFICANCE. This technique is valuable mostly for detection of monoclonal gammopathies.

Any sharp, well-defined peak (regardless of size) in the gamma region is a monoclonal gammopathy. After its detection by serum electrophoresis, immunoelectrophoretic methods, bone-marrow examinations, and a radiologic bone survey are necessary to further distinguish the disease.

Monoclonal gammopathies are rare in young adults; however, the incidence increases with age. Up to 4% of the "over-65" population exhibit a monoclonal peak. It is important from the prognostic standpoint to identify these people as early as possible in order to institute therapy (see the section on multiple myeloma).

MATERIALS AND REAGENTS

1. Electra HR buffer containing Tris barbital—Sodium barbital diluted to 750 ml in distilled water
2. Tital III cellulose acetate strips
3. Super Z applicator, sample well plates, and aligning base

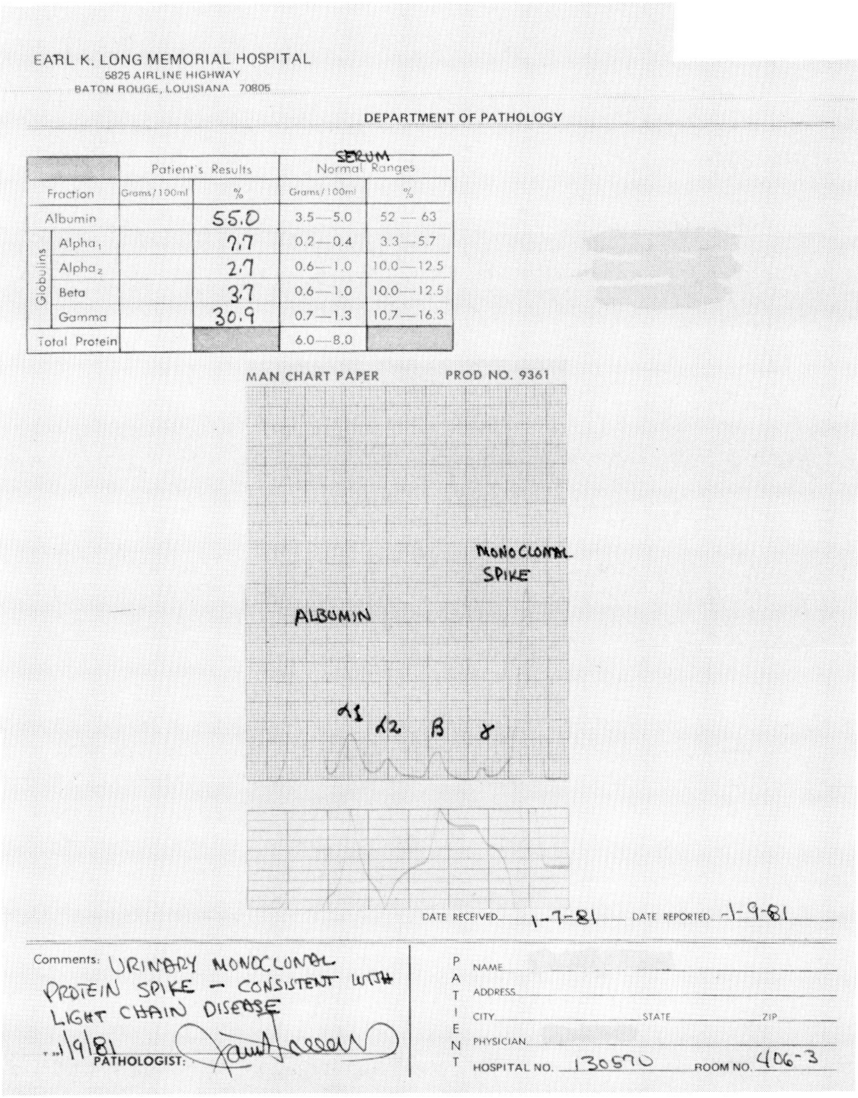

EARL K. LONG MEMORIAL HOSPITAL
5825 AIRLINE HIGHWAY
BATON ROUGE, LOUISIANA 70805

DEPARTMENT OF PATHOLOGY

	Patient's Results		SERUM Normal Ranges	
Fraction	Grams/100ml	%	Grams/100ml	%
Albumin		55.0	3.5—5.0	52—63
Globulins Alpha$_1$		7.7	0.2—0.4	3.3—5.7
Globulins Alpha$_2$		2.7	0.6—1.0	10.0—12.5
Globulins Beta		3.7	0.6—1.0	10.0—12.5
Globulins Gamma		30.9	0.7—1.3	10.7—16.3
Total Protein			6.0—8.0	

DATE RECEIVED 1-7-81 DATE REPORTED 1-9-81

Comments: URINARY MONOCLONAL PROTEIN SPIKE — CONSISTENT WITH LIGHT CHAIN DISEASE

1/9/81 PATHOLOGIST:

PATIENT NAME [redacted]
ADDRESS
CITY STATE ZIP
PHYSICIAN [redacted]
HOSPITAL NO. 130570 ROOM NO. 406-3

Fig. 1–25. Urine protein electrophoresis after dialysis.

4. Zip Zone chamber
5. Zip Zone chamber wicks
6. Microdispenser and tubes
7. Blotter pads
8. Zip Prep solution
9. Sharpie marker
10. Ponceau S dye
11. Acetic acid, 5% (w/v) (50 ml glacial acetic acid diluted to 1,000 ml with distilled water)
12. Methanol
13. Clearing solution containing 30 ml glacial acetic acid, 70 ml methanol, 6 ml Clear-Aid
14. Helena Flur-Vis Auto-Scanner

REFERENCES

1. Cawley, L.: Electrophoresis and Immunoelectrophoresis. Boston, Little, Brown, 1969.
2. Golias, T.: Helena Electrophoresis Manual. Vol. 5. Section 2, 1975.
3. Ritzmann, S.E., and Daniels, J.C.: Serum Protein Abnormalities—Diagnostic and Clinical Aspects. Boston, Little, Brown, 1975.

PROTEIN IMMUNOELECTROPHORESIS

METHOD. Agarose diffusion and immunoperception.

PRINCIPLE. The protein, previously concentrated in a diffusion chamber, is electrophoretically separated in agar or agarose and subsequently allowed to diffuse and to react with antiserum. The antiserum is placed in a trough parallel to the electrophoretically separated sample, and the antigen and antibody diffuse toward each other forming, upon confluence, well-defined precipitin lines. Visualization or photographic record can be made of antigen-antibody precipitin lines.

SAMPLE. Random urine or urine from refrigerated samples.

PROCEDURE

1. Preparation of the Immuno-tec II agarose plate
   a. Remove the plate from the aluminum foil envelope.
   b. Wipe any excess moisture from the plate.
   c. Holding the cassette between both hands with one thumb on the tab and the other thumb on the lid, gently pull the lid away from the bottom plate. Retain the lid for later use.
   d. Carefully remove water from the wells, if necessary, with absorbent paper.
   e. Do not remove the gel from the precut troughs at this time.
2. Application of the specimens
   a. The template illustrates the numbering sequence of the wells (1–7) on the template.
   b. The choice of antiserum filling pattern is dependent upon the requirements of the user (refer to Fig. 1–26).
3. Electrophoresis

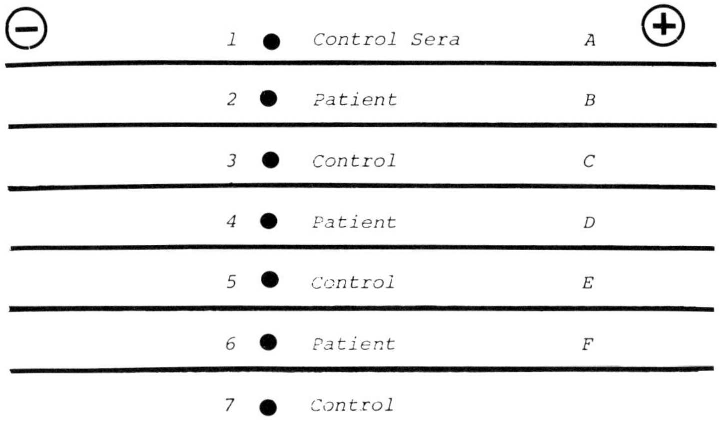

Fig. 1–26. Template for Immuno-Tec II agarose plate, prepunched for IEP.

a. Prepare the IEP Buffer: pH 8.2, 0.04 ionic strength barbital buffer, by dissolving the contents of one packet with distilled water to make a 1 L final solution. Fill the electrophoresis chambers with buffer (200 ml per chamber for the Behring Diagnostics IEP Cell).
b. Place the plate on the bridge of the electrophoresis cell with the "+" side facing toward the anode. If more than one plate is used, care must be taken to keep the plates separated.
c. Soak two precut sponges in the IEP Buffer and use as wicks. Assure complete contact of the sponges by pressing them firmly against the edge of the gel.
d. Turn on the power supply.
e. Conditions per plate for Helena Titan:
Voltage—100V
Time—Electrophoresis is complete when the bromphenol blue dye has migrated 5 to 10 mm before the end of the trough (approximately 45 to 55 minutes).
f. After electrophoresis is complete, turn off the unit and remove the plates.

4. Antiserum application and diffusion
a. Remove the gel from the precut trough with a 20-gauge injection needle or any other suitable device.
b. Dispense 90 μL of the desired antisera into the troughs. The figure on this page indicates the alphabetic labeling of the troughs (A–F).
c. Replace the lids on the plates and store at room temperature for 24 to 48 hours to permit the development of precipitin lines.

5. Examination of the plate
   a. Direct analysis: The IEP patterns should be interpreted directly without staining or drying. Examine the plate in a darkened room against a black background using a point source of light held behind the plate at an angle of approximately 45°. Although the plates can be discarded after direct analysis, permanent records may be obtained by photocopying or photographing the stained or unstained IEP patterns.
   b. Photography: Photographs of the plates are taken using the Cordis immunodiffusion camera. The magnification setting is on high and the exposure setting is 25. The film is allowed to develop for 45 seconds. The photographs are then labeled and affixed to an appropriate form.
   c. Staining: If staining is desired, the plate should be placed in 3 to 4 changes of normal saline for 24 to 48 hours to leach out soluble, nonprecipitated proteins. A distilled-water wash of 4 to 8 hours with agitation will remove the salt. The washed plate should be stained wet. Amido black, ponceau S, or other suitable protein dyes may be used. The stained plates may be retained as a permanent record if the following procedure is used. After destaining, rinse the stained plates in distilled water for 30 minutes and place in a 2% (w/v) glycerin solution for 30 minutes. After drying thoroughly (45 to 50° C in an oven or air-dry overnight), replace the lids and store.

INTERPRETATION. A positive reaction indicates the presence of a protein arc in the specimen of the same specificity as the antiserum. A negative result indicates the absence or decrease of this protein arc.

MATERIALS AND REAGENTS

1. Immuno-tec II agarose plates prepunched for IEP
2. IEP buffer; pH 8.2, 0.04 ionic strength diluted to 1 L
3. Bromphenol blue dye, 0.1%
4. Helena precut sponges
5. Antisera
6. Helena Titan power supply
7. Helena electrophoresis chamber/Behring IEP chamber
8. Control serum
9. MLA 100 μL pipette

NOTES

1. Sources of Error: Errors may be caused by imperfection or impurities in the agarose gel, unreliable or aged antisera, faulty techniques in applying the antigen or antibody solutions, insufficient electric contact, improper voltage control, too long or too short time periods for electrophoretic separation, unsuitable buffer, and unfavorable antigen-antibody ratios. In order to obtain reliable and

reproducible results and to avoid misinterpretation of precipitin patterns, meticulous technique is imperative.

2. Application of Antigen and Antibody Solutions: The improper application of antigen or antibody solutions may interfere with the development of precipitin patterns. The spilling of antigen or antibody solutions and their leakage under the agarose should be avoided. If spillage should occur, however, abnormally bent, blurred, diffuse, or dislocated precipitin arcs may appear. The electric current should be turned on within 10 minutes after application of the antigen, and antiserum should be added within 15 minutes after protein antigens have been separated.
3. Electrophoresis: Optimal electric contact between agarose and buffer is important. The sponge must be in contact with the agarose surface at both ends of the agarose plate. Insufficient contact may produce incomplete or uneven separation of serum proteins and may result in distorted or displaced precipitin arcs or a confusing precipitin pattern. Insufficient contact may be caused by an uneven or desiccated agarose surface. The electrophoresis time must be carefully controlled. Extended electrophoresis will result in elongated, flattened-out precipitin arcs, and "curling" of the precipitin lines (see "Sources of Error," in this section); shortened electrophoresis will not permit the proteins to migrate sufficiently, resulting in a telescoping of the bands of the precipitin lines.

REFERENCES

1. Behring Diagnostics brochure.
2. Helena Co. brochures.
3. Ritzmann, S.E., and Daniels, J.C.: Serum Protein Abnormalities—Diagnostic and Clinical Aspects. Boston, Little, Brown, 1975.
4. Laboratory Notes: Serum Proteins. Somerville, N.J., Behring Diagnostics, 1973, pp. 1–28.
5. Waldenstrom, J.: Monoclonal and Polyclonal Hypergammaglobulinemia. Nashville, Vanderbilt University, 1968.

PHENOLIC ACIDS (INCLUDING VANILMANDELIC ACID)

METHOD. Two-dimensional ascending paper chromatography, modified by Chrichton McNeil and Charles Berett.

PRINCIPLE. Phenolic acids are extracted with ethyl acetate from an amount of acidified urine containing 1 mg of creatinine. The dried extract is subjected to two-dimensional paper chromatography, and color is developed by spraying with diazotized paranitroaniline. The color and mobilities are used to identify VMA. Results may be quantitated by scanning in a densitometer.

PROCEDURE

VMA EXTRACTION

1. Transfer a volume of urine containing 1 mg of creatinine to a 15

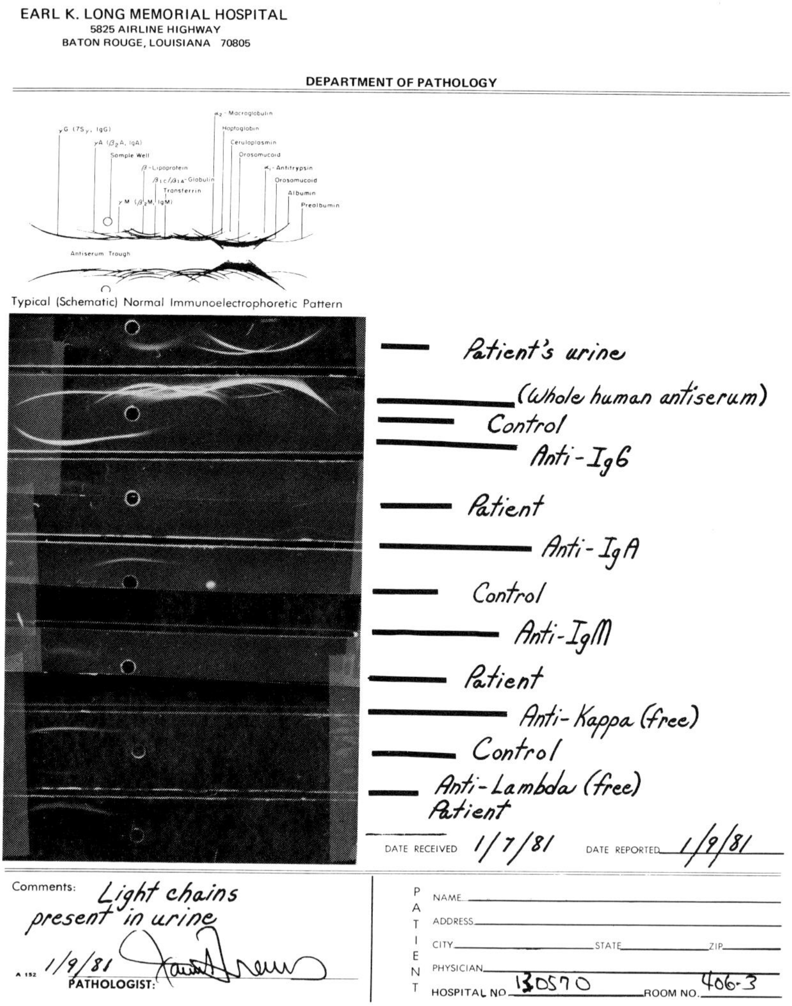

Fig. 1–27. Urine immunoelectrophoresis.

ml centrifuge tube and add enough distilled water to bring volume to 2 ml.

2. Add 0.2 ml of 3 N hydrochloric acid, followed by 4 ml ethyl acetate. Mix well.
3. Draw off ethyl acetate layer with small disposable pipette and bulb, and place in a clean 15 ml centrifuge tube.
4. Add 4 ml ethyl acetate to the original extraction tube. Mix again and draw off ethyl acetate and pool with first extraction.
5. In a stream of air with the tube placed in a water bath at 45° C, evaporate the ethyl acetate to dryness (this takes about 30 minutes).

6. Add 0.05 ml of absolute alcohol to the bottom of the tube. Wash down lower portion of tube.

PAPER CHROMATOGRAM

1. Prepare a sheet of Whatman no. 1 paper measuring 10″ × 11″ as indicated in figure below: Line A is 1″ from bottom, line B is 1/2″ from left, line C is 1/2″ from left border.

Some Phenolic Acids in Urine by Chromatography

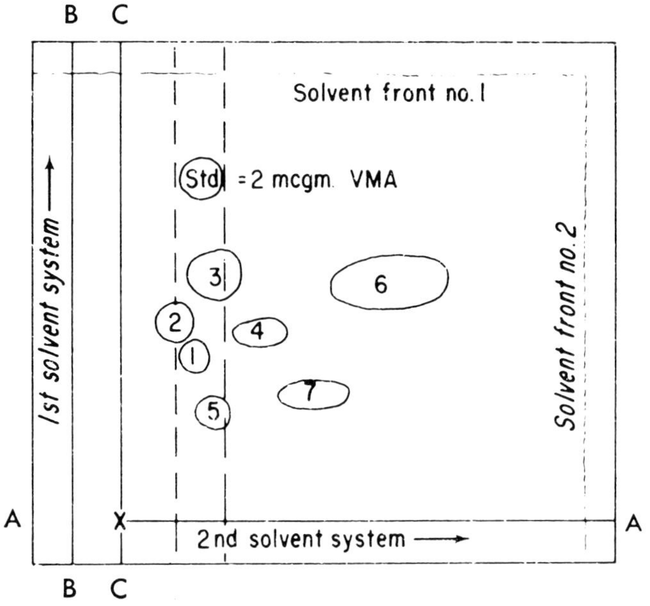

X=origin   Portion to cut to make strip for quantitation in Analytrol

Compound	Color with DpNA
1. Vanilmandelic acid (VMA)	strong purple
2. m-Hydroxyhippuric & p-Hydroxymandelic acids	dark rose, salmon
3. m-Hydroxyphenylhydracrylic acid	dark rose
4. 3-Methoxy-4-hydroxyphenylhydracrylic acid (dietary source)	purple
5. 5-Hydroxyindoleacetic acid (serotonin-carcinoids)	purple red
6. p-Hydroxyphenylacetic acid	purple
7. Salicyluric acid (aspirin)	salmon

Fig. 1–28. Some phenolic acids in urine by chromatography.

2. At intersection of lines "A" and "C," transfer with a finely drawn pipette and bulb the extract prepared in step 6 above. Keep the spot less than 1 cm in diameter by allowing small aliquots to dry before applying more. A hair dryer is useful for this purpose.
3. Four inches above applied spot on line "C," place a spot of standard VMA corresponding to 2 μg.
4. Make a cylinder of the paper with the axis along line "C" and staple.
5. Place cylinder in 6″ × 18″ jar containing 80 ml of freshly made no. 1 solvent solution. Put lid in place and allow to ascend for 15 hours (overnight).
6. Remove. Mark solvent front. Allow to dry. Remove staples. Cut off at line "B" and restaple, so that line "B" now forms the base of the cylinder.
7. Place in another 6″ × 18″ jar containing 80 ml of solvent no. 2, freshly made; allow to ascend for about 4 hours to within 1 cm of the top of the paper.
8. Remove, hang in hood, and allow to dry thoroughly.
9. Unstaple, hang on rack with clips, and spray with freshly made diazotized p-nitroaniline (mixed within the previous 2 minutes). Use Erlenmeyer-type fine sprayer with air pressure.
10. A colorful group of spots will appear almost at once when paper becomes damp with spray. Allow to dry.

READING CHROMATOGRAM. When first running this procedure, extract several normal urines so as to become accustomed to the results of the deep purple VMA. Usually the test VMA spot will be very nearly the size and depth of the standard of 2 μg.

CALCULATION. Simple quantitation is possible with a densitometer by cutting a strip 3 cm wide along the "C" axis so as to place VMA and the unknown VMA spots in the same straight line in the center. Place this in the slot and record the optical density. Match recording and the purple VMA spots on paper, then count blips under the standard and the unknown:

$$\text{VMA } (\mu\text{g/mg creatinine}) = \frac{2 \times \text{unknown blips}}{\text{standard blips}}$$

In the absence of a densitometer, an alternative method is to spot 2, 4, 6, and 8 μg at 4, 5, 6, and 7 inches above line "A" on the "C" axis. When completed, visually compare standards with unknown.

INTERPRETATION

Normal values	1.0 to 4.0 μg/mg creatinine
Doubtful values	4.0 to 8.0 μg/mg creatinine
Pheochromocytoma	9.0 to 25 μg/mg creatinine

DISCUSSION AND CLINICAL SIGNIFICANCE. This method was originally developed from the Armstrong procedure by Chrichton McNeil and is simple to perform. It has the advantage of allowing detection of possible interfering substances, and therefore represents one of the most specific of tests for VMA available.

Although relatively little technologist time is involved, the procedure extends over a 2-day period, and is therefore not well-suited to mass screening.

MATERIALS AND REAGENTS

1. Hydrochloric acid, 3 N
2. Ethyl acetate (reagent grade)
3. Whatman no. 1 paper, 28 × 22 cm
4. Solvent systems that are prepared fresh:

No. 1	Isopropyl alcohol	80 ml
	Distilled water	18 ml
	Ammonium hydroxide	2 ml
No. 2	Benzene	60 ml
	Propionic acid	40 ml
	Distilled water	2 ml

   Shake until haziness clears.

5. Diazotized p-nitroaniline
   a. 5% (w/v) sodium nitrite. Make fresh each time.
   b. 10% (w/v) potassium carbonate (anhydrous). Refrigerate.
   c. Add 10 ml concentrated HCl to 490 ml of distilled water and to this add 0.5 g p-nitroanaline. Mix.
6. Absolute ethyl alcohol (use as spray): Place 25 ml cold p-nitroaniline and 25 ml sodium nitrite in a 100 ml graduate and mix. Immediately add 50 ml cold potassium carbonate and mix, and pour into spray flask. Use within 2 minutes.
7. VMA standard (DL 3-methoxy, 4-hydroxy mandelic acid) Nutritional Biochemicals Corp.

   Stock VMA Standard. Dissolve 25 mg of VMA in 50 ml of ethyl acetate. Four μL (0.004 ml) will provide 2 μg for a standard spot (manufactured by Nutritional Biochemicals Corp.).

REFERENCES

1. Armstrong, M., Shaw, K., and Wall, P.: The phenolic acids of human urine. J. Biol. Chem., *218*:293, 1956.
2. McNeil, C.: Personal communication.

PHENOLIC ACIDS

METHOD. Chromatoelectrophoresis for phenolic acids (normetanephrine, metanephrine, 3-methoxy, 4-hydroxyphenolglycol, and VMA).

PRINCIPLE. Collect first voided morning specimen following 12-

hour restriction of fluid intake. Previous dietary and drug regulations should be accomplished, as noted previously.

PROCEDURE

1. Hydrolyze an aliquot of urine by placing in boiling water for 30 minutes at pH 1.0.
2. Apply an aliquot of urine equivalent to 0.2 mg of creatinine directly to Schleicher and Schuell no. 470 C filter paper strips and subject to chromatoelectrophoresis in barbital buffer, pH 8.6, ionic strength 0.1 at 600 volts for 3 hours at 4° C. Also run standards of metanephrine and normetanephrine, containing 0.25 to 1.0 μg in 200 μL of distilled water.
3. Following the run, remove strips from apparatus and spray with diazotized p-nitroaniline while still wet. The staining color is apparent right away, reaching full intensity in 1 hour.
4. Three characteristic bands of purple-blue color are present on the chromato-electrograms of urine samples from patients having pheochromocytoma which are not seen in samples from normal patients or from those with primary benign hypertension. The three purple-blue bands migrate approximately 7.8, 10.7, and 15.9 cm from the point of application, corresponding to the mobility of normetanephrine and metanephrine, 3-methoxy, 4-hydroxyphenylglycol, and VMA respectively.

Other urinary substances stain with diazotized p-nitroaniline and may have a mobility similar to that of VMA. For this reason, quantitation of the VMA may be difficult unless previous drug and dietary regulations have been enforced.

INTERPRETATION. In the series of patients with pheochromocytomas reported by the authors, normetanephrine plus metanephrine excretion was ± 25 μg/mg creatinine; and 3-methoxy, 4-hydroxyphenylglycol excretion was ± 19 μg/mg creatinine. These levels are normally not detectable by the method. VMA values for this method were not reported.

DISCUSSION AND CLINICAL SIGNIFICANCE. This test may be more suitable than previously described methods for screening. In addition, the authors claimed to have seen normal and hypertensive patients with elevated VMA levels; and some patients with pheochromocytoma with less than the usually quoted upper limit of normal for VMA.

REFERENCE

1. Wolf, R., Mendlowitz, M., Robz, J., and Gidlow, S.: Simultaneous urinary assays for the combined metanephrine and 3-methoxy, 4-hydroxyphenolglycol in patients with pheochromocytoma and primary hypertension. N. Engl. J. Med., *273*:1459, 1965.

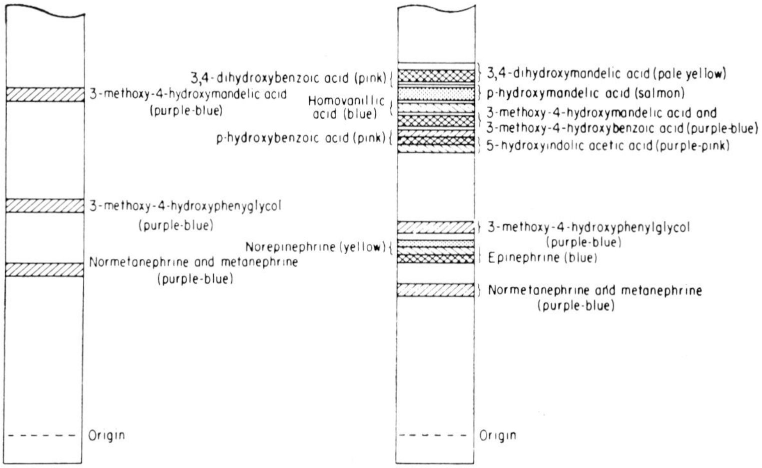

Schema of chromatoelectrophoretogram of urine sample obtained from patient with pheochromocytoma
Time of chromatoelectrophoresis is 30 hours
The chromatoelectrophoretogram is stained with diazotized p-nitroaniline

Schema of composite chromatroelectrophoretograms of catecholamines, catecholamine metabolites and various phenolic acids
The chromatoelectrophoretogram is stained with diazotized p-nitroaniline

Fig. 1–29. Some of the bands found in urine with chromatoelectrophoresis. (Modified from Wolf.)

PHENOLIC ACIDS (INCLUDING VANILMANDELIC ACID)

METHOD. KODAK CHROMAT/O/SCREEN (Thin Layer Chromatographic Analysis)

PRINCIPLE. Extracts of phenolic acids in urine are spotted on chromatographic Mylar strips and migrated in one dimension with butanol:ethanol:ammonium hydroxide in gel (rather than solvent) phase, along with known standards of phenolic acids. P-nitrobenzene-diazonium tetrafluoroborate is used to develop color for visual identification. Rf values can also be calculated.

SPECIMEN COLLECTION AND PRESERVATION. Certain precautions are usually required for the collection of urine specimens for VMA analysis. The patient is usually told he must abstain from all medication, chocolate, fruits, and any vanilla-containing substances for 48 hours before urine collection, but this is not absolutely necessary. (An early morning specimen can be taken for analysis, since VMA excretion varies diurnally and is lowest at noontime; however, a 24-hour urine collection is preferable.)

The urine must be kept acidic, since the catecholamines and phenolic and indolic acids are volatile at alkaline pH. This is done best by adding 1 ml of 6 N HCl to the colection bottle before it is used. If a 24-hour specimen is collected, add 10 ml of 6 N HCl to the collection bottle before use.

Pretreatment of the urine specimen by hydrolysis and extraction is not necessary since this is only a screening procedure, and quantitative results are not necessary. With active, secreting tumors, there are sometimes sufficient unconjugated catecholamines present in the urine for detection with the Chromat/O/Screen Analysis Kit; but it is relatively insensitive, and borderline-to-moderate elevations in VMA concentrations will be missed. We do not recommend the method for catecholamines.

PROCEDURE

1. Remove chromatographic sheet from package. Chromatographic sheets are wrapped in a shrink package and are stacked with the coated sides facing in one direction. The top sheet is a blank, protective piece of Mylar film. Use a sharp instrument to cut open the plastic shrink package on either the top or bottom. Remove a chromatographic sheet, being careful not to scratch or touch the coated side with the bare fingers. Always use the forceps provided for handling the sheets. Place the sheet on a clean horizontal surface.
2. Apply the sample using the pipette. Put a 1 μL pipette into the pipette holder. With the pipette in as nearly a horizontal position as possible, fill it completely by touching it to the surface of the urine sample. The liquid can be seen moving up the pipette as it fills the tube by capillary action. The liquid will stop when the pipette is full.

   To apply the sample, hold the pipette in a perpendicular position so that the tip just touches the chromatographic sheet between two of the cut-out circles. Do not scratch or break the coating by pressing the pipette on the sheet. Squeeze the holder and apply its entire volume in one application. The sample should spread to the edges of the circles.
3. Apply the standard solution. A vial containing a standard solution of catecholamine metabolites is included with the kit. This standard consists of:

4-hydroxy-3-methoxymandelic acid (VMA)	100 mg/dl
4-hydroxy-3-methoxyphenylacetic acid (HVA)	100 mg/dl
Dopamine	100 mg/dl

   Apply 1 μL of the standard to the chromatogram between two other circles in the same manner as the sample. To minimize the chances for error, always apply spots to the chromatogram in the same order—that is, left to right or right to left, with the standard in the same position. After chromatography, visual comparison of the sample with the standard will show any gross elevation of catecholamine levels.
4. Identify the specimen. Write the patient's name or identification

on the back of the developing chamber. The top of the chromatographic sheet can also be numbered with a sharp pencil.

5. Dry the sheet completely before proceeding. The sheet may be air dried. However, the use of a hair dryer will hasten the operation.

METHOD OF DEVELOPMENT

1. Fill the chamber trough with gel. Remove the cap and puncture the top of the tube of Kodak Chromat/O/Screen Gel. Caution: Care should be taken if the tube has been warmed, because a few centimeters of the gel may be expelled upon opening. After using the gel, replace the cap tightly to prevent any leakage or evaporation. (Do not open the second tube provided in the 150-test kit until the first tube has been completely used.) Completely fill the trough of the development chamber by squeezing the tube of gel into the trough until a peak projects just above the developing chamber floor. Use the special scraper to mold and remove excess gel; otherwise, the solvent will migrate in an uneven front causing Rf values to change.
2. Insert the spotted sheet and close the chamber.
   60-Analysis Kit: Place the opened chamber flat on a table or other horizontal surface with the trough toward you and your left and the door toward your right.
   150-Analysis Kit: Place the developing chamber on a horizontal surface with the trough away from you and the door open toward you.
   For either size kit: Insert the spotted, dried chromatographic sheet, coated side up, on the chamber door, with the spots toward you. With the door on the table, close the trough side over the door. Keep the chamber on the flat surface.
   Close the chamber tightly by pressing the edges with your thumb. For proper contact between the chromatographic sheet and the gel surface, gently tap the closed chamber, trough-side up, once or twice against a table edge. During development, the chamber may be left in a horizontal or vertical position (ascending or descending chromatography), or it may be transported with no change in results.
3. Develop the chromatogram. The advance of the solvent front can be seen by holding the chamber up to the light. It should reach the top in approximately 20 to 30 minutes. This will vary slightly, depending upon temperature and humidity. If the migration takes more than 45 minutes, it means that the gel has become dry. Good results can still be achieved, but care should be taken in interpretation, since Rf values may change.
4. Remove chromatogram from chamber. After the solvent front reaches the top, remove the sheet from the chamber with the

forceps. Air-dry the sheet until the solvents are completely evaporated.

VISUALIZATION. A spray bottle of a stabilized diazonium dye is supplied with this kit. The chromatogram must be free from any residual ammonium hydroxide from the solvent gel before applying the visualization spray. To visualize catecholamines with the reagent, place the chromatogram in an upright position in a hood or other well-ventilated area. Hold the spray bottle in a vertical position about 12″ from the chromatogram making sure that the nozzle is pointing toward the chromatogram. Depress the clamp completely and spray back and forth 2 or 3 times to cover the entire sheet. Best results can be achieved by spraying in a smooth, even motion. Do not overwet the chromatogram so that the reagent drips down the surface.

After spraying, expose the chromatogram to ammonia vapor; the separated zones will appear. The spots will disappear when the chromatogram is removed from the ammonia vapor, but will reappear when exposed to ammonia vapor again. A more permanent record of the spots is possible by spraying the chromatogram with a 10% (w/v) solution of either K_2CO_3 or Na_2CO_3. Colors and Rf values of the various catecholamines are listed below.

DISCUSSION AND CLINICAL SIGNIFICANCE. The main sources

TABLE 1–27. Characteristics of Catecholamines and Other Compounds That May Be Found in Urine.

Name	Abbreviations	Rf Value	Color after Visualization
Metanephrine	(MN)	95	Purple
Sympatol		90	Pink
5-Hydroxytryptamine		80	Brown-purple
o-Hydroxyphenylacetic acid	(o-HPAA)	75	Dark purple
Normetanephrine	(NMN)	70	Light purple
Imidazolelactic acid	(ILA)	60	Yellow
Dihydroxyphenylethylamine	(Dopamine)	60	Gray-purple
5-Hydroxyindoleacetic acid	(5-HIAA)	55	Brown-purple
p-Hydroxyphenylacetic acid	(p-HPAA)	55	Purple
p-Hydroxyphenyllactic acid	(p-HPLA)	55	Purple
Epinephrine	(E)	52	Brown-yellow
Tyrosine		50	Gray-purple
4-Hydroxy-3-methoxyphenylacetic acid	(HVA)	50	Blue
m-Hydroxybenzoic acid	(m-HBA)	50	Red
5-Hydroxytryptophan	(5-HT)	40	Brown-purple
Norepinephrine	(NE)	36	Brown-yellow
Histidine		35	Orange-brown
4-Hydroxy-3-methoxymandelic acid	(VMA)	30	Dark purple
p-Hydroxymandelic acid	(p-HMA)	30	Red
Vanillic acid	(VA)	20	Dark purple
3,4-Dihydroxyphenylacetic acid	(3,4-DHPAA)	10	Brown
Dihydroxyphenylalanine	(DOPA)	7	Light gray

NOTE: Detection of levels of 100–200 μg/ml urine is possible when 1 μL is chromatographed using this system.

of catecholamines in the body are the chromatin cells in the adrenal medulla, the heart, lungs, liver, intestines, prostate gland, the brain, and in the adrenergic nerves. Tyramine, octopamine, and N-methyloctopamine are also suspected as contributors to catecholamine levels in the human.

Four catecholamines are found in human nerve and adrenal tissue: dopamine, epinephrine, norepinephrine, and N-methylepinephrine. Excessive amounts of these compounds are produced by certain tumors and are excreted in the urine. Detection and identification of these catecholamines and their metabolites in the urine can often facilitate the diagnosis of neural and adrenal tumors. The determination of catecholamines and phenolic acids in the urine has been found very helpful in the differential diagnosis of several disorders (see "Catecholamines.") Perhaps most useful is the ability to rule out neural tumors as the cause of hypertension. Over 15% of the population suffers from hypertension due to one cause or another. However, less than 1.2% of the population suffers from neural tumors, and their presence must be determined before rational therapy can be initiated; thus, a simple, fast, and reliable screening test is valuable.

MATERIALS AND REAGENTS

1. KODAK CHROMAT/O/SCREEN Gel (butanol:ethanol:ammonium hydroxide:water)
   1 tube (60-test kit)　　2 tubes (150-test kit)
2. Chromatographic sheet, 30 two-channel sheets (60-test kit)
3. Chromatographic sheet, 15 ten-channel sheets (150-test kit)
4. Pipettes (1 μL)
5. Pipette holder, 1 pipette holder (60-test kit), 2 pipette holder (150-test kit)
6. Developing chamber, 30 chambers (60-test kit)
7. Developing chamber, 15 chambers (150-test kit)
8. Visualization spray (p-nitrobenzene-diazonium tetrafluoroborate)
9. Instruction booklet
10. Forceps
11. Standard
12. Scraper

TABLE 1–28. Catecholamine Metabolites.

Catecholamine	Major Metabolite
Norepinephrine	4-Hydroxy-3-methoxymandelic acid (VMA)
Dopamine	4-Hydroxy-3-methoxyphenylacetic acid (HVA)
Epinephrine	4-Hydroxy-3-methoxymandelic acid (VMA)
Tyramine	p-Hydroxyphenylacetic acid (p-HPAA)
Octopamine	p-Hydroxymandelic acid (p-HMA)
N-Methyloctopamine	p-Hydroxymandelic acid (p-HMA)

TABLE 1–29. Trouble Shooting.

Problem	Probable Cause	Remedy
Uneven advance of solvent front	1. Gel not leveled in trough 2. Chamber not tightly closed	1. Level gel with scraper 2. Tightly close chamber
Broad bands of separated catecholamines or long tails on either side (difficult to determine Rf values)	1. Sample has spread out too far on application 2. Too high a concentration of catecholamines	1. Spot urine in two applications of $^{1}/_{2}$ μL each 2. Use smaller sample
Long running time	Dried solvent gel	No effect on results if a standard is run along with unknowns
Smudged chromatograms, or specimens which do not run	Excess gel in trough is squeezed past sample when chamber is closed. Sample dissolves in gel	Level gel in trough
Large droplets of visualization reagent from spray bottle	Partial depression of button on aerosol can	Completely depress button on aerosol can

REFERENCES

1. Bjorklund, A., Falck, B., and Hakanson, R.: Microspectrofluorometric characterization of catecholamines and indolamine on silica gel thin-layer after formaldehyde condensation. Anal. Biochem., *35*:264, 1970.
2. Gitlow, S., Mendlowitz, M., and Bertani, L.: The biochemical techniques for detecting and estimating the presence of a pheochromocytoma. Am. J. Cardiol., *26*:270, 1970.
3. O'Neal, J., Traubert, T., and Meites, S.: Quantitative VMA by thin-layer chromatography. Clin. Chem., *43*:135, 1966.
4. Robinson, R., Ratcliffe, J., and Smith, P.: A screening test for pheochromocytoma. Clin. Path., *12*:541–543, 1959.
5. Young, R., Steiker, D., Bongiovanni, A., Koop, C., and Eberlein, W.: Urinary vanilmandelic acid (VMA) excretion in children: Use of a simple semiquantitative test. J. Pediatr., *62*:844, 1963.

VANILMANDELIC ACID

METHOD. Ion Exchange Column Elution, method of Kaplan and McIntosh.

PRINCIPLE. Vanilmandelic acid (VMA) is purified by resin absorption followed by elution with formate buffer. VMA in the eluate is converted to vanillin by periodate oxidation under alkaline conditions, and the vanillin concentration is measured by its absorbance at 350 nm.

PROCEDURE

VMA EXTRACTION

1. Label one 50-ml beaker for each urine sample "Test" and provide an identification number. Label only one beaker "Standard."

2. Add the following:

	Test Beaker	*Standard Beaker*
TRIS buffer solution	0.5 ml	0.5 ml
Urine sample	5.0 ml	—
Working VMA standard solution (1.2 mg/dl)	—	5.0 ml

3. Adjust pH of all beakers to 7.0 to 8.0 with small amount of 2 M NaOH.
   (To faciliate maximum absorption of the VMA on the resin, the pH must be slightly alkaline since acid conditions will reduce the efficiency of the resin.)
4. Assemble two columns with funnels. Remove column cap, snip column tip, plug funnel in top of column. Label one column "Test" and one column "Standard"; provide an identification number for each urine sample.
5. Insert a 21-gauge needle on tip of column.
6. Apply each beaker of solution to its respective column in 1.0-ml aliquots. Rinse beakers with a few milliliters of distilled or deionized water and apply the washing to the respective column. Drain completely to waste.
7. Remove the 21-gauge needle from the tip of the column.
8. Wash both "Test" and "Standard" columns with 10 ml of wash buffer and allow to drain completely to waste.
   (The wash buffer with low pH elutes impurities and prepares the column for elution of the VMA in the following step. Complete drainage is necessary to prevent alteration of the pH of the elution buffer.)
9. Label large test tubes. One should be labeled "Test Eluate" along with an identification number for each urine specimen and the other "Standard Eluate."
10. Place columns labeled "Test" and "Standard" over the respectively labeled tubes.
11. Add 15 ml elution buffer to each column and allow to drain completely by gravity, collecting eluates in the test tubes.
    (Forcing the elution buffer through the columns will excessively reduce the elution of the VMA from each resin column.)

VMA DETERMINATION

1. Label two test tubes. One should be called "Working VMA Standard Test" and the other "Working VMA Standard Blank." Add 2.0 ml standard eluate to each tube.
2. For each unknown specimen, label two tubes—one "Test" and the other "Unknown Blank," both with appropriate identification numbers. Add 2.0 ml of test eluate to each tube.
3. If you wish to calculate percent recovery, label a third set of tubes, one "Buffered VMA Standard Test" and the other "Buffered VMA

Solution" to each tube, "Test" and "Blank," as follows:

	Standard Test	Standard Blank
	Unknown Test	Unknown Blank
	Buffered Test	Buffered Blank
4. Then add saturated potassium carbonate	0.5 ml	0.5 ml

(The saturated K_2CO_3 provides the alkaline environment for oxidation of the VMA to vanillin by periodate in the following step.)

5. Periodate solution	0.2 ml	

6. Incubate all tubes, "Test" and "Blank," at 37° C for 20 minutes.
7. Remove all tubes from the water bath.

	Standard Test	Standard Blank
	Unknown Test	Unknown Blank
	Buffered Test	Buffered Blank
8. Sodium metabisulfite solution	0.2 ml	0.2 ml
9. Periodate solution	—	0.2 ml

(Suspension of oxidation process is effected by the metabisulfite and prevents any oxidation of the blank preparations by the addition of periodate solution in the following step.)

10. To each tube labeled "Blank," add 0.2 ml periodate solution and mix well. No oxidation of the contents of the "Blank" tubes can take place in the presence of the metabisulfite; therefore, it provides a blank analogous to the test solution.
11. Read and record absorbance of all tubes at 350 nm. Subtract appropriate "Blank" from "Test" figures and record.
12. Calculations:
    Calculate concentration from working standard results as described below. The buffered VMA standard results are used to calculate the percentage recovery of VMA from column and provide an indication of column and technical efficiency. If percentage of recovery is below 50%, results may be in error; procedure is not in control, and it should be reworked before reporting unknowns.

A. $$\frac{\text{Absorbance Unknown Test} - \text{Absorbance Unknown Blank}}{\text{Absorbance Working VMA Standard Test} - \text{Absorbance VMA Standard Blank}}$$

$$\times\ 1.2 = \text{mg/dl Urine Aliquot}$$

$$\text{mg/dl urine aliquot} \times \frac{\text{total urine volume (ml)}}{\text{dl}}$$

$$= \text{VMA in total urine volume}$$

$$\text{B.}\ \frac{\text{Absorbance Working VMA Standard Test} - \text{Absorbance Working VMA Standard Blank}}{\text{Absorbance Buffered VMA Standard Test} - \text{Absorbance Buffered VMA Standard Blank}} \times 100 = \%\ \text{of Recovered Standard}$$

INTERPRETATION. The normal adult value for 24-hour urine volume: mean is 4.9 mg/24 hours; standard deviation, 2.5 mg/24 hours; and range, 1 to 10 mg/24 hours.

DISCUSSION AND CLINICAL SIGNIFICANCE. Dowex I or II Resin is usually sold in the chloride form by suppliers. It can be converted to the acetate form by adding 3 M sodium acetate in 2 M acetic acid for 48 hours with at least six changes of solution, or until no precipitate forms when silver chloride is added to a portion of the solution that has been in contact with the resin. Wash the resin until free of acid. This will take about 3 days with at least 10 changes. The pH will be approximately neutral. Old resin can be rejuvenated by washing with 2 N NaOH until neutral, then 2 N HCl, followed by water until neutral, then treat as above.

This method has an advantage over many other methods in that no solvent extractions are required and the patient's diet does not have to be restricted. The authors report that the only intermetabolism present in some people will produce p-hydroxy-benzaldehyde detectable by the test conditions. This aldehyde has an absorption band at 330 to 340 nm.

Drug interference is reported to be limited: Clofibrate, which interferes with periodate oxidation of VMA; Aldomet, which prevents formation of catecholamines; and Imuran, which causes a depressed VMA value for unknown reasons.

MATERIALS AND REAGENTS

1. Wash buffer: 0.5 M sodium formate, pH 4.0, dissolve 34 g sodium formate in about 800 ml water; adjust pH with formic acid, make up to 1 L with demineralized water. Mix well.
2. Elution buffer: 1 M Na formate, pH 3.7, dissolve 68 g Na formate and 80 g NaCl in about 800 ml demineralized water; adjust pH with formic acid; make up to 1 L with demineralized water. Mix well.
3. Resin: Dowex II, acetate form, X2 crosslinkage, 200–400 mesh. 4 ml slurry used in 5 × 1 cm plastic column.
4. Alkaline buffer: Add 11 g KOH to 100 ml demineralized water, then saturate with K_2CO_3 by adding excessive reagent-grade crystals. Mix and allow to stand at room temperature for 1 day.

TABLE 1–30. VMA Recovery Experiment Illustrating Average Recovery of 87.5% with Test Conditions.

Number	Date	Urine Volume (ml)	Results of unknown (mg/total volume) (Sunderman method)	Results of unknown (mg/total volume) (Whale VMA method)	Amount VMA added to unknown (mg/total volume)	Actual results of recovery: VMA standard plus unknown value (mg/total volume)	Expected results of recovery: VMA standard plus unknown value (mg/total volume)	Percent recovery of VMA standard
1	8/3/72	1380	3.5	3.6	10.0	11.9	13.6	87.5
2	8/4/72	1040	5.1	5.0	5.0	8.5	10.0	85.4
3	8/4/72	1275	11.0	10.1	10.0	16.6	20.1	82.6
4	8/7/72	2160	5.3	5.3	10.0	13.6	15.3	88.9
5	8/7/72	1380	6.2	6.0	10.0	14.3	16.0	89.4
6	8/7/72	1050	6.3	6.2	5.0	9.89	11.2	88.3
7	8/7/72	320	1.8	2.0	5.0	6.35	7.0	90.7

$X = 87.5 \pm 2.5$

5. Sodium metaperiodate (2 g/dl): Dissolve 0.5 g in 25 ml of demineralized water. Make fresh each day. Mix well.
6. Sodium metabisulfite (10 g/dl): Dissolve 1 g in 25 ml of demineralized water. Make fresh each day. Mix well.
7. Stock VMA: Transfer 10 mg VMA to 24 ml demineralized water in a 25 ml volumetric flask; add 1 drop concentrated HCl acid; add demineralized water to make 25 ml. Mix well. Store frozen.
   Working VMA (elution standard): (1.2 mg/dl). Transfer 3 ml stock VMA solution to a 100 ml volumetric flask, add demineralized water to which one drop concentrated HCl acid has been added to make 100 ml.
   Buffered VMA (0.8 mg/dl): Transfer 1 ml stock VMA to a 50 ml volumetric flask and make up to 50 ml with elution buffer. Mix well. Make fresh each time new elution buffer is made.
8. TRIS buffer, 1 M, pH 7.4: Transfer 12 g TRIS to a 100 ml volumetric flask and fill to mark with demineralized water, then adjust to pH 7.4 with 6 N HCl.
9. Test tubes, 20 × 150 mm
10. Serologic pipettes, 10 and 20 ml
11. Spectrophotometer with 350 nm wavelength

REFERENCES

1. Kaplan, A. and McIntosh, J.: Personal communications and unpublished observations.
2. Stewart, T., and Freeman, J.: Vanilmandelic Acid and Catecholamines. 2nd Ed. Chicago, American Society of Clinical Pathologists, 1976.
3. Whale Scientific, Inc. (949 Ironton, Denver, Colo. 80239) brochure on test.

VANILMANDELIC ACID

METHOD. Sunderman and Sunderman (Quantitative extraction technique).

PRINCIPLE. After acidification of urine and removal of pigments and other interfering constituents by adsorption upon activated magnesium silicate, vanilmandelic acid is extracted with ethyl acetate, and recovered from the ethyl acetate extract by re-extraction with potassium carbonate. Vanilmandelic acid is then oxidized by vanillin with potassium ferricyanide at acid pH in the presence of zinc. Under these conditions, the ferrocyanide produced by the oxidation reaction is precipitated as potassium zinc ferrocyanide. Vanillin is extracted from the oxidation mixture with toluene, re-extracted from the toluene with potassium carbonate. The carbonate extract is acidified with sulfuric acid. Indole-phosphoric acid reagent is then added, producing a salmon-colored complex with vanillin. Photometric measurements are made at 495 nm. The optical density of the sample, minus that of a urine blank that has not been subjected to oxidation, yields the optical density attributable to vanilmandelic acid.

PROCEDURE

1. Collection of Urine: The patient is instructed to abstain from medications and from chocolate and vanilla-containing compounds for 2 days prior to collection of urine. A 24-hour specimen is collected in a brown glass bottle containing 25 ml of 6 N hydrochloric acid. The urine is stored in the refrigerator during collection. The urine volume is measured, and an aliquot is saved for analysis. The patient should be cautioned about the poisonous and corrosive nature of the preservative.
2. Adsorption of interfering constituents: Using two 125 ml Erlenmeyer flasks for each unknown, transfer the following:

Unknown Flask	*Unknown Recovery Flask*
50 ml urine	50 ml urine
5 ml concentrated HCl	5 ml concentrated HCl
	0.2 ml stock standard
Mix well	Mix well
5 g Florisil	5 g Florisil

   Swirl contents of the flask 10 minutes, then filter through Whatman no. 1 filter paper.
   (*NOTE:* The 0.2-ml stock standard added to the urine represents 0.4 mg/dl vanilmandelic acid present in the filtrate, in addition to the vanilmandelic acid already present in the urine.)
3. Extraction of vanilmandelic acid: Into 50 ml centrifuge tubes, transfer the following:

	Concentrated HCl	*H_2O*	*Dilute Standard*	*Filtrate*
Reagent blank	1 ml	9 ml	—	—
Standard (duplicate)	1 ml	8 ml	1 ml	—
Unknown blank	—	—	—	10 ml
Unknown	—	—	—	10 ml
Unknown recovery	—	—	—	10 ml

   (*NOTE:* If the urine volume is less than 1,500 ml, use 5 ml filtrate and 5 ml water in the blank, unknown and recovery tubes. Then in the calculations, multiply the factor by 2.)

   Add approximately 45 ml of ethyl acetate to each tube. Stopper the tubes, shake vigorously for 2 minutes, and centrifuge for 5 minutes to ensure separation of the aqueous and organic phases. Remove aqueous infranatant by aspiration and discard. Recentrifuge the tubes briefly, and aspirate the small amount of aqueous infranatant which usually collects at the tip of each tube. (Vanilmandelic acid is very unstable at an alkaline pH, so the next phase of extraction is done in a strictly timed interval. Between the addition of potassium carbonate and the addition of concentrated hydrochloric acid, allow only twenty minutes to elapse.)

Add 5 ml of potassium carbonate to each tube. Stopper, shake vigorously for 2 minutes, and centrifuge. Without delay, remove each supernatant organic phase by aspiration and discard. With careful technique, using gentle suction, the two phases may be separated quantitatively. Add 2.5 ml concentrated hydrochloric acid immediately to each carbonate extract. Shake the tubes and allow to stand for 5 minutes to ensure complete evolution of carbon dioxide.

4. Oxidation of vanilmandelic acid: Add 1 ml of 0.6% (w/v) potassium ferricyanide solution to all tubes except the urine blank.

   Add 1 ml zinc sulfate solution to all of the centrifuge tubes. Shake the centrifuge tubes and place those that contain ferricyanide in a 37° C water bath in the dark for 2 hours. Store the urine blanks in a refrigerator. The specimens should be protected from direct light throughout the entire period of oxidation.

5. Extraction of vanillin: Add approximately 45 ml of toluene to each centrifuge tube. Stopper the tubes, shake vigorously for 2 minutes, and centrifuge. Remove each aqueous infranatant by aspiration and discard. Recentrifuge the tubes briefly in order to pack the precipitated potassium zinc ferricyanide in the tips of the tubes, and to ensure separation of the aqueous and organic phases. Remove the small amount of aqueous infranatant, which usually collects at the tip of each tube, by aspiration.

   (The next extraction again involves the addition of potassium carbonate, so only 20 minutes must be allowed to elapse between the addition of potassium carbonate, and concentrated sulfuric acid.) Add to each toluene extract, 3.4 ml of potassium carbonate reagent. Stopper the centrifuge tubes, shake vigorously for 2 minutes, and centrifuge. Insert a 3-ml volumetric pipette through the toluene layer into each infranatant carbonate extract, and transfer 3 ml of each carbonate without delay to photometer cuvets.

6. Indole color reaction: Place the cuvets in an ice bath, and add 0.5 ml of concentrated sulfuric acid, very slowly, to each cuvet. Constant agitation of the cuvet during addition of sulfuric acid ensures evolution of carbon dioxide without heating or foaming.

   Add 4 ml of cold indole-phosphoric acid reagent to each cuvet. Stopper the cuvets. Mix by inversion. Replace the cuvets in the 12 to 15° C ice bath. Measure optical density at 495 nm precisely 5 minutes after addition of indole-phosphoric acid reagent. If measures of optical density exceed 0.800, repeat analyses upon smaller samples of urine.

7. Calculations: The concentration of vanilmandelic acid may be calculated from the following equation, which incorporates the factors for urine dilution and concentration of standard:

$$\text{VMA (mg/dl)} = \frac{\text{Absorbance (urine sample)} - \text{Absorbance (urine blank)}}{\text{Absorbance (standard)} - \text{Absorbance (reagent blank)}} \times 0.55$$

$$\text{VMA (mg/24 hrs.)} = \text{Value of VMA (mg/dl)} \times \frac{\text{volume (ml)}}{100}$$

The recovery is calculated in mg/100 ml, and the mg/100 ml of vanilmandelic acid extracted from the unknown urine is subtracted from the recovery result. There should be a difference of 0.4 mg/dl.

INTERPRETATION. Normal levels of VMA excretion are 1 to 8 mg/24 hours. Patients with essential hypertension may have higher levels than this. Values of 12 mg/24 hours or over are generally found in patients with pheochromocytoma.

DISCUSSION AND CLINICAL SIGNIFICANCE. Various studies have shown that measurements of the urinary excretion of catecholamines and of vanilmandelic acid have comparable clinical significance as aids in the diagnosis of pheochromocytoma. From the viewpoint of the clinical laboratory, determinations of vanilmandelic acid appear to have several practical advantages over estimations of urinary catecholamines.

For example, vanilmandelic acid has been reported to be more stable than catecholamines in urine; the amount of vanilmandelic acid present in urine is many times that of catecholamines; urinary excretion of

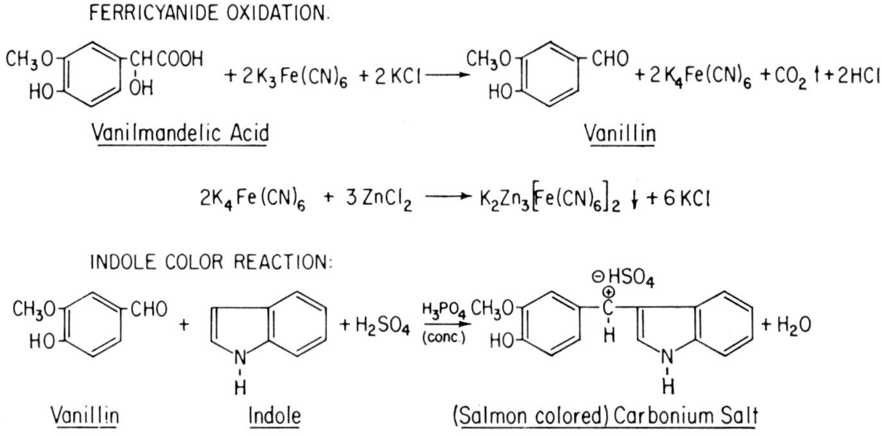

Fig. 1–30. Chemical reactions in determination of vanilmandelic acid (from Sunderman).

vanilmandelic acid is less subject to diurnal fluctuation than is excretion of catecholamines; the analytical method described is capable of greater precision and better recovery than usually obtainable with fluorometric procedures for urinary catecholamines; apparatus required for vanilmandelic acid determination is readily available in most laboratories. For these reasons, measurement of urinary excretion of vanilmandelic acid is probably more practical for most clinical laboratories than is estimation of catecholamines. The present procedure is considered to be the reference method. Unfortunately, it is too time consuming for use as a screening procedure. An experienced technologist will find analysis of six unknowns a full day's work.

MATERIALS AND REAGENTS

1. Vanilmandelic acid stock standard. Transfer 50 mg vanilmandelic acid (3-methoxy, 4-hydroxymandelic acid) to a 50 ml volumetric flask. Add 0.01 N hydrochloric acid to the mark. Mix to dissolve. Store in the refrigerator. (Solution is stable for at least 1 month.)
2. Vanilmandelic acid working standard. Transfer 5 ml of vanilmandelic acid stock standard to a 100 ml volumetric flask; dilute to the mark with distilled water. (One ml of the working standard contains 50 μg of vanilmandelic acid.) Store in the refrigerator. Prepare fresh each week.
3. Potassium carbonate (0.4 M). Transfer 55.3 g potassium carbonate (anhydrous, reagent grade) into a 1 L volumetric flask. Dissolve by adding distilled water to the mark. Mix well.
4. Potassium ferricyanide (0.6% w/v). Transfer 0.6 g of potassium ferricyanide (reagent grade) to a 100 ml volumetric flask; dissolve in distilled water; dilute to the mark. (Store in a brown glass bottle in the refrigerator. Stable for approximately 3 days.)
5. Zinc sulfate (1.2% w/v). Transfer anhydrous zinc sulfate, 1.2 g, to a 100 ml volumetric flask; dissolve in distilled water; dilute to the mark. Mix.
6. Ethanol indole reagent. Transfer 500 mg of indole (reagent grade) to a dl volumetric flask and dissolve by adding absolute ethanol. Dilute to the mark. Mix. Store in the refrigerator.
7. Phosphoric acid, 85% (w/v) (reagent grade). Store in refrigerator so that it is cold at the time of analysis.
8. Mixed indole-phosphoric acid reagent. Transfer 1 ml of indole reagent to a 50 ml glass-stoppered mixing cylinder and dilute to 40 ml with cold 85% (w/v) phosphoric acid. Mix. (This reagent is prepared immediately before use and kept chilled in an ice-bath.)
9. Hydrochloric acid, concentrated (reagent grade)
10. Sulfuric acid, concentrated (reagent grade)
11. Ethyl acetate (reagent grade)
12. Toluene (reagent grade)
13. Activated magnesium silicate (Florisil 60/100 mesh). Florisil, an

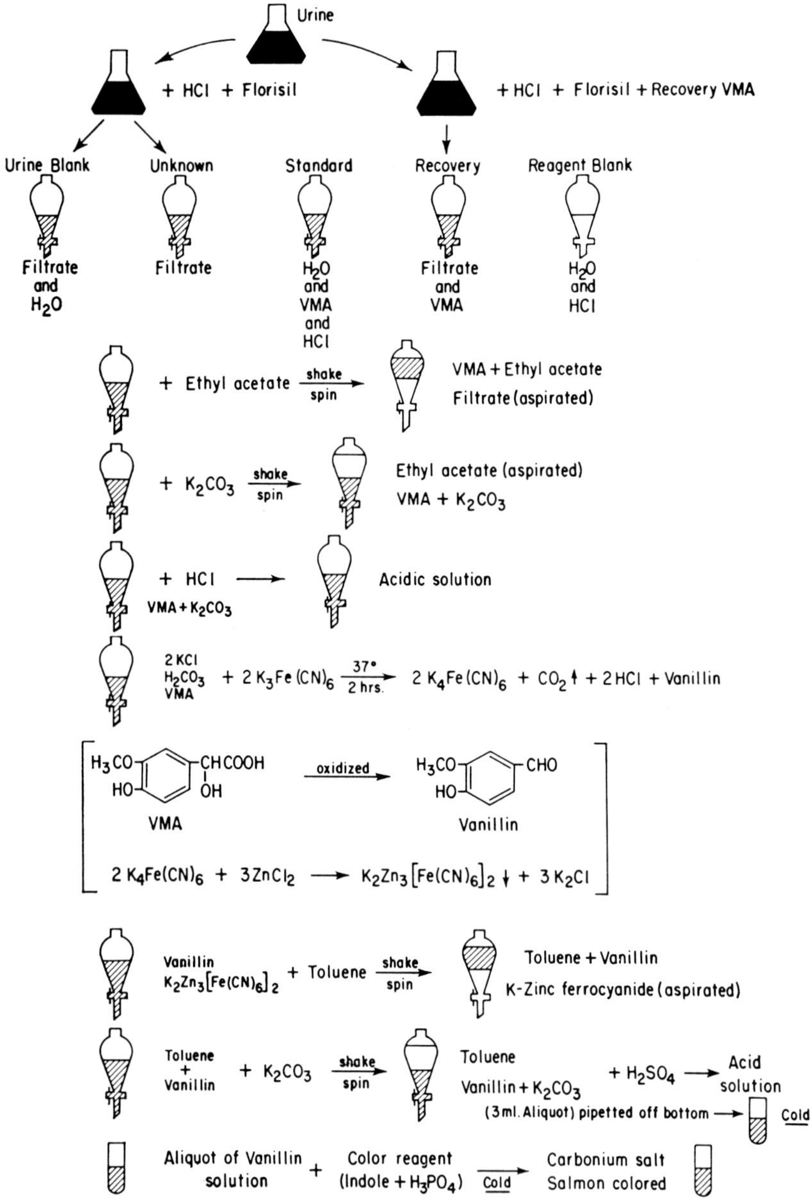

Fig. 1–31. Determination of VMA by the modified Sunderman extraction method.

activated magnesium silicate adsorbent, may be obtained from the Floridin Co., P.O. Box 989, Tallahassee, Fla. 32301.

14. Centrifuge tubes, 50 ml, with ground glass stoppers. (Centrifuge tubes, no. 45168, Kimble Glass Co., are suitable.)
15. Aspiration assembly. A Pasteur pipette with a fine bore, 6″ in length, is connected to suction by thin-walled rubber tubing. The rate of aspiration is regulated by digital pressure on the tubing.
16. Water bath, 37° C, fitted with cover
17. Spectrophotometer (Coleman Jr. suitable)
18. Centrifuge (International no. 2 or similar; check to see that tube stoppers do not break with centrifugation.)

REFERENCES

1. Stewart, T., and Freeman, J.: Vanilmandelic Acid and Catecholamines. 2nd Ed. Chicago, American Society of Clinical Pathologists, 1976.
2. Sunderman, F., Cleveland, P., Law, N., and Sunderman, F., Jr.: A method for the determination of 3-methoxy-4-hydroxy-mandelic acid (vanilmandelic acid) for the diagnosis of pheochromocytoma. Am. J. Clin. Path., *34*:293, 1960.
3. Sunderman, F., and Sunderman, F., Jr.: Urinary excretion of catecholamines and mandelic acid derivates. Trans. Stud. Coll. Physicians Phila., *27*:222, 1960.

VANILMANDELIC ACID

METHOD. Hycel Mandelic Acid Kit. The principle of this method is extraction followed by diazotization with p-nitroaniline and measurement of the diazotized complex spectrophotometrically at 530 nm. Recovery of VMA standard added in known amount to the urine, as in the Sunderman procedure, can be used as a quality control measure.

SPECIMEN. A 24-hour specimen is collected in a chemically clean brown bottle containing 25 ml of 6 N hydrochloric acid. It is important that the pH of the urine be less than 3. Check pH of the urine specimen with pHydrion paper. Except for freshly voided specimens (less than 6 hours old), do not perform the test if pH is above 3.0.

PROCEDURE

1. Pretreatment of Urine: Into a properly marked 25 × 100 mm test tube, place 1.0 ml of reagent grade concentrated hydrochloric acid. Add slowly, with gentle shaking, 10 ml of urine and mix well by flicking with the finger. Add one-quarter ($^1/_4$) teaspoon of magnesium silicate (reagent 1); cap tube with perforated cap; and shake gently for 10 minutes (swirling contents every 60 seconds will suffice). Centrifuge at high speed for 5 minutes and filter through Whatman no. 1 filter paper.
2. Extraction: Mark 50 ml conical screw-cap centrifuge tubes "B" for "blank" and "S" for "standard," and use numbers for the unknown specimens.
   To tube "B," add 2.0 ml distilled water.
   To tube "S," add 0.2 ml dilute mandelic acid standard.

Dilute 1.0 ml of mandelic standard concentrate (reagent 8) to 10.0 ml with distilled water. (The dilute mandelic acid standard is stable for 1 week if refrigerated.) To appropriately numbered tubes, add 2.0 ml of pretreated urine.

Add 20 ml ethyl acetate (reagent 2) to all tubes; cap tubes and mix contents of each tube vigorously by shaking, or with a mechanical mixer for 30 seconds.

Centrifuge at high speed in a clinical centrifuge for 3 minutes and gently remove the lower layer by aspiration. (Do not aspirate upper ethyl acetate layer!)

Add 2.5 ml sodium carbonate (reagent 3) to each tube, cap tubes, mix vigorously with mechanical mixer for 30 seconds, centrifuge at high speed for 1 minute, and carefully aspirate the major portion of the upper ethyl acetate layer without loss of lower layer.

Transfer 2.0 ml of the lower carbonate layer to marked cuvet.

3. Preparation of Diazo Reagent: Diazo reagent is prepared fresh before use by adding 1.0 ml of sodium nitrite solution to 8.0 ml of diluted p-nitroaniline solution. The diazo reagent must be used within 1 hour after its preparation.

   Prepare sodium nitrite solution by dissolving contents of vial (reagent 4) in 50 ml of distilled water. Store in amber bottle in refrigerator. (The sodium nitrite solution is stable for 60 days if refrigerated.)

   To prepare diluted p-nitroaniline solution, dilute 2.0 ml of stock p-nitroaniline (reagent 5) to 95 ml with distilled water. Add 5.0 ml concentrated hydrochloric acid and mix well by inversion. (The diluted p-nitroaniline solution can be stored in a 100 ml glass-stoppered graduated cylinder and should be refrigerated. Stability does not exceed 2 weeks.)

4. Color Reaction: Add 0.1 ml of the fresh diazo reagent to all cuvettes, mix by gentle swirling, and allow to stand at room temperature for 5 minutes.

   Add 5.0 ml ethyl acetate (reagent 2) to all cuvettes; mix and centrifuge at high speed for 1 minute, and carefully remove only lower layer by aspiration.

   Add 1.0 ml sodium hydroxide (reagent 6), mix, centrifuge at high speed for 1 minute, and carefully remove lower layer by aspiration.

   Repeat step 3 two times more. A total of 3 separate alkaline washings is required. Final aspiration of sodium hydroxide must be complete; if not, color reaction will be turbid.

   Add 2.0 ml methanol (reagent 7) to all tubes and mix by gentle swirling for a few seconds.

   Final color reaction should be clear and free of turbidity or particulate matter. Let stand for 5 minutes before spectrophotometric reading.

5. Spectrophotometry:
   a. Mix by gentle swirling to clear mixture of striated layers.
   b. Read standard and unknowns at 530 nm against blank set at zero Absorbance (100% T). Readings should be made within 30 minutes following color development.
6. Calculations:

$$\text{VMA (mg/24 hours)} = \frac{\text{Absorbance Unknown}}{\text{Absorbance Standard}} \times \text{volume urine}$$

(L) × 10 × 1.1
(1.1 = Urine dilution correction factor.)

INTERPRETATION (Hycel, Inc.). Normal range of VMA in urine is 0.5 to 12 mg/24 hours. The mean value of VMA in clinically normal adults is 5.0 mg/24 hours (± 1 S.D. 2.2 mg/24 hours).

DISCUSSION AND CLINICAL SIGNIFICANCE

1. Pretreatment of Urine: Subsequent to filtration, the sample should be clear or a pale yellow color. With heavily pigmented specimens, it may be necessary to repeat magnesium silicate treatment and centrifugation to remove discoloration.
2. Extraction: With forefinger, seal one end of a 2.0 ml volumetric pipette and introduce tip through ethyl acetate layer to bottom of tube in extraction procedure. Gently blow through pipette to clear any material trapped during passage through ethyl acetate. Wipe pipette carefully to prevent transfer of ethyl acetate to the tube for the diazo reaction.
3. General Comments: This method includes a shorter version of the Sunderman extraction technique. However, the VMA is diazotized with paranitroaniline for spectrophotometric quantitation, instead of the indole-complex as in the Sunderman procedure. Hycel, Inc., states that the spectral characteristics are such that best linearity is obtained at 530 nm, and the Absorbance follows Beer's law between 0 to 15 mg/L. Hycel, Inc., states that day-to-day reproducibility is: 13.6% at a 2.5 g/L level; 7.3% at a 10 mg/L level; and 6% at a 15 mg/L level. Recoveries are asserted to be 86–108% at the 2.5 mg/L level, and 75 to 94% at the 10 mg/L level.

In a parallel series of determinations on the same specimens, per cent recovery of VMA standard added to the urine with the Sunderman method ranged from 77.5 to 110% and with the Hycel Mandelic Acid Kit, ranged from 47.5 to 140%. The exact recovery values and percentages are recorded in Table 1–31. The poorest recoveries were obtained with low VMA levels; and in general, the lower the levels, the

TABLE 1–31. Comparative Results of Sunderman Method and Hycel Mandelic Acid Kit Method.

		SUNDERMAN METHOD					HYCEL MANDELIC ACID KIT METHOD				
Date	Urine volume (ml)	Results of unknown (mg/total volume)	Amount VMA standard added to unknown (mg/total volume)	Actual results of recovery: VMA standard plus unknown value (mg/total volume)	Expected results of recovery: VMA standard added plus unknown value (mg/total volume)	Percent recovery of VMA standard	Results of unknown (mg/total volume)	Amount VMA added to unknown (mg/total volume)	Actual results of recovery: VMA standard plus unknown value (mg/total volume)	Expected results of recovery: VMA standard plus unknown value (mg/total volume)	Percentage recovery of VMA standard
10/26/67	1330	4.7	5.32		10.02		8.4	5.32		13.72	
10/30/67	1010	3.0	4.04		7.04		5.6	4.04		9.64	
10/30/67	1730	3.8	6.92		10.72		5.1	6.92		12.02	
10/30/67	2120	3.9	8.48		12.38		12.9	8.48		21.38	
11/3/67	1310	1.9	5.4	7.53	7.14	108 %	5.4	5.24	11.03	10.64	108 %
11/13/67	630	5.6	2.52	7.74	8.12	85 %	2.7	2.52	2.83	5.22	50 %
11/15/67	675	5.3	2.7	7.66	8.0	87.5%	4.7	2.7	6.12	7.4	52.5%
11/15/67	4220	5.2	16.88	23.77	22.08	110 %	11.9	16.88	27.94	18.78	95 %
11/17/67	660	4.5	2.64	7.94	7.14	92.5%	6.3	2.64	7.55	8.94	47.5%
11/17/67	1080	4.8	4.32	8.2	9.12	92.5%	8.4	4.32	11.86	12.72	80 %
11/20/67	2300	5.8	9.2	13.85	15.0	92.5%	9.4	9.2	20.67	18.6	122.5%
11/20/67	950	3.4	3.8	6.63	7.2	85 %	6.4	3.8	10.2	10.2	100 %
11/20/67	990	3.0	3.96	6.37	6.96	85 %	6.1	3.96	11.64	10.06	140 %
11/20/67	3300	5.0	13.2	16.55	18.2	87.5%	10.9	13.2	25.75	24.1	112.5%
11/20/67	2830	4.0	11.32	14.47	15.32	92.5%	8.4	11.32	31.42	19.72	115 %
11/20/67	1950	7.1	7.8	13.15	14.9	77.5%	13.2	7.8	21.0	21.0	100 %
11/20/67	1370	2.7	5.48	8.45	8.18	105 %	5.1	5.48	8.8	10.58	67.5%
11/20/67	1920	5.6	7.68	12.32	13.28	87.5%	8.1	7.68	15.0	15.78	90 %

less the percentage recovery. Interfering substances might be present in urine samples that interfere with diazotization with paranitroaniline, but that do not interfere with determination of vanilmandelic acid by the Sunderman method (Campbell, Sherbaniuk, Rigby. False positive reaction due to methocarbamol in the screening test for vanilmandelic acid (VMA). Clin. Chem., *10*:447, 1964.) Some such substances that have been reported are mephenesin, methocarbamol, and glyceryl guaiacolate.

REFERENCE

1. Hycel, Inc., brochure on test (Hycel, Inc., Houston, Tex. 77042).

PHENOLIC ACIDS AND VANILMANDELIC ACID

METHOD. Cellulose acetate electrophoresis, with elution and spectrophotometric quantitation modified by Lee R. Morgan from Thorne Butler.

PRINCIPLE. This electrophoretic method utilizes cellulose acetate strips for support. About 0.1 ml urine is spotted and permitted to soak into minute filter paper strips, dried by forced air. The urine-impregnated strips are placed in the electrophoretic chamber, and migration proceeds for 2 hours. The purple VMA band is eluted with alkaline methanol and quantitated spectrophotometrically at 520 nm.

SAMPLE. The patient is instructed to abstain from medications and from vanilla-flavored foods (ice cream, etc.), chocolate, and citrus fruit for 2 days prior to collection of urine. A 24-hour urine sample is collected in a brown glass bottle containing 25 ml 6 N hydrochloric acid. The urine is stored in the refrigerator during collection. The urine volume is measured, and an aliquot is saved for analysis. The patient should be cautioned about the poisonous and corrosive nature of the preservative. No initial extraction of VMA from urine is necessary.

PROCEDURE

1. Preparation of urine-impregnated strips (standards and recovery experiments are included with each set of strips):
   A. Apply urine in 0.02 ml aliquots with a Sanz overflow pipette (or other appropriate pipette) to strips of filter paper cut to 25 × 3 mm, drying continually under a hot air blower until 0.1 ml urine is soaked into the strip.
   B. To filter paper strips identified by pencil markings as "4 mg" and "10 mg" standards, apply 0.04 ml proper working standards in the same fashion as the unknown urine. (If the strips cannot immediately be placed in the electrophoretic chamber, freeze them in tightly stoppered plastic test tubes.)
2. Electrophoresis:
   A. Presoak cellulose acetate strips in the electrolyte buffer. Blot thoroughly and place in electrophoresis chamber with strips

held taut. It is important that the cellulose acetate strips be free from water drops.

B. At the cathode end of properly marked cellulose acetate strips, place the 25 × 3 mm filter paper bands containing the dried urine and the standards. With a wet applicator stick, touch strip with enough drops of buffer to dampen the filter paper, making it obviously adherent to the cellulose acetate strips.

C. Cover the cell and let stand for 10 minutes. Electrophorese for 2 hours at 2 ma/strip. (The original recommendation was $1\frac{1}{2}$ to 2 hours with 250 volts across the strips and/or 2 ma/strip, but we find that 2 ma/strip gives the best separation of VMA).

D. The VMA band is located 6 to 6.5 cm from the origin. (Thorne Butler stained his strips with p-nitroaniline dye and estimated the amount of VMA visually by comparison with the 4 mg and 10 mg standards. The purple VMA bands are said to be able to be ranked visually to ± 0.02 mg, corresponding to ± 2 mg/ 1,000 ml urine, except when the quantity of VMA is greater than 1.5 mg. Normal urines require at least 100 ml of sample to obtain sufficient staining intensity for a reliable comparison.)

E. There are over 40 phenolic acids sometimes present in urine, varying in color reaction from red to yellow to orange to purple to blue. The purple VMA band is always accompanied by a yellow band on the anode side. Strips from persons taking salicylates show a deep salmon to orange salicyluric band located midway between the application site and the VMA band. Another purple band (vanillic acid) of varying intensity, depending on oral intake of vanillin, is located about 1 to 1.5 cm from the cathode.

3. Elution of VMA from cellulose acetate strips:

A. With scissors, cut the VMA band from the cellulose acetate strips unknown and standards; cut a similar section from a blank strip of cellulose acetate that has been wet with buffer and dipped in the staining solution. Extract VMA by placing

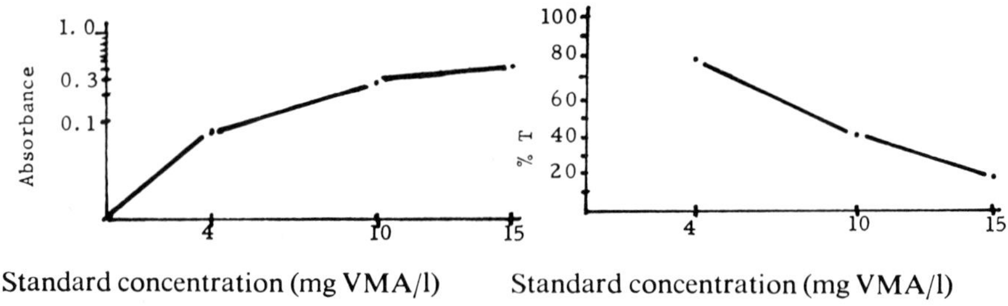

Fig. 1–32. Absorbance vs. % transmission with standard concentrations of VMA.

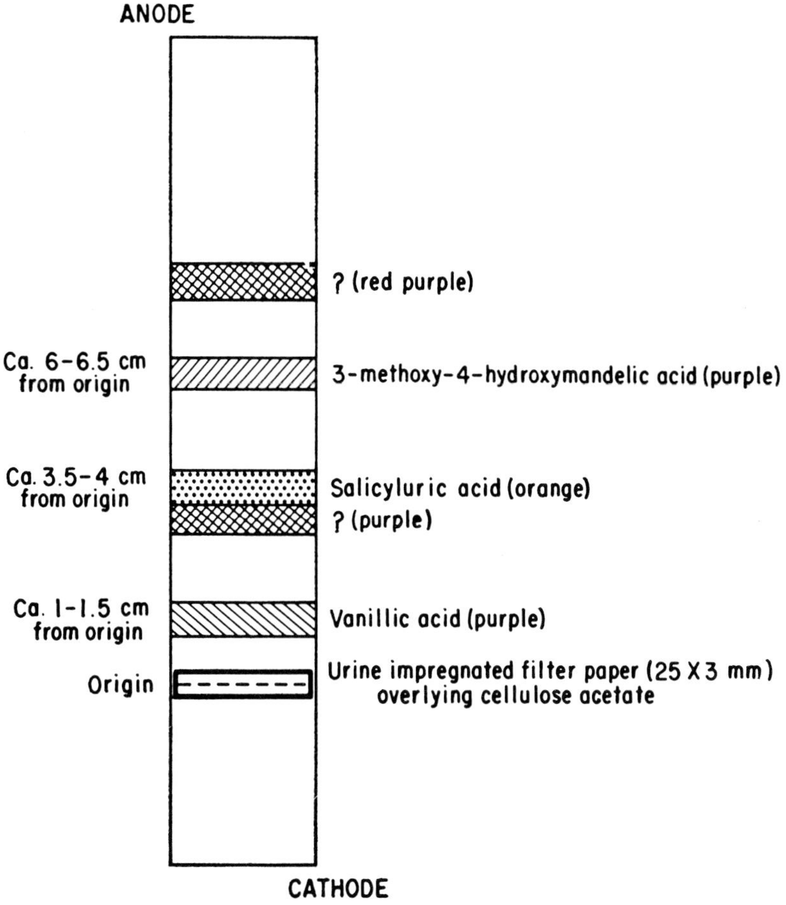

Fig. 1–33. Schema of an electrophoretogram (actual size 6¾″ × 1″) of urine sample obtained from a normal patient (after ingestion of aspirin). Electrophoresis was on Gelman Sepaphore III cellulose acetate strips at 2 ma for 2 hours.

cut portions each in a separate small test tube with 0.5 ml alkaline methanol solution and let stand 1 hour at room temperature with periodic shaking. Centrifuge mixture at 1500 rpm for 10 minutes.

4. Measure absorbances at 520 nm (or 505 nm), correcting for blank absorbance.
5. Calculations: Prepare a standard curve from 4 mg, 10 mg, and 15 mg VMA standards, plotting absorbance on the *abscissa* and concentration (mg) on the *ordinate:* then record concentration of unknown from curve.

   Calculate 24 hour excretion as follows:

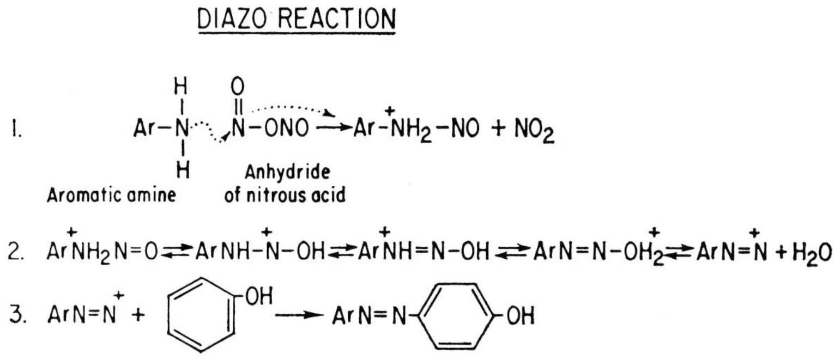

Fig. 1–34. Diazo reaction. In general terms, the process involves reaction of nitrous acid with a primary aromatic amine. The initial step is a nucleophilic attack of $-NH_2$ on N_2O_3 with displacement of NO_2. Subsequent proton exchange in the product of the initial attack, and loss of a water molecule lead to the formation of the diazonium ion, which then reacts with any phenolic acid. ("Ar" represents paranitroaniline.)

mg VMA/24 hours = Concentration (mg/L) × volume (expressed in L).

(If the unknown urine contains more than 1 μg/0.1 ml, it is best to repeat the procedure using a smaller volume of urine if p-nitroaniline staining is used.)

INTERPRETATION. Normal values have not yet been well established by the elution technique. From Thorne Butler's series of 400 specimens, using p-nitroaniline staining and visual estimation, the range of normal values was estimated to be 4.0 ± 2.0 mg/24 hour (with a high value of 11.0 mg/24 hour urine, and a low value of 1 mg/24 hour urine). Values ≥ 12 mg/24 hour urine are abnormal.

DISCUSSION AND CLINICAL SIGNIFICANCE. The technique is said to detect as little as 1 mg VMA/L, when 0.1 ml urine is applied to the filter paper strips. Since levels of VMA in urine of patients with catecholamine-secreting tumors are usually well above that level, averaging 12 mg/day, sensitivity is more than sufficient for recognition of abnormal elevations of VMA.

With this technique there is little interference by closely related urinary phenols. This permits elimination of time-consuming extraction procedures common to the Sunderman and Sunderman and the Hycel Mandelic Acid Kit methods. The method requires little technologist bench time; hence, it may be more adaptable to mass screening of hypertensive patients than any of the other methods described. (One can elute and measure only those specimens appearing elevated by visual estimate.)

MATERIALS AND REAGENTS

1. Sodium nitrite, 0.1% (w/v). Refrigerate.
2. Alkaline-methanol solution

   2% (w/v) sodium carbonate 100 ml

Methanol, absolute	100 ml

Refrigerate.

3. Acetic acid—pyridine buffer, pH 4.2 (need 300 ml for small Gelman chamber).

Glacial acetic acid	16.0 ml
Pyridine	3.5 ml
Distilled water, q.s. to	1,000 ml

Refrigerate.

4. Staining p-nitroaniline solution (prepare from refrigerated solutions. Make fresh solution for each cellulose acetate strip). To 5.0 ml stock p-nitroaniline solution, add sufficient 0.1% (w/v) sodium nitrite to decolorize the solution (about 5.0 ml). Add water to bring volume to 10 ml. Add 10 ml 10% (w/v) sodium carbonate; mix and immediately float strip into staining solution when strips are ready to stain.
5. Stock VMA standard, 10 mg/dl (Nutritional Biochemical Co.)

VMA	10 mg
Absolute ethanol, q.s. to	100 ml

Refrigerate

6. Working VMA standards (prepare fresh prior to use). Into two tubes, one labeled "4 mg" and the other "10 mg," add 0.1 ml and 0.25 ml, respectively, of stock VMA standard. Dilute each to 1.0 ml with absolute ethanol. (Standards will be 0.01 mg and 0.025 mg/0.1 ml equivalent to 4 mg VMA/L and 10 mg VMA/L.)
7. Concentrated hydrochloric acid (reagent grade)
8. Electrophoresis chamber (Gelman no. 51101) with power supply capable of 250 volts DC at 25 ma.
9. Sepaphore III cellulose acetate strips, $6^3/_4'' \times 1''$ (Gelman Instrument Co.)
10. Staining trays, 4 mm thick plexiglas, $8 \times 4 \times 1.5$ cm
11. Hot-air blower (home-style hair dryer)
12. Test tubes, 13×100 mm with plastic caps
13. Filter paper, cut into 25×3 mm strips (Schleicher & Schuell no. 2043A)

REFERENCES

1. Butler, T.: Electrophoretic determination of vanilmandelic acid (VMA) in urine by direct application to cellulose acetate. Clin. Chem., *13*:488, 1967. (Modified by Lee R. Morgan, Department of Pharmacology, LSU Medical Center, New Orleans, La.)
2. Stewart, T. and Freeman, J.: Vanilmandelic Acid and Catecholamines. 2nd Ed. Chicago, American Society of Clinical Pathologists, 1976.

AMINO ACIDS

METHOD. One-dimensional descending paper chromatography and ascending thin-layer chromatography.

PRINCIPLE. Urine is spotted on paper strips and allowed to descend in an atmosphere of butanol:acetic acid:water organic phase overnight; the strips are dried at room temperature or in an oven; they are stained with ninhydrin, and the amino acids are visualized. Alternatively, urine is spotted on cellulose acetate sheets, allowed to ascend in the same solvent system (which was described previously) for 2 hours, dried, rerun, dried, and stained with ninhydrin.

SAMPLE. A 24-hour urine specimen is preferred, collected in a chemically clean brown bottle, preferably kept under refrigeration. An amount of urine is spotted that contains about 5 mcg creatinine (previously determined chemically). Volume of urine sample spotted on the paper strips can also be based on total concentration of solids as determined by the TS meter (refractometer) according to the following schedule:

Total solids	*(Paper) urine volume (μL)*	*(TLC) urine volume (μL)*
Over 4%	5	1
3 to 3.9%	7.5	1.5
2 to 2.9%	10	2
1.5 to 1.9%	15	3
1.0 to 1.4%	20	4
1%	30	6

PROCEDURE

PAPER CHROMATOGRAPHY

1. Cut Whatman no. 3 paper into strips 9″ wide and 22″ long. Eight of these strips can be placed in the chromatank at one time. Spot urine on paper strips on a line 7″ from the top end. Place approximately 10 to 50 ml solvent in tank.
2. Arrange the strips for descending chromatography so that the sample spots are 1″ below the antisiphon rod.
3. Pipet 200 ml of solvent into the trough slowly.
4. Permit chromatograms to develop overnight until solvent front reaches the end of the paper.
5. Dry at room temperature or in a warm ventilating cabinet until all odor of solvent has been removed. (Heating above 80° C is unnecessary, and drying usually takes less than 10 minutes at this temperature.) If dry, dip into ninhydrin stain solution or spray with ninhydrin spray stain.
6. Compare chromatogram with normal urine chromatogram or standard migrated in same fashion.

THIN-LAYER CELLULOSE CHROMATOGRAPHY

1. Spot urine samples on a line 1.5 cm from edge of chromatogram sheet. Space samples at 1 cm intervals so that 19 can be placed on a sheet.
2. Draw a line across the sheet 10 cm above the sample line.
3. Sandwich the sheet between the chamber plates.

4. Add solvent to trough (same solvent as paper system).
5. Stand chamber plates on edge in solvent trough.
6. Permit to migrate 2 hours or until solvent front reaches line previously drawn.
7. Remove sheet and air dry.
8. Replace sheet between the chamber plates and develop a second time in the same direction with the same solvent. (This repeat procedure will create a remarkable improvement in the resolution of amino acids.)
9. Visualization is accomplished with the same stain used for the paper system.

INTERPRETATION. Amino acids appear as gray-violet, violet-to-yellow-to-green spots on the chromatogram (see Fig. 1–36).

DISCUSSION AND CLINICAL SIGNIFICANCE. In general, one-dimensional paper chromatographic systems have not provided sufficient resolution for separately identifying abnormal amino acids and normal constituents. This method appears to have overcome some of the previous difficulties, and the authors claim better resolution than with ascending paper chromatographic techniques. The ascending thin-layer techniques give comparable results.

MATERIALS AND REAGENTS

1. Shandon Model "500" "Panglas" Chromatank complete with two solvent troughs, two glass anchor rods, six anti-siphon rods and glass covers.
2. Whatman no. 3 chromatographic paper, 58 × 68 cm sheets. (Do not substitute 3M.)
3. Solvent: n-butanol:acetic acid:water (240 ml:60 ml:dl).
   Stain: (1) ninhydrin 0.25% (w/v); isatin 0.01% (w/v); lutidine 1% (w/v) in acetone OR
   (2) ninhydrin spray (Eastman-Kodak Company, Rochester, N.Y. 14650)
4. Eastman chromatogram cellulose sheets, 20 × 20 cm (no. 6064) without fluorescent indicator
5. Eastman chamber plate developing set no. 6071 with two recessed glass plates with clamps, solvent trough, and supporting wire frame.

REFERENCE

1. Jackson, S., Sardharwalla, I., and Evers, G.: Two systems of amino acid chromatography suitable for mass screening. Clin. Biochem., *2*:163, 1968.

AMINO ACIDS

METHOD. Two-dimensional ascending paper chromatography.

PRINCIPLE. Desalted urine specimens and standards are spotted on filter paper and allowed to develop in pyridine, acetone, and am-

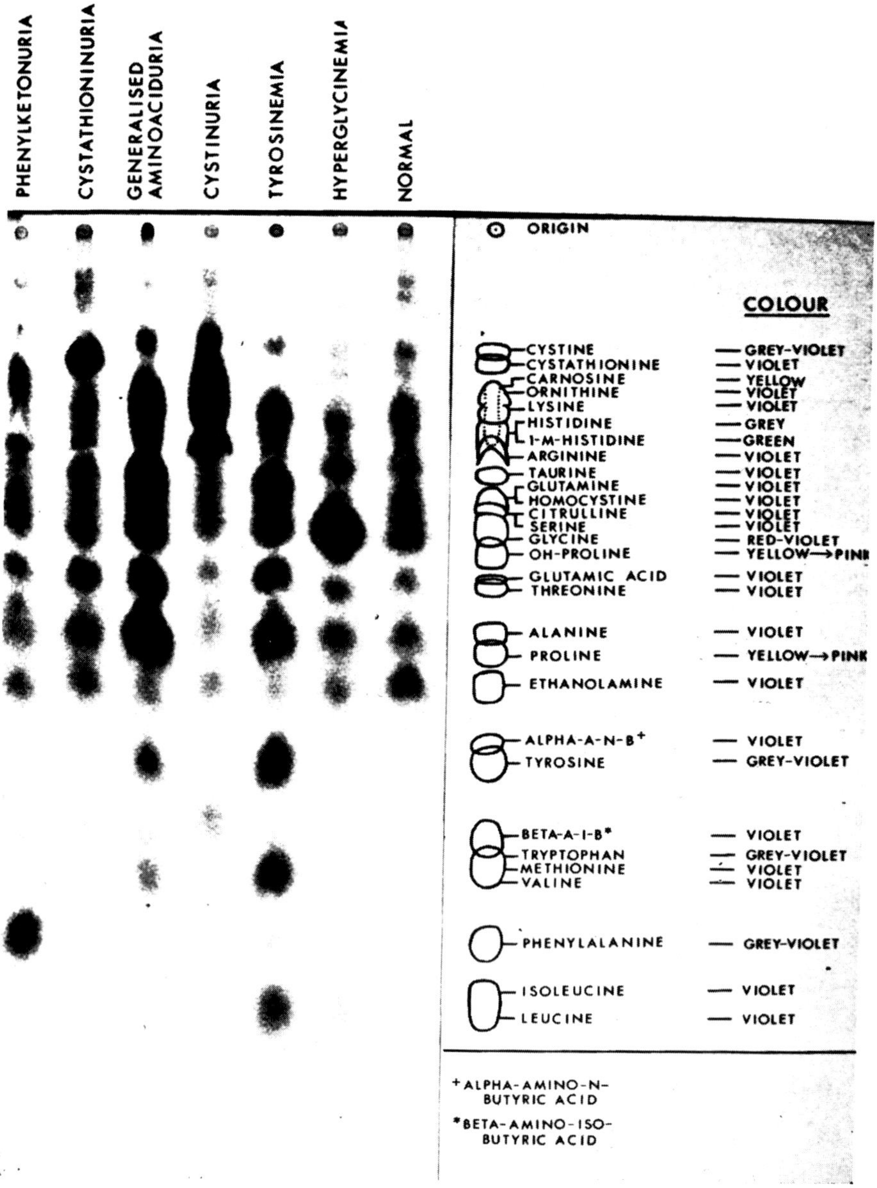

Fig. 1–35. Two-dimensional chromatogram of urine phenolic acid.

monium hydroxide for $1^1/_2$ hours. The specimens and standards are dried, allowed to develop at 90° angle to first run in isopropanol and formic acid and then dried again. Color is developed by spraying with ninhydrin, followed by drying, then heating. The chromatogram may be photographed or preserved by spraying with clear lacquer. Desalting

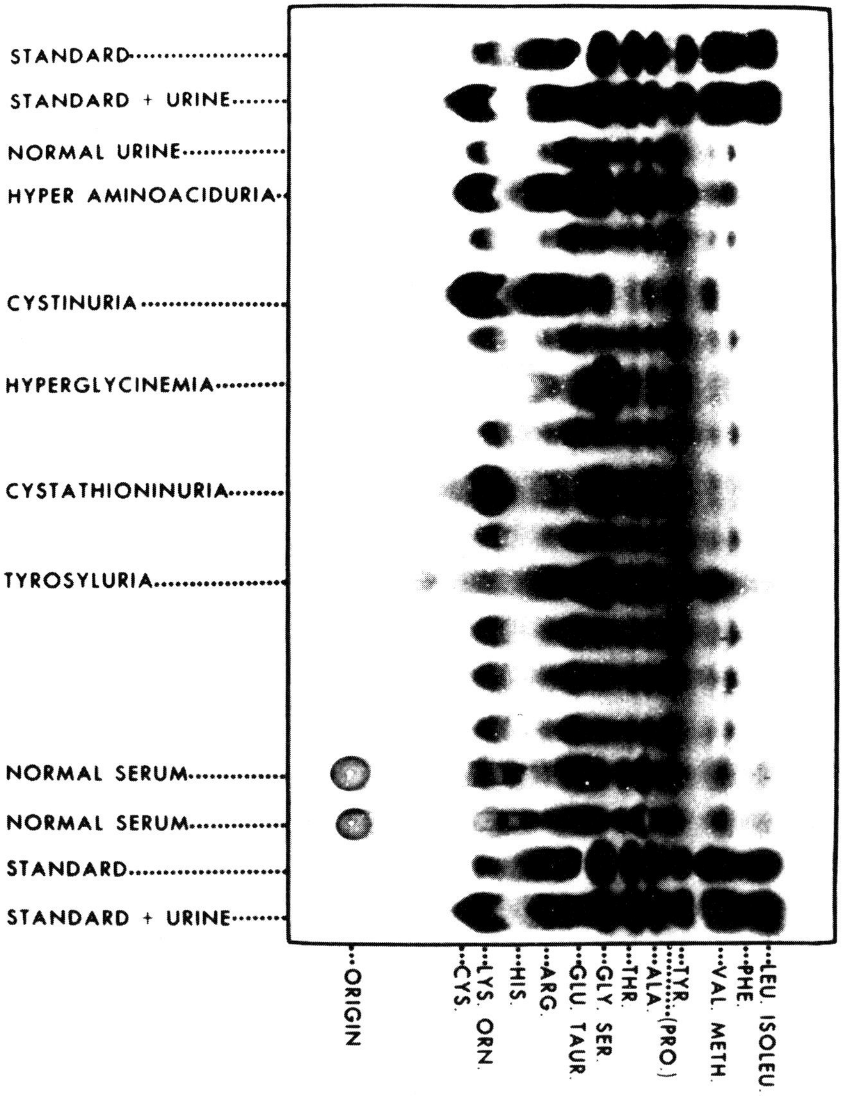

Fig. 1–36. Two-dimensional chromatogram of urine and serum amino acids.

is carried out at pH 5, 7, and 8 for better recovery of amino acids (tyrosine and protein are lost at pH 5; lysine and methionine, at pH 7).

SAMPLE. A 24-hour urine specimen is preferred, collected in a chemically clean bottle containing thymol crystals as a preservative. The bottle should be kept in the refrigerator during collection. The original or a 30 ml aliquot may be sent to the laboratory (also in a chemically clean container).

PROCEDURE

1. Pipet 1 ml urine into 1 ml compartment of Tobal desalter; 2 ml of urine brought to pH 5 with 1 N HCl in the 2 ml compartment; and 3 ml of urine brought to pH 8 with HK_2CO_3 into the 3 ml compartment.
2. Desalt at 80 ma until reading drops to 20 to 25 ma (usually 10 to 15 minutes).
3. Combine urine aliquots.
4. Prepare first developing solution and pour into chromatographic jar or cabinet. Allow to sit for 30 minutes for equilibration.
5. Draw two perpendicular pencil lines on Whatman no. 3 filter paper, each 2 cm from the edges, and shorter perpendicular lines on the opposite corner, 15 cm each from the first set of lines.
6. Spot 125 μL desalted urine, a little at a time, at the intersection of the first two perpendicular lines, keeping the wet circle smaller than 1 cm in diameter by drying after each spotting with a portable hair dryer. Proceed similarly with standard solution.
7. Clip paper in rack; place in tank so that lower edge is immersed in developing solution, and allow to develop to the 15 cm mark (approximately $1^1/_2$ hours).
8. About 30 minutes before this, equilibrate the second tank with the second developing solution.
9. Remove paper, air dry completely, rotate 90° and place in second tank until development to the 15 cm mark (approximately 3 hours).
10. Dry again in air. Spray with ninhydrin reagent. Air dry. Heat in 110 to 115° C oven for 1 to 3 minutes (for optimal color development).
11. Spray with clear lacquer and compare with standard.

INTERPRETATION. Amino acids appear on the chromatogram as purple-to-blue colored spots (see Fig. 1–37).

DISCUSSION AND CLINICAL SIGNIFICANCE. This has been discussed elsewhere to some extent. Aminoacidurias secondary to specific renal tubular transport defects include cystinuria, Hartnup disease, and proteinuria. Those secondary to generalized tubular dysfunction include the Lignac-Fanconi syndrome or cystinosis, adult Fanconi (no cystine deposits), Lowe's syndrome (generalized aminoaciduria, impairment in acidification, glaucoma, nystagmus, hypotonus), Wilson's disease, and heavy metal poisoning (lead, uranium, cadmiums). Overflow aminoacidurias include phenylketonuria, tyrosinosis, histidinemia, maple syrup disease, argino-succinic aciduria, homocystinuria (patients have vascular renal disease), and beta amino isobutyric aciduria).

MATERIAL AND REAGENTS

1. Acetone, pyridine, isopropanol, formic acid, ammonium hydroxide (analytic grade)

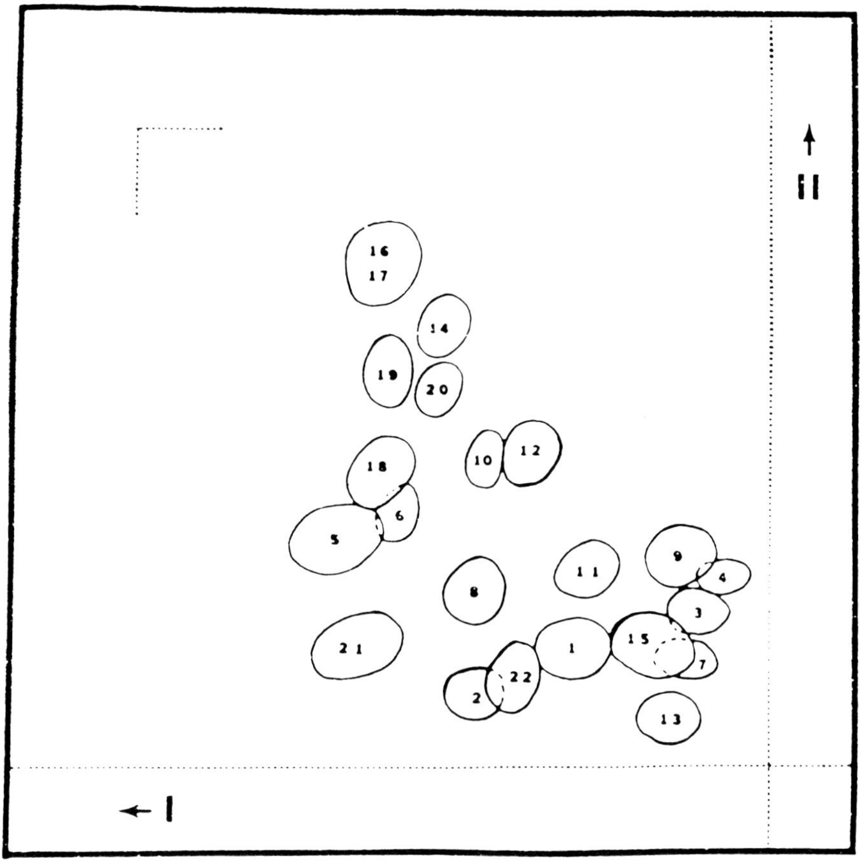

1. L-lysine
2. L-histidine
3. L-arginine
4. L-aspartic acid
5. L-threonine
6. L-hydroxyproline
7. L-homocystine
8. L-serine
9. L-glutamic acid
10. L-proline
11. Glycine
12. L-alanine
13. L-cystine
14 L-valine
15. L-methionine
16. L-isoleucine
17. L-leucine
18. L-tyrosine
19. L-phenylalanine
20. L-tryptophan
21. L-asparagine
22. L-glutamine

Fig. 1–37. Schematic drawing of a three-dimensional chromatogram of urine amino acids.

Solution no. 1: Pyridine, acetone, ammonium hydroxide, water (45, 30, 5, 20 ml)
Solution no. 2: Isopropanol, formic acid, water (75, 12.5, 12.5 ml)

2. Hydrochloric acid, 1 N
3. Potassium carbonate, 0.1 N
4. Stock amino acid standard calibration mixture, Beckman Instrument Co., Fullerton, California, containing 2,500 ± 0.05/g mole: lysine, histidine, arginine, aspartic acid, threonine, methionine,

serine, glutamic acid, proline, glycine, alanine, cystine, valine, isoleucine, leucine, tyrosine, phenylalanine, tryptophan. (The concentration of cystine is only half that of the others.)

5. Ninhydrin aerosol spray (Sigma Chemical Co., St. Louis, Mo.)
6. Working amino acid standard: Dilute standard 1:10 with water
7. Chromatography tanks, racks and clips
8. Whatman no. 3 filter paper (20 × 20 cm)
9. Tobal desalter, model CD-1
10. Hair dryer
11. Atomizer

(*NOTE:* Hydroxyproline, homocystine, asparagine, and glutamine are not present in standard.)

REFERENCE

1. Spinella, C.: Two-dimensional paper chromatographic determination of amino acids in urine. Clin. Chem., 45:1011, 1969.

AMINO ACIDS

METHOD. KODAK CHROMAT/O/SCREEN (thin-layer chromatographic analysis)

PRINCIPLE. Urine (or blood) is spotted on chromatographic strips and allowed to migrate in one direction with butanol:acetic acid:water in a gel (rather than solvent) phase along with known standards of amino acids. Ninhydrin in the gel stains the amino acids purple-to-blue after application of heat. Visual identification can then be made, or Rf values can be calculated. (Other differential amino acid staining procedures are described also.)

PROCEDURE

Sample Application

1. Remove chromatographic sheet from package. Chromatographic sheets are wrapped in a shrink package and are stacked with the coated sides facing in one direction. The topsheet is a blank, protective piece of Mylar film.

   Use a sharp instrument to cut open the plastic shrink package on either the top or bottom. Remove a chromatographic sheet, being careful not to scratch or touch the coated side with bare fingers. Always use the forceps provided to handle the sheets. Place the sheet on a clean horizontal surface.
2. Apply the sample using the pipette. Insert a 1 μL pipette into the pipette holder. With the pipette in as nearly a horizontal position as possible, touch it to the surface of the liquid sample. Then, either (1) half fill with plasma, or (2) fill completely with urine. The liquid can be seen moving up the pipette by capillary action. When filling with plasma, remove the tip of the pipette quickly when half filled. Otherwise, the liquid will stop when the pipette

is full (as is the objective with urine). To apply the sample, hold the pipette in a perpendicular position so that the tip just touches the chromatographic sheet between two of the cut-out circles. Do not scratch or break the coating by pressing the pipette on the sheet. Squeeze holder and apply its entire volume in one application. The sample should spread to the edges of the circles.

3. Apply the standard solution. A vial containing a standard solution of five amino acids is included with the kit. To simplify location and identification of the separated zones, concentrations of amino acids are several times greater than those found in normal urine or plasma. Composition of the standard solution is shown in the following chart:

Amino Acid	*mg/dl*
Alanine	50
Histidine	50
Leucine	75
Phenylalanine	100
Tyrosine	50

Apply $^1/_2$ μL of the plasma standard to the chromatogram between two other circles in the same manner as the sample. To minimize the chances of error, always apply spots to the chromatogram in the same order, *i.e.*, left to right or right to left, with the standard in the same position.

After chromatography, visual comparison of the sample with the standard will show any gross elevation of amino acid levels in plasma samples. In the case of urine, the standard will be helpful after comparison with several normal urine samples. Alternatively, normal urine (1 μL) can be used as a control instead of the standard included with the kit.

4. Identify the specimen. Write the patient's name or identification on the bottom of the developing chamber. The top of the chromatographic sheet can also be numbered with a sharp pencil.
5. Dry the sheet completely. Before proceeding, the sheet must be dried completely. It may be air dried. However, the use of a hair dryer will hasten the operation.

An advantage of the Chromat/O/Screen Analysis Kit is that no additional sample preparation is necessary. Urine requires no desalting; plasma requires no deproteinization.

METHOD OF DEVELOPMENT

1. Fill the chamber trough with gel. Remove the cap and puncture the top of the tube of Kodak Chromat/O/Screen Gel. **Caution:** Care should be taken, because some of the gel may be expelled upon opening if the tube has been warmed. After using the gel, replace the cap tightly to prevent any leakage or evaporation. (Do not open the second tube provided in the 150-test kit until the first tube

has been completely used.) Completely fill the trough of the development chamber by squeezing the tube of gel into the trough until a peak projects just above the developing chamber flood. Use the special scraper to mold and remove excess gel; otherwise, the solvent will migrate in an uneven front causing Rf values to change.

The gel contains ninhydrin, a reagent that will make the amino acids visible after heating the finished chromatogram. If ninhydrin comes in contact with the skin, it may cause a harmless purple stain resulting from amino acids contained in sweat.

2. Insert the spotted sheet and close the chamber.
60-Analysis Kit: Place the opened chamber flat on a table or other horizontal surface with the trough toward you and your left and the door toward your right.
150-Analysis Kit: Place the developing chamber on a horizontal surface, with the trough away from you and the door open toward you.
For either size kit: Insert the spotted, dried chromatographic sheet, coated side up, on the chamber door, with the spots toward you. With the door on the table, close the trough side over the door. Keep the chamber on the flat surface.

Close the chamber tightly by pressing the edges with your thumb. For proper contact between the chromatographic sheet and the gel surface, gently tap the closed chamber, trough-side up, once or twice against a table edge. During development, the chamber may be left horizontal or vertical (ascending or descending chromatography), or may be transported with no change in results.

3. Develop the chromatogram. The advance of the solvent front can be seen by holding the chamber up to the light. It should reach the top in approximately 20 to 30 minutes. This will vary slightly, depending upon temperature and humidity. If migration takes more than 45 minutes, it means that the gel has become dry. Good results can still be achieved, but care should be taken in interpretation, since Rf values may change.

In plasma samples, hemoglobin and its breakdown products may be drawn up in an irregular fashion from the origin. Although this may raise the Rf values of the lower amino acids, it will not interfere with visual interpretation of the chromatogram. If the amino acids are to be measured semiquantitatively by reflectance or by densitometry, hemolysis must be prevented.

After the solvent front reaches the top of the sheet, remove the sheet from the chamber with the forceps. Air dry the sheet until the solvents are *completely* evaporated.

METHOD OF VISUALIZATION

1. Heat the chromatographic sheet. The gel contains ninhydrin, a

reagent that stains the primary and secondary amine groups various shades of purple. Thus, for visualization, it is only necessary to heat the chromatographic sheet in an oven at 100° C (212° F) for 3 to 5 minutes.

Place the sheet on a solid support (such as a glass plate, aluminum tray, etc.) before placing in the oven. Putting the sheet directly onto the oven-grill shelves will cause uneven heating. Avoid heating at temperatures in excess of 100° C (212° F) since this may cause discoloration of the background.

Notes:

A. Ninhydrin colors may be bleached by strong acid fumes (HNO_3, HCl), ozones, organic peroxides, nitrogen oxides, or other similar oxidizing atmospheres.
B. The stained chromatogram will begin to fade within a few days. Colors can be preserved by dipping or spraying with a copper nitrate solution (1 ml saturated aqueous copper nitrate in 100 ml of ethanol plus 0.2 ml 10% (v/v) HNO_3). The colors change to pink-red, which is stable for many months.

2. Identification. The amino acids can be identified by comparison with the standard, and by referring to table below, which shows the Rf values of many amino acids. It is apparent from this table that some amino acids do not separate completely. Identification can be simplified in part by using further specific stains, as explained in the confirmative staining section.

   The specimen can also be analyzed quantitatively by automatic column chromatography if the amino acid concentration appears to be abnormal. The specimen may be further analyzed by two-dimensional thin-layer chromatography or by electrophoretic techniques. EASTMAN CHROMOGRAM Sheet 6064 (cellulose sorbent) is useful in these techniques.

   For additional information, request Kodak Publication no. JJ-47, Separation of Amino Acids by Thin-Layer Chromatography and Electrophoresis. This pamphlet is available from Dept. 412-L, Eastman-Kodak Company, Rochester, N.Y. 14650.

CONFIRMATIVE STAINING. Included with this kit is an aerosol spray bottle containing sodium bicarbonate. This may be used after observing the ninhydrin colors, to confirm the presence of phenylalanine. To do this, place the chromatogram in an upright position in a hood or other well-ventilated area. Hold the spray bottle in a vertical position about 8″ from the chromatogram, making sure that the nozzle is pointing toward the chromatogram. Depress the cap *fully*, and spray back and forth 2 or 3 times to cover the entire sheet. Best results can be achieved by spraying in smooth, even motions. Do not overwet the chromatogram so that the reagent drips down the surface.

Heat the chromatogram at 100° C for 3 to 5 minutes. Phenylalanine changes from purple to deep blue.

Several reagents may be sequentially applied over the ninhydrin stain for a more comprehensive confirmation of amino acids. Color reactions of amino acids with these stains are shown on the following chart. Most of these reagents are available as Eastman Organic Chemicals.

Isatin: 0.2% in acetone (w/v). Incorporate 2% (w/v) pyridine just before use. Dip the chromatogram in this solution, allow the solvent to evaporate, and dry the chromatogram in the oven at 100° C for 3 to 4 minutes.

Ehrlich's Reagent: Prepare 10% (w/v) of p-dimethylamino-benzaldehyde in concentrated HCl. Just before use, mix 1 volume of this solution and 4 volumes of acetone. Dip or spray the chromatogram and allow it to air dry.

Sakaguchi's Reagent: Dip the chromatogram in 0.1% (w/v) of 8-hydroxyquinoline in acetone and allow the solvent to evaporate. Dip the chromatogram in 0.3 ml liquid bromine in dl of 0.5 M NaOH.

Pauly's Reagent: Prepare stock solutions A and B as follows:

A. Dilute 9 g of sulfanilic acid and 90 ml concentrated HCl with 900 ml water.
B. Aqueous 5% sodium nitrite (made fresh daily), (w/v).
C. Mix equal volumes of solutions A and B, cool, and add an equal volume of 10% aqueous sodium carbonate, (w/v).

TABLE 1–32. Sequential Staining.*

AMINO ACID	VISUALIZATION REAGENT				
	Ninhydrin	Isatin	Ehrlich†	Sakaguchi‡	Pauly
Arginine	Purple	Violet		Orange-red	
Aspartic	Blue	Light Blue			
Citrunine	Purple	Violet	Orange		Yellow
Cysteine	Lavender	Lavender			Orange
Glutamic acid	Purple	Violet			
Glycine	Purple	Violet			
Histidine	Purple	Blue			Dark red
Hydroxyproline	Yellow	Blue	Purple		
Isoleucine	Purple	Violet			
Leucine	Purple	Violet			
Phenylalanine§	Purple	Violet			
Proline	Yellow	Blue	Violet-yellow		
Tryptophan	Purple	Violet	Dark purple		Dark red
Tyrosine	Purple	Blue			Pink
Valine	Purple	Violet			
Others	Purple	Violet			

*Adapted from Hsia
†Some colors may develop in 20 minutes and fade in 1 hour. Other colors take 1 day to develop.
‡Colors are unstable
§Free phenylalanine changes from purple to deep blue after spraying with sodium bicarbonate.

VISUALIZATION PROCEDURES (ADDITIONAL)

1. Aspartic acid appears as a pink spot after dipping the plate in 1 N HCl.
2. Homocystine will appear blue-brown after dipping the plate in 1% (w/v) of mercuric nitrate. This reagent is stable at room temperature, but must be prepared in a hood.
3. Proline gives a blue spot on a yellow background after dipping the ninhydrin-stained chromatogram in isatin (0.2% (w/v) in acetone), and heating it for 4 to 5 minutes at 100° C. If it is desirable to visualize hydroxyproline, dip the chromatogram in Ehrlich's reagent after proline appears. Hydroxyproline will appear as a pink spot.
4. Iodine-azide solution can be made by mixing equal volumes of 1.27 g iodine in 100 ml ethanol and 3.25 g sodium azide in 25 ml water plus 75 ml ethanol. Dip or spray the chromatogram with this mixture. White spots appear on the brown iodine background; the background very slowly fades as the iodine evaporates. The spots remain visible in ultraviolet light, even after the background has completely disappeared. All thiols (R-SH) and disulfides (R-S-S-R) react positively but thio-ethers (R-S-R; such as methionine) do not. If more than a visual comparison of spots is desirable, there are several published methods for the semiquantitation of amino acids on thin-layer chromatograms.

INTERPRETATION. The diagnosis of numerous pathological states can be made from knowledge of the identity and concentration of the free amino acids in plasma and urine. Current screening procedures use plasma almost exclusively because it is more easily collected from infants. Ideally, both plasma and urine should be examined, since there are a number of diseases that do not result in elevated plasma amino acid concentrations.

DISCUSSION AND CLINICAL SIGNIFICANCE. The amino acid composition of normal plasma does not vary as much as that of normal urine, so if a more intense band appears on the plasma chromatogram when compared to a standard run along side it, an amino acid defect is generally indicated. An exception to this rule is the glycine-serine band, which may be increased, due to a benign increase in serine. In rare instances, though, this may be due to glycinemia and should be positively identified by two-dimensional paper chromatography. Normally, the plasma has a prominent glutamine band, but this amino acid is hydrolyzed in the plasma with a corresponding increase in intensity of the glutamic acid band. Alanine is also prominent; glycine less so. Bands due to histidine, lysine, taurine, arginine, serine, threonine, glutamic acid, proline, valine, isoleucine, and leucine can also be seen in the chromatogram, but will not be as intense as the other amino acids.

Urine. The normal range of amino acid excretion is very wide, and

TABLE 1–33. Amino Acids Normally Occurring in Blood and Urine.

(This table shows the relative amounts of amino acids found in normal blood and urine. They are shown on a scale of 0 to 4, zero (0) indicating that amino acids are *never* present. Those not normally present are shown with an X.)

AMINO ACID	NORMAL URINE	Rf*	NORMAL BLOOD	RF*
Cysteic Acid	0	10	0	11
Cystine	X	11	0	9
Histidine	1	14	1	15
Ornithine	0	14	0	14
Lysine	0	14	0	14
1-Methyl-Histidine	X	14	0	16
Arginine	0	17	1	16
Homocystine	0	18	0	20
Taurine	2	20	1	21
Serine	1	23	1	24
Glutamine	1	21	4	22
Glycine	3	30	2	27
Hydroxyproline	0	27	0	30
Threonine	0	35	1	34
Glutamic Acid	0	35	1	32
Proline	0	37	1	38
Alanine	2	42	3	41
Tyrosine	0	51	1	52
Valine	0	61	1	61
Phenylalanine	0	63	1	64
Isoleucine	0	76	1	79
Leucine	0	78	1	79

NOTE: The Rfs may vary within a few percentage points, depending upon the humidity and temperature at which the chromatogram is run.

$$*Rf = \frac{\text{Distance (in cm) the amino acid travels}}{\text{Distance (in cm) solvent front travels}} \times 100$$

abnormality is usually associated only with the appearance of amino acids that are not normally present in the urine in sufficient concentration to show up in the chromatogram. Thus, spotting a moderate excess of a normal urine does not produce an abnormal chromatogram. With experience, the intensity, number, size, and shape of the amino acid bands become recognizable.

It is often desirable to use a standardized volume of urine for analysis. Several methods have been described to standardize the amount of urine applied to the chromatogram, including:

1. Creatinine concentration
2. Specific gravity or total solids
3. Timed collection
4. Color intensity
5. Alpha-amino nitrogen concentration
6. Urea concentration

The methods that depend upon creatinine, urea, and alpha-amino nitrogen concentrations are time-consuming and can be misleading when the cause of the aminoaciduria is renal tubular malfunction or liver disease. Alternatively, the method of Jackson, et al., as modified below, will be helpful in producing normal urinary chromatograms that are more or less similar.

Measure the total-solids content of one drop of urine. The amount of urine to be spotted can be determined from the following chart:

Total Solids	*Microliters of Urine*
Less than 1	1
1.0–1.9	$^3/_4$
2.0–2.9	$^1/_2$
More than 3	$^1/_4$

Normal physiologic variations in the urinary excretion of amino acids occur in pregnancy and early infancy. Benign forms of aminoaciduria may also occur. Moderate variations in levels of urinary glutamic acid, glutamine, glycine, alanine, serine, and taurine have no clinical significance.

In general, screening with the KODAK CHROMAT/O/SCREEN Analysis Kit will indicate whether an abnormal amino acid level exists. However, final diagnosis must be made on the basis of a quantitative analytical technique. A chromatogram of 1 μL of normal urine shows almost no cystine, no proline, and only traces of amino acids with Rf values greater than alanine (Rf 42). A chromatogram of normal urine will show a dominant spot for glycine, less analine, serine, and glutamine, and even less taurine, histidine, and methyl-histidine. Normal persons sometimes excrete taurine or aminoisobutyric acid in levels the same as or higher than glycine. Two chromatograms of normal urines are shown. In the normal adult, daily amino acid excretion is practically constant and independent of urine volume and dietary protein intake. A slight rise in amino acid output occurs postprandially, but gross aminoaciduria cannot be produced by excessive protein intake except in cases where intravenous amino acid solutions are administered. This therapy causes a 4- to 5-fold increase of amino acids normally present.

Normal, full-term babies have immature renal reabsorption mechanisms, and so, a higher level of amino acids in the urine. An intensified normal pattern may also be accompanied by appreciable amounts of cystine, asparagine, glutamine, glutamic acid, and often proline, hydroxyproline, and occasionally methionine, tyrosine, leucine, and valine.

Taurine, proline, and hydroxyproline excretion is very high at birth, but diminishes to the levels found in the adult by the sixth month.

Infants and children of school age show the same amino acid pattern as adults. Premature babies exhibit a generalized renal aminoaciduria, which may result in levels 5 times higher than in the adult. The amino acids most often encountered are glycine, alanine, threonine, serine, asparagine, and glutamine. Cystine, proline, and glutamic acid are also conspicuous. Tyrosine may be present in very high concentrations, with phenylalanine present in lower concentrations.

MATERIALS AND REAGENTS

1. Kodak Chromat/O/Screen Gel (Butanol:acetic acid:water. Ninhydrine included for visualization); one tube (60-test kit), two tubes (150-test kit)
2. Developing chamber, 30 chambers (60-test kit)
3. Developing chamber, 15 chambers (150-test kit)
4. Instruction booklet
5. Visualization spray (sodium bicarbonate)
6. Chromatographic sheet, 15 ten-channel sheets (150-test kit)
7. Chromatographic sheet, 30 two-channel sheets (60-test kit)
8. Pipette holder; one pipette holder (60-test kit), two pipette holders (150-test kit)

TABLE 1–34. Trouble Shooting.

Problem	Probable Cause	Remedy
Uneven advance of solvent front	1. Gel not leveled in trough 2. Chamber not tightly closed	1. Level gel with scraper 2. Tightly close chamber
Plasma chromatogram has vertical smudge	Presence of protein in sample	Spot sample completely across the narrow neck between holes on the chromatographic sheet
Broad bands of separated amino acids or long tails on either side (difficult to determine Rf values)	1. Sample has spread out too far on application 2. Too high a concentration of amino acids	1. Spot urine in two applications of $1/2$ μL each 2. Use smaller sample
Long running time	Dried solvent gel	No effect on results if a standard is run along with unknown
Smudged chromatograms, or specimens which do not run	Excess gel in trough is squeezed past sample when chamber is closed. Sample dissolves in gel	Level gel in trough
Large droplets of visualization reagent from spray bottle	Partial depression of button on aerosol can	Completely depress button on aerosol can
Final, visualized chromatogram has deep pink, purple, or brown background	Chromatogram heated too long or at too high a temperature	Warm chromatogram at 100 °C for 3 minutes

9. Scraper
10. Pipettes (1 μL)
11. Forceps
12. Standard

REFERENCES

1. Airaksinen, E., Farrel, G., and Johnson, R.: Congenital Mental Retardation. Edited by G. Farrel. Austin, The University of Texas Press, 1969, p. 191.
2. Baron, D., and Economidis, J.: Thin-layer chromatography for amino acids and sugars. J. Clin. Path., *16*:484, 1963.
3. Fahie-Wilson, M.: Routine investigation of amino acid patterns in blood serum and urine by thin-layer electrophoresis. J. Med. Lab. Tech., *26*:363,1969.
4. Ghadimi, H., and Shwachman, J.: Evaluation of amino-aciduria in infancy and childhood. Am. J. Dis. Child., *99*:457, 1960.
5. Hsia, D., and Inouye, T.: Inborn Errors of Metabolism. Chicago, Year Book Medical Publishers, 1966.
6. Jackson, S., Sardharwalla, I., and Ebers, G.: Two systems of amino acid chromatography suitable for mass screening. Clin. Biochem., *2*:163, 1968.
7. Kawerau, E., and Wieland, T.: Conservation of amino acid chromatogram. Nature, *168*:77, 1951.
8. Meyer, J., Droll, S., and Klingmuller, V.: Ein suchtest zur erkennung der phenylketonurie und eine semiquantitative bestimmung des phenylalins im blutplasma mit der dunnschicht chromatographie. Clin. Chim. Acta, *18*:69, 1967.
9. Samuels, S., and Ward, S.: Aminoaciduria screening by thin-layer high-voltage electrophoresis and chromatography on microplates. J. Lab. Clin. Med., *67*:669, 1966.
10. Spackman, D., Stein, W., and Moore, S.: Automatic recording apparatus for use in the chromatography of amino acids. Anal. Chem., *30*:490, 1958.
11. White, H.: Separation of amino acids in physiological fluids by two-dimensional thin-layer chromatography. Clin. Chim. Acta, *21*:297, 1968.
12. White, H.: Citation quoted in 3. p. 297.

PHENYLKETONES

METHOD. Folling ferric chloride method.

PRINCIPLE. Ferric ions chelate with the enol (–OH) group of phenylpyruvic acid, in an acid medium, to produce a green to green-gray colored complex.

SAMPLE. Since phenylpyruvic acid is unstable, fresh urine (or urine preserved by freezing) should be used for the test. Urine with an acid pH is preferable.

PROCEDURE

1. Place 5 ml urine in a test tube. Acidify with acetic acid if urine is alkaline.
2. Add ferric chloride drop by drop (a brown-white precipitate of ferric phosphate may appear. Continue adding until no more phosphates are precipitated; then, add more).
3. Observe for olive green-to-green-gray color in supernatant after 2 to 3 minutes, which fades rapidly or slowly in up to 1 to 2 hours;

OR

1. Add ferric chloride drop by drop (about 10 drops total) onto baby's urine-soaked diaper, and observe for olive green color.

INTERPRETATION. If phenylpyruvic acid is present, either immediately or within 3 minutes following addition of ferric chloride, the urine will become olive green or gray-green, and the color will fade after a few seconds to 2 hours (the latter depending on the level of phenylpyruvic acid and upon the concentration of ferric chloride). The diaper test color also will fade, and will not leave a permanent stain, although some phosphate and hydroxide may precipitate from urine with ferric ions.

DISCUSSION AND CLINICAL SIGNIFICANCE. The test will not detect phenylpyruvic acid in concentrations less than 5 mg/dl. Normally, phenylketones are not present in urine in amounts detectable by this test. The test is sometimes negative in *dilute urine* of patients with phenylketonuria, who, on a low-protein diet, may excrete less than 20 mg/dl, or in whom excretion is intermittent. Furthermore, phenylketonuric infants may not show a positive test until several weeks of age. Blood phenylalanine level about 3 mg/dl suggests the disease. Phenylpyruvic acid appears in the urine when blood levels reach 10 to 15 mg/dl. (It has been calculated that one in seven persons in the general population is a carrier. Consequently, about 5 in 100,000 infants born in the U.S. are expected to develop phenylketonuria.)

Premature newborn infants (less than 5 lb.) may have elevated phenylalanine and tyrosine levels without having the genetic disease, probably as a result of delayed development of appropriate enzyme activity in the liver. These patients will have a positive Guthrie bacteria inhibition test (a screening test based on ability of a phenylpyruvic acid-negative urine bacteria to grow on phenylpyruvic acid-free media only surrounding discs impregnated with phenylpyruvic acid-containing urine) but usually not a positive ferric chloride or Phenistix test. These patients also excrete phenylacetic acid (as do those with the genetic disorder), which gives the urine and sweat a "musty" or "athlete's" odor. Other substances react with ferric chloride producing colors as follows:

Bile: green
Homogentisic acid (alkaptonuria): green (fades very rapidly)
Diacetic acid (ketosis): red-brown "Bordeaux wine" color
Melanogen (malignant melanoma): gray (adherent to ferric phosphate); black (precipitate in alkaline urine)
Chloropromazine drugs: violet
Salicylates: red-brown to blue-purple
Para-aminosalicylic acid and lactic acid may also react, giving a red-brown to blue color

Positive and negative control should be examined at the same time.

MATERIALS AND REAGENTS

1. Aqueous ferric chloride, 10% (w/v) (store in polyethylene bottles)
2. Test tubes, 13 × 100 mm

3. Acetic acid, glacial
4. Dropping pipettes

REFERENCES

1. Centerwall, W., and Centerwall, S.: The Clinical Team Looks at Phenylketonuria. Rev. Ed. Children's Bureau Publication, DHEW, U.S. Government Printing Office, 1964.
2. Folling, A.: Excretion of phenylpyruvic acid in the urine as metabolic anomaly in connection with imbecility. Ztschr. Physiol. Chem., *227*:169, 1934.

PHENYLKETONES

METHOD. Phenistix test.

PRINCIPLE. Ferric ions in the test strip react with phenylpyruvic acid and other phenylketones in an acid medium to produce a green, gray, or blue color. Optimum acidity is provided by cyclohexysulfamic acid. Magnesium ions prevent phosphates from interfering with the color reaction.

SAMPLE. Fresh urine from patient (newborn) on a milk regimen (after 2 days of milk feeding as a minimum). Phenylpyruvic acid is unstable; therefore, fresh or frozen specimens should be used for testing.

PROCEDURE. Dip test strip into urine, remove immediately, and compare with color chart at 30 seconds.

INTERPRETATION. A color change of green-to-gray-to-blue appearing within 30 seconds is interpreted as a positive result. No observed color change is interpreted as a negative result. The test is negative in normal patients. (The test is often negative in newborns, and is usually used at the 4-week checkup!)

DISCUSSION AND CLINICAL SIGNIFICANCE. The Phenistix test will detect 75 to 80% of cases in which urine concentration of phenylketones is 8 mg/dl urine and 99.5% cases with concentration of 15 mg/dl. However, blood levels of phenylpyruvic acid have to reach 10 to 20 mg/dl to produce urine levels of 8 mg/dl. Since blood levels > 3 mg/dl in the first 2 to 3 days of life are considered suggestive of phenylketonuria, the test is obviously helpful only in those cases with high levels of phenylketones. However, the stick test is almost twice as sensitive as the ferric chloride test.

Beta-imidazolepyruvic acid is the only known substance that will give a strong positive Phenistix test within 30 seconds. (It is another hereditary disorder of children caused by deficiency of the enzyme histidine-alpha-deaminase.) Urinary metabolites of PAS, salicylic acid, and phenothiazides will produce a red-brown to pink color. The test is not affected by phenylacetate, pyruvate, phenylalanine, lactate, tyrosine, tryptophan, diacetic acid, thymol, homogentisic acid, or toluene. However, large amounts of ketones in urine will produce an atypical color reaction.

Confirmative tests for phenylketonuria are the Guthrie bacterial inhibition test, or the fluorescent determination of serum phenylalanine levels. Quantitative levels of urinary phenylpyruvic acid also can be determined by the Saifer-Harris modification of the Berry-Woolf method (Clin. Chem., *5*:203, 1959; and Nature, *169*:202, 1952.)

Positive and negative controls should also be tested.

MATERIALS AND REAGENTS. Phenistix (Ames Company, Elkhart, Ind. 46514).

REFERENCES

1. Ames Company brochure on tests.
2. Johnson, P., Free, H., and Free, A.: A simplified urine and serum screening test for salicylate intoxication. J. Pediatr., *63*:949, 1963.
3. Kark, R., et al.: A Primer of Urinalysis. 2nd Ed. New York, Hoeber Medical Division, Harper & Row, 1963, p. 57.
4. Knox, W.: Phenylketonuria. The Metabolic Bases of Inherited Disease. 2nd Ed. Edited by J. Stanbury, J. Wyngaarden, and D. Fredrickson. New York, McGraw-Hill, 1965.

PHENYLKETONURIA TESTING OF NEWBORN INFANTS

Laws have been passed by many state legislatures mandating routine screening of newborns for phenylketonuria. Such a law was passed by the state of Louisiana (1964) requiring that newborn infants have a phenylketonuria test (PKU) within the first 28 days of life. Consequently, testing by the Guthrie bacterial-inhibition test of blood samples from these infants has been made available by the State Department of Hospitals, Division of Laboratories, New Orleans.

The Louisiana State Board of Health provides the blotter-type cards and lancets for blood collection, and pre-addressed envelopes for mailing them to the Division of Laboratories, 325 Loyola Avenue, New Orleans, La. 70112.

If the infant is discharged from the hospital before blood can be collected for the Guthrie screening procedure, a form is provided to give to the mother or father instructing them to return. Additionally, at this institution (Earl K. Long Memorial Hospital) we stamp the back of the newborn sheet (footprint record) and have the parent sign a statement that instructions were given, to satisfy all legal requirements. This stamp was designed for our institution and use of it is not a standard procedure. The nurses in our nursery are responsible for instructing the parents.

The form shown is perforated, and the lower portion is detached and given to the parent. When the test is completed, the top portion of the form is filled out in its entirety. At the Earl K. Long Memorial Hospital, The Family Planning Clinic is responsible for sending the specimens to the State Board of Health laboratories. These laboratories mail results back to Family Planning, which, in turn, transmits the reports to the Medical Records section of our hospital.

LOUISIANA STATE BOARD OF HEALTH
Division of Laboratories
PKU SCREENING PROGRAM
INSTRUCTIONS FOR COLLECTING
BLOOD SAMPLE

After the skin is sterilized, the infant's heel is punctured with a sterile disposable lancet. If bleeding is slow, it is helpful to hold the limb dependent for a short period before spotting the blood on the filter paper. To insure an adequate test, each circle on the filter paper must be *filled completely* with a large drop of blood which has *soaked through* the paper. This can best be done by placing *this* side of the filter paper against the baby's heel and watching for the blood to appear on the front side of the paper and completely fill the circle.

The blank spaces are filled in with pencil (ball point pen or regular ink blurs and becomes illegible in the autoclaving that precedes the testing).

Only positive or suspicious results will be reported.

HOSPITAL PKU BLOOD TEST
Fill in all information with pencil only:

HOSPITAL ______________________

Baby's Name ______________________

Date of birth ....

Date 1st feeding ....

Bottle ☐; Breast ☐; Both ☐

Date of Sample ....

Premature? Yes ☐; No ☐

Baby's Doctor ....

Doctor's Address:

FILL 3 CIRCLES WITH BLOOD
(Be sure blood soaks through.)

○ ○ ○

Fig. 1–38. Blood collection card and instructions for PKU testing in Louisiana.

I HAVE ON THIS DATE ______________ RECEIVED AND UNDERSTAND INSTRUCTIONS CONCERNING PKU TEST ______________ ON MY BABY.
(done or to be done)

______________ WITNESS

______________ PKU FORM NUMBER

______________ SIGNATURE OF MOTHER

Fig. 1–39. Facsimile of medical record for signature of infant's mother to satisfy law requiring PKU testing in Louisiana.

PHENYLKETONURIA (PKU) TEST CARD

DATE OF DISCHARGE FROM HOSPITAL | RETURN APPT. DATE

NAME OF HOSPITAL OR PHYSICIAN | HOSPITAL NUMBER

BABY'S NAME | DATE OF BIRTH

PARENT'S NAME | PHONE NO.

ADDRESS - STREET (IF RURAL, GIVE LOCATION)

CITY OR TOWN | PARISH

DATE PKU TEST GIVEN | RESULTS ☐ POSITIVE ☐ NEGATIVE

MCH 39
REV. 11/67

(Send to Local Parish Health Unit, When Test Completed or 28 Days From Date of Birth, if Not Tested)

(OVER)

PHENYLKETONURIA (PKU) TEST

Baby's Name____________________

Dear Parent:

A law was passed by the 1964 Louisiana State Legislature requiring that all babies born in Louisiana have a phenylketonuria (PKU) test within the first 28 days of life. You should consult your physician regarding where this test should be done. If you have no physician, consult the nearest health unit.

Fig. 1–40. Instruction form for distribution to mothers of newborn infants in Louisiana.

PHENYLPYRUVIC ACID

METHOD. Saifer-Harris modification of Berry-Woolf method.

PRINCIPLE. Ferrous ammonium sulfate exerts a stabilizing effect on the colored complex formed by ferric chloride and phenylpyruvic acid at low temperature in the absence of light. Uranyl nitrate is used to precipitate any interfering phosphates.

SAMPLE. Phenylpyruvic acid is unstable; therefore, a fresh or frozen urine specimen should be tested.

PROCEDURE

1. Run a reagent blank using 1 ml water and 3 standards using 1 ml

solution of sodium phenylpyruvate (25, 50, 75 mg/dl standards) with the unknown.

2. Pipette 1 ml urine into 15 ml centrifuge tube
3. Add 4 ml glycine buffer to each tube
4. Add 1 ml uranyl nitrate reagent and mix by tapping with finger
5. Place tubes in ice bath (ca. 4° C) 10 minutes
6. Centrifuge at 3000 rpm for 5 minutes
7. Pipette 5 ml of the mixture from the centrifuge tubes into a separate 10 ml graduated cylinder
8. Cool ferrous ammonium sulfate and ferric chloride over 10 minutes in the ice bath
9. Add 1 ml cooled ferrous ammonium sulfate to each cylinder with the solution
10. Add 0.1 ml cooled ferric chloride
11. Cap with parafilm, mix well by inversion, and permit to stand in the ice bath *in the dark* for 30 minutes.
12. Read absorbance in spectrophotometer at 630 nm with reagent blank set to zero. Read again after 60 minutes.
    (Range of standards about 0.490 to 0.510)
13. Calculations:

$$\left[\frac{\text{A unknown}}{\text{A standard}}\right] \times [\text{C standard (mg/dl)}] \times 0.88 = \text{C unk (mg/dl)}$$

(The factor 0.88 is ratio of M.W. of phenylpyruvic acid and sodium phenylpyruvate—164.06/186.05)

INTERPRETATION. Normally, urine does not contain detectable amounts of phenylpyruvic acid (usually less than 5 mg/dl) with the ferric chloride test. Phenylpyruvic acid excretion ceases when blood phenylalanine levels are less than 10 to 15 mg/dl or 0.6 to 0.9 umol/ml. Phenylketonurics may excrete up to 180 mg/dl phenylpyruvic acid.

DISCUSSION AND CLINICAL SIGNIFICANCE. The test is alleged to be specific for phenylpyruvic acid. Homogentisic acid and p- or o-hydroxyphenylacetic acid will form a blue color, but the color fades within a minute. The stabilizing effects of low temperature and omission of light suggest that the Fe-PPA complex is in a delicate equilibrium.

MATERIALS AND REAGENTS

1. Sodium phenylpyruvate standards (Hoffman-La Roche, Nutley, N.J.)
2. 10% (w/v) aqueous $FeCl_3 \times 6H\ O$ (reagent grade)
3. Glycine-NaCl buffer (pH 2.2)

Glycine	4.35 g
NaCl	3.40 g

Dissolve in 400 ml distilled water (1,000 ml volumetric flask)
0.1 N HCl 420 ml
Distilled water q.s. to 1,000 ml

4. Ferrous ammonium sulfate
   $FeSO_4(NH)_2SO_4 \times 6H\ O$ 9.8 g
   Glycine buffer (prevents salt hydrolysis) 100 ml
5. 4% (w/v) uranyl nitrate reagent
   $(UO_2)\ (NO_3)_2 \times 6H\ O$ 4.0 g
   Glycine buffer 100 ml
6. Serologic pipettes, 1 ml and 5 ml and 0.1 ml
7. Clinical centrifuge
8. Ice bath
9. Graduated cylinder, 10 ml
10. Parafilm
11. Test tube rack
12. Centrifuge tubes, 15 ml
13. Spectrophotometer

REFERENCES

1. Berry, J., and Woolf, L.: Estimation of phenylpyruvic acid. Nature, *169*:202, 1952.
2. Saifer, A., and Harris, A.: Studies on the photometric determination of phenylpyruvic acid in urine. Clin. Chem., 5:203, 1959.
3. Stanbury, J., Wyngaarden, J., and Fredrickson, D.: The Metabolic Basis of Inherited Disease. 4th Ed. New York, McGraw-Hill, 1978, p. 240.

HOMOGENTISIC ACID

METHOD. Fishberg method.

PRINCIPLE. Homogentisic acid, which is 2, 5-dihydroxyphenylacetic acid, can cause development of photographic paper by reducing the silver salt. Addition of alkalinized urine containing homogentisic acid to photographic paper will, therefore, produce blackening (development) of the emulsion on photographic paper.

PROCEDURE

1. Make urine specimen strongly alkaline with sodium or potassium hydroxide. Watch for color formation (brown-black).
2. Place a drop of urine on sensitized photographic paper (this may be done in full daylight), and observe color for about 2 minutes.

INTERPRETATION. The paper, where spotted, turns coal black within 2 minutes if homogentisic acid is present. The test is reportedly specific for homogentisic acid; although, there is probably the possibility of drug interference.

DISCUSSION AND CLINICAL SIGNIFICANCE. Positive and negative controls should be tested at the same time. Homogentisic acid is a strong reducing agent (capable of reducing Benedict's and Fehling's reagent, with formation of a greenish-brown-black color, and eventually a black precipitate). Alkalinization of urine in the presence of atmospheric oxygen will result in formation of brown or black melanin-like pigments. Oxidation is more rapid at an alkaline pH, but does occur slowly even at an acid pH. Ascorbic acid can retard the oxidation.

The ferric chloride test applied to urine containing homogentisic acid may yield a transitory green color followed by development of a black precipitate (observed by one of the authors on a urine sample from a patient with the disease). Definitive identification can be made by two-dimensional paper chromatography. Homogentisic acid can be preserved in urine by adding 1 to 5 ml concentrated sulfuric acid/dl urine.

Homogentisic acid is present in the urine of patients with the metabolic defect known as "alcaptonuria." Other findings include development of degenerative changes and pigmentation of cartilage and calcification of the intervertebral discs, which develops slowly over the years.

MATERIALS AND REAGENTS

1. Sodium or potassium hydroxide, 10% (w/v)
2. Photographic paper

REFERENCES

1. Fishberg, E.: The instantaneous diagnosis of alkaptonuria on a single drop of urine. J.A.M.A., *119*:882, 1942.
2. Newberger, A.: The estimation of homogentisic acid. Biochem. J., *41*:431, 1947.
3. Newberger, A., Remington, C., and Wilson, J.: Studies on alkaptonuria. Investigations of a case of human alkaptonuria. Biochem. J., *41*:438, 1947.
4. Stanbury, J., Wyngaarden, J., and Fredrickson, D.: The Metabolic Basis of Inherited Disease. 4th Ed. New York, McGraw-Hill, 1978, p. 268.

CYSTINE

METHOD. Brand modification of Legal's test.

PRINCIPLE. The thiol (−SH) groups of cystine form a magenta-colored complex with nitroprusside in an alkaline medium. Cyanide prevents electrolytes from interfering with the reaction.

PROCEDURE

1. To 5 ml urine, add 2 ml sodium cyanide and mix by inversion.
2. Let stand 10 minutes.
3. Add a few drops of sodium nitroprusside solution.
4. Observe color.
5. Controls should be run.

INTERPRETATION. Cystine will cause formation of a stable magenta that will not be destroyed by boiling.

DISCUSSION AND CLINICAL SIGNIFICANCE. Nitroprusside is stable if kept in a dark bottle. The test is nonspecific and was originally devised for detection of acetone and acetoacetic acid (which give a ruby red that turns deeper following addition of acetic acid). Aspirin and salicylates (which give a positive Rothera test stable even after boiling) will not usually yield a positive Legal test result. If melanogens are present, the color after acidification is blue to blue-black, depending on concentration (due to formation of Prussian blue and melanin). Refer to the Thormählen test.

If positive, the test should be followed by a more definitive test for cystine, such as paper chromatography. In general, the Legal test has little value as urine with cystine in quantities sufficient to yield a positive test result usually contains microscopically visible cystine crystals. Cystine is present normally in urine; but only when present in abnormally excessive amounts is it in crystalline form. Spot tests are also available (Fischi, J., Sarson, L., and Segal, S.: A rapid spot test for the determination of cystinuria and aminoaciduria. Clin. Chem., 7:674, 1961).

MATERIALS AND REAGENTS

1. Sodium cyanide (NaCN), 5% (w/v)
2. Sodium nitroprusside ($Na_2FNO\ (CN)_5 \cdot 2H_2O$), 5% (w/v)
3. Test tubes, 13 × 100 mm
4. Dropper

REFERENCES

1. Brand, E., Harris, M., and Biloon, S.: Cystinuria: The excretion of a cystine complex which decomposes in the urine with the liberation of free cystine. J. Biol. Chem., *86*:315, 1930.
2. Isselbacher, K., et al.: Harrison's Principles of Internal Medicine. 9th Ed. New York, McGraw-Hill, 1979, p. 472.
3. Legal, E.: Ueber eine Neue acetonreaction und deren verwend barkeit zur harnuntersuchung. Bresl, Arztl, Ztschr., 5:25, 38, 1883.
4. Sullivan, M.: Studies on the biochemistry of sulfur. Further studies on the distinctive reaction for cystine and cysteine. Public Health Reports, *44*(Part 1-no. 1-26):1421, 1929.

ACID MUCOPOLYSACCHARIDES

METHOD. MPS screening test.

PRINCIPLE. The chondroitin sulfate A (chondroitin-4-sulfate) produces a visible metachromatic reaction with many dyes, especially azure A, in the MPS papers.

PROCEDURE

1. Prepare wash solvent by combining 0.1 ml glacial acetic acid, 20 ml anhydrous methanol, and 200 ml distilled water.
2. With forceps, transfer one MPS paper test square to a standard Petri dish.
3. Place one drop of well-mixed urine in center of test square. Urines that are cloudy or have been frozen must be centrifuged or filtered before testing. Wait 3 minutes.
4. Cover test square in Petri dish with wash solvent until dish is half full.
5. Rinse paper by gentle agitation for 10 minutes in solvent.
6. Remove test square with forceps and blot to remove excess solvent.
7. Interpret results.

INTERPRETATION

Negative: (AMPS within normal chemical range). No purple color seen, only pale blue background of paper. Any faintly blue spot not distinctly purple should be considered negative.

Positive: Distinct purple spot in center of paper where urine has been applied. Consider only purple color that forms on paper.

DISCUSSION AND CLINICAL SIGNIFICANCE. "Of all the acid mucopolysaccharidoses, among the many faults of human development, few equal in severity to changes wrought by the hereditable disorder known as the Hurler syndrome" (Andrew E. Lorintz, 1964). Basically, acid mucupolysaccharides are linear polyelectrolytes of high molecular weight consisting of repeating disaccharide units containing a sulfated hexosamine and a uronic acid group, in tissues attached to proteins through galactose and serine residues. Although the acid mucopolysaccharides are now called "glycosaminoglycoronoglycans," it is doutbful, according to Victor McKusick, that the term will ever become widely used, because of its complexity.

Hurler's syndrome is the most common acid mucopolysaccharide disorder; all forms of which, except Hurler's syndrome, are inherited as an autosomal recessive gene (Hurler's syndrome having a sex-linked recessive inheritance).

McKusick has classified the acid mucopolysaccharide disorders into six distinct clinical entities:

1. MPS I Hurler's syndrome
2. MPS II Hunter syndrome
3. MPS III Sanfilippo syndrome
4. MPS IV Morquio syndrome
5. MPS V Scheie syndrome
6. MPS VI Maroteaux-Lamy syndrome

Mucopolysaccharides were first recognized by John Thompson in 1900, and Hurler's syndrome was named in honor of Gertrude Hurler, who first published a description of patients matching those of Thompson. Hurler's syndrome is noted as "gargoylism," the latter being etymologically incorrect since the term "gargoyle" originally referred to "the person who carried rainwater away from columns," rather than to hideous chimeras.

The least acid mucopolysaccharide uronic acid that can be detected with MPS papers is about 0.2 mg/ml. Some urine specimens may induce a metachromatic reaction with MPS papers at low uronic acid levels when ionic content is diminished.

A number of related connective tissue disorders may or may not exhibit mucopolysacchariduria; including Marfan's syndrome, homocystinuria, alkaptonuria, Ehlers-Danlos syndrome, osteogenesis imperfecta, and pseudoxanthoma-elasticum (including the Grönblad-Strandberg syndrome).

MATERIALS AND REAGENTS

1. MPS strips (Ames Co.)
2. Wash solvent

Glacial acetic acid	1.0 ml
Methanol, anhydrous	20 ml
Distilled water	200 ml

3. Dropping pipette

REFERENCES

1. Ames Company brochure on test, and personal communications on July 11, 1973.
2. Berman, E., Vered, J., and Bach, G.: A reliable spot test for mucopolysaccharidoses. Clin. Chem., *17*:886, 1971.
3. Stanbury, J., Wyngaarden, J., and Fredrickson, D.: The Metabolic Basis of Inherited Disease. 4th Ed. New York, McGraw-Hill, 1978, p. 1282.

PORPHYRINS AND PORPHOBILINOGEN

METHOD. Anion resin exchange extraction, elution, and ultraviolet fluorescence and Ehrlich's aldehyde reaction.

PRINCIPLE. Urinary porphyrins are adsorbed to Dowex anion exchange resin, eluted with hydrochloric acid, and fluoresce red-pink when excited by ultraviolet light at 380 nm. Porphobilinogen can be similarly eluted with acetic acid, reacted with Erhlich's reagent and detected visually.

PROCEDURE

PORPHYRIN TESTING

1. Prepare the column by shaking vigorously until all the resin is resuspended. Allow the resin to settle in each column. Remove the caps and then snap off the tip, place in a test tube rack, and allow the columns to drain. Discard the runoff.
2. Add 4 ml aliquot of urine to each column and allow to drain. Discard the runoff.
3. Add a full reservoir (about 10 ml) of distilled water to each column and allow to drain. Discard the runoff. (Interfering materials are washed through the column in this step.)
4. Elute the porphyrins by adding 4 ml of 3 N HCl (in 2 ml portions for maximum porphyrin recovery). Collect the eluate in a test tube.
5. Examine the eluate under ultraviolet light.

PORPHOBILINOGEN TESTING

1. Prepare the column as above.
2. Wash in resin with 1 ml distilled water.
3. Add 4 ml aliquot fresh urine to the reservoir and allow to drain; discard the runoff.
4. Wash column with 7.5 ml distilled water.

5. Elute porphobilinogen with 2 ml 1 M acetic acid and 2 ml 0.2 M acetic acid; collect both eluate in same test tube.
6. Add 4 ml Ehrlich's reagent.
7. Observe for maximum color development in 5 minutes. (Distilled water can be used as a control.)

INTERPRETATION. A reddish-pink fluorescence indicates a positive test for porphyrins (uroporphyrins and coproporphyrins). A red color at 5 minutes with the Ehrlich's reagent is a positive test for porphobilinogen. This should be confirmed by extraction with chlorothen (urobilinogen complex is chlorothen extractable; porphobilinogen complex is not), followed by extraction with a butonal (melanogen complex is soluble, porphobilinogen is not).

DISCUSSION AND CLINICAL SIGNIFICANCE. All the usual variants of porphyria can be detected with this proposed scheme, including erythropoietic porphyria, porphyria cutanea tarda, and mixed varieties. The test for urinary porphobilinogen will detect acute intermittent porphyria and mixed porphyrias. If any of the screening tests are positive, appropriate quantitative procedures for urinary porphyrins, porphobilinogen, and delta-aminolevulinic acid should be performed.

MATERIALS AND REAGENTS

1. Dowex I-X8, 50/100 mesh chloride form, anion exchange resin in reservoirs (Bio-Rad Laboratories, Richmond, Calif. 94804)
2. Hydrochloric acid, concentrated and 3 N
3. Acetic acid, glacial, 1 M and 0.2 M
   (1M = 1:17.4 dilution glacial; 0.2 M = 1:5 dilution 1 M)
4. Distilled water
5. Test tubes, 15 ml conical (plastic tubes should not be used because some synthetic materials will interfere with observation of fluorescence)
6. Wood's ultraviolet light (emission about 380 μ)
7. Ehrlich's reagent III

p-dimethylaminobenzaldehyde, U.S.P.	15 g
concentrated hydrochloric acid	65.6 ml
Glacial acetic acid	194.4 ml

REFERENCES

1. Bio-Rad Laboratories technical bulletin on urine porphyrins. (Bio-Rad Laboratories, Richmond, Calif. 94804).
2. Castrow, F.: Complete office screening for porphyria. Cutis, 4:695, 1968.
3. Haining, R., Hulsch, T., and Labde, R.: Rapid porphyrin screening of urine, stool, and blood. Clin. Chem., 15:460, 1969.

DELTA-AMINOLEVULINIC ACID AND PORPHOBILINOGEN

METHOD. Double-column chromatography.

PRINCIPLE. Two-column chromatography procedure is used for the quantitative determination of both aminolevulinic acid (ALA) and

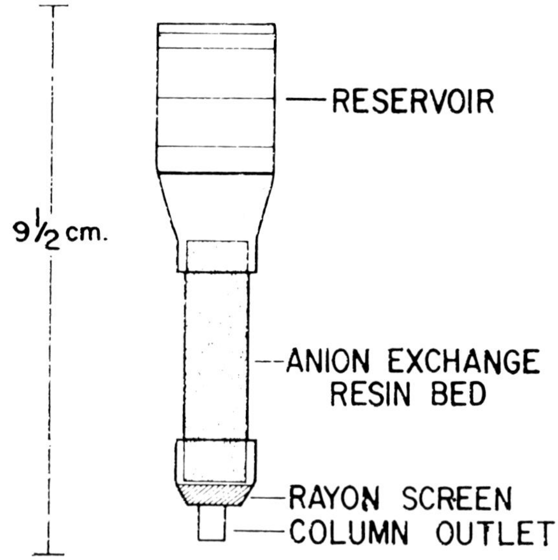

Fig. 1–41. Schematic diagram of disposable plastic column prepacked with anion exchange resin.

also porphobilinogen (PBG), the columns being used in a piggyback fashion (the top blue column removing PBG, and the bottom being clear, removing ALA). The Dowex resin is used to trap the compounds in addition to separating urea. The ALA is eluted then extracted with sodium acetate and reacted with acetylacetone; it is then coupled with Ehrlich's reagent to produce a faint yellow-to-pink color. Absorbance can be measured in a spectrophotometer at a wavelength of 555 nm.

SAMPLE. A random urine sample should be collected; however, it should not be the first morning voided specimen, the late evening specimens, or the specimen following excessive fluid intake. Urine should be acidified (acetic acid) and placed in the refrigerator or frozen. Frozen urinary ALA will remain constant up to 1 year, while frozen PBG will remain stable for 1 month.

ALA LEVELS

1. Collect fresh urine.
2. Add 0.1 ml of glacial acetic acid to 10 ml urine.
3. Freeze.

PBG LEVELS

1. Add approximately 10 ml random urine to an amber 15 ml screw-cap bottle without any fluid.

2. Add anhydrous powdered sodium carbonate to raise the pH to about 8.0. (Check with pH paper.)
3. Place the bottle in a dark refrigerator or freezer until ready to test. (The refrigerated urinary PBG will remain constant for 72 hours if it is unrefrigerated. Frozen, in alkaline urine, it will be constant for 8 months in the dark.)
4. When performance of porphobilinogen is desired, remove the bottle with urine from refrigerator and shake gently.

   Since urinary ALA is unstable at pH 8.0, the method of sample collection designed for the preservation or urinary PBG for 72 hours does not permit the measurement of urinary ALA in the urine specimen to which sodium carbonate has been added. Therefore, fresh urine must be used for ALA determinations.

PROCEDURE

ALA ANALYSIS

1. Place a blue Dowex exchange resin column on top of a clear column in piggyback fashion, after each has been shaken and resin resuspended.
2. Add distilled water to the column (approximately 10 ml), and allow to drain through both columns.
3. Pipette 0.5 ml random urine into the top column.
4. To each test add distilled water to the top of column, and permit to drain dry.
5. Do this two more times for a total of 30 ml wash volume/test. (It is important that all columns be completely drained.)
6. Remove and replace the top blue column into numbered test tubes if PBG result is desired, and save for PBG analysis. If only ALA is desired, discard the blue column.
7. The six aliquots of ALA-HCl stock solution can now be placed into test tubes as working standards as indicated in "Preparation of a Standard Calibration Curve."
8. Load the bottom clear columns of support rack into test tube racks.
9. Add 7 ml LM sodium acetate to each column and collect the drained liquid.
10. Remove and discard the bottom clear disposable column.
11. Pipette 0.2 ml acetylacetone to each test tube and mix.
12. Place test tubes in boiling water (90° C or greater) for 10 minutes; remove from water bath and allow to cool to room temperature.
13. Pipette 7 ml fresh Ehrlich's reagent to each tube and allow to stand 15 minutes.
14. If no color develops, test is negative and can be reported. If pink color develops, read absorbance of reaction at 555 nm and calculate from the standard curve.

PBG ANALYSIS

1. Remove the blue column from the wash rack as described above (step no. 6).
2. Add 10 ml 1 N acetic acid to each column.
3. Collect eluate.
4. Add 10 ml fresh Ehrlich's reagent to each test tube.
5. If no color develops, test is negative and can be reported. If pink color develops, read absorbance of reaction at 555 nm and calculate from the standard curve.

INTERPRETATION

Urinary ALA Range (ml/dl)	*Urinary ALA Code*	*Relationship to Lead Exposure*
0.00–0.54	Normal	None
0.55–0.99	Trace	Slight
1.00–1.49	1+	Moderate
1.50–1.99	2+	Heavy
2.00–2.99	3+	Severe
3.00–5.99	4+	Critical
6.00–10.00	5+	Overwhelming

Urinary PBG Range (ml/dl)	*Urinary PBG Code*	*Relationship to Porphyria*
0.00–0.03	Normal	None
0.04–0.19	Trace	Slight
0.20–0.49	1+	Moderate
0.50–1.99	2+	Heavy
2.00–3.99	3+	Severe
4.00–5.99	4+	Critical
6.00–10.00	5+	Overwhelming

The limit of detectability of PBG is 0.12 mg/dl.

DISCUSSION AND CLINICAL SIGNIFICANCE. The columns are capable of a 90% recovery of ALA and PBG, with a ±2% variation between samples.

The role of ALA testing in detecting industrial and general environmental lead poisoning has been clearly demonstrated. Cramer and Selander have investigated ALA testing in industry for several years. They comment on the urinary ALA test's economy and accuracy and particularly on its ability "to detect errors in the prophylactic measures at a very early stage before any symptoms have appeared." They further propose "that the ALA determination should be introduced into the regular statutory examination of lead workers, for it appears to give definite advantages in all cases."

In a survey publication from the State of California Department of Public Health, it was agreed that the concentration of blood lead in the population is now one-fourth to one-half of that recognized as hazardous to workers in industry. The margin of safety for workers in battery manufacturing, printing, and lead salvage, for example, is decreased by just this amount. The composite U.S. rural exposure to lead from the air is microgram per cubic meter and the composite urban exposure is 1.0 μg/M. However, several large increases from this level have been noticed recently. For example, a level of 25 μg/M has been determined over the Los Angeles freeways. Investigators in this field recommend that ALA in urine be used as a more sensitive test than blood lead. They further propose its use in future studies of lead distribution in the population.

The city of Chicago has paid particular attention to lead poisoning occurring in children who have ingested lead-containing paint and plaster. The Davis test for urinary ALA was developed with the active help of the Chicago Board of Health for the anticipated screening of large numbers of children under 7 years of age living in areas with high incidences of lead poisoning.

The major advantage of the urinary ALA test is that it is not just another measure of lead levels in the patient's system; it is, rather, the earliest measure of lead-induced metabolic derangement.

An article in the Lancet has discussed the detection of lead poisoning. Using the clinical symptoms of the disease as the primary criteria, several laboratory tests for lead poisoning are compared. The urinary ALA test showed by far the closest correlation with the clinical picture of lead poisoning of all major laboratory tests. Lancet also points out the poor correlation of urinary coproporphyrin and also urinary lead with the same clinical criteria.

The prolonged increase of urinary ALA due to lead exposure is a major advantage of testing for urinary ALA levels rather than blood lead. ALA levels remain increased for at least 1 year after lead exposure has been controlled. Blood-lead levels do not exhibit this constancy since lead exits the blood and is stored in the skeletal system. A random blood sample taken at this time can show a misleading normal lead level. When the stored lead is released, however, the dangerous effects of lead poisoning reappear. The detection of excessive lead exposure in asymptomatic individuals can be accomplished with a random sampling technique, if the urinary ALA test is used.

Davis and Andelman tested the urine of asymptomatic children who were positive for lead poisoning by urinary coproporphyrin standards; 85% of these coproporphyrin-positive children did not have elevated ALA levels and thus, were false-positive for lead poisoning. This high percentage of false-positive with the coproporphyrin test has been connected with iron-deficiency anemia rather than lead poisoning. Urinary ALA levels, on the other hand, are not elevated by iron-deficiency anemias. This lack of correlation between clinical symptoms and urinary coproporphyrin in adults and children has been noted by other investigators.

1.

Vol. of Standard Stock Solution (1 ml = 1.25 μg of ALA.HCl)	*μg of ALA Per Total Reaction Volume*	*Corresponding mg/dl Urinary ALA for 0.5 ml Sample of Urine Applied to the Column*
0.01 ml	1 μg	0.20 mg/dl
0.05 ml	5 μg	1.00
0.10 ml	10 μg	2.00
0.20 ml	20 μg	4.00
0.30 ml	30 μg	6.00
0.50 ml	50 μg	10.00

2. Dilute each of the six working standards to 7.0 ml mark with 1.0 M sodium acetate using graduated test tubes.
3. Pipette 7.0 ml of 1.0 M sodium acetate into an empty test tube to be used as a reagent blank.
4. Add 0.2 ml of acetylacetone to each tube and mix.
5. Place tubes in boiling water bath for 10 minutes, remove and cool to room temperature.

TABLE 1–35. Summary of the Primary Porphyrias and Their Clinical Aspects

Type	Synonyms	Clinical Manifestations	Laboratory Findings	Inheritance
Congenital (erythropoietic porphyria)	Congenital photosensitive; Gunther's disease	Photosensitivity hemolytic anemia with splenomegaly	Large amounts of uroporphyrin I and coproporphyrin I in bone marrow, erythrocytes, and urine	Homozygous for abnormal gene
	"Hydroa estivale" Erythropoietic protoporphyria	Solar urticaria or solar eczema	Increased protoporphyrin in bone marrow, erythrocytes, plasma and feces	Heterozygous for abnormal gene; latent cases frequent
Intermittent acute porphyria	Acute porphyria; porphyria hepatica; pyrro porphyria; Swedish type	Abdominal colics, hypertension, nervous system involvement; acute attacks frequent; photosensitivity absent	ALA and PBG in liver and urine	Heterozygous for abnormal gene; latent cases frequent
Photosensitive hepatic porphyria	Porphyria cutanea tarda hereditaria; mixed hepatic porphyria; South African genetic porphyria; variegate porphyria	Cutaneous abdominal, and neurologic. Acute attacks occur, usually precipitated by drugs	Copro- and protoporphyrin in liver and feces; during attacks, ALA, PBG, and porphyrins in urine	Heterozygous for abdominal gene; latent cases frequent

6. Add 7.0 ml of fresh Ehrlich's reagent to each tube, mix and let stand for 15 minutes for complete color development.
7. Set a colorimeter to 100% transmission at 555 nm using the reagent blank.
8. Read the optical density of the standards and unknowns.
9. Prepare a standard curve by plotting the concentrations of the standards against optical density.
10. Read the concentration of urinary ALA in the unknowns (0.5 ml urine sample applied to the column unit) in mg/dl from the standard calibration curve obtained.
11. To determine mg/dl PBG from the ALA standard calibration curve:
    A. Draw a horizontal line from the optical-density reading obtained with the PBG sample to the ALA standard calibration curve, which was previously plotted, and extend a line at right angles to the abscissa of the graph. This value of mg/dl should then be multiplied by the conversion factor of 3.53 in order to obtain the true value of mg/dl PBG in the 0.5 ml aliquot of urine applied to the column.
    B. Note: The conversion factor of 3.53 (mg/dl PBG = mg/dl ALA × 3.53) was obtained with authentic samples of PBG. Because of the difficulties involved in supplying authentic samples of PBG, however, it is recommended that ALA hydrochloride be used to plot an ALA standard calibration curve that, in conjunction with the conversion factor of 3.53, can be employed to calculate the mg/dl concentration of PBG in the 0.5 ml aliquot of urine applied to the column.

MATERIALS AND REAGENTS

1. Dowex I-X8, 50/100 mesh chloride form, anion exchange resin in reservoirs (Bio-Rad Laboratories, Richmond, Calif. 94804)
2. Hydrochloric acid, concentrated and 3 N
3. Acetic acid, glacial, 1 M and 0.2 M
   (1M = 1:17.4 dilution glacial; 0.2 M = 1:5 dilution 1 M)

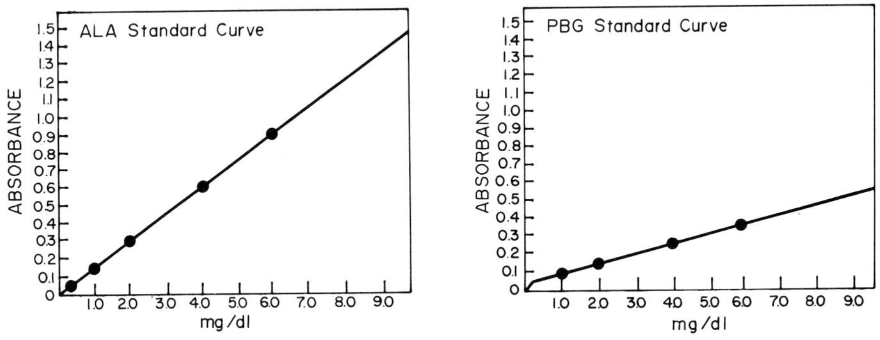

Fig. 1–42. Typical standard calibration curves.

4. Distilled water
5. Test tubes, 15 ml conical (plastic tubes should not be used because some synthetic materials will interfere with observation of fluorescence)
6. Spectrophotometer at 555 nm.
7. Ehrlich's reagent III

p-dimethylaminobenzaldehyde, U.S.P.	15 g
concentrated hydrochloric acid	65.6 ml
Glacial acetic acid	194.4 ml

REFERENCES

1. Bio-Rad Laboratories brochure on test.
2. Davis, J., and Andelman, S.: Urinary delta-aminolevulinic acid levels in lead poisoning. A modified method for the rapid determination of urinary delta aminolevulinic acid using disposable ionic-exchange chromatography columns. Arch. Environ. Health, *15*:53, 1967.
3. Needleman, H.: Preventing Lead Poisoning in Young Children. Atlanta, U.S. Department of Health, Education, and Welfare, Center for Disease Control, 1978.
4. Patterson, J., Catanzaro, C., and Dede, D.: Manual for Workshop on the Porphyrins and the Porphyrias. Chicago, ASCP Commission of Continuing Education, Council of Clinical Chemistry, 1966.

OCCULT BLOOD AND HEMOGLOBIN

METHOD. Benzidine test.

PRINCIPLE. Benzidine is oxidized to its blue form by oxygen liberated by the catalytic decomposition of hydrogen peroxide by the peroxidase activity of hemoglobin (or myoglobin or other similar substances).

PROCEDURE

1. Centrifuge 15 ml urine in a clinical centrifuge.
2. Decant supernatant.
3. Resuspend sediment in 0.5 ml remaining supernatant.
4. Mix equal quantities of benzidine and peroxide reagents in separate test tube.
5. Add 0.5 ml benzidine-peroxide mixture to test tube with supernatant and shake gently to mix.
6. Observe color.

OR

1. To 3 ml benzidine solution, add 2 ml urine.
2. Add 1 ml hydrogen peroxide.
3. Observe color.

INTERPRETATION. Blue developing within 1 minute is interpreted as positive for hemoglobin (and/or red blood cells).

DISCUSSION AND CLINICAL SIGNIFICANCE. Positive and negative controls should also be tested. Presence of detectable amounts of hemoglobin or blood in urine is abnormal. The test is highly sensitive, but not specific. The test is more sensitive than the Occultest tablet and guaiac tests, and is said to detect about 1 part blood in 64,000 parts urine. While these procedures can detect presence of red cells, the microscopic examination of urinary sediment remains the preferred method for red blood cell detection in urine, and is unsurpassed in sensitivity.

Caution should be employed in handling the reagent, as benzidine has been shown to be carcinogenic in animals.

MATERIALS AND REAGENTS

1. Benzidine dihydrochloride reagent

Benzidine dihydrochloride $(C_6H_4)_2(NH_2)_2 \cdot 2HCl$	1 g
Glacial acetic acid	20 ml
Distilled water	30 ml
95% (v/v) ethyl alcohol	50 ml

2. Hydrogen peroxide (fresh), 3% (v/v)
3. Test tubes, 15 ml conical
4. Clinical centrifuge
5. Serologic pipettes, 5 ml and 1 ml

REFERENCES

1. Derman, H., and Pauker, S.: Detection of occult blood in feces and urine. *In* Hemoglobin: Its Precursors and Metabolites. Edited by F. Sunderman and F. Sunderman, Jr. Philadelphia, J.B. Lippincott, 1964, p. 70.
2. Page, L., and Culver, P.: Syllabus of Laboratory Examinations in Clinical Diagnosis. Cambridge, Harvard University Press, 1961, p. 323.

OCCULT BLOOD AND HEMOGLOBIN

METHOD. Occultest method.

PRINCIPLE. Orthotolidine in the tablet is oxidized to its blue form by oxygen liberated by the catalytic decomposition of hydrogen peroxide produced by hemoglobin. Tartaric acid and calcium acetate in the tablet react with strontium peroxide to form the hydrogen peroxide. Sodium bicarbonate reacts with tartaric acid liberating carbon dioxide, which serves as an effervescent to facilitate solution of the reagents. A red dye is added to mask discoloration of the tablet by blood.

PROCEDURE

1. Place 1 drop of well-mixed centrifuged urine in the center of the filter paper.
2. Place Occultest tablet in center of moistened area.
3. Place 2 drops of water on tablet and allow water to run over edge of tablet.
4. Observe color on filter paper within 2 minutes.

INTERPRETATION. A diffuse blue on the filter paper around the tablet appearing within 2 minutes is a positive result. Disregard any color on tablet, or color on filter paper appearing after 2 minutes.

DISCUSSION AND CLINICAL SIGNIFICANCE. Positive and negative controls should also be tested. The test is specific for peroxidases, including hemoglobin, which have filtered through the glomerulus or been released from red cells in the urine by hemolysis. The manufacturer claims a sensitivity of 1 part blood in 100,000 parts of urine. Clinical investigators, however, have reported a sensitivity of 1 in 32,000 to 1 in 64,000 (corresponding to 10 to 15 RBC/HPF and 20 to 25 RBC/HPF, respectively). The test is one of the most sensitive of the chemical tests for hematuria, and is more sensitive than the Hemastix test. The microscopic examination of urinary sediment, however, is unsurpassed in detection of few (<10/HPF) red cells in the urine.

Iron and bismuth will not react with the tablets. Certain plant and bacterial components may produce a faint, transient blue color. When tablets become dark, discard them. If no gas bubbles form when 2 drops of water are placed on the tablet, decomposition of effervescent material has occurred, and sensitivity may be lost.

MATERIALS AND REAGENTS

1. Occultest tablets (Ames Company, Elkhart, Ind. 46514)
2. Dropping pipette

REFERENCES

1. Ames Company brochure on test.
2. Derman, H., and Pauker, S.: Detection of occult blood in feces and urine. *In* Hemoglobin: Its Precursors and Metabolites. Edited by F. Sunderman and F. Sunderman, Jr. Philadelphia, J.B. Lippincott, 1964, p. 70.
3. Kark, R., et al.: A Primer of Urinalysis. 2nd Ed. New York, Hoeber Medical Division, Harper & Row, 1963, p. 53.

OCCULT BLOOD AND HEMOGLOBIN

METHOD. Hemastix and Labstix tests.

PRINCIPLE. The stick contains orthotolidine, peroxide, and citrate buffers. Free heme derivatives are produced by the hemolytic action of reagents within the stick on impact with cells. The heme catalyzes oxidation of orthotolidine by oxygen received from hydrogen peroxide to its blue form. Optimum pH for the reaction is provided by citrate buffers.

PROCEDURE

1. Dip test end of strip into well-mixed urine or briefly pass strip through urine stream.
2. Observe color reaction 1 minute later.

INTERPRETATION. If the test end of the strip turns blue within 1 minute, the test is interpreted as positive. Although the manufacturer indicates that amounts of blood can be estimated semiquantitatively as "small," "moderate," and "large," the sensitivity of the test is so great that these designations have little clinical significance. It is, therefore, recommended that results be reported only if positive or negative. Absence of blue on the test strip at the end of 1 minute is interpreted as a negative test result.

DISCUSSION AND CLINICAL SIGNIFICANCE. Test positive and negative controls also. Positive results with Hemastix are specific for presence of red blood cells, hemoglobin, and/or myoglobin in the urine. No urinary constituent or drug metabolite has been found to date that will produce a false-positive reaction. Unlike some chemical tests for occult blood, Hemastix does not react with large quantities of iodine in the urine. Hemastix is more reactive in urine containing free hemoglobin than in urine containing intact red blood cells, inasmuch as hemoglobin directly catalyzes the oxidation, whereas the red cells must first be lysed. Ascorbic acid in high concentration may retard or inhibit the chemical reaction of hemoglobin with peroxide. Certain antibiotics (Terramycin, Achromycin, Panmycin, Tetracyn, and others) contain large amounts of ascorbic acid as a preservative. We do not know if the amount is sufficient to interfere with this test.

Orthotolidine has been reported to be 1 to 10 times more sensitive than benzidine reaction, which in turn is 10 to 1000 times more sensitive than the guaiac test, depending on test conditions. The test will detect blood diluted 1 to 8,000 with urine (corresponding to about 200 RBC/HPF), whereas the Occultest tablet detects blood in dilution of 1 to 32,000 (~20 RBC/HPF). The microscope, however, remains the primary instrument for red blood cell detection in urine and is unsurpassed in sensitivity.

The reagent strips are stable when stored away from high temperature and moisture.

MATERIALS AND REAGENTS

1. Hemastix reagent strips (Ames Company, Elkhart, Ind. 46514).

REFERENCES

1. Ames Company brochure on test.
2. Derman, H., and Pauker, S.: Detection of occult blood in feces and urine. *In* Hemoglobin: Its Precursors and Metabolites. Edited by F. Sunderman and F. Sunderman, Jr. Philadelphia, J.B. Lippincott, 1964, p. 70.

MYOGLOBIN

METHOD. Ammonium sulfate test.

PRINCIPLE. (Urine is first tested for protein with sulfosalicylic acid to be sure that some is present before proceeding with the test.) 80% (w/v) ammonium sulfate does not precipitate myoglobin, but does precipitate hemoglobin and other proteins, and denatured myloglobin. Saturated ammonium sulfate precipitates myoglobin as well as other urinary pigments, but not dyes.

SAMPLE. Test may be done on fresh urine or on refrigerated urine preserved by adjusting pH to 7.0 to 7.5 with dilute sodium hydroxide.

PROCEDURE

1. To 1.0 ml urine in a test tube, add 3.0 ml sulfosalicylic acid.
2. If a precipitate develops, continue test; if not, protein is not present, and the test is negative.
3. To a tube of 5 ml of fresh urine, add 2.8 g ammonium sulfate. Cap tube. Dissolve by shaking. (This brings urine to 80% (w/v) saturation.) To second tube, add 5 ml control urine and treat like unknown.
4. Filter both specimens, or centrifuge at 2500 rpm for 10 minutes (RCF about 1365).
5. Observe color of filtrate or supernatant as compared to control urine.

INTERPRETATION. The test is applied only if the urine is discolored red or brown-black. If the filtrate or supernatant is still red or brown-to-black, myoglobin or metmyoglobin, or both, are present. If the pigment has been precipitated and the filtrate is clear, the precipitated pigment is hemoglobin.

To confirm the presence of myoglobin (as opposed to dye, for example), add 0.8 g ammonium sulfate (or enough to get a supersaturated solution), shake, and centrifuge as above. The supernatant should be clear, since myoglobin will precipitate with saturated ammonium sulfate.

DISCUSSION AND CLINICAL SIGNIFICANCE. Myoglobinuria can be distinguished definitively from hemoglobinuria by spectroscopic (Bowden, et al.: Med., *35*:335, 1956) or electrophoretic (Prankard: Br. J. Hemat., *2*:80, 1956) methods; but, the present method may be useful for screening purposes. Porphyrins, homogentisic acid, drugs and dyes (pyridium) will color urine red, but will not precipitate with 3% (w/v) sulfosalicylic acid; hence, the reason for testing for protein before proceeding further.

MATERIALS AND REAGENTS

1. Ammonium sulfate, granular
2. 3% (w/v) aqueous sulfosalicylic acid
3. Test tubes, 13 × 100 mm
4. Serologic pipettes, 5 ml
5. Whatman no. 2 or no. 4 filter paper and filter funnel
6. Clinical centrifuge

REFERENCES

1. Blonheim, S., Margoliash, E., and Shafir, E.: A simple test for myohemoglobinuria (myoglobinuria). J.A.M.A., *167*:453, 1958.
2. Kagen, L.: Serum myoglobin. Arch. Int. Med., *139*:628, 1979.
3. Morgan, C.: Study on myoglobin. I. Solubility of myoglobin in concentrated ammonium sulfate solution. J. Biol. Chem., *112*:557, 1963.

BILE

METHOD. Foam test.

PRINCIPLE. Because lyophilic sols such as bile salts lower the surface tension, and because of the yellow color of bilirubin, urine containing these substances in increased amounts will readily form yellow foam when shaken.

PROCEDURE

1. Shake a small aliquot of urine vigorously in a test tube.
2. Observe for yellow foam.

INTERPRETATION. Copious yellow foam indicates pathologically increased concentration of bilirubin and bile salts.

DISCUSSION AND CLINICAL SIGNIFICANCE. This test is a relatively crude qualitative test for the presence of bile. Positive results should be confirmed by a specific test for bile. Proteins, mucoproteins, and mucin are the chief agents normally causing urinary foam (white foam). Phenylazodiaminopyridine, a urinary lyophilic azo dye antiseptic, will produce a yellow foam similar to that produced by bile pigments. Hay's test (sprinkling flowers of sulfur on urine and observing for sinking) is also dependent upon lowering of surface tension by bile salts. Normally, flowers of sulfur float on urine.

Only conjugated bilirubin can escape from the blood stream into the urine, so that increased concentrations of bile in urine suggest hepatic pathology or posthepatic obstruction to flow of bile, with serum concentration of bilirubin $\geq$4 mg/dl. At levels higher than this, urine concentration is usually 25 to 30% of serum concentration.

MATERIALS AND REAGENTS

1. Urine
2. Test tube

REFERENCES

1. Bodansky, M.: Biochemistry of Disease. New York, Macmillan, 1952, p. 408.
2. Newell, R., and Duke, B.: Workship on Urinalysis and Renal Function Studies. Chicago, American Society of Clinical Pathologists, 1962, p. 118.
3. Page, L., and Culver, P.: Syllabus of Laboratory Examinations in Clinical Diagnosis. Cambridge, Harvard University Press, 1961, p. 294.

BILE PIGMENTS

METHOD. Rosenbach's modification of Gmelin's reaction.

PRINCIPLE. Nitric acid (or sulfuric acid) oxidizes bilirubin into biliverdin (green), bilicyanin (blue), choletelin (yellow) and other derivatives, which appear as bands of rainbow colors at the junction of the acid and bile pigments.

PROCEDURE

1. Place 5 ml of urine in a clean test tube.

2. Overlay carefully with 1 to 2 ml concentrated nitric acid, so that two layers are formed.
3. Observe for a rainbow band of colors at the interface.

OR

1. Acidify 10 to 20 ml urine with 1 to 2 drops dilute (about 1 N) HCl, and filter through heavy filter paper (Whatman no. 4 is satisfactory).
2. Introduce 1 drop concentrated nitric acid into the apex of the paper, then unfold it.
3. Observe for rainbow band of colors.

INTERPRETATION. A rainbow of colors (succession of brown-red, red, purple, violet, blue, and green, from the center of the reaction outward) at the nitric acid-urine interface is produced by oxidation of bilirubin pigments (including monoglucuronides, diglucuronides, and sulfated esters).

DISCUSSION AND CLINICAL SIGNIFICANCE. The Gmelin reaction provides only a crude indication of the presence of bile pigments by their oxidative properties. Hematoporphyrin, a hematoidin-like compound which does not usually exist in the body, may give the same Gmelin reaction. Hematoidin, the iron-free molecule formed during the process of hemoglobin degradation, is related to bilirubin but will not give the same play of rainbow colors.

Quantitative determination of bile pigments in bile or urine may be performed in special instances (Schmidt, C., Jones, K., and Ivy, A.: method for determination of total pigments in bile which is applicable to "biliverdin biles." Proc. Soc. Exp. Biol. Med., *34*:17, 1937).

MATERIALS AND REAGENTS

1. Concentrated nitric acid
2. 1 N HCl
3. Test tubes, 13 × 100 mm
4. Filter paper (Whatman no. 4)
5. Dropping pipettes

REFERENCES

1. Kolmer, J., Spaulding, E., and Robinson, H.: Approved Laboratory Technic. 5th Ed. New York, Appleton-Century-Crofts, 1957, p. 162.
2. Lillie, R.: Histopathologic Technic and Practical Histochemistry. 4th Ed. New York, McGraw-Hill, 1976, p. 394.
3. Rosenbach, O.: Die chronsaure ais reagens auf eiweiss und gallenfarbstoff. Deutsche Med. Wschr., *18*:381, 1892.

BILE PIGMENTS

METHOD. Harrison test.

PRINCIPLE. Bile pigments are absorbed from urine onto barium chloride. The residue (barium plus pigments) is treated with a reagent consisting of ferric chloride in trichloracetic acid solution, which oxidizes bilirubin pigments (Gmelin reaction) to blue-colored (cholecyanin or bilicyanin), green-colored (biliverdin) or yellow-colored (choletelin) complexes.

PROCEDURE

1. Transfer 5 ml of urine to a small test tube.
2. Add 5 ml of barium chloride and mix well.
3. Filter through Whatman no. 2 filter paper. Fold filter paper and blot to get rid of excess fluid without losing residue. (Save the filtrate for urobilinogen or other determinations.)
4. Place the same folded filter paper containing the residue into an evaporating dish.
5. Add several drops of Fouchet's reagent to the center of the paper over residue and observe the colors.

INTERPRETATION. Development of a blue-to-green color is interpreted as indicating presence of bile pigments.

DISCUSSION AND CLINICAL SIGNIFICANCE. The normal concentration of bile pigments in urine (about 0.05 mg/dl) is not detectable by this method, which will detect about 3.0 mg bilirubin/dl urine; whereas, Ictotest tablets will detect about 0.05 to 0.1 mg bilirubin/dl. Salicylates and aspirin may react with Fouchet's reagent and give a false-positive test.

MATERIALS AND REAGENTS

1. Fouchet's reagent:

25% (w/v) trichloracetic acid	90 ml
10% (w/v) aqueous $FeCl_3$	10 ml

2. 10% (w/v) aqueous $BaCl_2 \cdot H_2O$
3. Test tubes, 13 × 100 mm
4. Filter paper (Whatman no. 2) and filter funnel
5. Droppers

REFERENCES

1. Godfried, E.: Clinical tests for bilirubin in urine. Biochem. J., *28*:2056, 1934.
2. Henry, J. (ed.): Clinical Diagnosis and Management by Laboratory Methods. 16th Ed. Vol. 1. Philadelphia, W.B. Saunders, 1979, p. 570.

BILIRUBIN

METHOD. Free and Free's Ictotest method.

PRINCIPLE. The reagent tablet contains p-nitrobenzene diazonium p-toluene sulfonate (bilazo) which couples with bilirubin to produce a blue to purple color. Sulfosalicylic acid in the tablet provides the proper pH; and sodium bicarbonate, together with the sulfosalicylic acid, acts as an effervescent.

PROCEDURE

1. Place 5 drops of urine on one square of the special test mat provided.

2. Place Ictotest tablet in center of urine-moistened area.
3. Allow 2 drops of water to flow onto tablet from dropper and observe color after 30 seconds.

INTERPRETATION. The reaction should be interpreted according to the color of the mat around the tablet as follows:

1. No color change or pink or red color: negative
2. Blue-to-purple color: positive

The speed of development and intensity of the color reaction may be roughly proportional to the amount of bilirubin present, although this is not consistently so.

DISCUSSION AND CLINICAL SIGNIFICANCE. Unlike the Harrison spot test (using Fouchet reagent), the tablets do not react with salicylates or aspirin. The tablets also will not react with urobilin. False-positive and false-negative reactions are rare. The test will reliably detect between 0.05 and 0.1 mg bilirubin/dl urine, which is just above the upper limit of normal.

The tablets are effervescent and hydroscopic and should be protected from moisture. The diazonium will decompose in light, so store in a brown bottle. The tablets will retain usefulness, even if they darken, as long as they are kept dry.

MATERIALS AND REAGENTS

1. Ictotest tablets and mats (Ames Company, Elkhart, Ind. 46514)
2. Dropping pipettes

REFERENCES

1. Ames Company brochure on test.
2. Free, A., and Free, H.: A simple test for urine bilirubin. Gastroent., *24*:414, 1953.
3. Godfried, E.: Clinical tests for bilirubin in urine. Biochem. J., *28*:2056, 1934.
4. Klatskin, L., and Klatskin, G.: An improved test for bilirubin in urine. N. Engl. J. Med., *248*:712, 1963.

PORPHOBILINOGEN AND UROBILINOGEN (QUALITATIVE)

METHOD. Watson-Schwartz.

PRINCIPLE. Porphobilinogen and urobilinogen form red pigments with Ehrlich's aldehyde reagent. The urobilinogen-aldehyde complex is soluble in chloroform; the porphobilinogen-aldehyde complex is insoluble in both chloroform and in n-butanol.

SAMPLE. The urine specimen to be tested should be fresh, since urobilinogen is converted to urobilin and porphobilinogen is converted to porphobilin on standing.

PROCEDURE

1. Transfer 54 ml of urine to a test tube.
2. Add 5 ml of Ehrlich's aldehyde reagent.
3. Mix and observe for development of red-to-pink color.
4. Add 10 ml saturated sodium acetate solution.
5. Mix and observe for development of pink or red color. If no color

develops, the test is negative. If color develops, follow steps 6 through 9.

6. Transfer to a small separatory funnel.
7. Add 10 ml chloroform, shake well, and allow to separate.
8. If chloroform becomes pink or red, and color remains in aqueous (lower) layer, remove chloroform and discard and re-extract with fresh chloroform, until no more color is extracted into the chloroform from the aqueous layer.
9. If pink color still remains in the aqueous layer, extract it with 10 ml of n-butanol. If color is extracted incompletely (into the lower, n-butanol layer), re-extract as in step 8, until no more color is extracted into n-butanol.

INTERPRETATION. Pink pigment extractable by chloroform is caused by the presence of urobilinogen. Pink pigment remaining in the aqueous layer after complete extraction with chloroform then with n-butanol is caused by porphobilinogen. Pink color remaining in the aqueous layer after extraction with chloroform, but extractable by n-butanol indicates presence of substances other than urobilinogen or porphobilinogen, such as melanogens.

DISCUSSION AND CLINICAL SIGNIFICANCE. Urobilinogen, porphobilinogen, and other substances can be detected by this benzaldehyde reaction. Positive reactions (may be red, orange, brown, or other off-colors), which indicate that the substances are chloroform-soluble, may also result from presence of indole derivates, sulfonamides, procaine, metabolic products of cascara sagrada. Chloroform-insoluble Ehrlich-reacting substances include melanogens and drugs (Sedormid). These and probably other Ehrlich-reacting substances are extracted by n-butanol.

When large amounts of urobilinogen are present, a single extraction with chloroform may not be sufficient, and the color remaining in the aqueous layer may mistakenly be regarded as a positive test for porphobilinogen. On the other hand, it is possible for both urobilinogen and porphobilinogen to be present in the same urine.

Bilirubin will interfere with the reaction by giving a green color with Ehrlich's reagent (remove by $BaSO_4$ precipitation-Gmelin test). Hyperlipemic or hyperalbuminemic serum will produce turbidity that will interfere with the photometric reading. Impure sodium acetate may not give proper reaction. Many drugs can color urine red to orange (see above).

Urobilinogen occurs in increased amounts in the urine of patients with hemolytic anemia, of those with liver disease, and in patients with intestinal stasis.

Presence of porphobilinogen suggests a diagnosis of acute intermittent porphyria.

MATERIALS AND REAGENTS

1. Ehrlich's aldehyde reagent, modified (Fisher Scientific Products, Pittsburgh, Pa. 15219)

Distilled water	100 ml
Conc. HCl (A.R. Grade)	150 ml
p-Dimethylaminobenzaldehyde	0.7 g

2. Saturated sodium acetate (199 g/dl at room temperature; 170 g/dl at 100° C).
   It is customary to allow solution to sit over excess crystals; in this case, care should be taken not to agitate when removing aliquot.
3. Chloroform (reagent grade)
4. n-butanol (reagent grade)
5. Test tubes, 13 × 100 mm
6. Volumetric pipettes, 10 ml and 5 ml
7. Separatory funnel, 50 ml
8. Propipettes

REFERENCES

1. Ludwig, G.: Urinary excretion of indole causing false-positive Watson-Schwartz for porphobilinogen. J. Clin. Invest., *37*:914, 1958.
2. Watson, C.J., and Schwartz, S.: A simple test for urinary porphobilinogen. Proc. Soc. Exper. Biol., *47*:395, 1941.
3. Watson, C., Bossenmaier, I., and Cardinal, R.: Acute intermittent porphyria. J.A.M.A., *175*:1087, 1961.
4. Watson, C., Taddeini, L., and Bossenmaier, I.: Present status of the Ehrlich-aldehyde reaction for urinary porphobilinogen. J.A.M.A., *190*:501, 1964.

UROBILINOGEN

METHOD. Urobilistix.

PRINCIPLE. Ehrlich's agent (paradimethylaminobenzaldehyde) will react with urobilinogen in a strongly acidic medium to form a reddish color.

SAMPLE. A fresh, random urine specimen.

PROCEDURE

1. Dip the strip into the fresh urine.
2. Tap the edges of the strip against the side of the container or against solvent paper to remove the excess.
3. At 60 seconds, compare the reagent area of the strip to color chart.

INTERPRETATION. The results are read directly in Ehrlich units/dl and no calculations are required when compared to the color chart. The normal urinobilinogen is less than 1 Ehrlich unit/dl. The reagent area will react in quantities as small as 0.1 Ehrlich unit/dl.

DISCUSSION AND CLINICAL SIGNIFICANCE. Urinobilinogen is very unstable when exposed to temperature and daylight; urine should be tested in the fresh state. Inasmuch as the reagent strips can oxidize, they should be kept in a tightly closed bottle and stored at room temperature, but not in a refrigerator.

The test area will react with interfering substances such as paraminosalicylic acid, porphobilinogen, azo dyes (as in drugs like Pyridium, Axo Gantrisin, and Azotrex used for treatment of urinary tract infections) giving a golden color and thus masking the reaction. The absence of urobilinogen cannot be confirmed with this test.

MATERIALS AND METHODS

1. Urobilistix (Ames Company, Elkhart, Ind. 46514)
2. Urine bottles

REFERENCES

1. Ames Company brochure on the test.
2. Hager, C., and Free, A.: Urine urobilinogen as a component of routine urinalysis. Am. J. Med. Tech., 36:227, 1970.
3. Henry, J. (ed.): Clinical Diagnosis and Management by Laboratory Methods. 16th Ed. Philadelphia, W.B. Saunders, 1979, p. 568.

UROBILINOGEN (QUANTITATIVE)

METHOD. Watson-Henry. There is a good review of the subject in the textbook Clinical Chemistry: Principles and Technics, by Richard J. Henry, M.D., published by the Hoeber Medical Division of Harper & Row, New York, on pages 608 to 617. According to Henry, color produced in the formerly widely employed Wallace-Diamond test is not due primarily to urobilinogen. For this reason, among others, we prefer the method of Watson, as modified by Henry, presented here.

PRINCIPLE. Urobilinogen and other reactive substances, including porphobilinogen and melanogens, react with Ehrlich's aldehyde reagent, producing a red color. Ascorbic acid acts as a reducing agent. Acidity of the mixture is decreased by subsequent addition of sodium acetate, which intensifies the urobilinogen-aldehyde color while inhibiting formation of indole and skatole derivatives. The blank is prepared by adding sodium acetate prior to addition of Ehrlich's reagent, preventing development of the urobilinogen-aldehyde pigment. Phenolsulfonphthalein is used as the standard, rather than the pontacyl dyes recommended by Watson.

SAMPLE. Because some authorities have found diurnal variation in urobilinogen output (the peak occurring in the afternoon between noon and 4 P.M.), it is usual to collect urine for a 2-hour period during midafternoon. Also, urobilinogen clearance varies with urinary pH, increasing from a rate of 2 ml per minute at pH 5, to a rate of 25 ml per minute at pH 8.0. Therefore, most reproducible results are obtained by alkalinizing the urine beforehand with oral administration of sodium bicarbonate. According to Milne, in many individuals the afternoon excretion rate may be 20 to 30 times that of the nocturnal excretion rate, and the direct swing may persist even after stabilization of urinary pH by sodium bicarbonate ingestion. Urobilinogen is not stable in urine at room temperature. Oxidation can be slowed by use of a dark collection bottle containing petroleum ether. Sodium carbonate must be added to prevent extraction of urobilinogen into the petroleum ether. According to Henry, samples may be stable for 1 month if frozen, but may show decreases ranging up to 60% following refrigerator storage for 18 hours. Sunlight or bright daylight speeds up the rate of oxidation and should be avoided.

PROCEDURE

1. At 1:00 P.M., have the patient drink a large glass of water containing a teaspoonful of sodium bicarbonate. At 2:00 P.M., have patient void, discard urine, and record exact time of voiding. Have patient void again at 4:00 P.M., collecting entire specimen. Record volume and exact time of collection.
2. Test urine for bilirubin. If more than a trace amount is present, remove by mixing 2.0 ml 10% (w/v) $BaCl_2$ with 8.0 ml urine and filtering. Final result must be corrected for dilution by multiplying by 1.25.
3. Dissolve 100 mg ascorbic acid in 10 ml clear urine, mix, and transfer 1.5 ml clear urine to each of two tubes, labeled "B" and "U," respectively.
4. To tube "B," add 3 ml standard sodium acetate, mix well, then add 1.5 ml Ehrlich's reagent and mix again.
5. To tube "U," add 1.5 ml Ehrlich's reagent, mix thoroughly, and immediately add 3.0 ml saturated sodium acetate.
6. Measure absorbance of "U" and "B" within 5 minutes, against distilled water at 560 nm (a 540 nm filter may be used).
7. Read PSP standard against distilled water at same wavelength.

CALCULATIONS:

$$\text{Ehrlich units per dl urine} = \frac{AU - AB}{AS} \times 0.346 \times \frac{6.0}{1.5}$$

$$\text{Ehrlich units per dl urine} = \frac{AU - AB}{AS} \times 1.38$$

Where AU equals absorbance of the unknown, AB equals absorbance of the blank and AS equals absorbance of the standard. One Ehrlich unit is equivalent to 1 mg urobilinogen.

NOTES. The spectral absorption of urine PSP is very similar to that of the urobilinogen-aldehyde complex between 530 and 570 nm. It is used because pure urobilinogen is not available commercially.

The method cannot be employed in presence of proteinuria because of formation of turbidity.

QUALITY CONTROL. Frozen urine with high concentration of urobilinogen may be used as a positive control.

INTERPRETATION. Henry found values for 11 healthy adult females to range from 0 to 1.1 Ehrlich units per 2 hours, while values for adult males ranged from 0.3 to 2.1 Ehrlich units. In our laboratory (Earl K. Long Memorial Hospital), results from a total of 29 tests on urine from healthy adults, largely male, ranged from 0.35 to 1.2 Ehrlich units per ml. A total of 27 tests of urine from patients with various diseases, including sickle cell disease, pernicious anemia, and infectious hepatitis, yielded results from 0.1 to over 9 Ehrlich units per ml.

DISCUSSION AND CLINICAL SIGNIFICANCE. According to Milne, in the reference cited, a high urinary output of urobilinogen may be the result of any of the following: (*a*) high production rate, as in hemolytic disease, erythropoietic porphyria or thalassemia; (*b*) colonization of small intestine by bacteria; (*c*) prolonged transit time in lower ileum and ascending color; (*d*) hepato-biliary disease with reduced capacity to re-excrete urobilinogen in bile, or with portal-systemic venous shunts allowing direct entry of urobilinogen into systemic veins; or (*e*) highly alkaline urine. Low urinary output of urobilinogen may result from (*a*) nearly complete or complete obstructive jaundice, preventing entry of bilirubin into lumen; (*b*) administration of broad-spectrum antibiotic, reducing bacterial content of gut; (*c*) rapid transit time in lower ileum and ascending colon; (*d*) reduced total renal function; (*e*) inhibitors of proximal tubular secretion (for example, probenecid), or (*f*) highly acid urine.

It should be remembered that the intestinal bacteria normally reduce bilirubin (conjugated and unconjugated) to a number of compounds that are reabsorbed into the blood stream and then are re-excreted into the bile, or (to a relatively small extent) pass into the urine. The term "urobilinogen" is used in a generic sense, as it includes numerous different degradation products of bilirubin.

The circadian rhythm seen in excretion of urobilinogen is very great, exceeding that for ammonia, sodium, potassium, phosphate, calcium, and magnesium.

The Ames Company, a division of Miles Laboratories, Inc., has developed a reagent-strip stick test for urobilinogen in urine. The dipsticks are provided 50 to a screw-cap jar with a label containing a color chart against which developing color on the stick is to be compared. Chart colors are provided equivalent to concentrations of 0.1, 4, 8, 12, and 16 Ehrlich units per 100 ml of urine. The test is rapid, simple, and correlates fairly well with results by the semiquantitative method described above. On the whole, results tend to be somewhat lower by the dipstick method. Out of 27 tests on urines from diseased patients, we encountered only 1 false-negative result (on a patient with pernicious anemia).

MATERIALS AND REAGENTS

1. Ehrlich's reagent: Dissolve 0.7 g p-dimethylaminobenzaldehyde in 150 ml concentrated HCl (AR grade). Add dl distilled water and mix. Reagent is stable if stored in brown glass bottle.

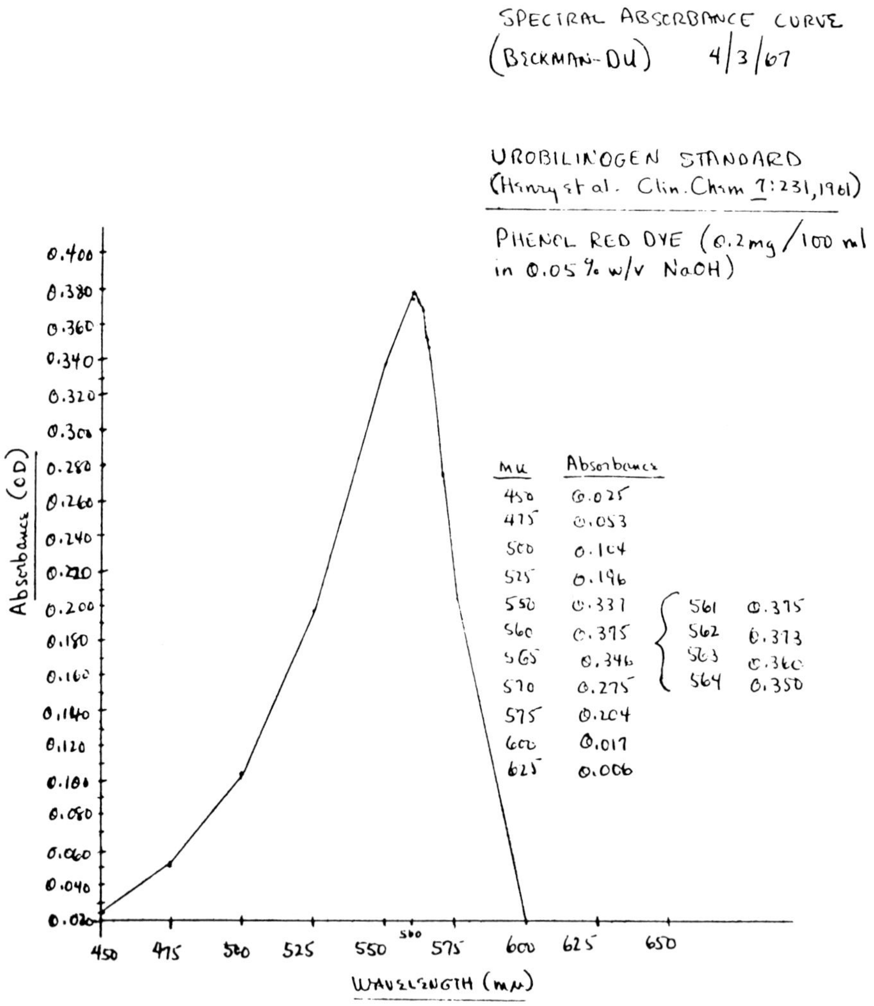

Fig. 1–43. Spectral Absorbance curve for urobilinogen ersatz standard using phenol red indicator dye.

2. Sodium acetate, saturated: Add 1000 g sodium acetate, AR triple hydrate, to 1 L of distilled water. Heat to approximately 60° C. When cooled, there should be an excess of crystals in the bottom.
3. PSP dye standard: Dissolve 20.0 mg phenolsulfonphthalein (PSP, phenol red) in dl 0.05% (w/v) NaOH. (The dye can be obtained from Eastman Kodak, British Drug Houses, La Motte and Mann.) Use the acid form. Dilute 1:100 with 0.05% (w/v) NaOH. Solution now contains 0.20 mg PSP per 100 ml colored solution, as read

in test. According to Henry, the working standard should have an absorbance 0.384 at 562 nm.

4. No special equipment other than spectrophotometer is needed.

REFERENCES

1. Bouchier, I., and Billing, B.: Bilirubin Metabolism. Philadelphia, F.A. Davis, 1967.
2. Henry, R.: Clinical Chemistry, Principles and Techniques. 2nd Ed. New York, Hoeber Medical Division, Harper & Row, 1974.
3. Moore, G., and Beeler, M.: Unpublished data.
4. Schwartz, C., Sborov, V., and Watson, C.: Studies of urobilinogen. The quantitative determination of urobilinogen by means of the Evelyn photoelectric colorimeter. Am. J. Clin. Path., *14*:598, 1944.
5. Watson, C., and Hawkinson, V.: Am. J. Clin. Path., *107*:108, 1947.
6. Watson, C., Schwartz, S., Sborov, V., and Bertiei, E.: Am. J. Clin. Path., *14*:605, 1944.

UROBILIN

METHOD. Schlesinger's test.

PRINCIPLE. After removal of bile pigments from the urine sample by barium chloride, and oxidation of urobilinogen to urobilin by addition of iodine, alcoholic zinc acetate is added to form a urobilin-zinc complex, producing green fluorescence in strong white light.

SAMPLE. Freshly voided urine.

PROCEDURE

1. Transfer 5 ml of urine, free of bile pigments (or $BaCl_2$ filtrate from urobilinogen determination) to a test tube.
2. Add 5 drops Gram's iodine solution.
3. Add 5 ml Schlesinger's reagent. (Shake reagent before using.)
4. Mix and filter or centrifuge. Filtrate should be clear.
5. Examine clear filtrate in strong white light.

INTERPRETATION. Presence of green fluorescence indicates more than normal amount of urobilin and urobilinogen in the urine. The minute amount of these substances normally present in urine is too small to be detectable by this test. (Urobilin may impart an orange tinge to urine when present in large amounts.)

DISCUSSION AND CLINICAL SIGNIFICANCE. This test will detect urobilin in concentration as low as 0.005 mg/dl urine and is 22.5 times more sensitive than determination by spectroscopic bands.

Normally, most urobilin is excreted in the feces, and the brown color of feces is thought to result, in part, from urobilin. Presence of urobilin in the urine has the same diagnostic significance as presence of urobilinogen. If the urobilinogen test is negative, urine should be checked for urobilin, since the former is oxidized to the latter upon standing. Pyridium will not interfere with the test.

The reaction, recorded by Jaffe, was applied to urine testing by Schlesinger. A similar reaction occurs with mercury. The zinc complex has absorption maxima at 637, 601, 551, and 521 nm; whereas, 1-stercobilin has absorption maxima at 638 and 520 nm only.

MATERIALS AND REAGENTS

1. 10% (w/v) barium chloride
2. Gram's iodine:

KI	2 g
Iodine	1 g
Distilled water	100 ml

3. Schlesinger's solution:

Zinc acetate (solid)	1 g
95% (v/v) ethyl alcohol	10 ml

4. Test tubes, 13 × 100 mm
5. Droppers
6. Strong white (fluorescent) light
7. Filter paper and filter funnel
8. Clinical centrifuge

REFERENCES

1. Jaffe, M.: Beitrag zur kenntnis der galeen-und ha pigments. Zentralbl. f. Med., 6:241, 1868.
2. Schlesinger, H.: Zum klinischen nachweis des urobilins. Deutsch. Med. Wschnschr., *32*:561, 1903.
3. Wallace, G., and Diamond, J.: Significance of urobilinogen in urine as a test of liver function. With a descriptive of a simple quantitative method for its estimation. Arch. Int. Med., *35*:698, 1925.

VERDOGLOBIN

METHOD. Visual inspection for color and ultraviolet-induced fluorescence.

PRINCIPLE. Verdoglobin may impart a bilious green to a tea color to urine. In addition, verdoglobin develops chalky-green fluorescence in ultraviolet light, and may be detectable by this before it is visually discernible in ordinary light.

PROCEDURE

1. To three 10 ml test tubes, add 1 ml urine.
2. To the first test tube, add 1 ml water; to the second test tube, add 1 ml glacial acetic acid; to the third test tube, add 1 ml ammonium hydroxide.
3. Examine test tubes in ordinary light and under ultraviolet light (Wood's lamp with a spectrum that includes wavelengths less than 380 nm).

INTERPRETATION. Verdoglobin is not normally present in urine, and when present, it is not detectable in ordinary light. A chalky-green fluorescence under ultraviolet light is suggestive of verdoglobinuria. By use of acid, neutral, and alkaline pH's, verdoglobin, pyocyanin, and fluorescin can be distinguished in urine under fluorescent light as follows:

	Acid (Acetic Acid)	*Neutral (Water)*	*Alkaline (Ammonia)*	
Pyocyanin	—	—	—	Staphylococcal septicemia
Fluorescin	—	green	green	Pseudomonas urinary tract infection
Verdoglobin	chalky-green	chalky-green	chalky-blue	Pseudomonas septicemia

DISCUSSION AND CLINICAL SIGNIFICANCE. Verdoglobin is a product of hemoglobin degradation in the reticuloendothelial system. In the case of pseudomonas infection of burned patients, it has been theorized that pseudomonas toxin (polysaccharide vs. endotoxin) inhibits degradation of hemoglobin after formation of verdoglobin. Therefore, verdoglobin accumulates in the blood and is excreted into bile. Pseudomonas organisms also contain potent hemolysins, which produce red cell destruction, thus making available hemoglobin for catalytic decomposition by the reticuloendothelial system.

Fluorescence in ultraviolet light appears to be a fairly accurate method for detecting verdoglobinuria days to weeks prior to the appearance of green urine and fatal gram-negative septicemia. The excretion may be intermittent, and increased by hydration enough to cause diuresis, or by a dressing change.

Fluorometric determination of the pseudomonas pigment, pyoverdin, has been used for many years to detect incipient pseudomonas spoilage of powdered eggs, but its value in assessing human infection is not great.

MATERIALS AND REAGENTS

1. Wood's lamp, or UV lamp with spectrum including wavelength less than 380 nm
2. Glacial acetic acid
3. 28% (v/v) ammonium hydroxide
4. Test tubes, 10 ml

REFERENCES

1. Polk, H., Jr., Ward, C., Clarkson, J., and Taplin, D.: UV light is said to spot infection of burn wounds. Medical Tribune, *8*:1, 1967.
2. Stone, H., Martin, J., and Graber, C.: Verdoglobinuria: an ominous sign of pseudomonas septicemia in burns. Ann. Surg., *159*:991, 1964.

MELANOGENS

METHOD. Thormählen test.

PRINCIPLE. Colorless chromogenic melanogens act as reducing agents, converting sodium nitroprusside to Prussian blue. In the process, the melanogens may be oxidized to black melanin-like pigment.

PROCEDURE

1. To 5 ml urine in a test tube, add a few crystals of sodium nitroprusside reagent and shake well.
2. Then add 20 drops sodium hydroxide until solution is strongly alkaline.
3. If a deep red color develops, acidify dropwise with glacial acetic acid and observe for the *immediate* development of a blue color.

INTERPRETATION. Deep ruby color will develop following addition of sodium hydroxide if melanogens, indole, acetone, or creatinine are present. A magenta color will appear if cystine is present. However, the immediate development of blue or black upon acidification indicates the presence of melanogens. After acidification:

Melanogen	Blue or black
Acetone/acetoacetic acid	Deep red
Creatinine	Yellow-green

DISCUSSION AND CLINICAL SIGNIFICANCE. The Watson-Schwartz test for urobilinogen, porphobilinogen and melanogen has already been described, as has the ferric chloride test (acetoacetic acid). Presence of melanogens in urine in sufficient quantities to detect by these simple tests occurs in only 20% of patients with malignant melanoma, and probably these all have widespread metastases. Melanogens do not give a positive Herter (naphthoquinone) test as does indole. Indican, an indole derivative, yields negative results with the Thormählen and Herter tests.

The ferric chloride test can detect melanogens, but is neither specific nor sensitive. The Ehrlich test is more sensitive, but it also is nonspecific. A more definitive test depends on extraction of urine with ethyl acetate, two-dimensional paper chromatography, and development of color with paranitrobromoaniline (Armstrong). Several urinary phenolic acids are consistently elevated in patients with pigmented melanomas, including homovanillic acid and, usually, vanilmandelic acid.

MATERIALS AND REAGENTS

1. Sodium nitroprusside reagent:

$Na_2FNO(CN)5 \cdot 2H_2O$	5 g
Ammonium sulfate crystals	100 g

2. 10% (w/v) aqueous sodium hydroxide
3. Glacial acetic acid
4. Test tubes, 13 × 100 mm
5. Dropper

REFERENCES

1. Armstrong, M., Straw, K., and Wall, P.: The phenolic acids of human urine. J. Biol. Chem., *218*:293, 1956.
2. Beeler, M.: Unpublished studies.
3. Beeler, M., and Henry, J.: Melanogenuria-evaluation of several commonly used laboratory procedures. J.A.M.A., *176*:136, 1961.
4. Rothman, S.: Studies on melanuria. J. Lab. Clin. Med., *27*:687, 1942.

5. Thormählen, J.: Mitteilunguber einen noch nicht bekannten Korper im pathologischen Menschenharn. Virchow's Arch. F. Path. Anat., *108*:17, 1887.

5-HYDROXYINDOLEACETIC ACID (5-HIAA)

METHOD. Sjöerdsma method.

PRINCIPLE. 1-Nitroso, 2-naphthol in presence of nitrous acid will form a purple complex with 5-hydroxytryptamine (serotonin) or 5-hydroxyindoleacetic acid (5-HIAA).

PROCEDURE

1. Run a negative and positive control for comparison.
2. Place 0.2 ml urine in a test tube.
3. Add 0.8 ml distilled water.
4. Add 0.5 ml 1-nitroso, 2-naphthol reagent and mix.
5. Add 0.5 ml nitrous acid and mix.
6. Let stand at room temperature (about 25° C) for 10 minutes.
7. Add 5 ml ethylene dichloride and shake with stopper on tube.
8. If turbid, centrifuge at 2500 rpm for 5 to 10 minutes in a clinical centrifuge.
9. Observe color of upper layer.

INTERPRETATION. A purple color in the upper layer is considered a positive reaction.

DISCUSSION AND CLINICAL SIGNIFICANCE. If 5-hydroxyindoleacetic acid is present in amounts greater than 8 mg/L, the upper layer turns purple. The test is for screening only. Substances known to or said to cause false-positive reactions include p-hydroxyacetanilide (a metabolite of acetanilide), some fruits, such as ripe bananas (in large quantities), and some tranquilizers. Color formation may be inhibited by large amounts of keto acids.

Normally, the liver metabolizes serotonin, and its principal urinary metabolite, 5-HIAA, is excreted (in amounts ranging from 2 to 8 mg/24 hours). In patients with argentaffine cell (Kutchitsky cell) or "carcinoid" tumors, excretion may exceed 25 mg/day (although excretion is variable diurnally and from day to day. Two-thirds of carcinoids metastasize very slowly and 15 to 25 years may elapse between appearance of the primary and appearance of metastases or death. Excessive serotonin excretion from carcinoids, especially when there are liver metastases, produces the carcinoid syndrome—skin flushing, patchy cyanosis, hypertension, right heart valvular (tricuspid) disease, congestive heart failure, asthma, and watery diarrhea. Mild-to-moderate elevations of 5-HIAA also may be seen in patients with adult celiac disease.

MATERIALS AND REAGENTS

1. 1-nitroso, 2-naphthol in 95% (v/v) ethanol, 0.1% (w/v)
2. Nitrous acid reagent:

2.5% (w/v) sodium nitrate (fresh)	0.2 ml
2 N sulfuric acid (prepare fresh daily)	5.0 ml

3. Ethylene dichloride, reagent grade
4. Propipette
5. Test tubes, 13 × 100 mm
6. Serologic pipettes, 1 ml, 5 ml

REFERENCES

1. Boutwell, J.: Clinical Chemistry, Laboratory Manual and Methods. Philadelphia, Lea & Febiger, 1961, p. 286.
2. Page, L., and Culver, P.: Syllabus of Laboratory Examination in Clinical Diagnosis. Cambridge, Harvard University Press, 1961, p. 286.
3. Path. Capsule no. 5, Chicago, College of American Pathologists, 1965.
4. Sjöerdsma, A.: Serotonin. N. Engl. J. Med., *261*:181 and 231, 1959.
5. Sjöerdsma, A., Weissbach, H., Udenfriend, S.: A simple test for diagnosis of metastatic carcinoid (argentaffinous). J.A.M.A., *159*:397, 1955.

INDICAN

METHOD. Obermayer test.

PRINCIPLE. Indican (potassium indoxyl phosphate) is oxidized to indigo blue (or red) by Obermayer's reagent. Bile pigments, which interfere with the reaction, are removed by barium absorption; and the red-violet generated by oxidation of iodides or thymol is suppressed with the reducing agent, thiosulfate.

PROCEDURE

1. Place 10 ml patient's urine in one test tube, and 10 ml normal urine (control) in another test tube.
2. Add 2 ml barium chloride, mix, and filter each specimen.
3. Transfer 5 ml of filtrate to separate clean test tubes.
4. Add 5 ml Obermayer's reagent to each tube and mix.
5. Add 2 ml chloroform to each tube and mix by inversion.
6. Allow specimen to settle and layer.
7. If lower (chloroform) layer is colorless, the test is negative.
8. If blue to red develops in lower layer, transfer it to another tube; add small crystal of thiosulfate, mix, and again observe for color.

INTERPRETATION. If blue or red color disappears, the test is negative. If color of control and patient's specimen are same, test is negative. If color of patient's specimen is more intense than control, test is positive.

DISCUSSION AND CLINICAL SIGNIFICANCE. Normal concentrations of indican in urine (2 to 4 mg/24 hours) are not detectable by this test.

Indole, skatol, cresol, and phenol arise from bacterial action (especially E. coli) on tyrosine and tryptophan, or from ingestion of benzene or other phenolic compounds. Large amounts of indole produced because of increased intestinal putrefaction are absorbed, oxidized in the body to indoxyl, esterified to indoxyl sulfuric acid and excreted in the urine as the potassium salt. Melanogens and indole will not give positive tests (since there is no substituted-C- on the pyrole ring to react).

Indole may cause interference in the tests for urobilinogen and porphobilinogen. Other than this, its presence in increased amounts in the urine is of little significance.

MATERIALS AND REAGENTS

1. Barium chloride, 10% (w/v)
2. Chloroform
3. Sodium thiosulfate crystals
4. Obermayer's reagent:

Ferric chloride ($FeCl_3$)	0.3 g
Conc. HCl	100 ml

5. Test tubes, 13 × 100 mm
6. Filter paper and funnel
7. Serologic pipettes, 10 ml

REFERENCES

1. Böhm, F.: Beitrag zur Kenntnis der Thormählenschen reaktion. Ztschr. f. Physiol. Chem., *258*:108, 1939.
2. Everett, M.: Medical Biochemistry. 2nd Ed. New York, Hoeber Medical Division, Harper & Row, 1946, p. 430.
3. Kolmer, J., Spaulding, E., and Robinson, H.: Approved Laboratory Technic. 5th Ed. New York, Appleton-Century-Crofts, 1951, p. 160.

CALCIUM

METHOD. Sulkowitch test.

PRINCIPLE. Calcium in the urine specimen reacts with ammonium oxalate to form insoluble calcium oxalate. The degree of precipitation is roughly proportional to the amount of calcium in the specimen. The additional chemicals in the Sulkowitch reagent prevent precipitation of phosphates and other urinary substances by providing a barely acid pH (although Hirsch Sulkowitch originally used 50% (w/v) acetic acid for this purpose).

SAMPLE. The patient should be on a neutral, low-calcium diet for at least 1 day before urine collection is made. A 24-hour urine specimen is preferable.

PROCEDURE

1. If urine is not clear, centrifuge or filter.
2. Place 3 ml of urine in a test tube, and add 3 ml of Sulkowitch reagent.
3. Mix and allow to stand for a few minutes.
4. Note the density of the precipitate.

INTERPRETATION. The turbidity is reported as follows:

Negative	No precipitate (Less than 5 mg/dl)
1+	Slight clouding (5–10 mg/dl)
2+	Definite clouding (10–15 mg/dl)
3+	Clouding throughout but not totally opaque (15–20 mg/dl)
4+	Opaque precipitate (over 20 mg/dl)

DISCUSSION AND CLINICAL SIGNIFICANCE. A negative test (0) suggests hypocalcemia (serum calcium less than 7.5 mg/dl). A constant 3+ to 4+ reaction suggests hypercalcemia (serum calcium greater than 11.0 mg/dl). If the serum calcium determination is not available, this test can be used in an emergency, especially when hypercalcemia is suspected, since this can be life-threatening.

MATERIALS AND REAGENTS

1. Sulkowitch reagent:

Oxalic acid	2.5 g
Ammonium oxalate	2.5 g
Glacial acetic acid	5.0 ml
Distilled water q.s. to	150 ml

2. Test tube, 13 × 100 mm
3. Filter paper and filter funnel
4. Clinical centrifuge

REFERENCES

1. Air Force Manual, Laboratory Procedures in Clinical Chemistry and Urinalysis. Gunter AFB, Alabama, pp. 18–4, March 15, 1962.
2. Barney, J., and Sulkowitch, H.: Progress in the management of urinary calculi. J. Urol., 37:746, 1937.
3. Latner, A.: Cantarow and Trumper Clinical Biochemistry. 7th Ed. Philadelphia, W.B. Saunders, 1975.

HEMOSIDERIN

METHOD. Lillie's Stain Technique (slightly modified).

PRINCIPLE. Fe^{++} is oxidized to Fe^{+++} by ferricyanide in an acid environment. In the process, ferricyanide is reduced to Prussian blue. Ferrocyanide reacts with Fe^{+++}.

PROCEDURE

1. Centrifuge 15 ml urine to obtain sediment, and decant supernatant.
2. Add 2 ml ferrocyanide-ferricyanide and 2 ml hydrochloric acid to sediment and mix.
3. Let stand 10 minutes, centrifuge, and decant supernatant.
4. Examine with microscope.

INTERPRETATION. Hemosiderin stains blue.

DISCUSSION AND CLINICAL SIGNIFICANCE. Hemosiderin is not normally found in urine. It may be present in urine of patients with hemolytic anemias, transfusion reactions, hemochromatosis, or hemosiderosis. With low concentrations of iron, low pH is essential for staining, but a green color may be produced at pH 3 to 4.

Hemosiderin consists of ferritin, the molecule of which has been assigned the formula $(FeOOH)_8\ FeOPO_3H_2$ and has a weight of about 460,000. Fe^{++} is demonstrated as Turnbull's blue; Fe^{+++}, as Prussian blue.

MATERIALS AND REAGENTS

1. Hydrochloric acid, 3% (v/v)
2. Ferricyanide-ferrocyanide solution

$K_4Fe(CN)_6 \cdot 3H_2O$	2.0 mg (for Fe^{+++})
$K_3Fe(CN)$	3.2 mg (for Fe^{++})
Distilled water q.s. to (mix fresh daily)	100 ml

3. Centrifuge
4. Microscope and microscopic slides

REFERENCES

1. Air Force Manual, Laboratory Procedures in Clinical Chemistry and Urinalysis. Gunter AFB, Alabama, Section 18–5. March 15, 1962.
2. Lillie, R.: Histopathologic Technic and Practical Histochemistry. 4th Ed. New York, Blakiston Division, McGraw-Hill Book Co., 1976, p. 454.

LIPID

METHOD. Sudan staining.

PRINCIPLE. Except for lipids and lipoids of high melting point (cholesterol, carotenoid, and paraffin), most lipids, including most neutral fats (triglycerides and tristearin) stain with oil-soluble dyes. Staining is based on the partition coefficient between solvent and lipid—that is, greater solubility of the dye in the lipids than in other solvents.

PROCEDURE. Place 1 drop of saturated Sudan III or IV at the edge of the coverslip and permit it to mix with urinary sediment by capillary action.

INTERPRETATION. Presence of fat indicated by yellow-orange to orange-red globules, which tend to collect at the edges of the coverslip.

DISCUSSION AND CLINICAL SIGNIFICANCE. Globules of stainable fat rarely appear in the urinary sediment unless they are in cells, since fat floats. (We have found no good normal studies recorded in the literature.) Lipemia is not usually accompanied by lipuria. Embolism from bone marrow fat causes lipuria if there is glomerular infarction. Renal tubular epithelial cells containing fat may be seen in urine of patients with degenerative tubular disease, the so-called "oval fat bodies," and in fatty casts. Probably the most common cause of "chyluria" is retroperitoneal malignancy, causing rupture of renal lymphatics distended because of obstruction, which releases fat into the urine. Unclean collection containers or oiled catheters, or soaps may contaminate urine with stainable fats or lipoids. Unstained droplets appear microscopically as round, highly refractile areas that may appear black under low-power examination with subdued light.

Some of the lipid seen in urine of patients with the nephrotic syndrome exhibits anisotropism—that is, it rotates a beam of polarized light and appears as shining maltese crosses against a dark field. Waxy casts may also exhibit anisotropism. Cholesterol esters are anisotropic, and so it has been assumed that maltese crosses are cholesterol esters. Neutral fats and fatty acids do not exhibit anisotropism.

MATERIALS AND REAGENTS

1. Sudan III and IV (saturated solution in 95% (v/v) ethyl alcohol)
2. Microscope and microscope slides
3. Dropping pipettes

REFERENCES

1. Lillie, R., and Fullmer, H.: Histopathologic Technic and Practical Histochemistry. 4th Ed. New York, McGraw-Hill, 1976.
2. Lippman, R.: Urine and the Urinary Sediment. A Practical Manual and Atlas. 2nd Ed. Springfield, Charles C Thomas, 1957, p. 26.

METACHROMATIC GRANULE DETECTION

METHOD. Toluidine Blue O Stain.

PRINCIPLE. Cerebroside sulfuric acid esters (sulphatides) formed in a demyelinating disease of the central nervous system and by alterations of epithelium (renal, biliary, etc.) stain brown with Toluidine Blue O. The reaction has yet to be fully characterized.

SAMPLE. Fresh, clean, uncontaminated urine sample is essential.

PROCEDURE

1. Examine a control specimen using fresh, "normal" urine.
2. Place 10 ml urine in a centrifuge tube.
3. Centrifuge 2500 rpm (RCF ca. 375) for 5 to 10 minutes. Decant and discard supernatant.
4. Add 2 drops aqueous Toluidine Blue O.
5. Mix well; transfer a drop of urine to a glass microscope slide; apply coverslip.
6. Examine under microscope (10X and 43X).

INTERPRETATION. Golden brown granules or granular bodies either singly (3 to 5 μ) or in "mulberry" clusters (10 to 25 μ), free or in cells or casts are "metachromatic bodies."

DISCUSSION AND CLINICAL SIGNIFICANCE. The test is only a screening procedure and is suggestive but not diagnostic of hereditary metachromatic leukodystrophy. Confirmation of excess sulfatide excretion should be made by chemical determination of arylsulfatase A activity. The granules, in polarized light, are doubly refractile ("Maltese-cross" effect), and migrate to the anode at pH 12. Metachromatic granules also stain with PAS, aniline, methylene blue (red color), thionine, and other dyes. The granules will not stain with Sudan IV or Turnbull blue.

MATERIALS AND REAGENTS

1. Toluidine Blue O, 2% (w/v) aqueous
2. Test tube, 15 ml, conical
3. Clinical centrifuge

4. Dropper
5. Microscope, slides and coverslips

REFERENCES

1. Austin, J.: Metachromatic form of diffuse cerebral sclerosis. Diagnosis during life by urine sediment examination. Neurol., 7:415, 1957.
2. Helfant, M., Borgeson, M., and Hellstrom, B.: The value of urinary sediment examination as a screening method in suspected cases of metachromatic leukodystrophy. Acta Pediatr. Scand., 51:49, 1962.

URINARY SEDIMENT STANDARDIZED CONCENTRATION

METHOD. Kova system for microscopic examination.

PRINCIPLE. Centrifugation of a standardized amount of urine and then aspiration of a fixed amount of sediment is placed in a plastic chamber of constant volume for microscopic evaluation. This permits reproducible results in urinary microscopic evaluation; thus, there is "quality control assurance" in the urinalysis laboratory.

SAMPLE. Random urine specimen.

PROCEDURE

1. Label the Kova-Tube (plastic graduated centrifuge tube) with the patient's name.
2. Fill the tube with urine to the 12-ml graduation (Fig. 1–44A).
3. Centrifuge tube at a relative centrifugal force (RCF) of 400 for 5 minutes (about 1500 rpms for 5 minutes with a 6-inch motor radius).
4. Remove tube from centrifuge and insert Kova-Petter into tube to bottom until it is firmly seated (Fig. 1–44B).
5. Decant and discard supernatant from tube, 11 ml (Fig. 1–44C).
6. Remove Kova-Petter from tube.
7. Add 1 drop of Kova-Stain to the remaining 1 ml of urine and sediment in the tube (Fig. 1–44D).
8. Replace Kova-Petter and mix well by using Petter as a squeeze dropper and agitator.
9. Squeeze Kova-Petter several times and allow specimen to be drawn into Kova-Petter.
10. Using the Kova-Petter, transfer one drop of specimen to area adjacent to appropriate covered chamber on Kova-Slide. Allow specimen to be drawn into chamber by capillary action (Fig. 1–44E).
11. Allow specimen to stand for 1 minute to permit settling.
12. Place Kova-Slide on a microscope stage under objectives (Fig. 1–44F).
13. Read and record results.

INTERPRETATION. The specimen is examined microscopically in the usual manner. This technique permits the evaluation of the elements present in a standardized amount of urine (i.e., 12 ml); therefore, it affords the opportunity to provide accurate and reproducible results.

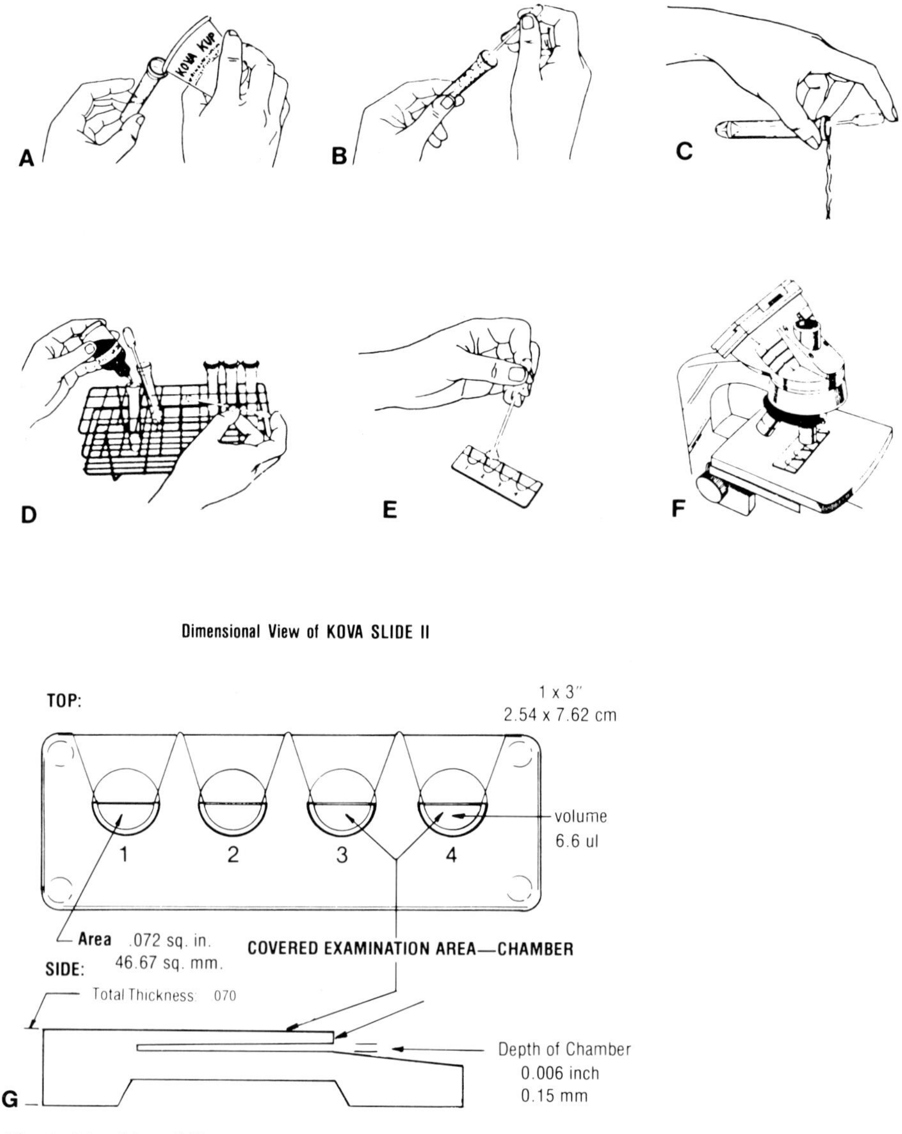

Fig. 1–44. Use of Kova system.

DISCUSSION AND CLINICAL SIGNIFICANCE. The ability of a physician not only to make a diagnosis, but also to follow a patient's course after therapy, is of vital importance in the practice of medicine. This is facilitated by offering urine sediment evaluations that are precise and reproducible. This system provides for additional "quality assurance" in the laboratory for this examination. Standardization and quality control in urinalysis have lagged behind those of the rest of the clinical laboratory, but are important nonetheless. The ability to make data comparisons between performances of laboratories and also between individual technologists is a major advantage.

MATERIAL AND METHODS

1. Kova system (ICL Scientific, 18249 Euclid, Fountain Valley, Calif. 92708)
2. Microscope
3. Centrifuge

REFERENCES

1. Freeman, J.: Clinical Laboratory Manual. Baton Rouge, Earl K. Long Memorial Hospital, 1978.
2. Gadeholt, H.: Quantitative estimation of urinary sediment with special regard to sources of error. Br. Med. J., *1*:1547, 1964.
3. ICL Scientific brochure on the test.
4. Thomas, M.: A rapid slide method for urine cell counts. Med. Lab. Tech., *28*:38, 1971.
5. Haber, M.: *A Primer of Microscopic Urinalysis.* Fountain Valley, Calif., ICL Press, 1978.

URINARY SEDIMENT

METHOD. Microscopic examination (Addis count and routine screening).

PRINCIPLE. Sediment is examined for formed elements which are identified and the numbers present are roughly estimated. Alterations from the normal are present in many patients with urinary tract disorders and in some with systemic disorders.

SAMPLE

1. Addis Count: Place patient on a dry diet (nothing that can be poured) from 8:00 A.M. of the day prior to the test to 8:00 A.M. the day following the test, with normal solid intake. Discard first 8:00 A.M. to 8:00 P.M. specimens. Collect 12-hour night specimen, including final complete voiding at 8:00 A.M. or collect a midnight to noon specimen. Use container with 0.5 ml 10% (v/v) formalin.
2. Routine: It is preferable to collect a first morning voiding when the urine can be examined promptly. If forced to make a choice, a fresh specimen is often preferable later in the day to an old first morning specimen.

PROCEDURE

ROUTINE SCREENING

1. Pour a 10-ml aliquot of fresh urine into a clean conical centrifuge tube and centrifuge at 2,000 rpm for 5 minutes (exact relative centrifugal force not critical).
2. Decant the supernatant, permitting 0.5 ml of residual urine to remain above the sediment. Results will be more reproducible if this amount of residual urine is kept fairly constant (0.5 ml).
3. Resuspend the sediment by agitation.
4. Transfer a drop of suspension to a microscope slide.

5. Apply coverslip and scan entire specimen under low magnification to determine the presence or absence of casts. Study thoroughly before turning to higher power.
6. Using the high-dry objective, examine at least ten representative fields. Identify, count, and record all significant formed elements. Report the average number of each element per high power field. Fecal contamination or menstrual material renders the specimen unsuitable for examination.

ADDIS COUNT

1. Measure volume of urine and record.
2. Mix urine thoroughly.
3. Transfer 10 ml to an Addis sediment tube, allow to stand 10 minutes. Centrifuge for 10 minutes at 2,000 rpm. (Centrifugal force is not critical.)
4. Remove supernatant with a pipette until meniscus is at the 0.5 ml mark. (If sediment is heavy, supernatant may be removed.)
5. Resuspend sediment and transfer to hemocytometer counting chamber. Count entire ruled areas of both chambers until 25 casts or the contents of 12 counting chambers have been counted. Count white cells (including round epithelial cells), until 50 cells or contents of 2 chambers have been counted. Count red cells similarly.
6. Calculations:

$$\text{Casts/12 hour} = \frac{\text{no. casts counted} \times 0.05 \text{ (dilution factor)} \times \text{volume (ml/12 hour)}}{\text{no. chambers counted} \times 0.0009}$$

OR

$$\text{Cells/12 hour} = \frac{\text{no. cells counted} \times 0.05 \times \text{volume}}{\text{no. large squares counted} \times 0.001}$$

(1 chamber = 0.0009 ml; 1 large square = 0.0001 ml)

INTERPRETATION. Many techniques described for Addis counting are very insensitive and will miss small-to-moderate increases in numbers of casts, especially. It is instructive to calculate the least number of casts detectable with the technique you employ.

Normally the following values may be obtained:

	Routine	*Addis*
Total red cells	0–2/HPF	0–500,000/12 hours
Total white cells	0–5/HPF	10,000–3,000,000/12 hours
Total casts	0–1 (hyaline casts)	0–5,000/12 hours

TABLE 1–36. Comparison of Addis Counts and Routine Examination of the Sediment.

Formed element	Semiquantitative Addis count (Total excretion per 12 hours)	Corresponding results of routine screening examination (per high power field)
Casts	6,700 to 79,000	0 or 1 to 2
	122,000 to 1,000,000	1 to 2
	6,000,000 to 15,000,000	10 to 20
Red cells	220,000 to 2,400,000	0 to 10
	2,500,000 to 8,200,000	1 to 20
	190,000,000 to 570,000,000	5 to 60
Leukocytes and epithelial cells	Less than 1,000,000	0 (occasional pt.) 3 to 5 (usual pt.) 10 to 20 (rare pt.)
	1,000,000 to 10,000,000	5 to 10
	10,000,000 to 75,000,000	10 to 20 (clumped)

DISCUSSION AND CLINICAL SIGNIFICANCE. See text discussion.

MATERIALS AND REAGENTS

1. Microscope
2. Microscope slides (1″ × 3″) and coverslips
3. Centrifuge tubes, conical, 15 ml
4. Clinical centrifuge

REFERENCES

1. Addis, T.: Glomerular Nephritis. New York, Macmillan Publishing Co., 1950, p. 10.
2. Addis, T.: The number of formed elements in urinary sediment of normal individuals. J. Clin. Invest., 2:409, 1926.
3. Davidsohn, I., and Wells, B.: Clinical Diagnosis by Laboratory Methods. 13th Ed. Philadelphia, W.B. Saunders, 1962, p. 40.
4. Haber, M.: Urine Casts: Their Microscopy and Clinical Significance. 2nd Ed. Chicago, American Society of Clinical Pathologists, 1976.
5. Haber, M.: Interference contrast microscopy provides 3-D images of urine sediment. Lab. Med., 2:9, 1971.
6. Kark, R., et al.: A Primer of Urinalysis. 2nd Ed. New York, Hoeber Medical Division, Harper & Row, 1964, p. 60.
7. Kern, W.: Epithelial cells in urine sediment. Am. J. Clin. Path., 56:67, 1971.
8. Page, L., and Culver, P.: Syllabus of Laboratory Examinations in Clinical Diagnosis. Cambridge, Harvard University Press, 1961, p. 310.

URINARY SEDIMENT STAINING

METHOD. Sternheimer-Malbin stain.

PRINCIPLE. Some formed elements, especially casts, can be more easily recognized by microscopic examination after differential staining with crystal violet and safranin dyes.

SAMPLE. A fresh concentrated first morning specimen with an acid pH is preferred inasmuch as it is more likely to contain casts than a dilute alkaline afternoon specimen.

PROCEDURE

1. Centrifuge 10 ml urine in a test tube in a clinical centrifuge at 2000 rpm for 5 minutes.
2. Pour off supernatant fluid leaving about 0.5 ml sediment in the bottom of the test tube.
3. To the sediment, add 1 drop of stain; mix by flicking with the finger; pour sediment on a microscope slide.
4. Examine under the microscope for formed elements.

INTERPRETATION, DISCUSSION AND CLINICAL SIGNIFICANCE

1. Red blood cells: In acid or neutral urine, the red cells often remain intact and colorless or stain slightly purple. In alkaline urine, the red cells are usually lysed and alkaline hematin forms, which stains dark purple.
2. White blood cells: The nuclei of ordinary leukocytes usually stain a dark orange-purple, and there is significant granularity of the cytoplasm discernible. Some cells may be intermediate between light and dark forms.
3. Granular motility cells ("glitter cells"): These are large polymorphonuclear leukocytes, that appear pale light blue to almost colorless. The cells are larger than dark-staining cells. Cytoplasmic granules with or without Brownian movement may be noted. (These cells are frequently seen in urine from patients with pyelonephritis, as previously mentioned.)

Epithelial Cells

1. Renal tubular epithelial cells: The nucleus stains dark purple with small rim of orange-purple cytoplasm.
2. Bladder epithelial cells: Round cells with a blue nucleus and a large surrounding border of pale blue cytoplasm.
3. Squamous vaginal and/or urethral cells: Cells with ragged and irregular shape with orange-to-purple nuclei and extensive blue or purple cytoplasm.

Casts

1. Hyaline casts: Much of the value of differential staining lies in the ease with which casts can be recognized. Hyaline casts appear pink to light purple with homogeneous matrices.
2. Red blood cell casts: They have a pale pink hyaline matrix with unstained or pale lavender red blood cells enmeshed within the matrix.
3. Pigmented (hemoglobin) casts: They are deep purple and coarsely granular with mixtures of hemoglobin, red blood cells, and fibrin. In stained sediment, they are hard to differentiate from clumped materials, and are best identified in unstained sediment.

4. White blood cell casts: Purple to orange-white blood cells can be seen enmeshed in pale pink hyaline matrix. With "glitter cell" casts, the cells are pale blue with a granular cytoplasm surrounded by the pink hyaline matrix.
5. Renal epithelial cell casts: The cells are small with purple nuclei in a pale pink hyaline matrix.
6. Bacterial casts: Bacteria stain purple and may be visualized enmeshed in pale pink hyaline matrix.
7. Granular casts: They may appear as granules staining light purple (finely granular) or dark purple (coarsely granular) enmeshed in a pale pink hyaline matrix.
8. Fatty casts: The highly refractile globules will be unstained in pale pink hyaline matrix. They may be seen as doubly refractile "Maltese crosses" under polarized light.

MATERIALS AND REAGENTS.

1. Sternheimer-Malbin stain:

Solution I:		*Solution II:*	
Crystal violet	3.0 g	Safranin O	1.0 ml
95% (v/v) ethyl alcohol	20.0 ml	95% (v/v) ethyl alcohol	40.0 ml
Ammonium oxalate	0.8 g	Distilled water	40.0 ml
Distilled water	80.0 ml		

Mix 3 parts of Solution I and 97 parts of Solution II. Filter. Refilter every 2 weeks. Make fresh every 3 months. The separate Solutions I and II keep indefinitely.

OR

The pre-prepared stain can be purchased commercially. Other stains based on the Sternheimer-Malbin formula are marketed, such as Sedi-Stain (Clay-Adams Co., Inc., Parsippany, N.J. 07054).

2. Clinical centrifuge
3. Microscope, slides, and coverslips
4. Dropping pipettes
5. Dilute hydrochloric acid, about 6 N

REFERENCES

1. Haber, M.: Urine Casts: Their Microscopy and Clinical Significance. Chicago, American Society of Clinical Pathologists, 1975, p. 91.
2. Schreiner, G.: The urinary sediment. Ciba Clinical Symposia, *13*(2):35, April-May-June, 1961.
3. Schreiner, G.: Identification and significance of casts. A.M.A. Arch. Int. Med., *99*:356, 1957.
4. Sternheimer, R. and Malbin, B.: Clinical recognition of pyelonephritis with new stain for urinary sediments. Am. J. Med., *11*:212, 1951.

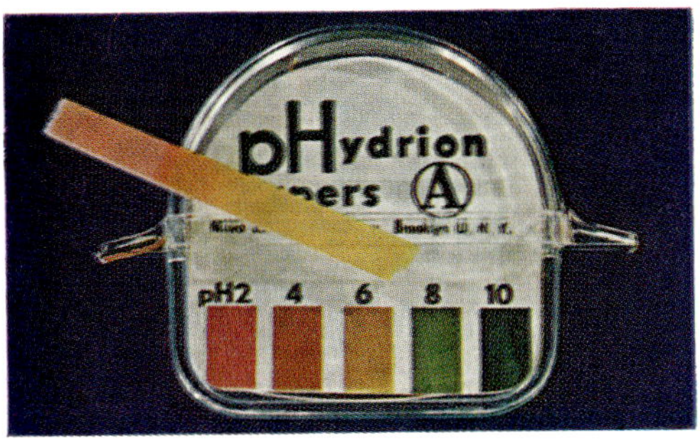

Fig. 1–45. pHydrion paper for urinary pH determination.

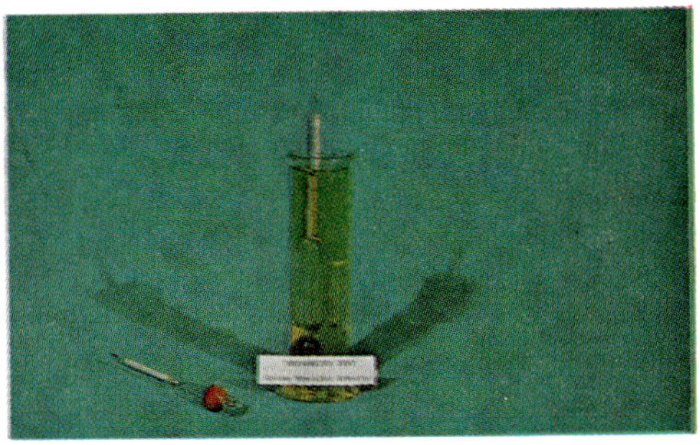

Fig. 1–46. Urinary specific gravity by hydrometer method.

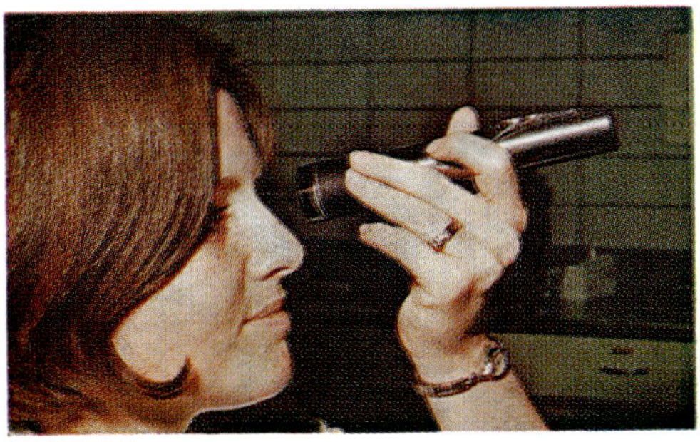

Fig. 1–47. Urinary "specific gravity" by refractometry.

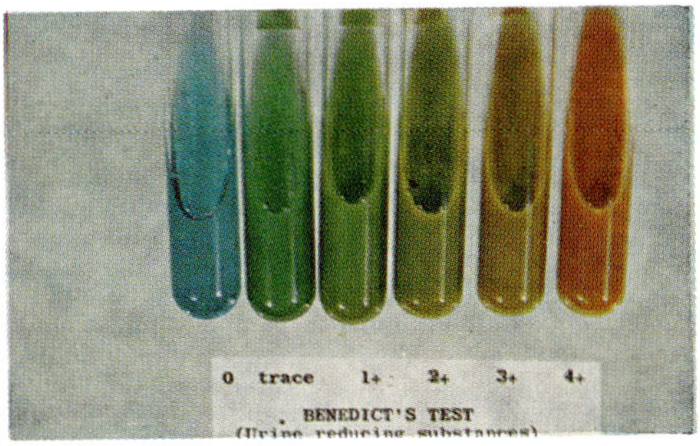

Fig. 1–48. Urine: Benedict's test for reducing substances.

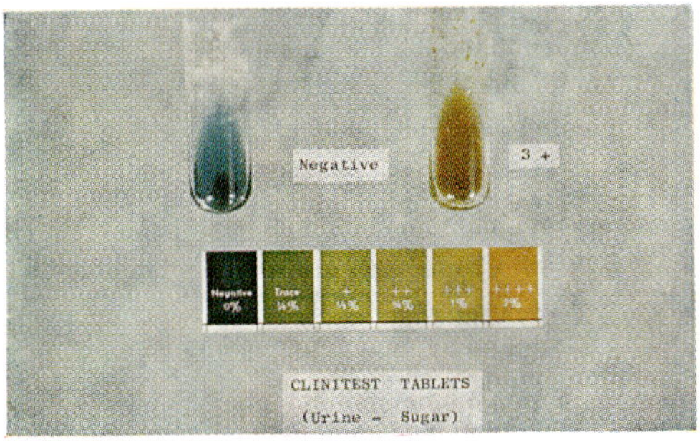

Fig. 1–49. Urine: Clinitest determination.

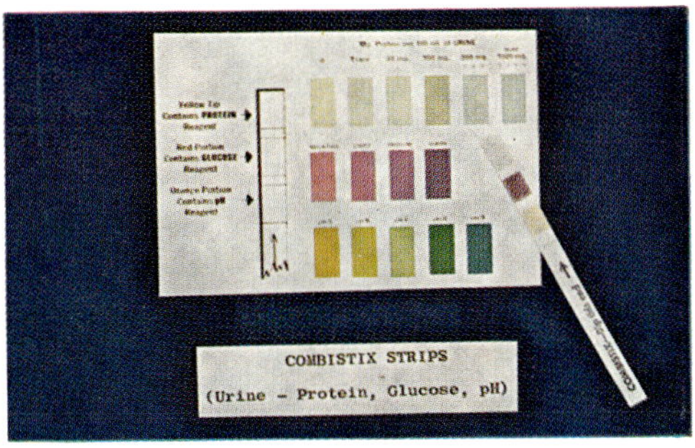

Fig. 1–50. Urine: Combistix determination.

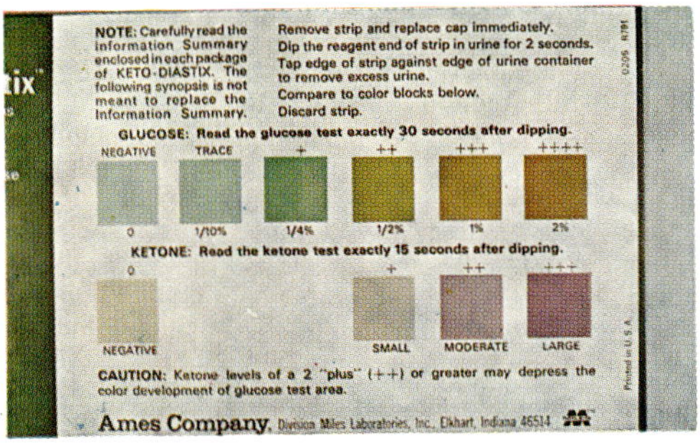

Fig. 1–51. Urine: Ketodiastix.

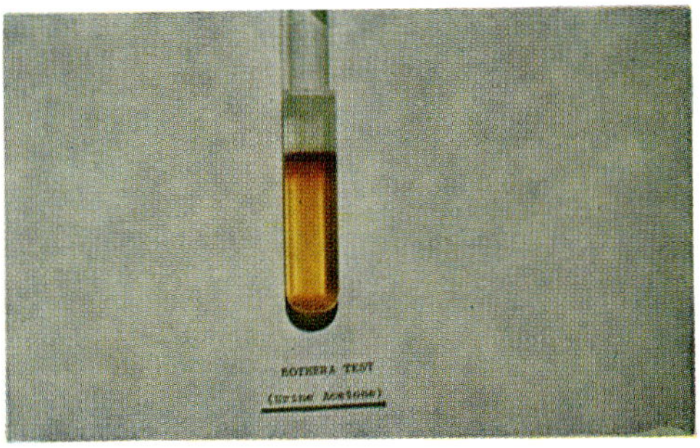

Fig. 1–52. Urine: Rothera test for acetone.

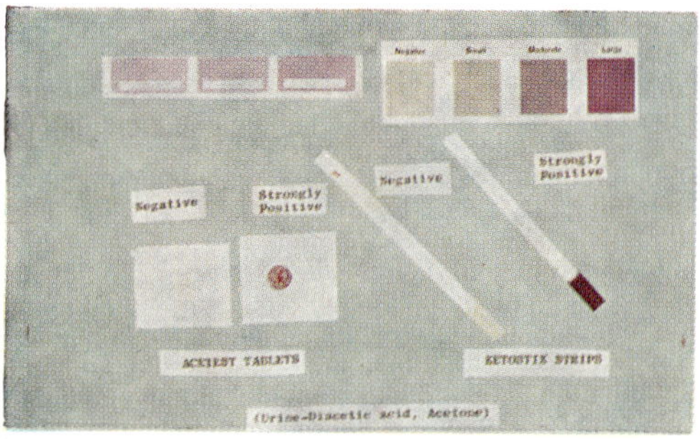

Fig. 1–53. Urine: Ketostix test for acetone.

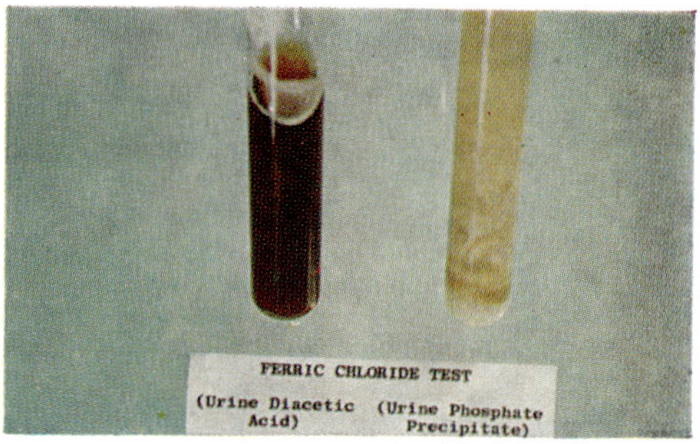

Fig. 1–54. Urine: Ferric chloride (diacetic acid and phosphates).

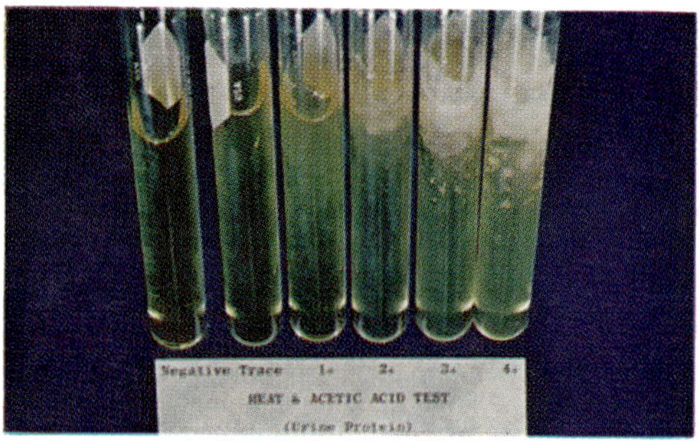

Fig. 1–55. Urine: Heat and acetic acid test for protein.

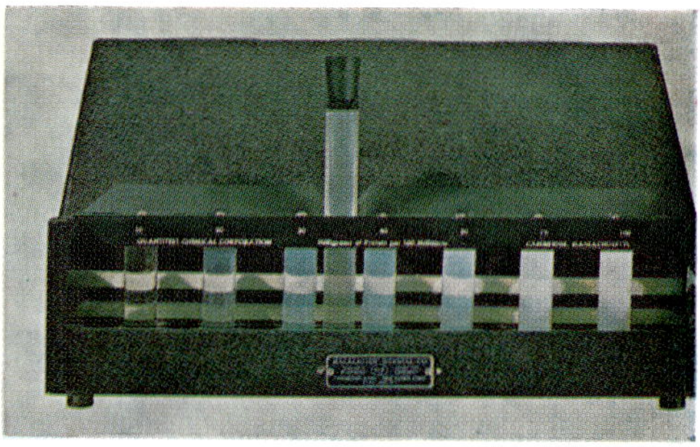

Fig. 1–56. Urine: Kingsbury's sulfosalicylic acid method for protein.

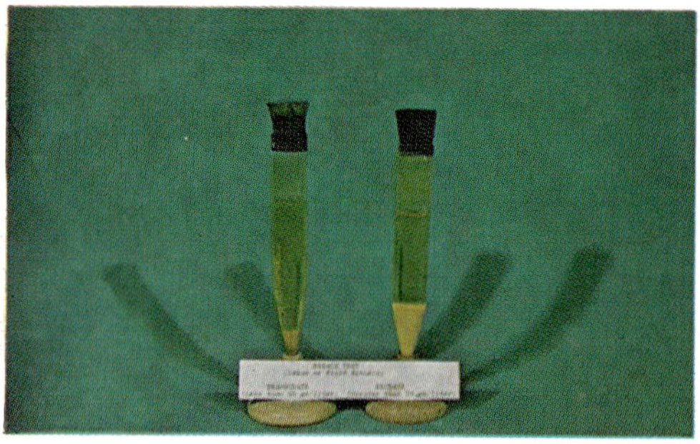

Fig. 1–57. Urine: Esbach's quantitative test for albumin.

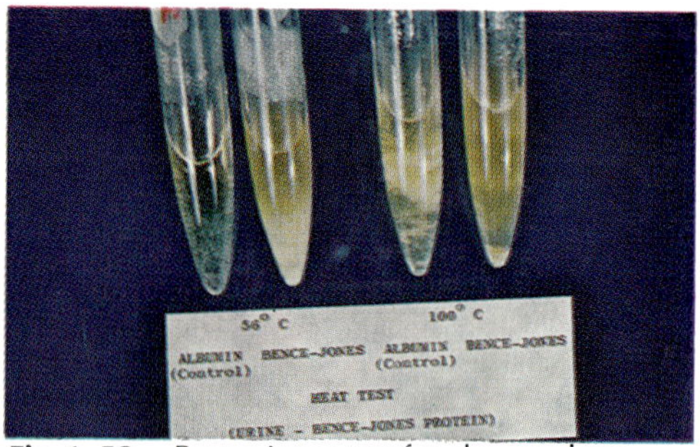

Fig. 1–58. Bence Jones test for abnormal protein. (Inasmuch as the protein is not visible at 100 C, the specimen was permitted to cool just slightly to show a precipitate and such precipitate at 100 C is artifactual).

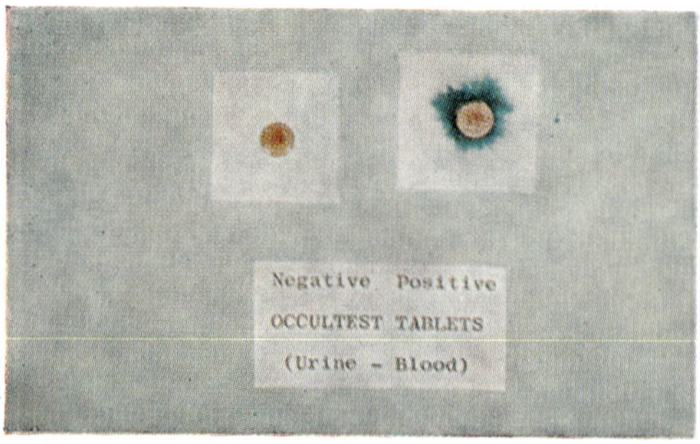

Fig. 1–59. Urine: Occultest tablets for blood.

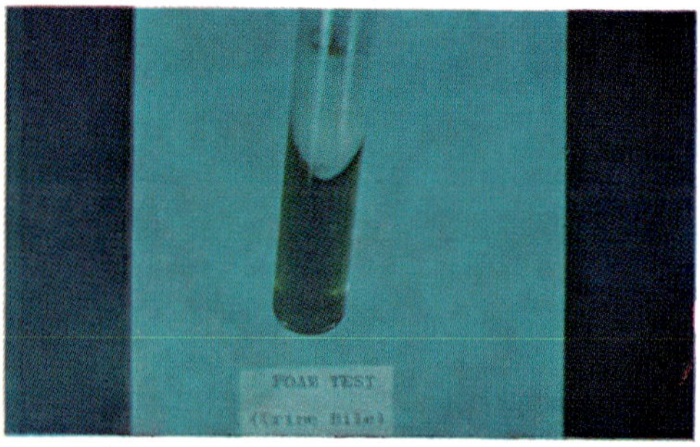

Fig. 1–60. Urine: Foam test for bile.

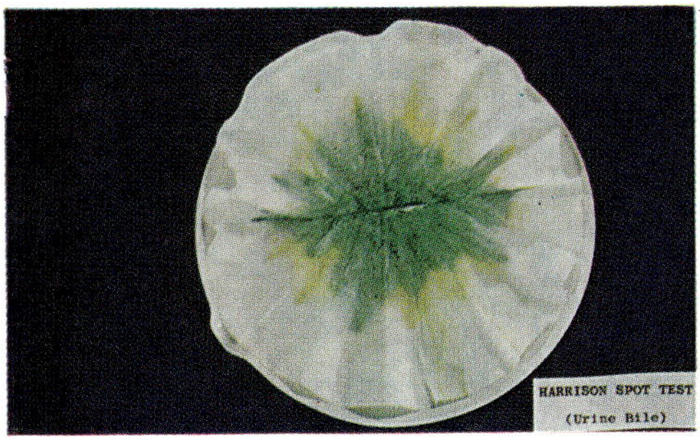

Fig. 1–61. Urine: Harrison spot test for bilirubin pigments.

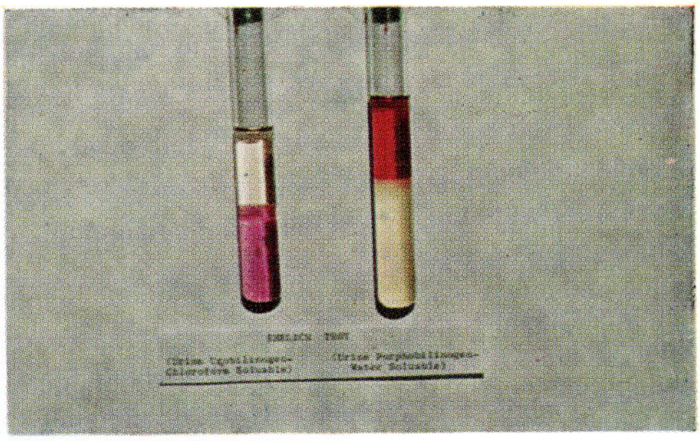

Fig. 1–62. Urine: Urobilinogen and porphobilinogen.

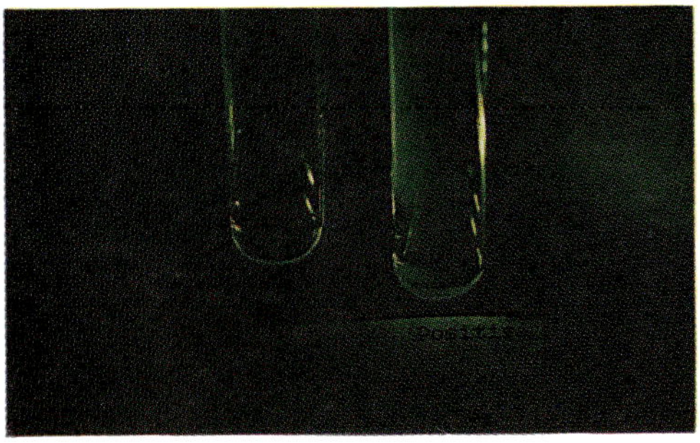

Fig. 1–63. Urine: Schlesinger's fluorescent test for urobilin.

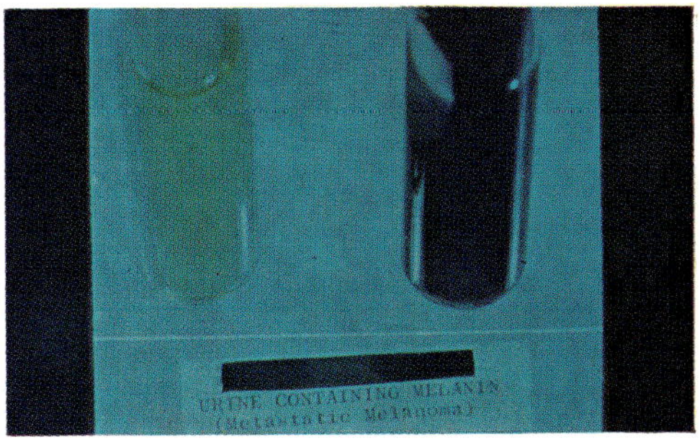

Fig. 1–64. Urine: Melanin determination.

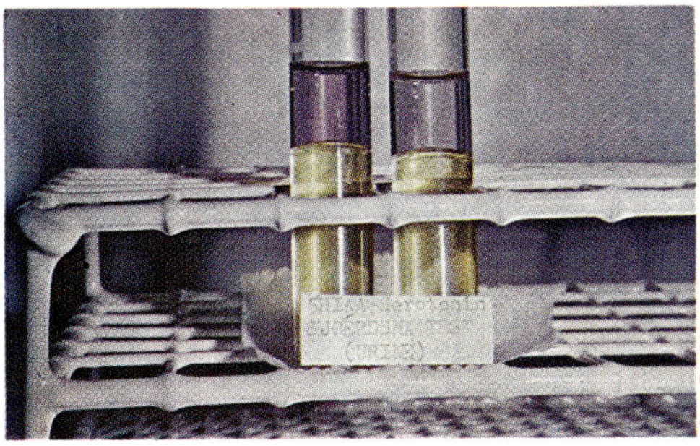

Fig. 1–65. Urine: Sjoerdsma's test for 5-HIAA acid and serotonin. Positive test on left; negative test on right.

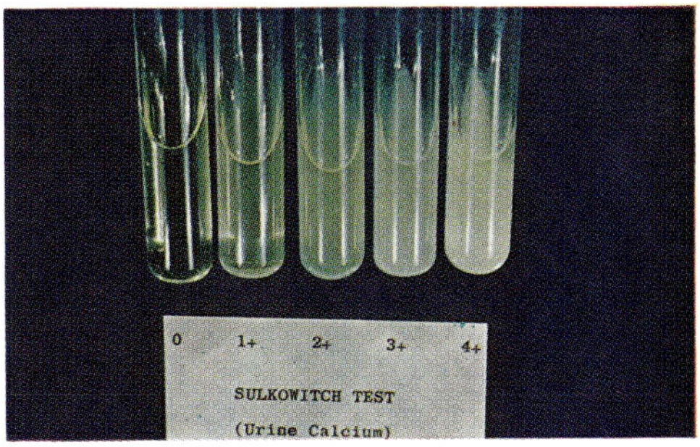

Fig. 1–66. Urine: Sulkowitch quantitative test for calcium.

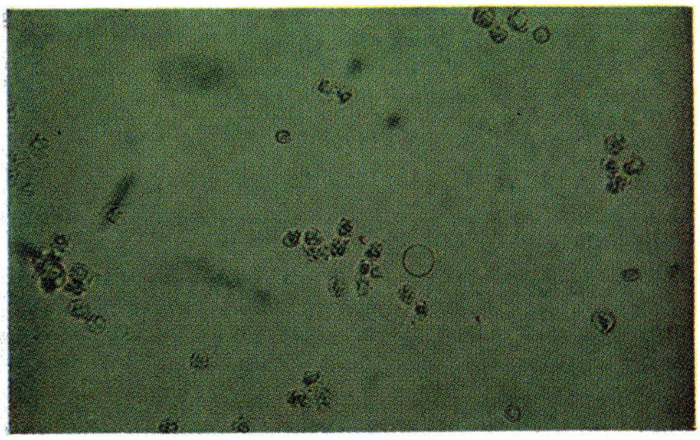

Fig. 1–67. Urine sediment: White blood cells (unstained).

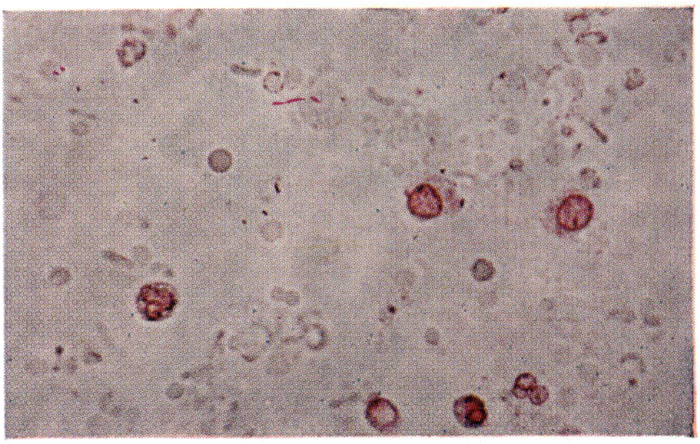

Fig. 1–68. Urine sediment: Red blood cells, white blood cells and casts (Sternheimer-Malbin stain).

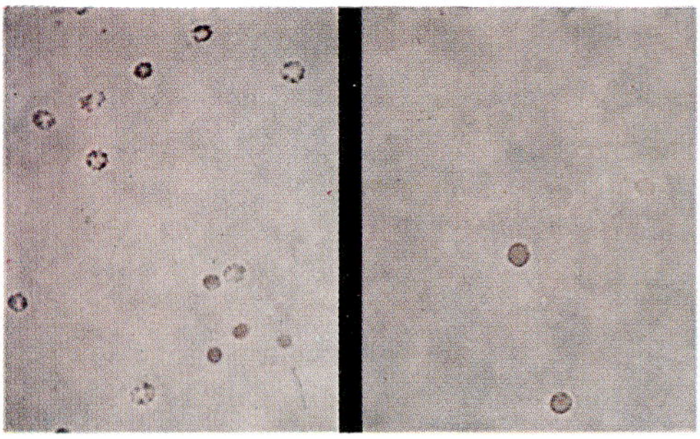

Fig. 1–69. Urine sediment: Red blood cells in urine with high osmolality (left) and low osmolality (right) (unstained).

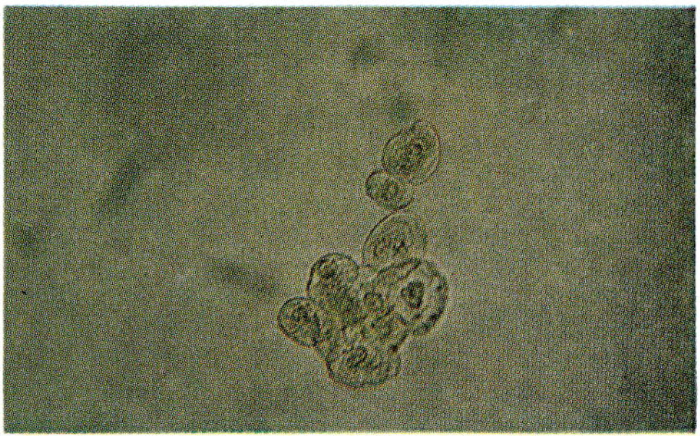

Fig. 1–70. Urine sediment: Renal epithelial cells (unstained).

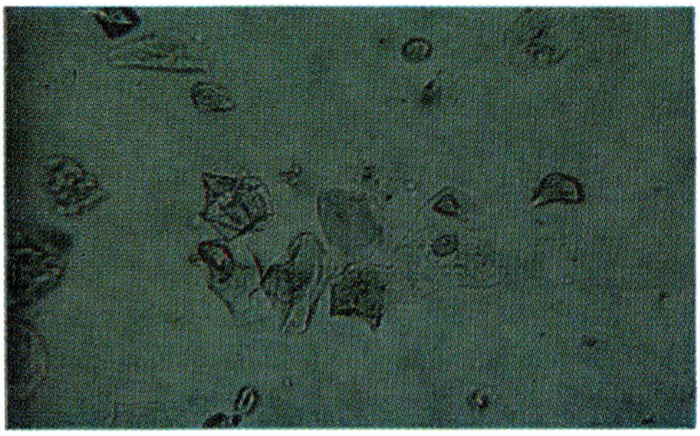

Fig. 1–71. Urine sediment: Squamous epithelial cells (unstained).

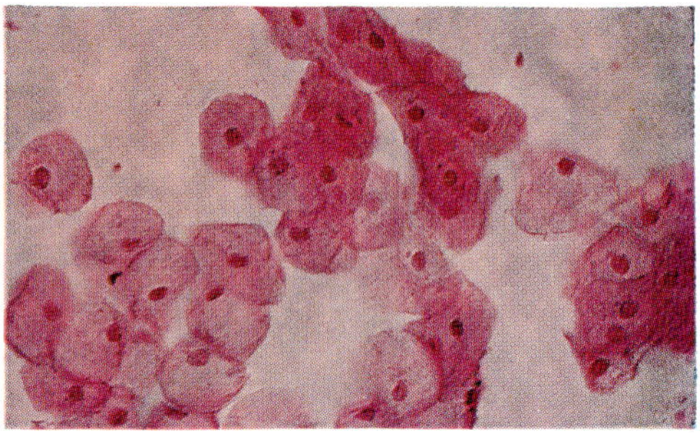

Fig. 1–72. Urine sediment: Squamous cells (Sternheimer-Malbin stain).

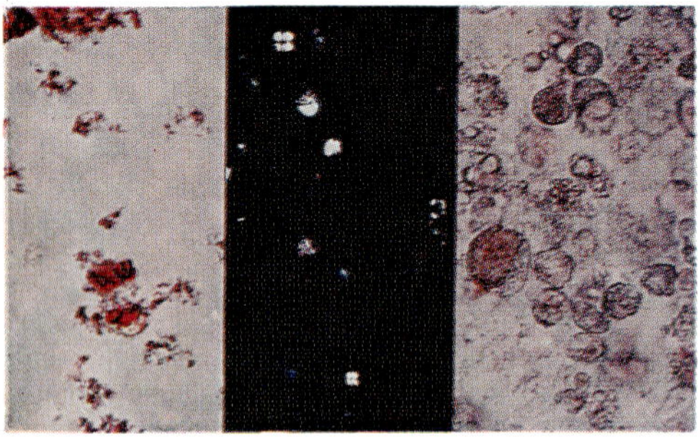

Fig. 1–73. Urine sediment: Oval and free fat, unstained (left), polarization microscopy (center) and ORO stain (right).

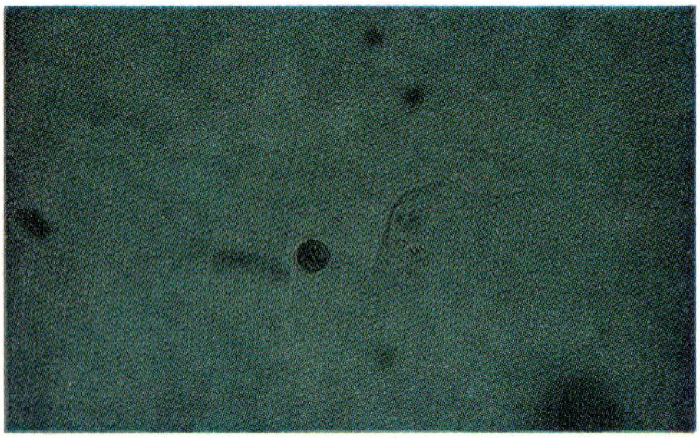

Fig. 1–74. Urine sediment: Glitter cells (unstained). Of course, the glitter is produced by Brownian movement that cannot be properly depicted in a still photograph.

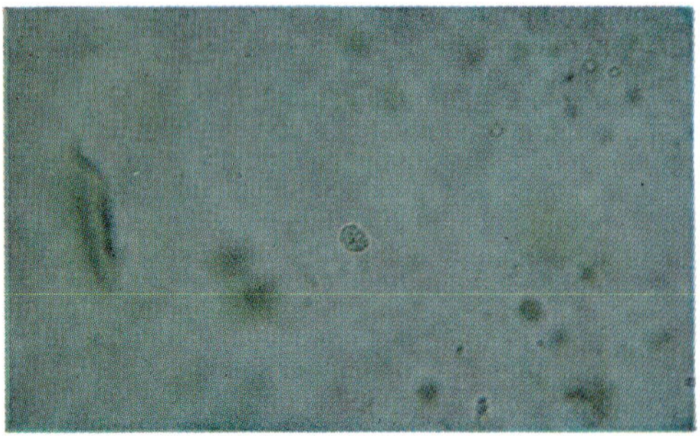

Fig. 1–75. Urine: Trichomonads (unstained).

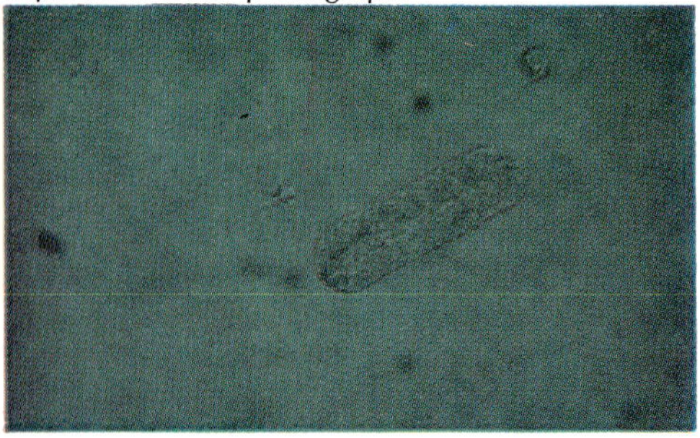

Fig. 1–76. Urine sediment: Hyaline casts (unstained).

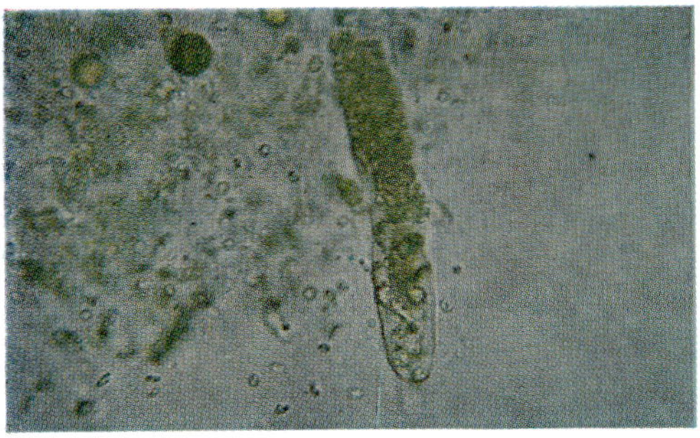

Fig. 1–77. Urine sediment: Hyaline casts with WBC's (unstained).

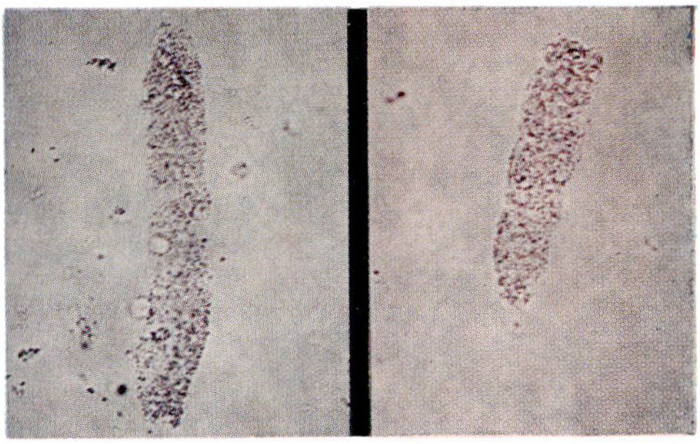

Fig. 1–78. Urine sediment: Degenerative cellular casts and granular casts (unstained).

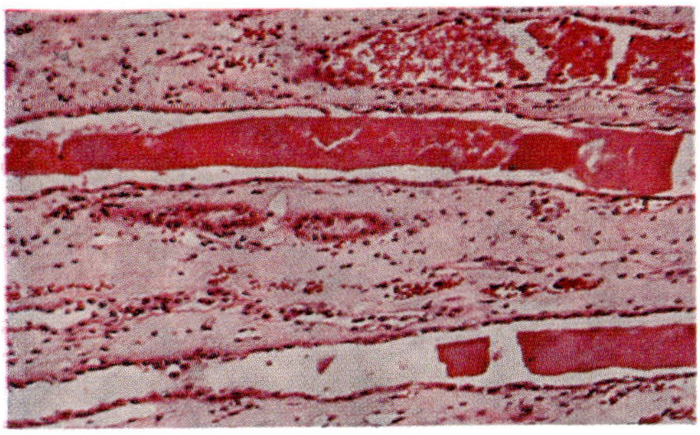

Fig. 1–79. Kidney biopsy: Hyaline casts (hematoxylin and eosin stain of paraffin-impregnated section).

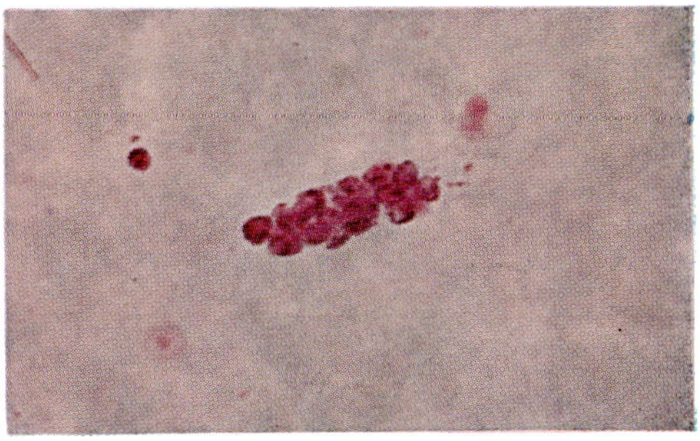

Fig. 1–80. Urine sediment: WBC casts (unstained).

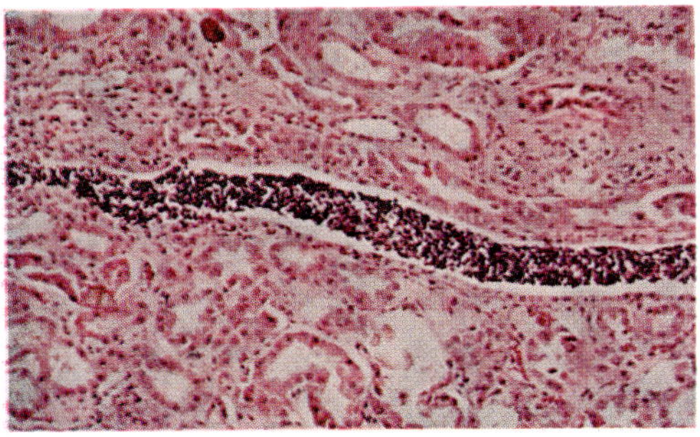

Fig. 1–81. Kidney biopsy: WBC casts and sulfonamide crystals (hematoxylin and eosin stain of paraffin-impregnated section).

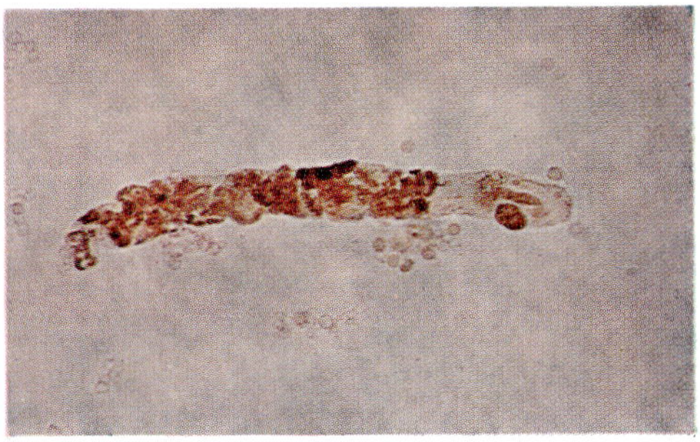

Fig. 1–82. Urine sediment: Bile-stained renal cell casts (unstained).

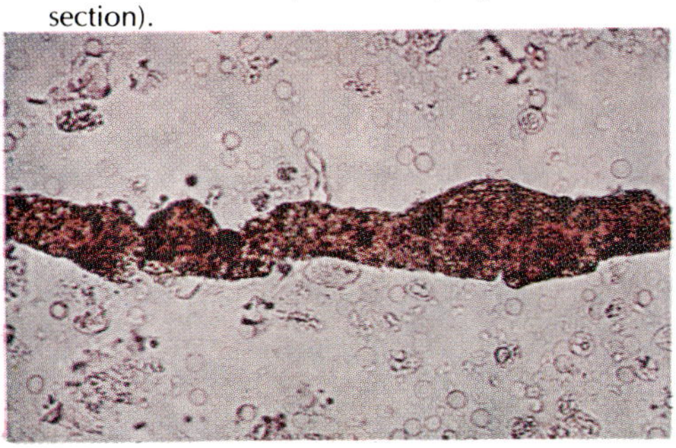

Fig. 1–83. Urine sediment: Red blood cell casts (unstained).

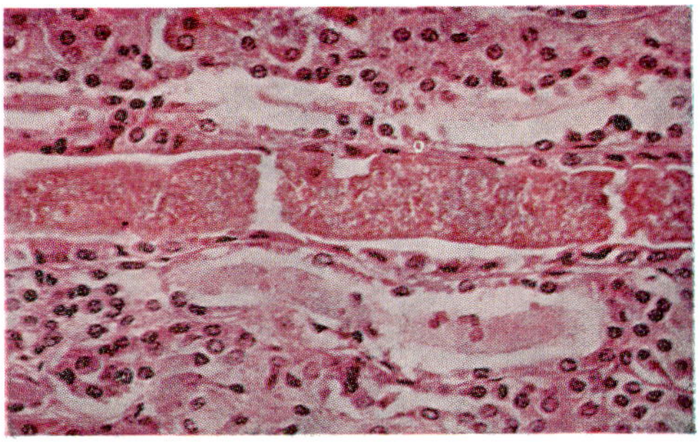

Fig. 1–84. Kidney biopsy: Red blood cell casts (hematoxylin and eosin stain of paraffin-impregnated section).

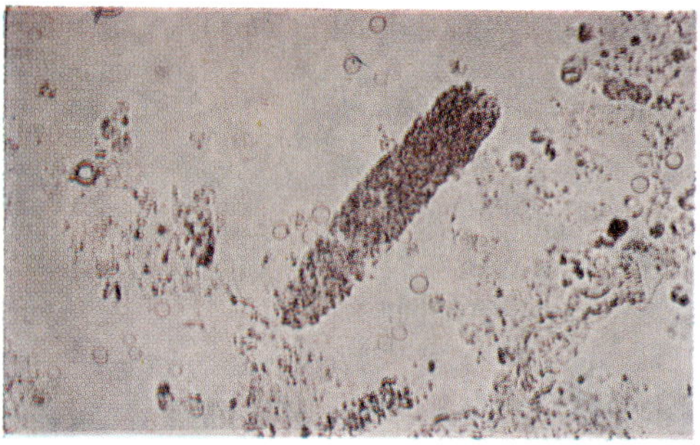

Fig. 1–85. Urine sediment: Granular casts (unstained).

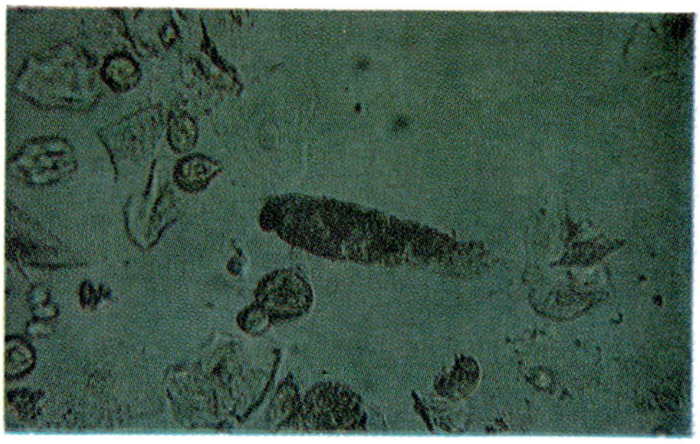

Fig. 1–86. Urine sediment: Coarsely granular casts (unstained).

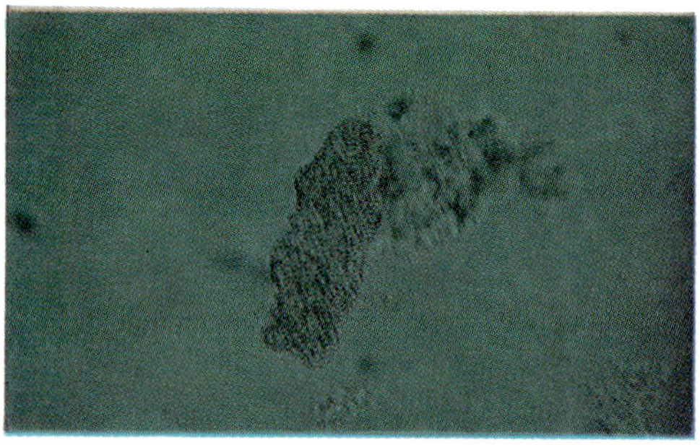

Fig. 1–87. Urine sediment: Coarsely granular casts (unstained).

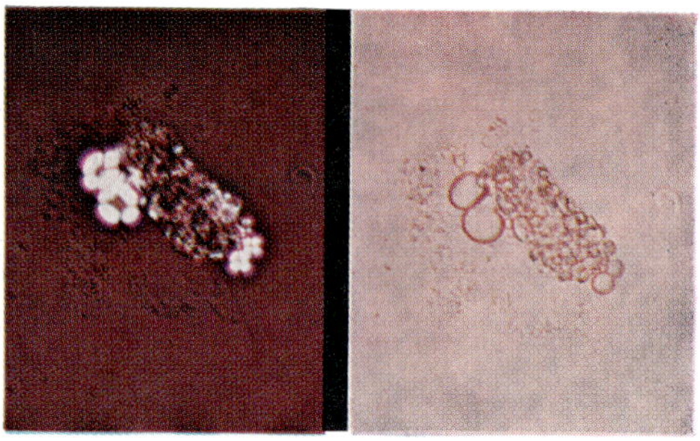

Fig. 1–88. Urine sediment: Fat and fatty casts, polarizing microscopy (left) and visible microscopy (right), unstained.

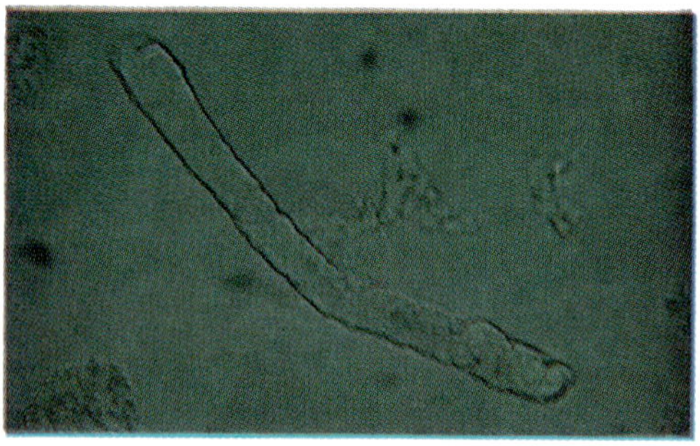

Fig. 1–89. Urine sediment: Waxy casts (unstained).

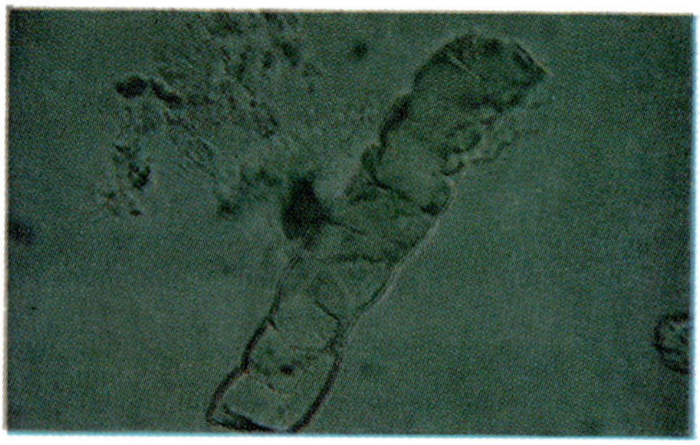

Fig. 1–90. Urine sediment: Broad waxy casts (unstained).

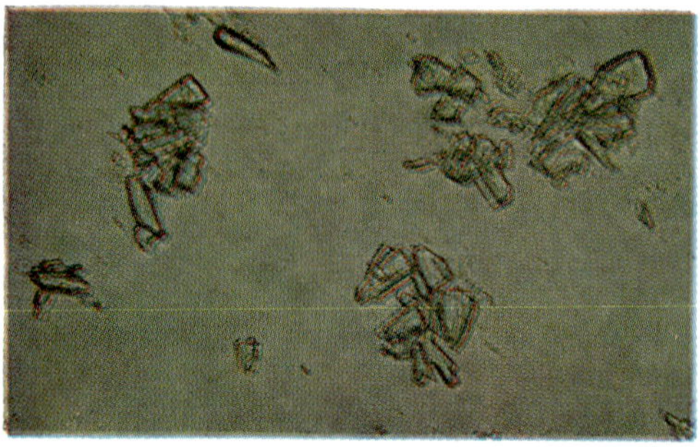

Fig. 1–91. Urine sediment: Triple phosphate crystals (unstained).

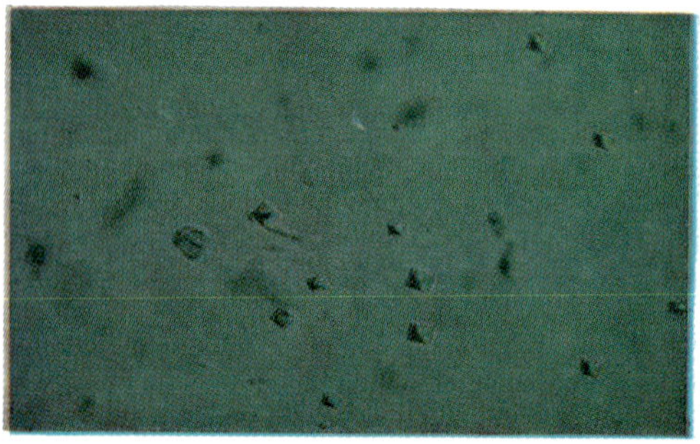

Fig. 1–92. Urine sediment: Calcium oxalate crystals (unstained).

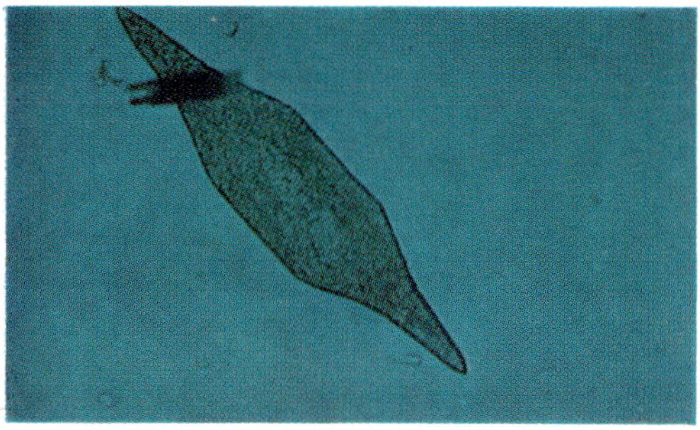

Fig. 1–93. Urine sediment: Uric acid crystals (unstained).

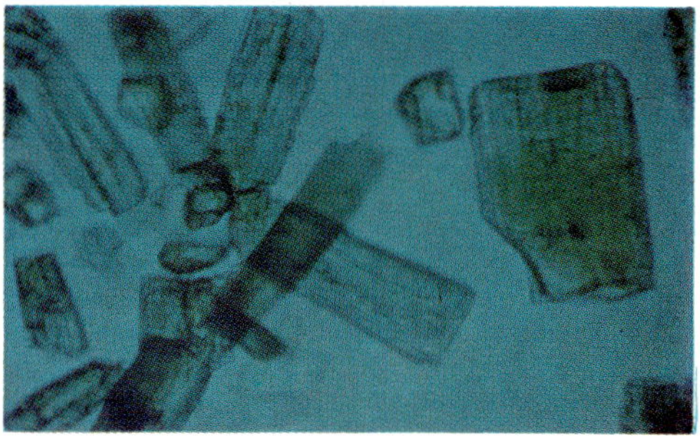

Fig. 1–94. Urine sediment: Uric acid crystals (unstained).

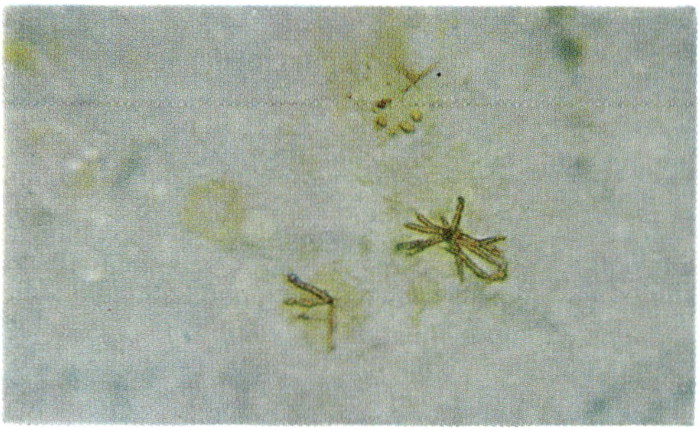

Fig. 1–95. Urine sediment: Tyrosine crystals (unstained).

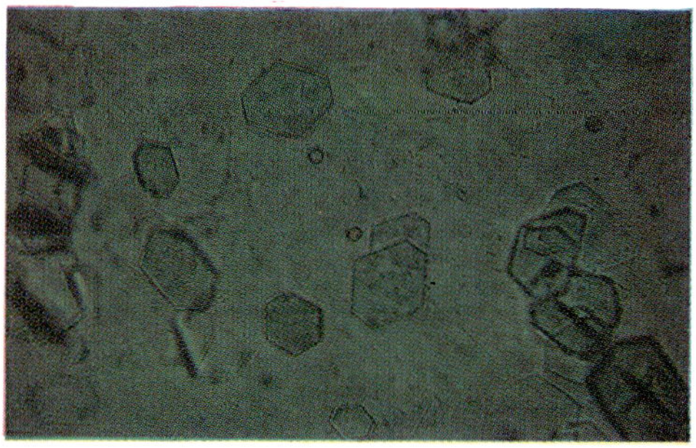

Fig. 1–96. Urine sediment: Cystine crystals (unstained).

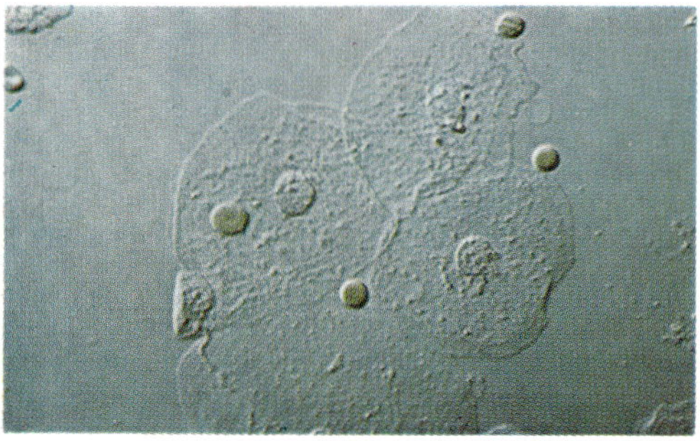

Fig. 1–97. Urine sediment: Squamous cells, phase microscopy (unstained).

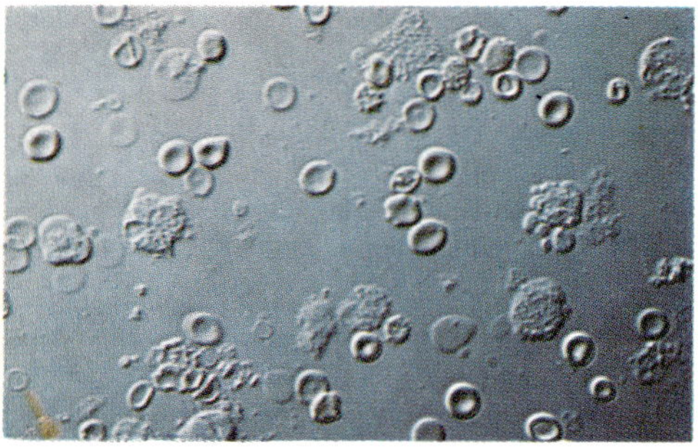

Fig. 1–98. Urine sediment: Red blood cells, white blood cells, phase microscopy (unstained).

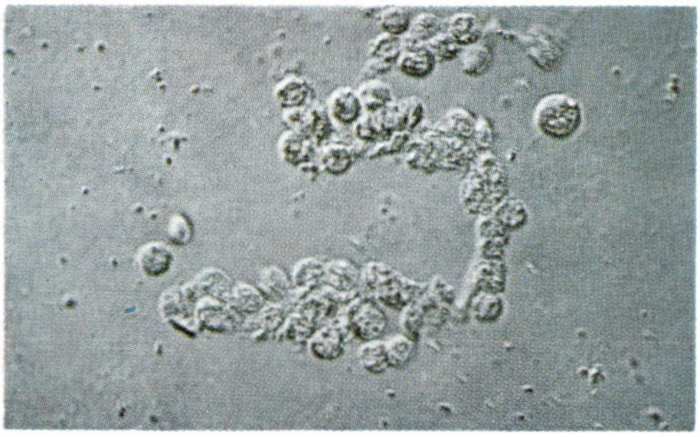

Fig. 1–99. Urine sediment: White blood cell casts, phase microscopy (unstained).

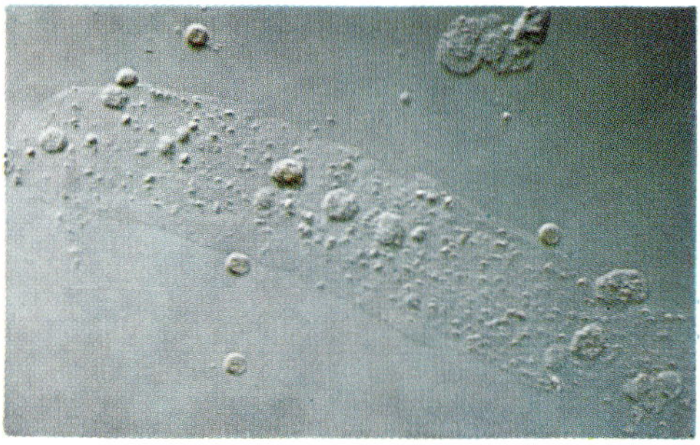

Fig. 1–100. Urine sediment: Granular casts with white blood cell inclusions, phase microscopy (unstained).

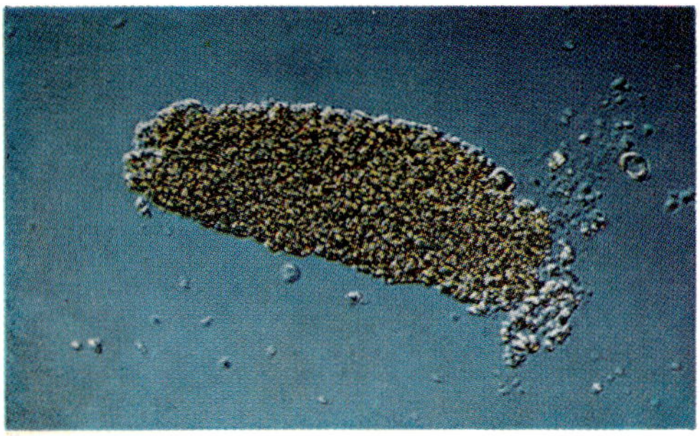

Fig. 1–101. Urine sediment: Finely granular casts, phase microscopy (unstained).

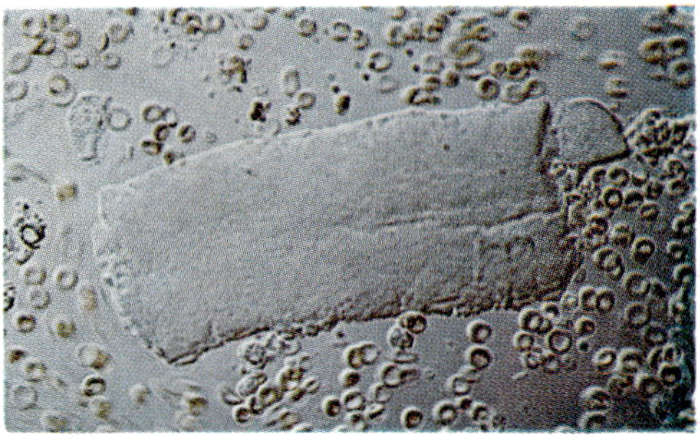

Fig. 1–102. Urine sediment: Broad waxy casts, phase microscopy (unstained).

Figures 1–68, 1–69, 1–72, 1–73, 1–78 through 1–85, and 1–88 are reproduced with permission from Lancaster, R., Cannon, D., Freeman, J., and Lehman, R.: Urinary Sediment: Formed Elements and Casts. Vol. 1. Chicago, American Society of Clinical Pathologists, Commission on Continuing Education, 1970.
Figures 1–97 through 1–102 are reproduced with permission from Haber, M.: Interference Contrast Microscopy Provides 3-D Images of Urinary Sediment. Lab. Med., *2*:9, 1971.

Chapter

2 Fecal Analysis

MYRTON F. BEELER
JAMES A. FREEMAN

Examination of feces is often approached with reluctance because of the offensive nature of the material. This reaction of aversion was played on in the 11th Canto of Dante Alighieri's Commedia, in which, abandoning his usual symbolic rhetoric, he stated "thence in the ditch beneath, I saw a people dipped in excrement, that seems as it had flowed from human privies," in reference to a disheveled strumpet being scourged by horned demons and driven naked into the Eternal Pit.[1] The Scotsman James Hamilton in his book (1805), which came to be known as Hamilton on Purgatives, also recognized it by stating, in his preface, that "Peculiarities of my practice have passed silently into the world. . . and (been) made the subject of hasty and mistaken criticism. . . ."[2]

This attitude, although prevalent, has not always prevailed. Thus, the sometime status of excreta is reflected in an inscription found on the tomb of a 4000-year-old Egyptian Pharaoh-physician: "Guardian of the Royal Bowel Movement"—a degree of medical specialization at least equal to that which we have achieved.[3] The Pharaoh's name, appropriately enough, was Erj. A glance at the Papyrus Ebers reveals at once that constipation is an ancient scourge.[4] Purchased from a wealthy Egyptian of Luxor near Thebes by George Ebers in 1872, the Papyrus, the most ancient complete book in the world, has a slightly greater amount of text devoted to the alimentary system than to cos-

This chapter was revised, expanded, and reproduced (and illustrations added) with permission from Rencher, L., and Beeler, M.: The examination of feces. Clinical Diagnosis by Laboratory Methods. 14th ed. Edited by J. Davidsohn and J. Henry. Philadelphia, W.B. Saunders, 1969.

metics (Fig. 2–1). One passage describes inspection of "not only the sick man's body but also what came out of it, urine, feces, what is lifted by cough, or blood." The feces, in the case of an intestinal obstruction, are described as being "like hog's blood when it is cooked."[4] In fact, visual examination of stool antedated Egyptian medicine by a millennium and might be considered the earliest documented form of the practice of clinical pathology. The writings in the Papyrus Ebers recommend oil of the kiki (castor oil plant) for constipation.[4]

A curious outgrowth of the belief in sorcery was the practice of burying women's hair in horse feces, in the belief that snakes would emerge. The colorful alchemist physician Theophrastus Bombastus von Hohenheim of the 16th century (who modestly renamed himself Phillipus Aureolus Paracelsus after the master physician Celsus) viewed this as nonsense long before the idea of spontaneous generation was finally discredited, summing up in his words: "Nihil est sine spermate" (Nothing exists without sperm).[3]

We find some mention of purgatives in Macbeth who replies to a physician's mention of mental ailment, "Throw physik to the dogs"; he than asks, "What rhubarb, senna, or what purgative drug would scour these English hence?" Baron Richelieu, Cardinal during the reign of Louis XIV of France, on his deathbed was fed horse feces mixed with white wine—a therapeutic remedy of the day.[3] "There have been many speculations concerning the cause of a frantic upsurge of interest in

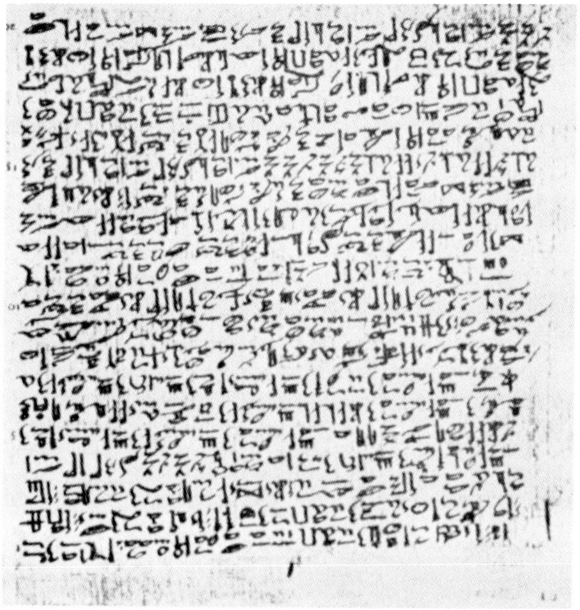

Fig. 2–1. Papyrus Ebers.

obnoxious medicinal mixtures during the 16th and 17th centuries," related Richard Mathison in The Shocking History of Drugs, "none of (the reasons) explain the penchants for fried feces, crushed lice, dried toads"—which could all be found in the family medicine chests of the day.[3] Medication was even retrieved from the stool to be swallowed over and over again. Such was the case of the nonabsorbable pellets of antimony, sold in the 17th century as "everlasting pills," inasmuch as a single pill, by judicious retrieval from the stool after oral ingestion, could be reused by a family for years.[3] The importance of stool examination in earlier American medicine is mirrored in the recommended analysis of stool even before diagnosis of such an entity as gras fondure, mentioned in The Cyclopedia of Practical Medicine (1845).[5]

Even in our times, use of poultices of cow feces, originally a popular Hindu remedy for injured muscles or bites, lingers on in European and American farm areas as a readily available remedy for minor bruises; although substitution of the constituent benzoic acid and phosphates—the major remedial constituents of cow feces—would be, at least, more aesthetic by our standards.

SPECIMEN COLLECTION

It is easy to obtain feces on a finger cot or glove during digital rectal examination and proctosigmoidoscopy. Demonstration of gastrointestinal bleeding is usually of considerable diagnostic significance, and fecal specimens so collected may help to expedite the clinical study of a patient. Transfer of fecal material in these cases can be accomplished by merely smearing the feces on a piece of filter paper. Paper towels should not be used for the purpose, since many of them contain vegetable fibers with peroxidase activity that may give false positive tests for occult blood. Specimens collected within 72 hours after a barium enema or a barium swallow usually are unsatisfactory for examination. Similarly, stools from patients taking mineral oil are undesirable for microscopic examination, as the oil may mimic findings of steatorrhea.

A well-rinsed bedpan is a convenient collection vessel. If the patient does not own one, a carefully cleaned, rinsed, and boiled glass jar provides a satisfactory alternate. Patients, especially females, should be warned against urinating into the bedpan, because among other things, urine has a harmful effect upon protozoa. The feces can be transferred by tongue depressors or pieces of cardboard from bedpan to containers for transport to the hospital laboratory. We prefer 2-ounce ointment jars with screw caps because they are odor-free, leakproof, and easy to transport. Patients should be instructed not to contaminate the outside of the container, and not to overfill the container. Gas, which frequently accumulates in the jar, should be released gradually by careful loosening of the cap! Failure to observe this simple precaution, especially in the case of an overfilled container, can result in an explosive release of contents, with unaesthetic results.

INSPECTION OF FECES

Volume

The quantity of feces (stool) excreted/24 hours is so variable from one individual to another, from infancy to adulthood, and from diet to diet that no didactic statement can be made regarding normalcy. The "healthy" adult may defecate at frequencies varying from 3 times a day to once a week; the common pattern is once a day. Infants usually defecate after every feeding, inasmuch as they have an active gastrocolic reflex promoting rectocolic peristalsis. Infants may excrete anywhere from 4 to 120 g (wet weight) feces/24 hours. Young children may excrete up to 150 g/24 hours. Adults in the United States, consuming a mixed diet with vegetables, meats, and other foodstuffs may excrete from 60 to 250 g/24 hours, or a comparable amount over a longer period if they do not defecate daily. On a pure vegetable diet this may increase to 370 or more g/24 hours; while on a pure meat diet, the quantity of feces excreted daily may drop to 60 or so. In malabsorption states involving fat, the amount of feces excreted may rise to more than 1,200 g/day. In the latter case, the usually neutral to alkaline feces—pH 4.6 to 8.8 observed in healthy individuals—may become more acid.

Color

The usual color of feces is caused chiefly by stercobilin, and other substances as yet of undetermined origin. Stercobilin is formed from urobilinogen, which, in turn, is formed in the intestine by bacterial action on conjugated bilirubin compounds. Feces will darken on exposure to air with oxidation of urobilinogen to stecobilin. The feces may become dark on a low residue meat diet or may become lighter on a high residue vegetable diet. Golden yellow or yellowish-white feces, seen chiefly in infants, is caused partly by a milk diet, and partly by absence of stercobilin. Infant stools may be green when containing much biliverdin, and frequently as a result of ingestion of chlorophyll (in spinach and other leafy vegetables). Green stools are not uncommon in children with severe diarrhea, and they may be passed alternately with yellow stools. However, they may also be passed sometimes by healthy infants and are relatively of little diagnostic importance. Certain chromogenic bacteria can also produce green stools. Cocoa and chocolate produce dark gray stools; while dietary blueberry juices, carbon, iron, and bismuth can cause gray to pitch black feces. Light gray stool also may result from undigested fats, following inadequate bile secretion, or in malabsorption syndromes. The neutral fats and calcium soaps formed in these conditions produce this color. Light yellow or "clay"-

colored (acholic) stools are characteristic, in adults, of lack of bilirubin derivatives and may occur following obstruction to the biliary outflow tract as a result of stones, carcinoma of the ampulla of Vater, the bile ducts, or of the pancreas, or other disease states. They, therefore, are indicative of deficient biliary secretion. Consequently, in such a case, as a result of incomplete digestion of fat, the stool may be yellow (fatty) and greasy. The color in such a case may result more from the presence of fat than from the absence of bilirubin pigments. Fatty and greasy stools also occur in patients with certain intra-abdominal processes, such as tuberculous peritonitis, and pancreatic disease when there is fat malabsorption and steatorrhea. Large amounts of blood produce tarry stools when the bleeding is from high enough in the gastrointestinal tract for the hemoglobin to undergo alteration by the time it reaches the rectum. Red streaks of blood on the outside of the stool are usually caused by fresh blood from hemorrhoids, fissures, and other diseases that produce bleeding in the rectum or anus (see discussion on blood). Beets may produce a reddish color in the stool.

Many drugs affect the feces as follows:

Color Imparted to the Feces	*Drug(s) Responsible*
Pink to red to black (some color resulting from internal bleeding)	Salicylates, anticoagulants
Orange-red	Phenazopyridine (Pyridium)
Whitish discoloration or speckling of feces	Aluminum hydroxide preparations; barium
Blue	Dithiazinine (Delvex); methylene blue
Red	Pyrvinium pamoate (Povan); bromsulfalein dye; carmine dye
Black	Bismuth salts (Bistrimate, Milibis, Peptobismol, etc.), iron preparations (ferrous sulfate, etc.), charcoal
Dark brown to black	Manganese dioxide
Reddish brown	Hematoxylin
Brownish staining of the rectal mucosa	1, 8-Dihydroxyanthraquinone (Dorbane; Doxan)
Green	Calomel
Yellow	Senna extracts, santonin, rhubarb extracts

Mucus

Large amounts of mucus, whether admixed with the feces or on the surface, are abnormal and usually occur with colonic diseases, the most notable of which are mucus colitis and villous adenomas (the latter disease being a premalignant tumor).

Presence of recognizable mucus in a stool specimen is abnormal and should be reported. Translucent gelatinous mucus clinging to the surface of the formed stool suggests spastic constipation or mucus colitis. It is seen in stools of emotionally disturbed patients and may result from excessive straining. Bloody mucus clinging to the fecal mass suggests neoplasm or inflammatory processes of the rectal canal. Mucus associated with pus and blood is found in ulcerative colitis, bacillary dysentery, ulcerative carcinoma of the colon, and more rarely, acute diverticulitis or intestinal tuberculosis. Patients with villous adenoma of the colon may pass copious quantities of mucus aggregating up to 3 to 4 L in 24 hours. These patients frequently develop severe dehydration and electrolyte disturbances, especially hypokalemia.

Odor

The odor of stools results from bacterial conversion of tryptophane to indole and skatole depending largely on the amount of meat in the diet and the putrefactive bacteria present in the intestine. A sour odor caused by the presence of fatty acids is normal for nursing infants, but in adults usually indicates steatorrhea. In severe diarrhea of childhood, the sour odor may change to a putrid odor.

ROUTINE FECAL ANALYSIS

Laboratory examination of feces is most commonly employed for

1. Detection of gastrointestinal bleeding
2. Confirmation of steatorrhea
3. Detection and identification of parasites

Inasmuch as parasitology is a separate discipline and since excellent texts are already available, we have confined our discussion to chemical and microscopic examination of feces. Detection of occult blood in the stool by methods suitable for routine screen can be of considerable diagnostic value, pointing to the need for further investigation of the patient for gastrointestinal neoplasm or other pathologic condition. Confirmation and differential diagnosis of steatorrhea can be accomplished by relatively simple screening tests suitable for performance in any clinical microscopy laboratory, although results may need confirmation by more definitive tests.

BLOOD

Of one group of patients with significant gastrointestinal bleeding, 18% were found to have malignant tumors and 30% benign peptic ulcers.[7] In over one-half of the patients, the bleeding source was in the esophagus, stomach, or duodenum; in 45%, it was in the colon and rectum. Bleeding from the jejunum and ileum was found in very few of the patients. Blood arising in the upper gastrointestinal tract is relatively uniformly mixed throughout the specimen, but blood from the lower gastrointestinal tract is likely to be segmental in distribution within the stool, or it may only coat the surface. The presence of focally distributed blood should be reported after chemical verification. (In routine testing, an attempt is made to use an aliquot from the center of the formed stool.)

Drugs administered orally, particularly salicylates, steroids, rauwolfia derivatives, indomethacin, thiazide diuretics, and colchicine, have been associated with gastrointestinal blood loss in normal subjects, and more pronounced increases in patients with bleeding from pathologic sources. This effect may even follow parenteral administration of some of these drugs. Bromides, iodides, and potassium permanganate have also been said to be able to produce false positive benzidine tests.

Gross Blood

Visible bleeding is usually caused by minor pathologic conditions such as hemorrhoids and anal fissures. Blood from the anorectal region frequently causes red streaking of the surface of the stool. It indicates the need for investigation because, obviously, patients with carcinoma of the rectosigmoid can also have bleeding hemorrhoids.

Loss of more than 50 to 75 ml of blood from the upper gastrointestinal tract generally imparts a dark red to black, tarry appearance to the stool. It is this appearance, along with the dark urine of blackwater fever, that the medical historian Henry Sigerist believes led to postulation of the existence of the fourth humor, "black bile," which is so frequently mentioned in the works of ancient medical practitioners. Somewhat similar quantities entering the lower gastrointestinal tract may produce similarly appearing stools or may appear as bright red blood. Such stools should be considered grossly bloody only after verification with chemical tests to avoid confusion with coloring from dietary substances or medications.

Occult Blood

Smaller increases in blood content may not alter appearance of the stool. Such stools are said to contain occult blood.[6,7] (Passage of 2.8 ml of blood per day is taken to be the upper limit of normal.) It is in the detection of increased (occult) bleeding that examination of feces may be most useful in uncovering gastrointestinal disease. Negative tests for occult blood in the presence of hypochromic anemia, otherwise unexplained, should not prevent a thorough search for gastrointestinal tract malignancy, because false-negative test results may occur.

TESTS FOR OCCULT BLOOD

The commonly applied tests for detection of occult blood depend on determination of peroxidase activity as an indication of hemoglobin content.[5,6] Reagents used include guaiac, benzidine, orthotolidine, and orthodianisidine (Figs. 2–3, 2–4, and 2–5). Peroxidases, including hemoglobin (which can act both as a catalase and as a peroxidase), release oxygen (from hydrogen peroxide), which then oxidizes the test substances, causing development of various shades and intensities of blue that depend on the reagent, concentration of hemoglobin or other catalases and peroxidases, presence of other coloring matter, and presence or absence of inhibiters.

The amount of peroxidase activity in the stool produced by a given amount of bleeding varies with the location of the bleeding and the intestinal transit time. Another variable is the level of digestive enzyme activity in the bacterial flora of the gastrointestinal tract. Although most of the hemoglobin entering the gastrointestinal tract reaches the stool in the form of hematin, which has peroxidase activity, a large amount of activity may be lost through further degradation to inactive materials. One investigator found a marked decrease in the peroxidase activity of blood passing through the gastrointestinal tract as compared to blood added directly to the feces. Furthermore, because of inhibiting substances in the stool, a similar loss of activity may be found after adding blood to feces, as compared with adding similar quantities of blood to water. Franklin Ebaugh and his associates suggested that this inhibition results from masking of indicator color by the added coloration of the feces. Another factor may be competition for the oxygen by reducing substances in the feces.

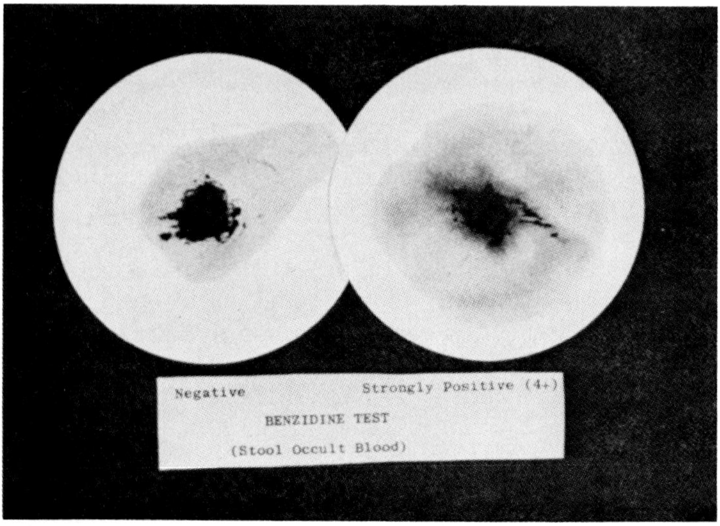

Fig. 2–3. Benzidine.

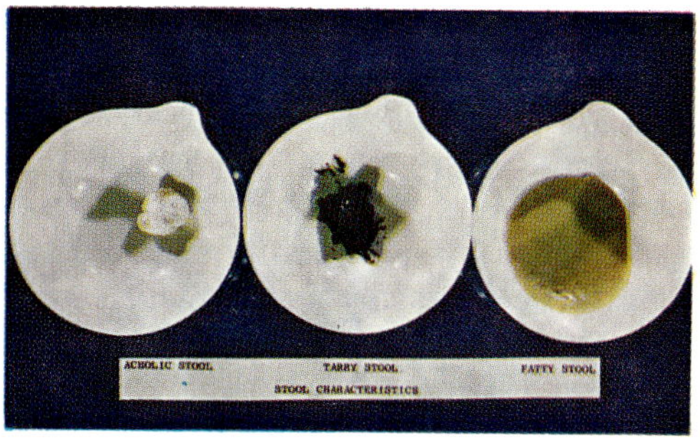

Fig. 2-2. Clay-colored, tarry, and fatty stools.

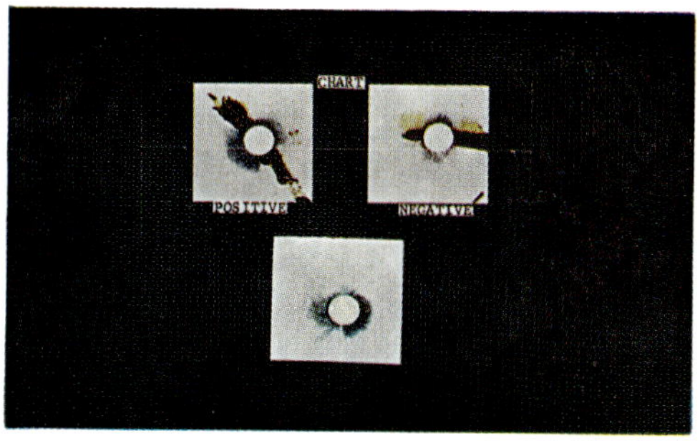

Fig. 2-4. Stool Hematest® for occult blood.

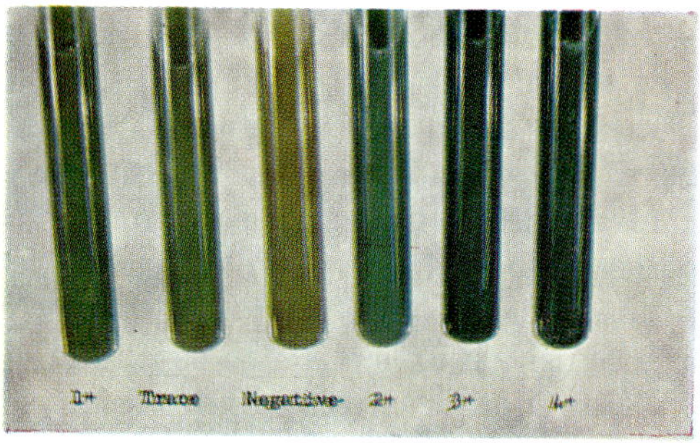

Fig. 2-5. Stool guaiac testing for occult blood.

peroxide in the same guaiac procedure, one obtains approximately the same sensitivity. We advise use of a saturated guaiac solution because of the tendency of some strongly positive reactions to fade with the weaker solutions presently available commercially. Addition of extra powdered guaiac will restore the color in these cases. This problem may be overcome by constantly observing for maximal color development.

The APT test represents a method of detecting alkali-resistant hemoglobin F, thus permitting evaluation of melena in the stool of the fetus to differentiate intestinal fetal blood (a common occurrence during delivery) from maternal blood that may have been swallowed during in vivo placental bleeding.

In recent years quantitative methods have been evolved for the study of gastrointestinal bleeding using radioactive ^{51}chromium and gamma ray quantitation. The methods can be combined with other techniques to determine the actual location of bleeding, when present. Inasmuch as these tests involve considerable time, effort, and expense, their use should be reserved for patients presenting special diagnostic problems. Procedures are based on the ability of ^{51}chromium to be bound to red blood cells, and on the fact that ^{51}chromium is not reabsorbed from the gastrointestinal tract, but is excreted in the feces, where it can be measured by gamma radiation detectors. For this purpose a sample of blood is withdrawn from the patient, mixed with citrate solution containing ^{51}chromium as sodium chromate, and then reinjected into the patient. Most of the sodium chromate is bound to the red blood cells and remains bound until the cells are destroyed or lost through hemorrhage. Subsequently, stools contain quantities of ^{51}chromium quantitatively related to the blood content. Gamma ray activity of the stool specimen is determined and the blood loss is calculated by comparison with activity of patient's blood. The bleeding source may be localized by similarly examining aspirate from the various levels within the gastrointestinal tract removed through a Miller-Abbott tube.

FAT

Healthy individuals on a normal fat intake excrete daily up to 5 g of lipid (measured as fatty acids)/24 hours in the stool. While the source of fecal lipid is largely dietary, gastrointestinal excretion, cellular desquamation, and bacterial metabolism also contribute. Lipids are normally present as soaps and triglycerides. In addition, lipoids are present, including high alcohols, paraffins, and vegetable carotenoids. Although diet has some effect on it, the pattern of lipids excreted may be very different from that of the diet, and the quantity of fat ingested by the normal individual has a relatively small effect on his total output of fat. According to one study, the fecal lipid is equal to a constant

(2.93 g) plus 2.1% of the dietary fat intake.[6] On a fat-free diet, the output of fat usually varies from 1 to 4 g/day.

The amount of fat in the feces may be expressed as percent by weight of dry stool, percent of ingested fat retained (absorbed), and weight (usually as fatty acids) per 24-hour stool collection. Because of wide variation in water content of the stool, wet weight concentrations are uninformative and so not recommended. Dry weight concentrations are only slightly less variable because of the effect of diet on bulk. Weight of fat excreted per 24 hours, based on analysis of an aliquot of at least a 3-day stool collection, is the most meaningful expression. For this purpose the patient is placed on a standard diet containing 100 g fat/day. (In infants and children for whom the standard 100 g diet cannot be used, percent coefficient of fat retention is the more useful expression. This is the difference between fecal fat and ingested fat, expressed as a percentage of the ingested fat. The coefficient of fat retention of normal children and adults is 95% or higher, although in premature infants it may be much lower than this.) Greater than normal fat excretion is steatorrhea. If the screening tests are positive, a quantitative determination of fecal fat provides the definitive diagnostic test for it. These are also useful for following effects of treatment.

It is convenient to consider steatorrhea according to the area of disease: *pancreatogenous*, caused by deficiency of pancreatic digestive enzymes; *hepatogenous*, caused by deficiency of bile salts; and *enterogenous*, in which absorption is impaired (sometimes referred to as "malassimilation," as opposed to "maldigestion"). Enterogenous steatorrhea includes such conditions as gluten-induced enteropathy (celiac disease, nontropical sprue, tropical sprue), abetalipoproteinemia, lymphangiectasis, intestinal lipodystrophy, amyloidosis, lymphoma, surgical loss of bowel function, and the "blind-loop" and diverticulum syndromes. Recent studies also suggest the presence of significant steatorrhea in acute diarrheal syndromes. The problem with these patients generally is not with digestion but rather with transference of materials from the gut lumen to the lymphatics and bloodstream. Hepatogenous steatorrhea results from interference with bile flow, as already mentioned. Loss of bile salts interferes with emulsification of fat, diminishing the surface area available for lipolytic action. In addition, there is loss of bile salt activation of lipase activity. The patients are usually jaundiced, excrete dark urine, and have other signs of deranged liver function. Hepatogenous steatorrhea may coexist with pancreatic steatorrhea, as, for example, in the case of neoplasm obstructing both the common duct and the pancreatic duct. In children, pancreatogenic steatorrhea most frequently results from fibrocystic disease of the pancreas (mucoviscidosis). In adults the most common causes are chronic pancreatitis and carcinoma of the head of the pancreas. It is generally associated with creatorrhea, evidenced by presence of undigested meat fibers in the feces and by an increase in neutral fat (triglycerides) in the stool, because of the lack of lipase (Fig. 2–6).

When the diagnosis of steatorrhea has been established, differential diagnosis becomes important for determining treatment. The usual problem is differentiation of pancreatogenous from enterogenous steatorrhea. In the case of children, the definitive test for mucoviscidosis (fibrocystic disease of the pancreas) is the sweat electrolyte determination (especially chloride). This test should be used whenever clinically warranted, although screening tests are available based on absence of stool trypsin and on semiquantitative demonstrations of increased sweat chloride (Fig. 2–7). Patients with steatorrhea, regardless of etiology, are liable to develop deficiencies of fat-soluble vitamins; hence, they may have low serum carotene levels.

Pancreatic lipase is necessary for hydrolysis of triglycerides to free acids and glycerides, and in these forms, absorption occurs into the intestinal epithelial mucosal cells. In patients lacking pancreatic enzymes, hydrolysis does not occur; hence, there is malabsorption of fat. Simple microscopic examination of stool stained for fat can detect pancreatogenous steatorrhea. In patients with clinical steatorrhea, every high power field may be filled with globules ranging up to 75 μ in size. Fatty acid crystals will not take up fat stains. In this case, stool must first be heated with acetic acid for fat stains to work.

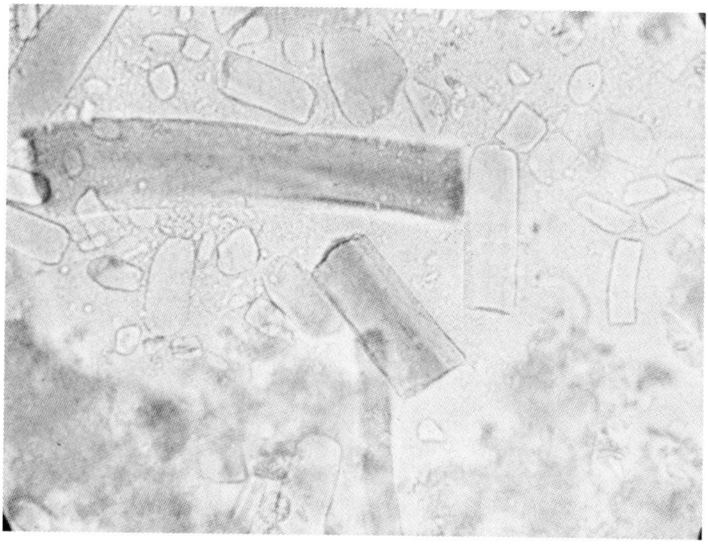

Fig. 2–6. Meat fibers.

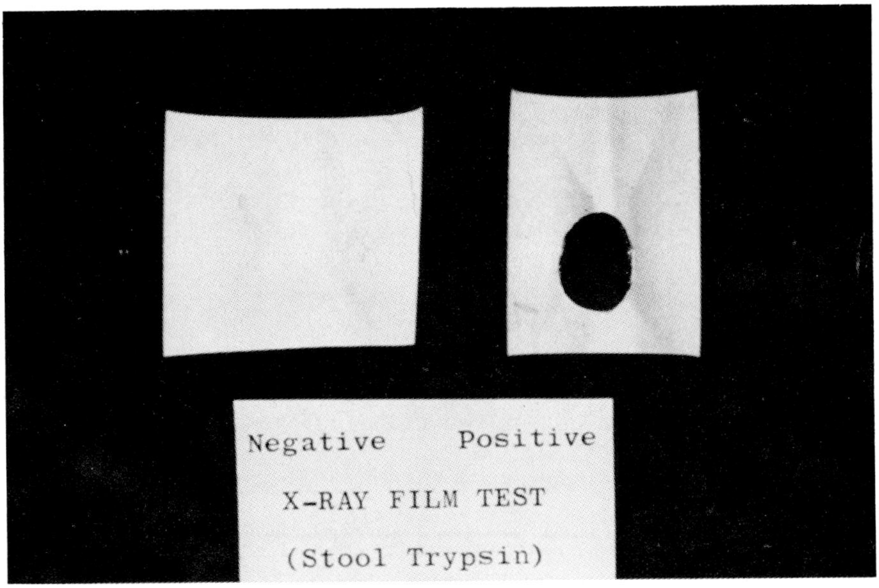

Fig. 2–7. Trypsin.

Malabsorption Tests

Laboratory investigation of patients with steatorrhea may involve examination of stool for undigested or unabsorbed foods or examination of blood and urine for presence of orally administered substances. Most of the tests suitable for the average clinical microscopy laboratory are simple screening procedures.

Screening tests for detection of pathologic increases in stool fat (steatorrhea) include:

1. Microscopic examination of the stool for fat globules
2. Microscopic examination of the stool for undigested meat fibers
3. Detection of urinary iodine excreted after ingestion of iodinated fat compounds
4. Measurement of previously ingested d-xylose in serum or urine
5. Testing for proteolytic enzyme (trypsin activity) in stools of young children
6. Measurement of serum turbidity at timed intervals following a fat meal
7. Determination of serum carotenoids
8. Glucose and lactose tolerance tests (primarily for detection of malabsorption of disaccharides and related carbohydrates)

FAT STAINS (MICROSCOPIC)

Microscopic examination is a procedure often performed for semi-quantitative estimation of fecal fat, because of the simplicity of the test. This usually involves use of Sudan III or Sudan IV, or Oil Red O stains (Fig. 2–8). Staining with these dyes depends upon the partition coefficient of dye between solvent and lipid; that is, the greater solubility of the dye in lipid substances than in other solvents. (Firm chemical union does not occur between the Sudan dye and lipids.) A rough estimate of the quantity of fat in the stool can be made visually after staining. Fatty acids appear as lightly staining flakes or as unstained needle-like crystals that may be missed (Fig. 2–9). Soaps, also, do not stain, but appear as well-defined amorphous flakes or as rounded masses or coarse crystals. Neutral fats, however, appear as large orange or red droplets, about 1 to 4 μ in diameter. In a normal stool there are less than 50 fat globules/high power field by microscopic examination, equivalent to less than 6 g fat (expressed as fatty acids)/24 hours (Fig. 2–8). Steatorrhea may be associated with large numbers of fat globules, some up to 75 μ in diameter. When 60 or more stained droplets of fats are seen per high power field, one may be reasonably certain that the patient has steatorrhea. Caution is advisable in interpretation, since mineral oil, castor oil, and other oily laxatives may stain and thereby, mimic neutral fat. After acidification and heating of stained fecal fat, the triglycerides (neutral fats) will be hydrolyzed to fatty acids and the fatty acids will melt into droplets that will stain strongly with Sudan III or other fat stains. After this procedure, up to 100 stained droplets

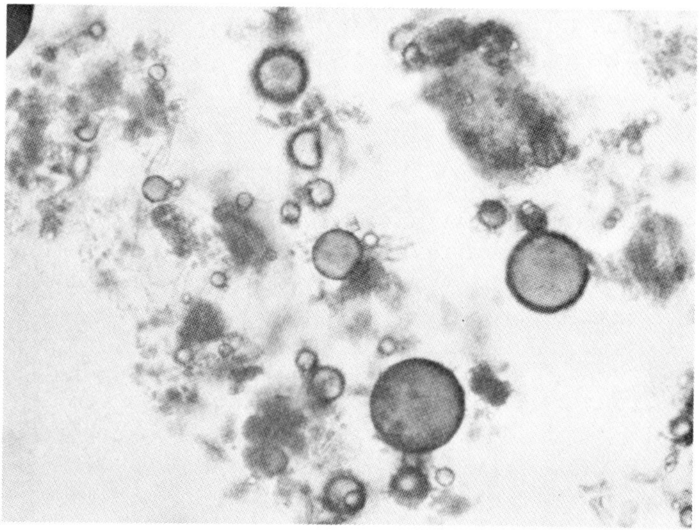

Fig. 2–8. Fat droplets in the stool.

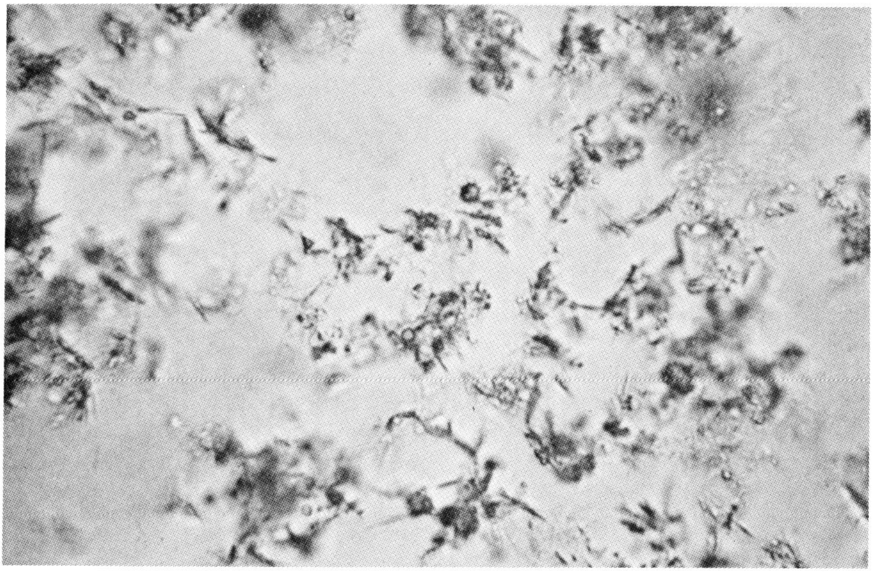

Fig. 2–9. Fatty acid crystals.

per high power field (about 1 to 4 μ in diameter) are considered normal. When the slide cools, fatty acids may crystallize in the form of needles (Fig. 2–9). (Use of Oil Red O has been advocated by some because it permits substitution of isopropanol, a less expensive alcohol that is not federally controlled, for ethanol.)

LIPIODOL ABSORPTION

We have found the Lipiodol absorption test to be useful as a screening test for lipid malabsorption and steatorrhea. Normal individuals readily absorb Lipiodol (an iodinated poppyseed oil composed of oleic, linoleic, linolenic, and other unsaturated fatty acids) through the intestinal epithelium. Iodine is split off and excreted via the kidneys.The iodine can be detected in the urine by its blue reaction with starch. In patients with steatorrhea, the Lipiodol is not absorbed; hence, little or no iodine is demonstrable in the urine. Peak urinary excretion of iodine in normal subjects occurs between 12 and 18 hours after oral ingestion of the dye. Lipiodol dye used for radiologic intravenous injection is used, but given orally. The consistency is "greasy" but patients will accept it without too many complaints. Patients should not be on a fat-restricted diet for at least 2 days prior to and on the day of testing, since even patients with malabsorption syndromes may then absorb more fat, giving false normal test results.

There is excellent correlation between the 24- and 72-hour quantitative fecal fat determination and the Lipiodol absorption test. In one study, patients with steatorrhea, as defined by quantitative fecal fat determination (over 5 g fat/24 hours), were found to have negative test results, or a positive reaction only in test dilution up to 1 in 2. Urine from healthy persons gave a positive Lipiodol reaction in dilutions of 1 in 8 or 1 in 32, corresponding to quantitative fecal fat excretions below 5 g/24 hours. The test is a very useful screening procedure inasmuch as a normal response may obviate need for a quantitative chemical determination. Positive test results following Lipiodol absorption are not specific for any particular disease, but can result from any disorder leading to impaired intestinal fat absorption regardless of etiology. Not all patients with fibrocystic disease will have abnormal test results; but those with steatorrhea will, even if some tryptic activity is present in their duodenal secretions. A positive test result, however, does not replace the more definitive diagnostic tests: analysis of sweat from children with suspected fibrocystic disease, or electrolyte determinations of duodenal drainage.

d-XYLOSE EXCRETION

One of the most valuable of the differential diagnostic tests, in adults especially, has been the d-xylose absorption test. Xylose is a pentose that is passively absorbed primarily in the duodenum and jejunum. Since it is a monosaccharide, no digestion is necessary prior to absorption. Xylose, unlike glucose, is not normally present in blood in detectable quantities and is not metabolized by the liver or peripheral tissues. In the preferred procedure, a 25-g dose of the sugar is administered orally in water, and the amount excreted in the urine during the following 5-hour period is determined. Excretion of 5 g or more in the test period is regarded as a normal response. Excretion of less d-xylose than this occurs in patients with enterogenous malabsorption, but not in those with pancreatogenous malabsorption (inasmuch as pancreatic enzymes are not required for absorption of d-xylose). Patients with sprue or sprue-like syndromes, therefore, have low values, usually excreting less than 10% of the 25-g dose in 5 hours. The finding of normal excretion in symptomatic patients eliminates sprue as a diagnostic possibility. The test is often abnormal even in asymptomatic patients with sprue. Patients with Whipple's disease may have abnormal d-xylose tests even in the presence of normal small bowel roentgenograms. Excretion is abnormal in postgastrectomy patients in whom the Höfmeister technique was used. Elevated urinary excretion values have been observed in hyperthyroid patients. Because the standard 25-g dose may produce borborygmus, abdominal cramping, diarrhea, nausea, and vomiting in some patients, investigators have resorted to a 5-g test dose, which is normally followed by a similar percentage excretion of d-xylose, but has fewer undesirable side effects. It is probably less sensitive, however. Since d-xylose is excreted by the kidney, renal function should be investigated prior to the test, inasmuch as poor kidney function may result in a low excretion. For the same reason, serum levels may also be determined. *High serum values coupled with low urine values suggest renal disease.* Low serum levels still suggest malabsorption.

D-xylose administration to small rodents has been shown to be cataractogenic, even though the cataracts are reversible. The only known human side effects are generally no more severe than similar side effects seen in glucose tolerance tests. The test appears still to be in widespread use throughout the United States, probably because *it remains the most useful single test for differentiating pancreatogenous and enterogenous steatorrhea.* The drug was not licensed for use in the United States until 1974.

DISACCHARIDE EXCRETION

In patients with intestinal malabsorption syndromes produced by carbohydrate intolerance, primary disaccharide deficiency is the most common etiology. When an offending sugar is fed to such a patient, diarrhea is rapidly produced. Screening laboratory tests using Clinitest (Ames Company) may be positive in such patients, obviating the need for more sophisticated chromatographic screening. Stool is emulsified in water, placed in a test tube, and the Clinitest tablet added. The chemical reaction is similar to that of urine containing glucose; therefore, the result can be semiquantitated by visual reference to the color chart provided for urine testing. (A result of 0.25% is considered negative; 0.25 to 0.50% is regarded as suspect; and greater than 0.50% is considered an abnormal amount of sugar present.) This test is not intended to provide conclusive evidence of defective disaccharide absorption, but will cull out those patients who should be investigated more intensively for carbohydrate malabsorption. (Kerry, K., and Anderson, C.: Lancet: 981, May 2, 1964.)

PROTEOLYTIC ENZYMES (TRYPTIC ACTIVITY)

Testing for tryptic activity in the stool by digestion of gelatin on x-ray film has been widely used as a screening test for cystic fibrosis in children (Fig. 2–7).

Trypsin and chymotrypsin are nearly always present in grossly measurable quantities in the stools of normal young children (Fig. 2–7). There is frequently much less activity detectable, however, in the adult stool, except when there is rapid transit through the gastrointestinal tract. The enzymes are apparently partially destroyed by bacteria within the gastrointestinal tract. Activity is seldom detectable at all by the cruder tests when there is constipation. The simple x-ray film test, therefore, is not very useful for adults. On the other hand, many bacteria produce proteolytic enzymes which have gelatinase activity and may give positive tests in the absence of pancreatogenous enzymes. For this reason, also, results must be interpreted with caution. In spite of these drawbacks, the tests have gained wide popularity. A number of other methods have been devised for detecting and measuring proteolytic activity in stools and duodenal fluid. These include ability of stool solutions to digest such substrates as serum proteins, hemoglobin, and casein, but most methods lack specificity and precision.

Recently, quantitative assays for trypsin and chymotrypsin activity have been developed, using more specific substrates. In these methods, such as that described by Bernard Haverback in 1963, the stool is incubated with substrate at 37° C at pH 8.2; the pH is maintained by automatic titration with sodium hydroxide. The quantity of sodium hydroxide used over a known period of time to neutralize the amino acids formed can be used to calculate trypsin or chymotrypsin activity in the stool. Substrates commonly used are para-toluenesulfonylarginine methyl ester (TAME) for trypsin determinations, and N-acetyl-L-tyrosine ethyl ester (ATEE) for chymotrypsin. The test is standardized with crystalline trypsin and chymotrypsin.

With these quantitative tests, it has been found that the stools of normal adults usually contain the equivalent of 20 or more mg trypsin/g of feces, and 74 or more mg of chymotrypsin per g of feces. Patients with exocrine insufficiency of the pancreas generally have values far below these. The correlation with chymotrypsin activity is better than that with trypsin. Because of their specificity, the tests are useful for the differential diagnosis of malassimilation disorders.

There are no fully satisfactory alternatives for these determinations for the differential diagnosis of pancreatic and enterogenous malabsorption, although isotopic techniques are of some use, and a *starch tolerance test* has been used by some workers for this purpose. In the latter, serial blood glucose determinations are performed following ingestion of starch, and are compared with those obtained following a glucose tolerance test. Theoretically, if the patient lacks pancreatic amylase, the glucose tolerance test will result in higher blood sugar values than will the starch tolerance test. Probably the most reliable alternative laboratory diagnostic aid, although unpleasant for the patient, is duodenal intubation and examination of duodenal contents.

MISCELLANEOUS

In addition to the usual screening tests, a number of procedures of lesser clinical usefulness are available, or are of interest primarily for research or other purposes. They are often performed in the clinical chemistry, rather than the clinical microscopy laboratory, and they include tests for nitrogen, porphyrins, sodium, calcium, magnesium, and chloride. Nitrogen determinations have been used for diagnosing malabsorption, as fecal nitrogen, as well as fecal fat, may be increased in these conditions because of difficulty with protein digestion and absorption. However, nitrogen content varies markedly with bacterial flora; the finding is less constant than steatorrhea, so the clinical usefulness of this determination is limited. Fecal calcium tends to vary with diet and is seldom determined except in special balance studies. Assays of stool for other electrolytes have not proven clinically useful.

Stool urobilinogen assays, however, have been used to confirm diagnosis of complete obstruction to bile flow. For the purpose, after emulsification of stool, urobilins are reduced to urobilinogens by ferrous sulfate. Then the urobilinogens are reacted with Ehrlich's aldehyde reagent (paradimethyl-aminobenzaldehyde) to form a red urobilinogen-aldehyde complex, which can be measured semiquantitatively by visual comparison with standards (prepared with pontacyl dyes or with phenolsulfonphthalein dye), or by measurement of absorbance in a spectrophotometer at 560 nm.

MICROSCOPIC EXAMINATION FOR MEAT FIBERS

Undigested food remnants may frequently be seen during microscopic examination, including vegetable particles, seeds, bone, cartilage, and some meat fibers. The amount of undigested particles or their degree of digestion depends on prior cooking, mastication of food, exposure to enzymes, pH of secretions, gastric hydrochloric acid, intestinal motility, intestinal bacterial flora, intestinal transit time, and a host of other factors. Consequently, it is difficult to assess the significance of undigested food. Also, in the feces of children, it is common to see grossly visible whole kernels of corn and other vegetables. Nevertheless, excretion of large numbers of undigested meat fibers (creatorrhea) is abnormal and usually associated with diarrhea or steatorrhea (Fig. 2–6). In adults, creatorrhea frequently accompanies the pancreatogenic steatorrhea of carcinoma of the pancreas or pancreatitis.

REFERENCES

1. Caryle-Wicksteed translation, The Divine Comedy of Dante Alighieri. New York, The Modern Library (#208), 1932.
2. Hamilton, J.: Observations on the Utility and Administration of Purgative Medicines in Several Diseases. 5th ed. Philadelphia, Thomas Kite, 1829.
3. Mathison, R.: The Shocking History of Drugs. New York, Ballantine Books, 1958.
4. Bryan, C.: The Papyrus Ebers. New York, D. Appleton & Co., 1931.
5. Forbes, J., Tweedie, A., and Conolly, J. (ed.): The Cyclopedia of Practical Medicine. Vol. 1. Philadelphia, Lea & Blanchard, 1845.
6. Beeler, M., Kao, Y., and Scheer, W.: Malabsorption diarrhea and examination of feces. *In* Clinical Diagnosis and Laboratory Methods. Edited by J. Henry. 16th Ed. Philadelphia, W.B. Saunders, 1979.
7. Derman, H., and Pauker, S.: Detection of occult blood in feces and urine. *In* Hemoglobin: Its Precursors and Metabolites. Edited by F. Sunderman and F. Sunderman, Jr. Philadelphia, J.B. Lippincott Co., 1964, p. 70.

OCCULT BLOOD

METHOD. Guaiac method.

PRINCIPLE. Hemoglobin, myoglobin, and other substances having peroxidase activity will, in the presence of hydrogen peroxide, oxidize colorless guaiacol to green-blue tetraguaiacol.

PROCEDURE 1. Run a control using feces known to contain enough occult blood to produce 4+ peroxidase activity.

1. Place about 5 g feces in a 15-ml test tube.
2. Add 2 ml water and mix well, using applicator stick.
3. Add 0.5 ml glacial acetic acid and mix well, as above.
4. Add about 2 ml guaiac solution and mix well, as above.
5. Add about 2 ml hydrogen peroxide, mix well, and start timer.
6. Observe for color development within 2 minutes.

PROCEDURE 2

1. Spread feces on filter paper.
2. Place guaiac tablets on feces.
3. Add 2 drops glacial acetic acid onto tablet.
4. Add 2 drops hydrogen peroxide.
5. Observe for color development within 2 minutes.
6. Positive control is run by dropping 2 drops 1:500 control solution on filter paper, placing guaiac tablet onto area, and continuing test procedures as above.

INTERPRETATION. Green-blue developing within 2 minutes is interpreted as a positive test result. The reaction can be interpreted semi-quantitatively as follows:

Trace	Tan (or barely perceptible blue)
1+	Pale tan-blue
2+	Blue
3+	Moderately dark blue
4+	Very dark blue

Strongly positive reactions may fade rapidly, and should be read according to maximal color development, rather than by color present at the end of 2 minutes.

DISCUSSION AND CLINICAL SIGNIFICANCE. Positive reactions by this method are abnormal. The benzidine test and orthotolidine tests (including Hematest and Occultest) have greater sensitivity and may yield an unacceptable number of false positive reactions. The guaiac method represents a compromise, suitable for routine screening, that does not require a meat-free diet. The test will detect about 70 to 100 mg hemoglobin/100 ml solution of feces or 0.5 to 1.0 mg hemoglobin/ml of aqueous solution (whereas the Occultest and Hematest techniques are said to detect as little as 1 to 10 mg hemoglobin/dl fecal suspension). Ingested iron will not give a positive test result. Fat may interfere, imparting an unusual appearance to a positive test.

Fat can be removed by shaking the specimen (after step 2 in the above procedure) with an equal volume of ether. If this is done, allow the ether layer to separate, then discard. Add a volume of glacial acetic acid about equivalent to a third of the remaining emulsion. Extract the acidified mixture with one volume of ether. Proceed with steps 4 and 5. Blue develops quickly if hemoglobin is present.

In the case of dried stains on cloth, wood, or other material, dissolve the stain with distilled water and test the solution, or press a piece of moist filter paper against the stain and add drops of the guaiac solution and hydrogen peroxide to the paper. False negatives can occur in the presence of large amounts of vitamin C. Laxatives and barium do not interfere with the performance of the test.

MATERIALS AND REAGENTS

1. 1 in 60 (w/v) solution gum guaiac in 95% (v/v) ethyl alcohol (a saturated solution is preferable, if available)
2. Glacial acetic acid
3. 3% (v/v) hydrogen peroxide
4. Guaiac tablets (Cambridge Chemical Products, Inc., 6880 N.W. 17th Avenue, Fort Lauderdale, Fla. 33009. Catalog no. 1003)
5. Test tubes, 15 ml
6. Test tube rack
7. Wooden applicator sticks
8. Positive control solution—1:500 dilution whole blood in distilled water

REFERENCES

1. Barnett, R.: The guaiac test: correlation with clinical findings. Gastroenterology, *21*:540, 1952.
2. Derman, H., and Pauker, S.: Detection of occult blood in feces and urine. *In* Hemoglobin: Its Precursors and Metabolites. Edited by F. Sunderman and F. Sunderman, Jr. Philadelphia, J.B. Lippincott Co., 1964, p. 70.

OCCULT BLOOD

METHOD. Benzidine test (not recommended; Benzine is carcinogenic)

PRINCIPLE. Hemoglobin (and other substances with peroxidase activity) in the presence of hydrogen peroxide cause oxidation of benzidine to benzidine blue.

PROCEDURE. (Run a control, using feces known to contain enough occult blood to produce 4+ peroxidase activity.)

FILTER PAPER METHOD

1. Spread a thin layer of stool specimen in the center of a piece of filter paper.
2. Add 4 drops of benzidine reagent.
3. Mix well with applicator stick.
4. Add 4 drops of hydrogen peroxide.

TEST TUBE METHOD

1. Emulsify about 1 part feces in 40 parts of water (about 0.25 g/10 ml water) in a 15-ml test tube.
2. Add 1 ml benzidine reagent to 1 ml 1 to 40 emulsion of feces.
3. Add 1 ml hydrogen peroxide

INTERPRETATION. Green-blue developing at 1 minute (and persisting with agitation in the test tube method) is interpreted as a positive result for peroxidase activity.

DISCUSSION AND CLINICAL SIGNIFICANCE. With the filter paper technique the test is said to be able to detect 50 to 100 mg hemoglobin/100 g feces. The test tube method is said to be able to detect about 100 to 300 mg hemoglobin/dl of a 1 to 40 emulsion.

Refer to an earlier section of this chapter for a more complete discussion. Presence of detectable blood in the feces of patients who have been on a meat-free diet for at least 3 days prior to the test is abnormal, and usually denotes gastrointestinal bleeding. Iron ingestion does not interfere with the reaction. However, as already mentioned, the test lacks specificity. Peroxidases from dietary meat, and perhaps from vegetables, may produce a positive reaction. Modifications of the test intended to destroy plant peroxidases by boiling also destroy some of the peroxidase activity of hemoglobin, and therefore are not recommended. The test is subject to numerous errors arising from inconsistencies in amount of feces used, variable absorption of material into filter paper, improper timing of reaction, lack of uniform mixing of blood from lower gastrointestional tract, etc. In addition, benzidine has been reported to be carcinogenic and is not even available for use in the British Isles for this reason.

MATERIALS AND REAGENTS

1. Benzidine dihydrochloride reagent

Benzidine dihydrochloride $(C_6H_4)_2(NH_2)_2.2HCl$	1g
Glacial acetic acid	20 ml
Distilled water	30 ml
95% (v/v) ethyl alcohol	50 ml

2. 3% (v/v) hydrogen peroxide
3. Filter paper
4. Test tubes, 15 ml
5. Wooden applicator sticks

REFERENCES

1. Derman, H., and Pauker, S.: Detection of occult blood in feces and urine. *In* Hemoglobin: Its Precursors and Metabolites. Edited by F. Sunderman and F. Sunderman, Jr. Philadelphia, J.B. Lippincott Co., 1964, p. 70.
2. Kark, R., et al.: A Primer of Urinalysis. 2nd ed. New York, Hoeber Medical Division, Harper & Row, 1963, p. 53.

OCCULT BLOOD

METHOD. Hematest method.

PRINCIPLE. Orthotolidine in the tablet is oxidized to toluidine blue in the presence of hydrogen peroxide and hemoglobin. Sodium bicarbonate and tartaric acid act as effervescents. Hydrogen peroxide is produced by the reaction of tartaric acid and calcium acetate with strontium peroxide.

PROCEDURE. (Run a control using feces known to contain enough occult blood to produce 4+ peroxidase activity.)

1. Smear an aliquot (from the central portion) of the stool specimen on filter paper using applicator sticks. (Do not use an emulsion.)
2. Place Hematest tablet in center of specimen.
3. Place 1 drop of water on tablet, wait 5 to 10 seconds, and add a second drop on the tablet so that it runs down the sides onto the filter paper.

INTERPRETATION. The moistened area on the filter paper turns blue within 2 minutes if hemoglobin, myoglobin, or other peroxidases are present in detectable amounts. Disregard any color change on the tablet, or any color change after 2 minutes on the filter paper.

DISCUSSION AND CLINICAL SIGNIFICANCE. The test has been claimed to detect as little as 0.1 mg hemoglobin/dl of aqueous solution of feces. As previously mentioned, most of the blood and hemoglobin reach the stool in the form of hematin, which has peroxidase activity, and hence gives a positive test. Bismuth will not give a positive reaction, but ferric chloride may produce a blue color.

The tablets are stable for 3 or more years if kept tightly sealed. Sensitivity decreases with extreme heat and humidity. Although the tablets darken with age, moderate color change is not accompanied by a perceptible change in sensitivity. Paradoxical negative or trace results may occur with tarry stools, as previously mentioned. An unacceptable number of false positives are encountered in patients not placed on a meat-free diet. We prefer the guaiac test.

MATERIALS AND REAGENTS

1. Hematest tablets and paper (Ames Company, Elkhart, Ind. 46514)
2. Wooden applicator sticks

REFERENCES

1. Ames Company brochure on test.
2. Derman, H., and Pauker. S.: Detection of occult blood in feces and urine. *In* Hemoglobin: Its Precursors and Metabolites. Edited by F. Sunderman and F. Sunderman, Jr. Philadelphia, J.B. Lippincott Co., 1964, p. 70.
3. Rencher, J., and Beeler, M.: Stool examination. *In* Clinical Diagnosis by Laboratory Methods. 14th ed. Edited by I. Davidsohn and J. Henry. Philadelphia, W.B. Saunders, 1968.

MELENA NEONATORUM (DIFFERENTIATION OF SWALLOWED MATERNAL BLOOD FROM FETAL BLOOD)

METHOD. Apt test.

PRINCIPLE. Hemoglobin prepared from maternal blood is changed to a brown-yellow color in 1 to 2 minutes after the addition of an alkali, the latter of which causes conversion of oxyhemoglobin to alkaline hematin. The color change can be visualized grossly. (It is important that the stool be bloody and red and not tarry, because oxyhemoglobin has already been converted to hematin in a tarry stool.)

PROCEDURE

1. Mix a small amount of stool with distilled water in a test tube to lyse the erythrocytes (usually 1 part of stool to 5 to 10 parts of water).
2. Mix well with applicator sticks.
3. Centrifuge at 2000 RPM's for 2 minutes to separate the fecal material.
4. Filter or decant the supernatant.
5. To 5 ml of the supernatant, add 1 ml of sodium hydroxide.
6. Observe the color change after 2 minutes.

INTERPRETATION. If maternal blood has been swallowed by the neonate and is present in the feces, the pink supernatant hemoglobin solution will turn to brown after 2 minutes. If fetal blood is present, it resists denaturation of the red cells by alkali; hence, there is no conversion of the oxyhemoglobin to hematin.

DISCUSSION AND CLINICAL SIGNIFICANCE. Neonatal infants may have grossly blood stools as a result of bleeding internally or as a result of swallowing maternal blood during delivery. Prompt identification of the adult type hemoglobin, presumably swallowed maternal blood, would spare the newborn infant from undergoing unnecessary and sometimes detrimental examination to determine whether there is, in fact, intestinal bleeding.

While spectrophotometry is a more precise method of distinguishing two types of hemoglobin, this particular test is rapid, simple, and gives useful clinical information. When only a blood-stained diaper is available, the test can be modified by adding sodium hydroxide directly to the stain on the diaper to detect the type of pigment present.

MATERIALS AND REAGENTS

1. Centrifuge, clinical
2. Test tubes, 15 ml
3. Serological pipettes, 1 ml
4. Sodium hydroxide, 0.25 N; add 9.5 ml H O and 0.5 ml of 5 N NaOH.
5. Applicator sticks

REFERENCES

1. Apt., L., and Downey, W.: Melena neonatorum: The swallowed blood syndrome. J. Pediatr., 47:6,, 1955.
2. Schaffer, A., and Avery, M.: Diseases of the Newborn. 4th Ed. Philadelphia, W.B. Saunders, 1977, p. 317.

NEUTRAL FAT ESTIMATION

METHOD. Sudan III staining.

PRINCIPLE. Except for lipoids of high melting points (cholesterol, carotenoids, paraffins) most lipids, including most neutral fats (triglycerides), stain with oil-soluble dyes (Sudan III, Oil Red O). Staining with these dyes depends upon the partition coefficient of dye between solvent and lipid; that is, greater solubility of the dye in lipid substances than in other solvents. (Firm chemical union does not occur between the Sudan dye and lipids.) A rough estimate of the quantity of fat in the stool can be made visually after staining.

PROCEDURE

1. Mix stool specimen thoroughly with an applicator stick.
2. Place a small amount (2 to 3 mm^3) on a clean stick. Emulsify with a drop of ethyl alcohol.
3. Add 2 drops of Sudan stain.
4. Mix well and apply coverslip.
5. Let stand for 5 minutes and examine microscopically.

INTERPRETATION. Presence of neutral fat droplets is indicated by yellow-orange to red globules (about 1–4 μ in diameter), which tend to collect at the edges of the coverslip. In normal stools, there are less than 50 fat globules/high power field by microscopic examination, equivalent to less than 5 g fat (expressed as fatty acids)/24 hours.

DISCUSSION AND CLINICAL SIGNIFICANCE. Pancreatic lipase is necessary for hydrolysis of triglycerides to free fatty acids and glycerides, which are absorbed. Lack of pancreatic enzymes causes maldigestion, and therefore, malabsorption, leading to steatorrhea. The test described may not detect enterogenous malabsorption, since fatty acids are not stained unless previously heated. Oily laxatives may cause false positive test results. Oil Red O is taken up fairly readily by mineral oil, for example. Steatorrhea is associated with large numbers of fat globules, some up to 75 μ in diameter.

MATERIALS AND REAGENTS

1. 95% (v/v) ethyl alcohol
2. Sudan III, saturated solution in 95% (v/v) ethyl alcohol
3. Microscope, slides, and coverslips
4. Wooden applicator sticks
5. Medicine dropper

REFERENCES

1. Beeler, M., Kao, Y., and Scheer, W.: Malabsorption diarrhea and examination of feces. *In* Clinical Diagnosis and Laboratory Methods. Edited by J. Henry. 16th Ed. Philadelphia, W.B. Saunders, 1979.
2. Lillie, R.: Histopathologic Technic and Practical Histochemistry. 3rd ed. New York, McGraw-Hill, 1965, p. 454.
3. Page, L., and Culver, P.: A Syllabus of Laboratory Examinations in Clinical Diagnosis. Cambridge, Harvard University Press, 1961, p. 378.

TOTAL FAT ESTIMATION

METHOD. Sudan III staining.

PRINCIPLE. Fatty acids can be stained with oil-soluble fat stains when warm. Heating stool with acid hydrolyzes triglycerides to fatty acids and glycerol and melts the fatty acid crystals, allowing them to coalesce into droplets.

PROCEDURE

1. Place a small amount (2 to 3 mm^3) of stool on a glass slide.
2. Emulsify with 2 drops of acetic acid.
3. Add 2 drops of Sudan stain and mix well; cover with a coverslip.
4. Gently heat the slide over a low flame until there is boiling under the coverslip (repeat this 2 or 3 times to assure complete hydrolysis)
5. Examine specimen microscopically while it is still warm.

INTERPRETATION. Fatty acids will appear as orange globules while the preparation is still warm. As the preparation cools, fatty acids may recrystallize into colorless needle-like crystals in sheaths.

DISCUSSION AND CLINICAL SIGNIFICANCE. The test is positive in enterogenous and hepatogenous as well as in pancreatogenous steatorrhea. In stools from patients with severe steatorrhea, every high power field may be filled with globules ranging up to 75 μ in size.

"Total fat" includes neutral fat, free fatty acids, and combined fatty acids (soaps). Fat appears in feces even during starvation and during fat-free diets. According to one study already referred to, fecal fat excretion is relatively constant at 2.93 g/day plus 2.1% of dietary intake.

MATERIALS AND REAGENTS

1. Sudan III (saturated solution) in 95% (v/v) ethyl alcohol
2. 36% (v/v) acetic acid
3. Microscope, slides, and coverslips
4. Bunsen burner
5. Wooden applicator sticks
6. Medicine dropper

REFERENCES

1. Halstead, J., and Halstead, C.: The Laboratory in Clinical Medicine: Interpretation and Application. 2nd Ed. Philadelphia, W.B. Saunders, 1981.
2. Isselbacher, K., et al.: Harrison's Principles of Internal Medicine. 9th Ed. New York, McGraw-Hill, 1980, p. 1396.

3. Lillie, R., and Fullmer, H.: Histopathologic Technic and Practical Histochemistry. 4th Ed. New York, McGraw-Hill, 1976, p. 459.

LIPIODOL ABSORPTION

METHOD. Jones and di Sant'Agnese modification of Lipiodol absorption test.

PRINCIPLE. Iodine excreted in the urine of normal patients after ingestion of Lipiodol can be detected by its blue reaction with starch and may be estimated semiquantitatively by serial dilutions of the urine.

SAMPLE. Since the peak excretion of iodine in urine occurs between 12 and 18 hours after administration of test Lipiodol, urine should be collected during this time interval. There is no time limitation for performance of the test after specimen collection. (It is imperative that patients be on an unrestricted fat diet for at least 2 days prior to and on the day of testing, because even patients with the malabsorption syndrome may have better fat absorption following a period of dietary fat restriction, and may thus have a normal test result.)

PROCEDURE

1. Place seven 10-ml test tubes in a rack and label "1" through "7."
2. Pipette 0.5 ml distilled water into tubes "2" through "7," and 0.5 ml of urine into tubes "1" and "2."
3. After mixing by shaking the tube, transfer 0.5 ml urine from tube "2" to tube "3." Repeat with each successive tube. Discard 0.5 ml from tube "7" (this will produce 0.5 ml volumes of undiluted urine, and urine dilutions of 1 in 2 through 1 in 32).
4. Place tubes in ice bath for 10 minutes.
5. Add 0.2 ml of nitric acid to each tube.
6. Shake tubes and allow to stand at room temnperature for 5 minutes.
7. To each tube, add 3 drops of fresh starch suspension.
8. Shake all tubes and allow to stand for 5 minutes.
9. Observe precipitate at the bottom of the tubes for blue indicative of the starch-iodine complex.
10. Record the tube of greatest dilution with perceptible blue.

INTERPRETATION. Even the faintest tinge of blue should be considered a positive reaction. Tubes containing large amounts of iodine may turn black or dark brown. (Observe tubes against a white background.)

DISCUSSION AND CLINICAL SIGNIFICANCE. Patients with steatorrhea have negative test results or positive reactions only up to a dilution of 1 in 2, while urine from healthy individuals gives positive reactions in dilutions of 1 in 8 to 1 in 32. The test is useful as a screening procedure for malabsorption. It is abnormal in all disorders leading to impaired intestinal absorption of fat, regardless of etiology. The definitive test for fibrocystic disease of the pancreas is the sweat sodium determination.

Erroneous results may be obtained in patients receiving iodinated medications, or in those with impaired renal function.

MATERIALS AND REAGENTS

1. 8 N Nitric acid
2. 1% (w/v) starch (solution of buffered starch substrate for amylase procedure, type s. Dade Reagents Inc., Miami, Fla.)
3. Test tubes, 13 × 100 mm
4. Serologic pipettes, 1 ml
5. Ice bath
6. Test tube rack

REFERENCES

1. Jones, W., and di Sant'Agnese, P.: Laboratory aids in the diagnosis of malabsorption in pediatrics. Lipiodol absorption as a simple test for steatorrhea. J. Pediatr., *62*:44, 1963.
2. Silverman, F., and Shirkey, H.: Fat absorption test using iodized oil, with particular application as a screening test in the diagnosis of fibrocystic disease of the pancreas. J. Pediatr. *15*:143, 1955.

FECAL TRYPSIN DETERMINATION

METHOD. Schwachman, Patterson, and Laguna, modified by Johnstone.

PRINCIPLE. X-ray film strips are immersed in serially diluted fecal emulsions. Proteolytic activity (of trypsin and chymotrypsin) there causes digestion of the gelatin emulsion on x-ray film. This permits semiquantitative estimation of enzyme activity.

SAMPLE. A freshly collected stool or duodenal aspirate (not more than a few hours old) is necessary, since enzymatic activity decreases with time. If necessary, the stool can be frozen for preservation.

PROCEDURE. Test as a control an x-ray strip immersed in 1 ml buffer only.

1. Make a 1 in 5 (v/v) dilution of stool (1 ml stool, 4 ml buffer), by placing 4 ml buffer in a large test tube (16 × 125 mm), marking level of fluid on tube, then adding stool until fluid level rises 20% higher (visual estimate). Mix well with applicator sticks.
2. Label 12 small test tubes (13 × 100 mm) "1" through "12."
3. Place 1 ml buffer into tubes "2" through "12."
4. Place 1 ml 1 in 5 stool emulsion into tube "1," and 1 ml into tube "2," using a propipette and a broken tipped 10 ml serologic pipette.
5. Serially dilute, starting with tube "2" (1 in 10 dils), up to 1 in 10,240 (tube "12") by transferring 1 ml to the next tube; mixing; then transferring again.
6. Add a strip of x-ray film to each tube, including the control tube.

7. Incubate for 1 hour at 37° C.
8. Remove strips, wash *gently* in running tap water, and observe.

INTERPRETATION. Complete digestion of gelatin is recognized by complete clearing of x-ray film (the blue tint of the film base should become apparent). Partial digestion is indicated by a mixed clear and cloudy film. When there is no digestion, the gelatin remains intact, and it has the same appearance as the control.

DISCUSSION AND CLINICAL SIGNIFICANCE. Complete digestion of the film occurs up to at least a 1 in 100 dilution of feces of normal children. Stools from patients with fibrocystic disease (mucoviscidosis) are usually negative; or are positive only in the lower dilutions. Many intestinal bacteria produce gelatinase, which may digest gelatin in the absence of fecal trypsin and chymotrypsin. However, the amount of bacterial gelatinase normally present is rarely sufficient to produce positive clearing in as high as the 1 in 96 dilution. Whenever it is uncertain whether clearing has been produced by tryptic activity or by bacterial gelatinase, soybean trypsin inhibitor (2 mg/ml) can be added to the stool specimen. This should inhibit tryptic activity, but not bacterial gelatinase activity. In one series, 96% of 9,600 tests on postmeconium infant stools yielded positive results in dilution of 1 in 96 or higher.

There is much less trypsin activity in adult feces, except when there is rapid intestinal transit. The enzymes are apparently destroyed by bacteria. Whatever result is obtained in a patient whose symptoms are suggestive, a sweat electrolyte (Na^+, Cl^-) determination should be performed.

Stools negative for trypsin in the first 24 hours should be retested after 24- to 48-hour storage at 37° C. Hard stools indicate that there has been slow intestinal passage and dehydration of bowel content, hence trypsin activity may be completely expended prior to testing.

MATERIALS AND REAGENTS

1. Barbital buffer, pH 8.0

Sodium diethylbarbiturate	20g
Distilled water q. s.	1,000 ml

Adjust with 0.1 N HCl to pH 8.

(Requires about 3 volumes HCl for each 7 volumes barbital.)

2. Undeveloped x-ray film (cut into 3 × 120 mm or 5 × 120 mm strips)
3. Wooden applicator sticks
4. Test tubes, 13 × 100 mm and 16 × 125 mm
5. Serologic pipettes, 5 ml with broken tips
6. Water bath or incubator at 37° C
7. Propipette

REFERENCES

1. Johnstone, D.: Studies on cystic fibrosis of the pancreas. Role of various diluents and the dilution factor in the interpretation of the x-ray film test for fecal trypsin. Am. J. Dis. Child., 84:191, 1952.
2. Meites, S. (ed.): Pediatric Clinical Chemistry. 2nd Ed. Washington, D.C., American Association for Clinical Chemistry, 1981, p. 417.
3. Shwachman, H., Patterson, P., and Laguna, J.: Studies in pancreatic fibrosis: A simple diagnostic gelatin film test for stool trypsin. J. Pediatr., 4:222, 1949.

D-XYLOSE ABSORPTION TESTS

PRINCIPLE. Xylose is given to the patient; and the subsequent urine voided is collected; and a blood specimen is taken. The xylose concentrations in the 5-hour urine specimen and in the blood specimen are determined by treating the diluted urine and a protein-free filtrate of the blood with p-bromoaniline in an acid medium. Xylose, when heated with acids, will form furfural, which reacts with p-bromoaniline. A pink color is produced in this reaction. The concentrations of xylose in blood and urine are calculated on the basis of a standard xylose solution.

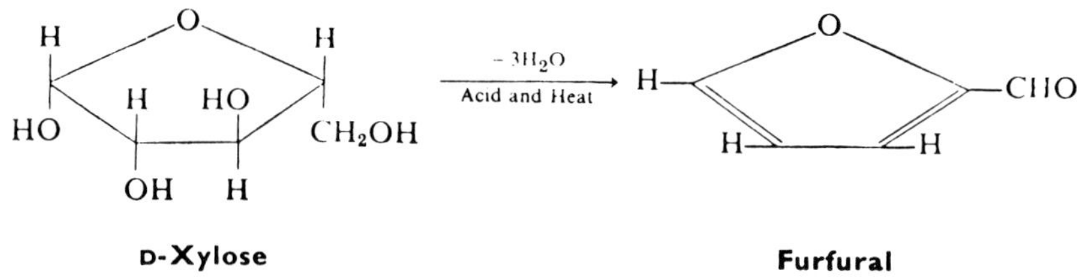

SAMPLE COLLECTION
ADULTS

1. Keep patient fasting overnight and during test period.
2. In the morning (for example, at 7 AM), have the patient empty his bladder completely and discard this urine. Some investigators recommend checking a fasting urine and blood sample for nonspecific chromogens that react with p-bromoaniline; such interferences have been reported in some cases. Correction may be made by subtracting the base value from that found in test specimen.
3. Give 25 g (or 5 g, if so specified by the physician) of d-xylose dissolved in 250 ml of water, followed immediately by an additional 250 ml of water.
4. Collect and pool all urine specimens voided during the next 5 hours, including the 5-hour specimen.
5. After approximately 2 hours, collect a blood sample, preferably in a tube containing sodium fluoride.

CHILDREN

1. Keep patient fasting overnight and during test period.
2. In the morning (for example, 7 AM), have the patient empty his bladder completely.
3. Give 0.5 g of d-xylose/lb of body weight (up to 25 g), cutting the amount of water according to the weight of the patient.
4. Collect and pool all urine specimens during the next 5 hours.
5. Collect a blood sample approximately 60 minutes after xylose administration. The time of blood collection is different from that in adults, because the peak of absorption in children is reached sooner.

PROCEDURE

1. *Urine:* If 5 to 15 g of xylose is given, dilute the urine to 500 ml; if 15 g or more of xylose is given, dilute the urine to 1,000 ml (freeze a part of the first diluted urine for possible repeat). Further dilute a convenient portion of the urine 40-fold.
2. *Blood:* Deproteinize the blood by using 1 ml blood, $ZnSO_4$•$7H_2O$, (10.5 g/L) and 1 ml $Ba(OH)_2$•$8H_2O$ (9.5g/L). Mix after each addition and centrifuge.
3. Add the following amounts (in ml) of blood filtrate, urine, standard solutions, and p-bromoaniline to a set of test tubes as indicated.

	Blood		Urine		Standard (0.1 mg/ml)		Standard (0.2 mg/ml)	
	Test	Blank	Test	Blank	Test	Blank	Test	Blank
Supernatant	0.5	0.5	—	—	—	—	—	—
Diluted urine	—	—	0.5	0.5	—	—	—	—
Xylose (0.1 mg/ml)	—	—	—	—	0.5	0.5	—	—
Xylose (0.2 mg/ml)	—	—	—	—	—	—	0.5	0.5
p-Bromoaniline	2.5	2.5	2.5	2.5	2.5	2.5	2.5	2.5

4. Place all tests into a 70° C water bath for 1 minute, and all blanks in the dark room temperature.
5. Cool the incubated tubes and place all test tubes in the dark. After 70 minutes, read the test against the blank, using a spectrophotometer or colorimeter at a wavelength of 520 nm. Alternatively, all tests and blanks may be read against a water blank.
6. Calculation: Blood

$$\text{mg xylose/dl} = \frac{A(\text{test})}{A(\text{standard, 0.1 mg/ml})} \times 10 \times 10$$

If all test and blank tubes are read against water:

$$\text{mg xylose/dl} = \frac{\text{A(test)} - \text{A(blank)}}{\text{A(standard)} - \text{A(blank)}} \times 10 \times 10$$

Calculation: Urine

If urine was diluted to dl:

$$\text{g xylose excreted} = \frac{\text{A(test)}}{\text{A(standard, 0.2 mg/ml)}} \times \frac{20 \times 40}{100} \times \frac{1{,}000}{1{,}000}$$

If urine was diluted to 500 ml:

$$\text{g xylose excreted} = \frac{\text{A(test)}}{\text{A(standard, 0.2 g/dl)}} \times \frac{20 \times 40}{100} \times \frac{500}{1{,}000}$$

If all test and blank tubes were read against water, the absorbance of the blank must be subtracted from the absorbance of the test as indicated under blood.

INTERPRETATION. Adults, after a 25 g dose of xylose, should excrete more than 4.0 g of xylose/5 hour urine specimen. In patients over 65 years of age, the minimum excretion is 3.5 g/hour. Blood values are normally more than 25 mg xylose/dl blood. Normal children excrete 16 to 33% of the ingested xylose and their blood xylose level is more than 30 mg/dl.

DISCUSSION AND CLINICAL SIGNIFICANCE. Xylose is a pentose not normally present in significant amounts in blood. When given orally, it is passively absorbed in the proximal small (duodeno-jejunal) intestine, passes unchanged through the liver, and is excreted by the kidneys. The xylose absorption test is considered a reliable index of the functional integrity of the jejunum (in the absence of massive bacterial overgrowth). Low absorption of xylose is observed in intestinal malabsorption, but not in malabsorption caused by pancreatic insufficiency. In the latter condition, the absorption of xylose will be essentially normal provided that there is no significant increase in intestinal motility. Therefore, the test is of some help in distinguishing between these two types of malabsorption. The test findings are abnormal in 80% of patients with malabsorption syndrome.

The accuracy of the procedure depends not only on the rate of absorption but also on the rate of excretion of xylose by the kidneys. Thus, patients with renal insufficiency will excrete a decreased amount of xylose. One can eliminate misinterpretations because of renal retention, myxedema, or incomplete urine collection, and thus prevent invalid tests. Aspirin decreases the excretion of xylose by the kidneys, and indomethacin depresses intestinal absorption.

Some abdominal discomfort or slight diarrhea may be observed in certain patients. These symptoms can be minimized by use of the 5-g-xylose dose. Normal urinary excretion of xylose after a 5-g dose is more than 1.2 g/5 hours. Kendall recommends the 5-g dose because it is easier to take and much less likely to cause abdominal distension and diarrhea. The author also suggests reducing the collection period to 2 hours to minimize any possible metabolism of xylose by microorganisms.

There is only slight decrease in values obtained when the urine is refrigerated at 37° F for 12 hours; however, values will be markedly lowered in urine stored 72 hours or more at room temperature.

MATERIALS AND REAGENTS

1. Zinc sulfate ($ZnSO_4 \cdot 7H_2O$); 10.5 g/L
2. Barium hydroxide. Dissolve 9.5 g of $Ba(OH)_2 \cdot 8H_2O$ in water and dilute to 1000 ml with water. Boil for a few minutes, stopper, cool, and filter.
3. p-Bromoaniline reagent. Prepare a saturated solution of thiourea in glacial acetic acid by shaking about 4 g of thiourea/dl of glacial acetic acid, and decant the supernatant. Dissolve 2 g of p-bromoaniline in dl of the decanted thiourea solution.
4. Stock standard, 200 mg of xylose/dl. Place 200 mg d-xylose into a deciliter volumetric flask, dissolve in and fill up to volume with benzoic acid (0.3 g/dl).
5. Working standard (0.1 mg/ml). Dilute stock standard 20-fold with saturated benzoic acid.
6. Working standard (0.2 mg/dl). Dilute stock standard 10-fold with saturated benzoic acid.

REFERENCES

1. Benson, J., et al: The d-xylose absorption test in malabsorption syndromes. N. Engl. J. Med., *256*:335, 1957.
2. Kendall, M., Nutter, S., and Hawkins, C.: Bacteria and the xylose test. Lancet *1*:1017, 1972.
3. Reiner, M., and Cheung, J.: Xylose. *In* Standard Methods of Clinical Chemistry. Vol. 5. New York, Academic Press, 1965, pp. 257.
4. Roe, J., and Rice, E.: A photometric method for the determination of free pentoses in animal tissue. J. Biol. Chem., *173*:507, 1948.
5. Sheehy, T., and Flock, M.: The Small Intestine: Its Function and Diseases. New York, Hoeber Medical Division, Harper & Row, 1964, p. 51.
6. Tietz, N.: Fundamentals of Clinical Chemistry. Philadelphia, W.B. Saunders, 1976, p. 1091.

Chapter

3 Gastric Analysis

DONALD C. CANNON
JAMES A. FREEMAN

Interest in gastric function and stomach pathology is deeply rooted in ancient history. In the doctrine of Yin and Yang, before 1000 B.C., the ancient Chinese recognized the functional capacity and expansibility of the stomach in the expression, "It can stretch itself until it will hold 5 tou of rice or 1 tou and 5 sheng of water" (1 sheng = 1.035 L; 1 tou = 10 sheng).[1] T'sang Kung, the great Chinese physician of the Han Dynasty (206 B.C. to 220 A.D.), actually recorded visual observations of carcinoma in the stomach. The more recent history of gastric analysis has been comprehensively reviewed by Hollander and Penner.[2,3,4] During the seventeenth and eighteenth centuries, investigators obtained gastric-fluid specimens from experimental animals by retrieving swallowed sponges or from human beings by induced vomiting.

As a result of serendipity, gastric activity was first visualized in vivo in 1822 by army surgeon William Beaumont. Serving at Fort Michilimackinac in northern Michigan, Beaumont was called upon to administer to a French Canadian fur trader, Alexis St. Martin, who had been struck in the left side by a shotgun blast at close range. Beaumont, thinking his patient would die within a few days, merely dressed the wound and left the outcome to Providence. St. Martin fully recuperated and was able to resume his usual pursuit; however, a fistula had formed and persisted from the external abdominal wall to the stomach. Beaumont seized this opportunity for repeated visualization of gastric activity and reported his findings in 1833 in his book, Experiments and Observations on the Gastric Juice and the Physiology of Digestion.[5] Ironically, St. Martin did not die until 1880 and outlived Beaumont by 27 years.

Gastric intubation was first practiced in antiquity, largely for therapeutic purposes (such as lavage following ingestion of poison). For routine medical applications, gastric intubation was not practical until the discovery of vulcanization of rubber by Charles Goodyear in 1844. Intubation for diagnostic purposes was first performed in 1883 by Wilhelm von Leube, who was primarily interested in the gastric residue following ingestion of a test meal but also in quantitating the gastric acid and pepsin.[6] During the next decades, clinical interest in gastric secretion was heavily focused on the introduction and evaluation of various test meals, each of which carried the name of its originator. These concoctions, which continued in common use until about 20 years ago, included the Riegel meal (steak, beef broth, white bread, and water), the Ewald meal (bread and water), and the von Leube meal (soup, beefsteak, and white bread). A significant advance in the technique of gastric intubation occurred with the introduction of an improved tube by Martin Rehfuss in 1914.[7] At the same time, Rehfuss introduced the concept of fractional gastric analysis, which dominated clinical gastric analysis for the next 40 years or so. In this approach, small aliquots (10–15 ml) of gastric fluid are removed at designated time intervals for chemical analysis.

During the first half of the twentieth century, more potent stimuli to gastric secretion were introduced. These stimuli included ethanol, caffeine, and later, histamine. The concept of maximal secretory stimulus was introduced in 1953 by Kay, who recommended a dose of histamine acid phosphate that would effect maximal acid output by the stomach and, thus, conclusively distinguish acid-secretors from nonsecretors.[8] This test, known as the augmented histamine test, soon became the standard reference test in gastric analysis and remained so until it was largely replaced by pentagastrin as a stimulus in the late 1960s in Europe and subsequent to 1975 in the United States, when it was finally approved for routine clinical use by the Food and Drug Administration.

The identification of gastric acid as hydrochloric acid was made by English chemist William Prout, who unfortunately—from the standpoint of current physiochemical knowledge—introduced the concepts of "free acid," "combined acid," and "total acid."[9] These terms were probably adapted from the nomenclature of contemporary chemists, but they remained ingrained in gastric analysis for the next 140 years or so. In 1926, Michaelis presented data from extensive titration studies of gastric secretion, which appeared to support the concepts of free and combined acid.[10] Unfortunately, however, these studies are invalid, because Michaelis analyzed gastric contents obtained after test-meal stimulation, which were thus diluted with buffers inherent in the food itself. It was not until 1962 that Bock recommended discarding the terms "free acid" and "total acid" in favor of expressing gastric acid simply in terms of meq of hydrochloric acid/L.[9]

PHYSIOLOGY OF GASTRIC SECRETION

The stomach has basically three major physiologic functions. First, the stomach acts as an expansible reservoir that temporarily stores ingested food so that it can be partially dissolved and liquefied while it is mixed with gastric secretion. Second, protein digestion is initiated in the stomach through the secretion of gastric proteolytic enzymes termed, collectively, "pepsin." This initial phase of proteolysis is not particularly important in the overall digestive process. Third, the gastric mucosa secretes intrinsic factor, which is essential for the subsequent absorption of vitamin B_{12} in the ileum and, thus, for the prevention of pernicious anemia.

Gastric secretion is classicially represented as occurring in three phases based on the origin of the excitatory stimuli, but the three phases are interrelated. The cephalic, or neurogenic, phase involves transmission of excitatory stimuli from the brain to the stomach via the vagal nerves. The vagal nerves originate from the vagal nuclei in the medulla oblongata just beneath the fourth ventricle of the brain. The vagal nuclei are susceptible to various neural stimuli including those initiated by the taste, sight, smell, or anticipation of food, as well as by excitatory and inhibitory stimuli that originate from other centers of the brain (depression, anger, and fear, for example). Vagal stimulation has four effects on the stomach. The most important consequence of vagal stimulation is secretion of gastrin into the blood by specialized cells (G cells) located in the pyloric glands. Gastrin reaches the more proximal body and fundus of the stomach through the bloodstream and stimulates the parietal cells of the gastric glands in these regions to secrete hydrochloric acid and the chief, or peptic, cells to secrete pepsin. Gastrin is thus a true endocrine hormone and is the most potent known stimulus to gastric secretion. Gastrin is a polypeptide, which consists of two molecular species in the circulating blood, a 17-amino-acid molecule and a 34-amino-acid molecule, which is often termed, "big gastrin." Although it constitutes only about one third of the total gastrin in blood, the small species exhibits the greatest increase in response to vagal stimulation and is about six times as potent as its larger counterpart. Vagal excitation also lowers the threshold of the parietal cells to gastrin stimulation and directly stimulates the parietal cells to secrete hydrochloric acid. The fourth vagal effect is maintenance of gastric tone and motility, which together promote gastric peristalsis and emptying.

The gastric phase of secretion includes those stimuli originating in the stomach itself. Distention of the stomach with food or fluid and contact of amino acids and various protein breakdown products, collectively termed "secretagogues," with the gastric mucosa stimulate antral G cells to secrete gastrin and probably also directly stimulate the parietal and chief cells to secrete. In view of this effect of gastric distention, it is obvious that simple vagotomy can be a self-defeating procedure for treating peptic ulcer. Consequently, vagotomy is ordinarily combined with antrectomy or a drainage procedure, such as gastroduodenostomy or gastrojejunostomy.

The intestinal phase of gastric secretion is the least significant. It also involves the secretion of gastrin by G cells located in the duodenal glands and perhaps other hormones in response to distention and contact of acid contents and protein products with the duodenal mucosa.

Several mechanisms inhibit gastric secretion in addition to the psychogenic stimuli previously mentioned (fear or depression, for example). Acidification of gastric contents to a pH of less than 3.0 decreases the responsiveness of gastrin release by the antral G cells, and this inhibition is virtually complete when the pH falls to 1.5. Enterogastrone is the name given to hormonal substances released by the duodenum in response to contact of its mucosa with fat or fatty acid breakdown products that inhibit gastric-acid secretion and gastric motility. Further investigations have led to the purification and characterization of a polypeptide hormone, gastric inhibitory polypeptide (GIP), which is responsible for most of the enterogastrone activity.[11] GIP is produced by specialized cells (K cells) located in the intestinal glands of the mid and distal duodenum and proximal jejunum. GIP is secreted into the blood in response to contact of various substances with the duodenal mucosa, including fats, glucose, and amino acids. In addition to suppressing gastric motility, GIP inhibits both pepsin and hydrochloric-acid secretion by direct effect on the chief and parietal cells and by inhibiting gastrin release.

Other intestinal hormones also inhibit gastric-acid secretion.[12] Vasoactive intestinal polypeptide (VIP) is a polypeptide hormone produced by H cells, which are widely distributed in the intestinal mucosa and by certain nerve cells including those in the brain. Although very little is known about its physiologic release mechanisms, it has a broad spectrum of physiologic and metabolic effects, including inhibition of acid and pepsin secretion, inhibition of gastrin release, and inhibition of gastric motility. Increased blood levels of VIP have been implicated in a rare syndrome of watery diarrhea, hypokalemia, and achlorhydria (WDHA syndrome). The importance of the hormones secretin and cholecystokinin-pancreozymin, both produced by cells in the mucosa of the small intestine, is debatable. Both have an inhibitory effect on gastric secretion, but this is probably a minor role under physiologic conditions.

CHEMICAL COMPOSITION OF GASTRIC FLUID

In view of the diversity of cell types that contribute to gastric secretion and the wide range of physiologic influences that control the secretory process, it is not surprising that the net result is a complex chemical mixture that varies considerably in its composition. Attempts to define the overall process by which gastric fluid is compounded have proved to be oversimplifications. The best known of these is the two-component hypothesis of Franklin Hollander, who proposed that gastric fluid is basically a mixture of acid secretion from the parietal cells, of more or less fixed composition, with an alkaline component of varying composition secreted by other cells, including the chief and mucus cell.[13]

Hydrochloric Acid

The parietal cells, located in the fundus and body of the stomach, can secrete hydrogen ion under conditions of maximal stimulation against a gradient of about one million times the hydrogen-ion concentration of plasma. In terms of any direct participation in the digestive process, hydrochloric acid has a minor role. It major function is to activate the conversion of pepsinogen to the proteolytic enzyme, pepsin, but it also directly hydrolyzes polypeptides and disaccharides to a very limited extent.

Pepsin

Pepsin is the generic term for similar proteolytic enzymes that are derived from precursors (pepsinogens) upon contact with acid. The various pepsinogens have pH optima varying from 1.6 to 3.6.[14] Small amounts of the pepsinogens diffuse into the blood, but only one of these, pepsinogen 1, occurs in the urine. Attempts have been made to relate blood and urine pepsinogen activity with gastric secretory activity, but the correlation is not reliable. Pepsin catalyzes the proteolysis of all soluble native proteins, except mucins, and has a special affinity for peptide bonds involving leucine, tyrosine, or phenylalanine. Pepsin will curdle milk and, thus, is responsible for the activity formerly ascribed to rennin, which does not occur in the gastric secretion of primates. The oligopeptides resulting from pepsin proteolysis are more potent stimuli for gastrin secretion than either intact proteins or oligopeptides produced by other proteolytic enzymes.

Pepsin is secreted in response to the same stimuli as is hydrochloric acid-vagal stimulation, stomach distention, mucosal contact with secretagogues, and gastrin. Consequently, it is generally believed that no additional useful information is to be gained by analysis of peptic activity. There are, however, some quantitative differences in the responses to the various secretory stimuli. For example, gastrin stimulates secretion of hydrochloric acid to a greater degree than secretion of pepsin.

Mucus

Gastric mucus is a complex mixture of mucoproteins and mucopolysaccharides secreted by cells distributed throughout the entire gastric mucosa. The major function of mucus appears to be to protect the mucosa of the stomach from autodigestion. Slight changes in mucus do occur in various disease states, but analysis of mucus is not warranted for diagnostic purposes.

Miscellaneous Substances

Various nondigestive enzymes are found in gastric fluid and reflect the active metabolism of the stomach: isocitric dehydrogenase, alanine aminotransferase, lactic dehydrogenase, aspartate aminotransferase, beta-glucuronidase, phosphohexose isomerase, alkaline phosphatases, and ribonuclease. Lactic dehydrogenase, beta-glucuronidase, and phosphohexose isomerase have increased activity in the gastric fluid of patients with gastric carcinoma, but this is not useful for diagnostic purposes.[15,16]

Small amounts of plasma proteins, especially albumin and gamma globulin, are detectable in gastric fluid. Increased amounts of plasma proteins occur in conditions involving loss of selective permeability of the microvasculature or in frank blood loss—giant hypertrophic gastritis, peptic ulcer, or gastric carcinoma, for example. Electrophoretic evaluation of gastric-fluid proteins has no clinical value.

Secretor substance is present in gastric fluid as well as in other body fluids of the 80% of individuals who are either homozygous or heterozygous for the secretor gene.

Intrinsic factor is a very minor component of gastric fluid from the standpoint of concentration, but it is the most important component in relation to total body physiology, because of its role in facilitating the intestinal absorption of vitamin B_{12}. It is a glycoprotein of molecular weight 17,000.

INDICATIONS FOR GASTRIC ANALYSIS

Gastric analysis is performed far less frequently today than it was only several decades ago, and there are several reasons for this decline. Most important is the fact that the scope of gastric analysis has not changed appreciably while numerous procedures have been introduced that greatly enhance the diagnosis of gastric disease, including improved radiologic techniques, fiberoptic gastroscopy, exfoliative cytology, in vivo and in vitro assays for intrinsic factor, and radioimmunoassays for vitamin B_{12} and gastrin. General awareness of the fact that anacidity occurs in a minority of cases of stomach carcinoma—and then, only in the advanced stage—has finally eliminated gastric analysis as a screening test for this disease. An important factor of considerable good fortune to medicine is that the incidence of both peptic ulcer and stomach carcinoma has decreased dramatically in the past 25 years for reasons that are unknown. Also, the improved diagnostic procedures and medical therapy, including the recent introduction of the H_2 receptor antagonist, cimetidine, along with the general availability of improved surgical care have reduced both the morbidity and mortality of peptic-ulcer disease but, unfortunately, have only slightly decreased the mortality of stomach carcinoma.

Although there is some difference of opinion, there are four reasonably well established diagnostic applications for conventional gastric analysis. First of all, gastric analysis is the sine qua non for diagnosing gastric anacidity. Anacidity is an essential feature of the syndrome of adult pernicious anemia, which also includes megaloblastic bone-marrow morphology with macrocytic anemia, absence of intrinsic-factor secretion, low plasma concentration of vitamin B_{12}, high plasma concentration of gastrin, and degenerative changes of the central nervous system as well as of peripheral nerves. Interestingly, immunoglobulin IgG or IgA antibodies to gastric parietal cells occur in 70 to 90% of affected patients. Although all of these manifestations need not be demonstrated to make the diagnosis of pernicious anemia, many physicians perform conventional gastric analysis to demonstrate anacidity in the augmented stimulation test in order to substantiate the diagnosis. Gastric analysis is indicated particularly in suspected cases in which the anemia and megaloblastic bone-marrow changes have been corrected by recent administration of vitamin B_{12}. Anacidity in a maximal gastric-stimulation test also effectively excludes the possibility of benign peptic ulcer to explain an ulcerating lesion of the stomach, but this is not a very useful finding for diagnostic purposes.

Gastric analysis is of value in determining the surgical procedure to be used for peptic ulcer.[17] The maximal acid output in the augmented histamine test or pentagastrin test provides an estimate of the number of functioning parietal cells in the gastric mucosa, a concept sometimes termed the parietal cell mass. Surgeons who utilize this concept recommend that patients with normal or only slightly increased acid output be treated with limited gastric resection or vagotomy with a drainage procedure. In contrast, patients with a significantly elevated acid output, which indicates an increased parietal cell mass, require a more extensive procedure, such as subtotal gastric resection with vagotomy.

Gastric analysis is useful in diagnosing the Zollinger-Ellison syndrome, which consists of greatly increased gastric secretion in terms of both acid and secretory volume, intractable peptic ulceration, and high plasma concentration of gastrin as a consequence of a neoplasm usually in the pancreatic islets.

Determination of gastric-acid secretion in response to insulin-induced hypoglycemia is useful in assessing the completeness of surgical vagotomy. Complete vagotomy in patients other than those with the Zollinger-Ellison syndrome will result in a low basal acid output that does not increase significantly with the central vagal stimulation provided by hypoglycemia.

PERFORMANCE OF GASTRIC ANALYSIS

Specimen Collection and Intubation of Patients

The great majority of patients subjected to gastric analysis are outpatients or ambulatory inpatients. This is fortunate because better recovery of gastric contents is achieved when the patient is able to sit upright and thus create a more optimal sump along the distal greater curvature of the stomach for gastric fluid to accumulate for aspiration. The patient who is bedfast and cannot sit upright should be placed on his left side with the head of the bed inclined 45° in order to optimize the pooling of gastric fluid. In either case, care should be taken to protect the patient's clothing with towels, aprons, or other suitable drapes in the event of gagging and regurgitation. Intubation can be performed either orally or nasally, but most patients will exhibit better tolerance for nasal intubation. Prior chilling of the tube has been recommended to decrease the gagging and nausea that some patients experience during intubation. Lubrication of the tip of the tube with K-Y jelly or glycerin may assist passage, but some lubricants will interfere with acid-fast staining for tubercle bacilli. The tube that is chosen for oral or nasal intubation should have a radiopaque tip, so that fluoroscopic monitoring of the tube placement can be readily achieved. The most dependent portion of the stomach and, thus, the sump, in which gastric fluid will accumulate will ordinarily be in the antrum, if the patient is sitting, and in the middle of the greater curvature or somewhat more distally, if the patient is positioned on the left side. Although many tubes are precalibrated with distances from the tip, placement by such measurements or by clinical judgment will be found to be suboptimal in at least half of the attempts, thus allowing gastric fluid to escape into the duodenum.

For oral intubation, any suitable tube, such as a Rehfuss tube, can be used provided that it has a radiopaque tip. In the sitting position, the patient should lean forward slightly with the chin forward and inclined slightly upward. This position facilitates tube passage by providing a straighter pathway from the mouth to the stomach. The tube is placed on the posterior part of the tongue and gently directed to the pharynx. Contact with the uvula and soft palate is to be avoided because extensive gagging can be triggered. Once the tube has reached the posterior pharynx, the patient should partially close his or her mouth so that the tube can be advanced at intervals while the patient swallows. Deep breathing by mouth should be encouraged.

For nasal intubation, the patient should be similarly positioned. A 14F or 16F Levin tube is commonly employed. Some prefer double-lumen tubes, such as Einhorn, Cleland, or Salem tubes, because blockage of the tube with mucus is more readily avoided. Two barriers to nasal passage can be encountered—the nasal concha and the epiglottic opening. The nasal concha can most effectively be bypassed by directing the tube horizontally and slightly downward into the nostril (Fig. 3–1). The epiglottis can best be passed by having the patient swallow while the tip of the tube passes (a helpful approximation is that the distance from the nares to the glottis is about the same as the distance from the nares to the external ear canals).

Once the position of the tube tip is optimized under fluoroscopic monitoring, the free end can be taped to the patient's face with surgical Scotch tape. Ordinary Scotch tape or adhesive tape should not be used, because they may cause considerable discomfort during removal and skin irritation can result. Suction can be performed either with an aspiration pump or by simply attaching a syringe to the tube. Actually, the best recovery of gastric fluid is achieved by gentle continuous suction with a glass or plastic syringe.[18] Cooperative patients will usually be able to maintain the suction process by themselves with assistance only for the periodic detachment and emptying of the syringe. The syringe contents can be emptied into any clean container, such as a disposable, plastic urine container. Patients should be instructed to expectorate saliva while gastric contents are being collected.

Although unpleasant at best, gastric intubation is a relatively benign procedure. Nausea and gagging are common but usually of brief duration. Nosebleeds rarely result from nasal intubation. Occasionally, a stomach tube enters the trachea, but this will usually be evident immediately by the paroxysms of coughing that ensue. There are a few contraindications to gastric intubation: esophageal varices, carcinoma, diverticulum, stenosis, aortic aneurysm, recent gastric hemorrhage, congestive heart failure, and pregnancy.

Basal Gastric Secretion Test

The basal gastric-secretion test is intended to represent the gastric secretion in the interdigestive period. Consequently, patients must be fasting (a 12-hour overnight fast with water allowed until 8 hours before the test is preferable). All other liquids are prohibited during the 12-hour fast, particularly coffee, tea, colas, and alcohol, because these are stimuli for gastric secretion. Twelve hours is more than adequate time for the normal stomach to purge itself of ingested contents. All medications that can influence gastric secretion (antacids, anticholinergic drugs, cimetidine, caffeine, reserpine, and adrenocorticosteroids, for example) should be withheld for at least 48 hours prior to the test. The patient should not engage in any vigorous physical activity immediately prior to the test and should be protected from stressful encounters. The test should be conducted in a tranquil atmosphere, but obviously, many patients are anxious because of their anticipation of the procedure.

The basal gastric-secretion test has now been reasonably well standardized as a 1-hour collection of secretion in four 15-minute specimens.

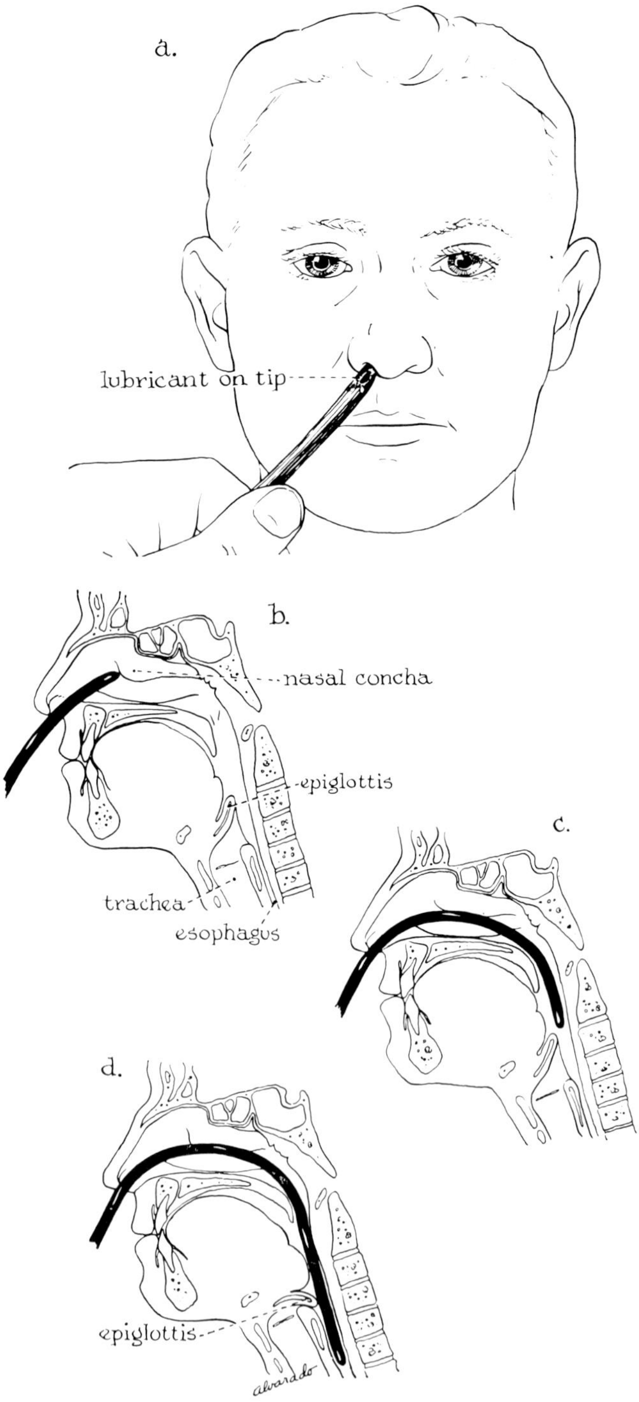

Fig. 3–1. Intubation of patients for collection of gastric contents (a). Two barriers to passage may be encountered: the nasal concha (b), which may be bypassed by passing the tube downward into the nostril with the head tilted forward (c); and the epiglottis (d), which may be bypassed by insertion of tube at height of deglutition (d).

Unfortunately, the 12-hour overnight collection continues to be used in spite of the fact that the 1-hour test has been shown to be representative of gastric secretory activity and has a diagnostic reliability at least equal to the 12-hour test.[19] Devotees of the 12-hour test claim that its greater sampling period more effectively integrates fluctuations in gastric secretion, but any such advantage is more than outweighed by the requirements for overnight hospitalization and mechanical suction, less complete collection of secretion, and generally cumbersome nature of the test.

The 1-hour basal test is ordinarily begun after 15 to 30 minutes have elapsed following intubation, in order to allow the patient to adjust physiologically and psychologically to the intubation process. The following parameters are measured:

1. Volume
2. pH
3. Titratable acidity
4. Acid output

The volume, pH, and titratable acidity are measured for each specimen and the acid output is calculated. The total volume and total acid output for the entire hour are calculated by simply adding the four 15-minute values.

Augmented or Maximal Stimulation Tests

These tests are characterized by their performances under conditions designed to result in maximum stimulation of gastric secretion. Prior to Andrew Kay's introduction of the augmented or maximal histamine test in 1953, various test meals, caffeine, alcohol, and low doses of histamine were used as gastric stimulants. All of these agents, however, resulted in a submaximal secretory response.

The augmented or maximal histamine test uses a subcutaneous dose of histamine acid phosphate (0.04 mg/kg body weight) that was found experimentally by Kay to be the smallest dose of histamine that produced maximum acid secretion.[8] The test was eventually adapted as the standard test for quantitating gastric-acid secretion until it was replaced by the pentagastrin test in the later 1960s in Europe and in 1975 in the United States. The augmented histamine test is usually performed as a 1-hour collection of gastric fluid segregated into four 15-minute specimens immediately following the 1-hour basal secretion test. This test does require the parenteral administration of an appropriate antihistamine [for example, 10 mg chlorpheniramine maleate (Chlor-Trimeton) or 50 mg diphenhydramine hydrochloride (Benadryl)] 30 minutes before the injection of histamine to suppress, if not totally obviate, the serious side effects of histamine, which include hypotension, headache, cutaneous erythema, tachycardia or bradycardia, lacrimation, and nasal obstruction. Nevertheless, these side effects do occur frequently in varying degrees of severity. The classic antihistamines do not interfere with gastric secretion because they block the actions of histamine only at the H_1 receptor sites—that is, those responsible for vasodilation, contraction of nonvascular smooth muscle, and increased capillary permeability.

Histalog (betazole, 3 beta-aminoethylpyrazole dihydrochloride), a synthetic histamine analog introduced in 1949, has had considerable application in gastric analysis, because of its ability to stimulate gastric secretion while largely avoiding the unpleasant side effects of histamine.[20] The stimulatory effect of Histalog on gastric secretion is quantitatively similar to histamine in that the peak acid outputs are similar if not identical, but the secretory responses to the two drugs are qualitatively different, in that Histalog has a longer latency period and a longer duration of action. Consequently, the stimulated secretion test with Histalog is ordinarily extended to 2 hours and eight, segregated 15-minute specimens. A prior injection of antihistamine is not needed. Analogous to the determination of histamine dosage required to cause maximal gastric secretion, the augmented Histalog dose is 1.7 mg/kg body weight administered intramuscularly.[21]

Pentagastrin is a synthetic pentapeptide composed of the four C-terminal amino acids of gastrin linked to a substituted alanine derivative. Because it retains much of the biologic activity of intact gastrin, pentagastrin has been used extensively in gastric analysis since it was introduced in Europe in 1966. Unfortunately, it was not approved by the Food and Drug Administration for routine clinical use until 1975 in the United States, where it is now commercially available as Peptavlon. Pentagastrin has a stimulatory effect on gastric-acid secretion that is quantitatively and qualitatively very similar to histamine except that it has minimal residual stimulatory effect after the first postinjection hour, which is actually an advantage.[22] Side effects are slight and include transitory dizziness, faintness, flushing, and numbness of the extremities in some patients. Maximal acid secretion is achieved by a subcutaneous dose of 6 mg/kg body weight.[23] Otherwise, the test is conducted in an identical manner to the augmented histamine test, except that no antihistamine is required. Because of its simple protocol and relative freedom from side effects, the pentagastrin test should replace all others for routine stimulated gastric analysis.

Insulin Hypoglycemia Test

The use of insulin-induced hypoglycemia as a test for completeness of vagotomy was first reported by Hollander in 1946.[24] In the subsequent 30 years, numerous protocols were introduced for performing the test.[25] Hypoglycemia directly stimulates the vagal nuclei of the brain to transmit excitatory stimuli via the vagal nerves to cause increased gastric acid secretion. Complete transection of the vagal nerves obviously interrupts this sequence of events. Actually, the effect of hypoglycemia on the normal stomach with intact vagal nerves is complex and not completely explained.

During the first 30 minutes or so after insulin injection, there is often a slight and unexplained decrease in gastric secretion. The major effect on gastric secretion during the first two postinsulin hours is, however, a marked increase in both the volume of secretion and the acid output as a direct consequence of vagal stimulation. A later stimulatory effect ordinarily occurring after 2 hours results from hypoglycemia-induced secretion of corticotrophin-releasing factor (CRF) by the hypothalamus. CRF increases the secretion of adrenocorticotrophic hormone (ACTH) by the anterior pituitary. The net effect is an increased plasma concentration of adrenocortical hormones, which directly stimulate the parietal cells to secrete acid.

Among the many protocols for performing the insulin hypoglycemia test, the procedure of Steven Stempien has considerable merit.[26] After an overnight (12 hours) fast, a 2-hour basal secretory test is performed followed by insulin injection and a 2-hour postinsulin secretion test. Both tests are collected as 15-minute segregated specimens for measurement of volume, pH, and titratable acidity and calculation of acid output. Blood specimens are collected immediately prior to insulin injection and at 30, 60, and 90 minutes thereafter to ascertain that plasma glucose falls to 50 mg/dl or less at some point in the test, most often in the 30-minute specimen. The dose of insulin is either 0.20 units/kg body weight or a fixed dose of 15 or 20 units administered intravenously in either case. The risk of serious hypoglycemia is real, so the test should be performed only when a physician, as well as a 50-ml syringe of 50% (w/v) glucose solution, are readily available. A number of side effects are, unfortunately, an integral part of the hypoglycemic response: hunger, thirst, diaphoresis, tachycardia, increased pulse pressure, and palpitations—all of which usually peak at about 45 minutes after insulin administration. These signs and symptoms are often followed by drowsiness, a subjective feeling of warmth, and continued diaphoresis. Severe hypoglycemic reactions can be promptly abated by the intravenous administration of glucose, preferably a 50% (w/v) solution.

Tubeless Gastric Analysis

In 1950, Harry Segal, Leon Miller, and John Morton introduced the use of an orally administered ion-exchange resin to detect the presence of hydrogen ions in gastric fluid.[27] The test was eventually marketed under the trade name, Diagnex Blue. The test is based on the use of a carboxylic-acid cationic resin (amberlite XE-96) with an innocuous indicator dye, azure A, coupled to it. Hydrogen ions in gastric secretion combine with the resin, thereby liberating the azure-A ions, which are then absorbed into the bloodstream in the small intestine and subsequently excreted in the urine.[28] In principle, the presence of hydrogen ions in the gastric fluid can be determined by an estimate of the urine azure A. Because some of the azure-A dye is converted to its reduced, colorless form, oxidation of the urine specimen by boiling with copper sulfate is often necessary. Caffeine sodium benzoate was ordinarily used as a gastric stimulant.

Although a novel approach to the detection of gastric acid, the tubeless procedure is fraught with many sources of false-positive as well as false-negative results. It is largely discredited for this reason as well as for the fact that quantitation of gastric-acid secretion is not possible.

PHYSICAL EVALUATION OF GASTRIC FLUID

Appearance

Gastric fluid collected after a 12-hour fast will be translucent, pale grey, and slightly viscous under normal circumstances. The presence of food particles indicates either a failure to adhere to the fasting regimen or delayed gastric emptying, which most commonly occurs as a consequence of pyloric obstruction from either a peptic ulcer, neoplasm, or inflammatory scarring. Flecks of blood commonly occur as a result of minor trauma during intubation. A large amount of blood is obviously an untoward finding and an indication for withdrawal of the stomach tube and termination of the procedure.

Bile is not usually found in gastric fluid, but reflux from the duodenum into the stomach can occur if intubation is accompanied by severe or prolonged retching or gagging. A large amount of bile can occur in association with intestinal obstruction distal to the ampulla of Vater. Intubation of patients with partial gastrectomies and gastroduodenostomies or gastrojejunostomies will regularly contain bile. Bile is readily identified by its yellow-to-green tint.

Volume

In the fasting state, the stomach usually does not contain more than 50 to 75 ml of gastric fluid. More than 1 dl is definitely abnormal, if it can be ascertained that the patient did not swallow excessive amounts of saliva during intubation.

Odor

Normal gastric juice has a faint, pungent odor reflecting its acid nature. Absence of this odor should suggest the possibility of anacidity. Reflux of colonic and even distal jejunal contents causes the fetid odor characteristic of lower-bowel obstruction. A putrid odor can often be detected from stomach contents of patients with advanced ulcerating carcinoma of the stomach, particularly if obstruction has supervened.

Mucus

The quantity of mucus varies considerably. Large amounts of mucus are often swallowed during intubation. Mucus from the mouth and nasopharynx appears as stringy clumps, which float on the surface of the gastric fluid. Gastric mucus is miscible with the remainder of the gastric fluid.

Microscopic Examination

There is very little information to be gained from microscopic examination of gastric contents. Red blood cells in small numbers have no pathologic significance, because, as previously noted, small amounts of blood can result from the trauma of intubation. White blood cells are frequently present but are usually in a state of poor preservation because of the cytolytic effect of hydrochloric acid. Even large numbers of leukocytes are not necessarily of significance, because they can originate from the nasopharynx or paranasal sinuses and become incorporated with swallowed mucus. Squamous cells are always present and originate from the mouth, pharynx, or esophagus as a consequence of sloughing or traumatic release during intubation. Desquamated gastric columnar epithelial cells are difficult to identify without careful cytologic preparation and appropriate staining, as with the Papanicolaou technique.

Parasites are rarely recovered from gastric fluid. It is possible, however, to find Giardia lamblia cysts or trophozoites, rhabditiform larvae of Strongyloides stercoralis, and ascaris or hookworm ova, especially when duodenal contents reflux into the stomach.

MEASUREMENT OF GASTRIC ACID

Because hydrochloric-acid secretion is easy to measure and has proven to be a clinically valid index of gastric secretory function, it is ordinarily the only component that is measured in gastric fluid. As previously mentioned, Prout, in 1924, introduced the terms of "free," "combined," and "total" acid when he discovered hydrochloric acid as the acid component of gastric secretion. These terms and the analytic procedures that purportedly were required to distinguish them dominated gastric analysis until the 1960s. Thre is nothing inherently wrong with these terms or the concepts that they represent—that is, free acid, when used to represent free or dissociated hydrogen ion; combined acid, to represent the undissociated hydrogen ion that occurs when hydrogen is combined with the anion of a weak acid, as in a buffer system; and total acid, to represent the sum of the previous two species. In gastric fluid, the buffer anions consist of mucus and various other proteins secreted by the stomach. Nevertheless, there are several, basic, scientific objections to the manner in which the terms "free" and "combined" acid have been applied in practice and in theory, so that it is desirable to avoid these terms altogether and instead refer to the two species as hydrogen ion and undissociated hydrogen ion. For example, no diagnostic importance has been demonstrated for the relative amounts of hydrogen ion and undissociated hydrogen ion. Earlier studies greatly overemphasized the amount of undissociated hydrogen ion, partly because the gastric contents were typically contaminated with the components of various test meals, which acted as buffer anions with which the hydrogen ions could combine. Furthermore, the classic analytic method for distinguishing free from combined acid is scientifically incorrect. The distinction was made titrimetrically. Free hydrogen was determined by titrating an aliquot of gastric fluid to the endpoint of a suitable indicator with a color change at a pH of approximately 3.5, because it was believed that hydrogen ions were largely dissociated below this pH and undissociated above this pH. Dimethylaminoazobenzol (Topfer's reagent), which has a color change from red to salmon-yellow as the pH is increased in the range 2.8 to 3.5, was used frequently. Total acid was determined by titrating to the endpoint of phenolphthalein (pH 8.2–10) while combined acid was calculated as the difference between these two values. Collateral units of measure were devised to quantitate the gastric acidity—that is, clinical units or degrees of acidity representing the number of ml of 0.1 N sodium hydroxide required to titrate 1 dl of gastric fluid to an endpoint, either that of Topfer's reagent or phenolphthalein.

It has now been clearly established that gastric fluid has an acid-base titration curve closely resembling that of pure hydrochloric acid with slight buffering largely restricted to pH values above about 4.0.[29] Most gastroenterologists and clinical chemists now agree that quantitation of gastric acid secretion can best be represented by measuring the pH of the specimen with a glass electrode and calculating the acid output in a defined time interval. The acid output is calculated by multiplying the titratable acidity expressed in meq per L times the volume of the specimen in ml divided by 1,000 (to convert ml to L). Titratable acidity is readily determined by titrating an aliquot of gastric fluid with 0.1 N sodium hydroxide to neutrality and monitoring the endpoint of titration potentiometrically (with a glass electrode). Some difference of opinion exists as to precisely what pH should be designated as neutrality—pH 7.0, which is chemical neutrality, or 7.4, which is physiochemical neutrality, at least insofar as extracellular fluid is concerned. Because acid output theoretically means the acid secreted by the stomach against a physiochemical gradient, the pH of extracellular fluid would seem most appropriate. However, the very small difference that will result in measured acid output between the two pH endpoints, 7.0 and 7.4, is negligible for clinical purposes.

One interesting approach to the measurement of gastric acid that was introduced by Edward Moore and Robert Scarlata has gained sufficient acceptance to merit discussion.[29] This procedure utilizes hydrogen-ion-activity coefficients and pH measurement to calculate hydrogen-ion concentration. As originally defined by Sorenson in 1909, pH refers to the negative logarithm of the hydrogen-ion concentration. When determined with the glass electrode, however, pH represents the negative logarithm of the hydrogen ion activity:

$$pH = -\log_{10} a_{H^+}$$

Electrode potentials are generated by differences in ionic activities at the glass-solution interface. In ideal (infinitely dilute) solutions, ionic activity and molal concentration are equal, but in more concentrated solutions, such as gastric fluid, this relationship does not hold. In nonideal solutions, therefore, the hydrogen-ion activity differs from the hydrogen-ion concentration by a fraction known as the hydrogen-ion-activity coefficient (γ_{H^+}) so that:

$$C_{H^+} \text{ (meq/L)} = \frac{a_{H^+}}{\gamma_{H^+}}$$

Activity coefficients for the hydrogen ion as well as for other ions vary inversely with the total-ion concentration in solution represented by the ionic strength:

$$\mu = 1/2 \, \Sigma \, m_i z_i^2$$

in which m_i is the molality of each ionic species, *i*, of valence z. Because γ is always less than 1.0 except in ideal solutions, the hydrogen-ion activity is always less than the hydrogen-ion concentration of physiologic fluids. Obviously, ions other than hydrogen and chloride will contribute significantly to the ionic strength of gastric fluid.

Moore and Scarlata determined the hydrogen-ion-activity coefficients for gastric fluids at varying pH and with varying concentrations of sodium and potassium (Fig. 3–2). From this figure, it can be seen that a gastric fluid with a pH of 2.0, corresponding to a hydrogen-ion activity of 10 meq/L and a combined concentration of sodium and potassium of 50 meq/L would have a hydrogen-ion-activity coefficient of 0.817 and an actual hydrogen-ion concentration of 12.2 meq/L. For practical purposes, Moore and Scarlata concluded that the combined concentration of sodium and potassium could be assumed to be 50 meq/L, thus

[Na + K] concentration (mEq/L)

		0		20		40		50		60		80		100	
pH	HYDROGEN ION ACTIVITY (a_{H^+})	γ_{HCl}	c_{H^+}	γ_{HGJCl}	c_{H^+}	γ_{HGJCl}	c_{H^+}	γ_{HGJCl}	c_{H^+}	γ_{HGJCl}	c_{H^+}	γ_{HGJCl}	c_{H^+}	γ_{HGJCl}	c_{H^+}
14.0	0.0	1.0	0.00	0.873	0.00	0.837	0.00	0.827	0.00	0.816	0.00	0.800	0.00	0.788	0.00
↓	↓	↓	↓	↓	↓	↓	↓	↓	↓	↓	↓	↓	↓	↓	↓
5.00	0.01	-	-	0.873	0.01	0.837	0.01	0.827	0.01	0.816	0.01	0.800	0.01	0.788	0.01
4.00	0.10	-	-	"	0.11	"	0.12	"	0.12	"	0.12	"	0.12	"	0.13
3.50	0.32	-	-	0.872	0.37	"	0.38	"	0.39	"	0.39	"	0.40	"	0.41
3.00	1.00	0.966	1.04	0.871	1.15	0.836	1.20	0.826	1.21	0.815	1.23	"	1.25	"	1.27
2.90	1.26	0.961	1.31	0.870	1.45	"	1.51	"	1.52	"	1.55	"	1.58	"	1.60
2.80	1.58	0.955	1.65	"	1.82	"	1.89	0.825	1.92	"	1.94	0.799	1.98	"	2.00
2.70	2.00	0.950	2.10	0.868	2.30	0.835	2.40	"	2.42	"	2.45	"	2.50	"	2.54
2.60	2.51	0.947	2.65	0.867	2.90	0.834	3.01	0.824	3.05	0.814	3.08	"	3.14	0.787	3.19
2.50	3.16	0.944	3.35	0.865	3.65	"	3.79	"	3.83	"	3.88	0.798	3.96	"	4.02
2.48	3.31	0.942	3.51	"	3.83	0.833	3.97	0.823	4.02	0.813	4.07	"	4.15	"	4.20
2.46	3.47	0.940	3.69	0.864	4.02	"	4.16	"	4.22	"	4.27	"	4.35	"	4.41
2.44	3.63	0.938	3.87	"	4.20	"	4.36	"	4.41	"	4.46	"	4.55	"	4.61
2.42	3.80	0.937	4.06	"	4.40	"	4.56	"	4.62	"	4.67	"	4.76	"	4.83
2.40	3.98	0.935	4.26	"	4.61	"	4.78	"	4.84	"	4.90	0.797	4.99	0.786	5.06
2.38	4.17	0.934	4.46	"	4.83	0.832	5.01	0.822	5.07	0.812	5.14	"	5.23	"	5.31
2.36	4.36	0.933	4.67	0.863	5.05	"	5.24	"	5.30	"	5.37	"	5.47	"	5.55
2.34	4.57	0.932	4.90	"	5.30	"	5.49	"	5.56	"	5.63	"	5.73	"	5.81
2.32	4.79	0.931	5.14	0.862	5.56	"	5.76	"	5.83	"	5.90	0.796	6.02	"	6.09
2.30	5.01	0.928	5.40	"	5.81	0.831	6.03	0.821	6.10	"	6.17	"	6.29	"	6.37
2.28	5.25	0.926	5.67	0.861	6.10	"	6.32	"	6.39	"	6.46	"	6.60	"	6.68
2.26	5.50	0.925	5.94	"	6.39	"	6.62	"	6.70	"	6.77	"	6.91	0.785	7.01
2.24	5.75	0.923	6.23	0.860	6.69	"	6.92	"	7.00	0.811	7.09	"	7.22	"	7.32
2.22	6.03	0.922	6.54	0.859	7.02	0.830	7.26	"	7.34	"	7.44	0.795	7.58	"	7.68
2.20	6.31	0.921	6.85	"	7.34	"	7.60	"	7.68	"	7.78	"	7.94	"	8.04
2.18	6.61	0.919	7.19	0.858	7.70	0.829	7.97	0.820	8.06	0.810	8.16	"	8.31	"	8.42
2.16	6.92	0.917	7.55	0.857	8.07	"	8.35	"	8.44	"	8.54	"	8.70	"	8.82
2.14	7.24	0.915	7.91	"	8.45	"	8.73	"	8.83	0.809	8.95	"	9.11	0.784	9.23
2.12	7.59	0.914	8.30	0.856	8.87	0.828	9.17	0.819	9.27	"	9.38	"	9.55	"	9.68
2.10	7.94	0.912	8.71	0.855	9.29	"	9.59	"	9.69	"	9.81	0.794	10.0	"	10.1
2.08	8.32	0.910	9.14	"	9.73	0.827	10.1	0.818	10.2	0.808	10.3	"	10.5	"	10.6
2.06	8.71	0.907	9.60	0.854	10.2	"	10.5	0.818	10.6	"	10.8	"	11.0	0.783	11.1
2.04	9.12	0.905	10.1	"	10.7	0.826	11.0	"	11.1	"	11.3	"	11.5	"	11.6
2.02	9.55	0.903	10.6	0.853	11.2	"	11.6	"	11.7	0.807	11.8	0.793	12.0	"	12.2
2.00	10.00	0.902	11.1	"	11.7	"	12.1	0.817	12.2	"	12.4	"	12.6	"	12.8
1.98	10.47	0.900	11.6	0.852	12.3	0.825	12.7	"	12.8	"	13.0	"	13.2	0.782	13.4
1.96	10.96	0.898	12.2	"	12.9	"	13.3	0.816	13.4	"	13.6	"	13.8	"	14.0
1.94	11.48	0.896	12.8	0.851	13.5	0.824	13.9	"	14.1	0.806	14.2	0.792	14.5	"	14.7
1.92	12.02	0.894	13.4	0.850	14.1	"	14.6	"	14.7	"	14.9	"	15.2	0.781	15.4
1.90	12.59	0.893	14.1	0.848	14.8	0.823	15.3	0.815	15.4	0.805	15.6	0.791	15.9	"	16.1
1.88	13.18	0.891	14.8	0.847	15.6	"	16.0	"	16.2	"	16.4	"	16.7	"	16.9
1.86	13.80	0.889	15.5	0.846	16.3	0.822	16.8	0.814	17.0	0.804	17.2	"	17.4	"	17.7
1.84	14.45	0.888	16.3	0.845	17.1	"	17.6	0.813	17.8	"	18.0	0.790	18.3	"	18.5
1.82	15.14	0.885	17.1	0.843	18.0	0.821	18.4	"	18.6	0.803	18.8	"	19.2	"	19.4
1.80	15.85	0.882	18.0	0.842	18.8	0.820	19.3	0.812	19.5	"	19.7	"	20.1	0.780	20.3
1.78	16.60	0.880	18.9	"	19.7	0.819	20.3	"	20.4	0.802	20.7	0.789	21.0	"	21.3
1.76	17.38	0.878	19.8	0.841	20.7	0.818	21.2	0.811	21.4	"	21.7	"	22.0	"	22.3
1.74	18.20	0.876	20.8	0.840	21.7	0.817	22.3	0.810	22.5	0.801	22.7	"	23.1	0.779	23.4
1.72	19.05	0.873	21.8	0.839	22.7	"	23.3	0.809	23.5	0.800	23.8	"	24.1	"	24.4
1.70	19.95	0.871	22.9	0.837	23.8	0.816	24.4	0.808	24.7	0.799	25.0	0.788	25.3	0.778	25.6
1.68	20.89	0.869	24.0	0.835	25.0	0.815	25.6	"	25.8	0.798	26.2	"	26.5	"	26.8
1.66	21.88	0.867	25.2	0.834	26.2	0.814	26.9	0.807	27.1	"	27.4	0.787	27.8	0.777	28.2
1.64	22.91	0.864	26.5	0.833	27.5	0.813	28.2	0.806	28.4	0.797	28.7	"	29.1	"	29.5
1.62	23.99	0.862	27.8	0.832	28.8	0.812	29.5	0.805	29.8	0.796	30.1	0.786	30.5	0.776	30.9
1.60	25.12	0.860	29.2	0.831	30.2	0.811	31.0	0.804	31.2	"	31.6	"	32.0	"	32.4
1.58	26.30	0.857	30.7	0.830	31.7	0.810	32.5	0.803	32.8	0.795	33.1	0.785	33.5	0.775	33.9
1.56	27.54	0.855	32.2	0.829	33.2	0.809	34.0	0.802	34.3	"	34.6	0.784	35.1	0.774	35.6
1.54	28.84	0.852	33.8	0.827	34.9	0.808	35.7	0.801	36.0	0.794	36.3	0.783	36.8	"	37.3
1.52	30.20	0.849	35.6	0.825	36.6	0.807	37.4	0.800	37.8	0.793	38.1	"	38.6	0.773	39.1
1.50	31.62	0.847	37.3	0.823	38.4	0.806	39.2	0.799	39.6	0.792	39.9	0.782	40.4	0.772	41.0
1.48	33.11	0.845	39.2	0.822	40.3	0.805	41.1	0.798	41.5	"	41.8	0.781	42.4	0.772	42.9
1.46	34.67	0.842	41.2	0.821	42.2	0.803	43.2	0.797	43.5	0.791	43.8	0.781	44.4	"	44.9
1.44	36.31	0.840	43.2	0.819	44.3	0.802	45.3	0.796	45.6	0.790	46.0	0.780	46.6	0.771	47.1
1.42	38.02	0.837	45.4	0.817	46.5	0.801	47.5	0.795	47.8	0.789	48.2	0.779	48.8	0.771	49.3
1.40	39.81	0.834	47.7	0.816	48.8	0.800	49.8	0.794	50.1	0.788	50.5	0.778	51.2	0.770	51.7
1.38	41.69	0.832	50.1	0.813	51.3	0.798	52.2	0.793	52.6	0.787	53.0	0.778	53.6	0.770	54.1
1.36	43.65	0.829	52.7	0.812	53.8	0.797	54.8	0.792	55.1	0.786	55.5	0.777	56.2	0.769	56.8
1.34	45.71	0.827	55.3	0.810	56.4	0.795	57.5	0.791	57.8	0.785	58.2	"	58.8	"	59.4
1.32	47.86	0.824	58.1	0.808	59.2	0.794	60.3	0.790	60.6	0.784	61.0	0.776	61.7	0.768	62.3
1.30	50.12	0.822	61.0	0.806	62.2	0.792	63.3	0.788	63.6	0.783	64.0	"	64.6	"	65.3
1.28	52.48	0.820	64.0	0.804	65.3	0.791	66.3	0.787	66.7	0.782	67.1	0.775	67.7	0.767	68.4
1.26	54.95	0.818	67.2	0.802	68.5	0.790	69.6	0.786	69.9	0.781	70.4	0.774	71.0	0.766	71.7
1.24	57.54	0.815	70.6	0.800	71.9	0.788	73.0	0.785	73.3	0.780	73.8	0.773	74.4	"	75.1
1.22	60.26	0.811	74.3	0.798	75.5	0.787	76.6	0.784	76.9	0.779	77.4	0.772	78.0	0.765	78.8
1.20	63.10	0.809	78.0	0.796	79.3	0.785	80.4	0.783	80.6	0.777	81.2	0.771	81.8	0.764	82.6
1.18	66.07	0.807	81.9	0.794	83.2	0.784	84.3	0.782	84.5	0.776	85.1	0.770	85.8		
1.16	69.18	0.804	86.0	0.792	87.3	0.783	88.4	0.780	88.7	0.775	89.3	0.769	90.0		
1.14	72.44	0.802	90.3	0.790	91.7	0.782	92.6	0.778	93.1	0.774	93.6	0.768	94.3		
1.12	75.86	0.799	94.9	0.788	96.3	0.780	97.2	0.777	97.6	0.773	98.1	0.767	98.9		
1.10	79.43	0.796	99.8	0.786	101.0	0.779	102.0	0.776	102.4	0.772	102.9	"	103.6		
1.08	83.18	0.793	104.9	0.784	106.1	0.778	106.9	0.775	107.3	0.771	107.9				
1.06	87.10	0.791	110.1	0.782	111.4	0.776	112.2	0.774	112.5	0.770	113.1				
1.04	91.20	0.788	115.7	0.780	116.9	0.774	117.8	0.773	118.0	0.769	118.6				
1.02	95.50	0.786	121.5	0.779	122.6	0.773	123.5	0.772	123.7	0.768	124.3				
1.00	100.0	0.784	127.6	0.778	128.5	0.772	129.5	0.771	129.7	0.767	130.4				
0.99	102.3	0.783	130.6	0.777	131.7										
0.98	104.7	0.782	133.9	0.776	134.9										
0.97	107.2	0.781	137.2	0.775	138.3										
0.96	109.6	0.780	140.5	"	142.0										
0.95	112.2	0.779	144.0	0.774	145.0										
0.94	114.8	0.778	147.6	"	148.3										
0.93	117.5	0.777	151.2	0.773	152.0										
0.92	120.2	0.776	154.9												
0.91	123.0	0.775	158.7												
0.90	125.9	0.774	162.7												
0.89	128.8	0.773	166.6												
0.88	131.8	0.772	170.7												
0.87	134.9	0.771	175.0												
0.86	138.0	0.770	179.2												
0.85	141.3	0.769	183.7												

Fig. 3–2. Moore and Scarlata's nomogram for conversion of glass electrode pH values to hydrogen ion concentration (c_{H^+}) in gastric juice at 25° C. Inasmuch as the mean concentration of sodium ion (c_{Na^+}) and potassium ion (c_{K^+}) in gastric juice is usually about 50 mEq/L, for clinical purposes this value suffices for conversion of gastric juice pH to hydrogen ion concentration (c_{H^+}). (Reproduced with permission of Edward Moore and Robert Scarlata.)

obviating the need for these measurements and resulting in the concentrations of hydrogen ion at various pH values listed in Table 3–1.

The approach of Moore and Scarlata thus requires only a single pH measurement to determine hydrogen-ion concentration. It is not, however, a completely valid way to estimate acid output. Furthermore, it

TABLE 3–1. Conversion Values of Glass Electrode pH to Hydrogen-Ion Concentration (C_{H^+}) in Gastric Juice at 25 C with (C_{Na^+} and C_{K^+}) Value of 50 meq/L.

pH	CH_+ (meq/L)	pH	CH_+ (meq/L)
1.00	129.70	1.84	17.80
1.02	123.60	1.86	17.00
1.04	118.00	1.88	16.20
1.06	112.50	1.90	15.40
1.08	107.30	1.92	14.70
1.10	102.40	1.94	14.10
1.12	97.60	1.96	13.40
1.14	93.10	1.98	12.80
1.16	88.70	2.00	12.20
1.18	84.50	2.02	11.70
1.20	80.60	2.04	11.10
1.22	76.90	2.06	10.60
1.24	73.30	2.08	10.20
1.26	69.90	2.10	9..69
1.28	66.70	2.12	9.27
1.30	63.60	2.14	8.83
1.32	60.60	2.16	8.44
1.34	57.80	2.18	8.06
1.36	55.10	2.20	7.68
1.38	52.60	2.22	7.34
1.40	50.10	2.24	7.00
1.42	47.80	2.26	6.70
1.44	45.60	2.28	6.39
1.46	43.50	2.30	6.10
1.48	41.50	2.32	5.83
1.50	39.60	2.34	5.56
1.52	37.80	2.36	5.30
1.54	36.00	2.38	5.07
1.56	34.30	2.40	4.84
1.58	32.80	2.42	4.62
1.60	31.20	2.44	4.41
1.62	29.80	2.46	4.22
1.64	28.40	2.48	4.02
1.66	27.75	2.50	3.38
1.68	25.80	2.60	3.05
1.70	24.70	2.70	2.42
1.72	23.50	2.80	1.92
1.74	22.50	2.90	1.52
1.76	21.40	3.00	1.21
1.78	20.40	3.50	0.39
1.80	19.50	4.00	0.12
1.82	18.60	5.00	0.01

is probable that hydrogen-ion activity is a more physiologically accurate expression of the gastric-acid secretory gradient than is the hydrogen-ion concentration.

MEDICAL INTERPRETATION OF GASTRIC-ANALYSIS RESULTS

Definition of Terms

Although the definition of anacidity would appear to be a simple one, the term has been complicated by various definitions and interpretations. Furthermore, the term "achlorhydria" has been used as a synonym for anacidity by most physicians, but some have rendered other definitions. Thus, one definition of achlorhydria that continues to be used is that it represents a failure of the pH to fall below 3.5 and at least 1 pH unit following maximal gastric stimulation.[30] In this same system of nomenclature, hypochlorhydria is defined as a failure of the pH to fall below 3.5 provided that it does decrease at least 1 pH unit following maximal gastric stimulation. In view of the fact that the pH of 3.5 has no particular chemical, physiologic, or diagnostic significance, it is recommended that these definitions be discarded. Although any pH below 7.0 is acidity in the strict, chemical sense of the term, an equally cogent argument can be made that any pH below 7.4 is acidity in reference to body physiology. Actually, the most useful definition of anacidity is an empirical one—that is, anacidity represents failure of the gastric fluid pH to fall below 6.0 in a maximal gastric stimulation test. With this definition, all adult patients with pernicious anemia will exhibit anacidity because some such patients will secrete gastric fluid with a pH below 7.0 but not below 6.0.[30] Achlorhydria should be used as a synonym of anacidity if it is to be used at all.

Hyposecretion and hypersecretion are frequently used terms, that are intended to be semiquantitative but are, in fact, inherently imprecise. This is a consequence of the fact that the normal ranges for gastric-acid secretion have not been rigorously defined because of wide variations among healthy individuals; multiple population subsets based on age, sex, behavioral factors and probably other determinants; considerable overlap between healthy and diseased individuals (except for anacidity and the marked hypersecretion of the Zollinger-Ellison syndrome); and a continuing paucity of totally reliable data in the medical literature.

Several terms have been introduced in relation to the augmented histamine test, but these can apply to the maximal pentagastrin stimulation test as well. Maximal acid output was originally defined by Kay as the acid output in the 30-minute period from 15 to 45 minutes after injection of histamine.[8] Kay chose this time interval because his data indicated that it encompassed the highest sustained secretion of acid following a single dose of histamine. Confusion has been engendered by the fact that Kay and other authors later referred to this as the maximal histamine response or the augmented histamine response and some chose to multiply the value by 2 so that results could be expressed as an hourly rate.[22] As a further complication, maximal acid output was also defined as the meq of acid secreted during the entire 60-minute period following histamine.[31] Baron found that the period from 15 to 45 minutes after histamine represented the maximum 30-minute acid output in fewer than half of all cases and consequently introduced the term "peak acid output," which was defined as two times the highest sum of two consecutive 15-minute acid outputs in the hour following maximal histamine stimulation.[32] The peak acid output thus defined was also found to be the most reproducible expression of acid output. Obviously, considerable caution must be exercised in the use of any of these terms.

Stimulation Tests

There are rather wide variations reported in various investigations of the gastric fluid of normal individuals in both the basal secretory test and the maximal secretory (pentagastrin or histamine) test. Some of these differences are no doubt attributable to such factors as the geographic location, sex, and age of the population studied, and perhaps also to the particular technique employed (for example, the care with which the placement of the stomach tube was monitored, which obviously governs the completeness of collection of the gastric fluid). Most healthy individuals will secrete between 0 and 6 meq of acid in the 1-hour test. This should not be considered to be the equivalent of a rigorous normal range, however, because of the continuing paucity of reported data. As a group, women secrete less acid than do men; thus, Marks et al. reported a range for basal-acid output of 0 to 13.8 meq/hour with a mean of 4.0 meq/hour for 20 healthy males (age range from 27 to 57 years with a mean age of 45) and a range of 0 to 6.5 meq/hour with a mean of 1.9 meq/hour for 15 healthy females (age range from 18 to 68 with a mean age of 46).[33] These results are somewhat higher than those reported by Baron, who studied 16 healthy males and 15 healthy females age 30 or older and found a range for acid output in the basal secretory test of 0 to 3.8 meq/hour for males (mean of 1.0 meq/hour) and 0 to 2.1 meq/hour for females (mean of 0.5 meq/hour).[34] Interestingly, both male and female medical students were reported to have somewhat greater acid secretion in the basal secretory test than other healthy individuals, but this may be in part a reflection of the younger ages of the students.[33] Indeed, it is generally accepted that older age groups have a lower acid output.

The total volume and titratable acidity of the individual specimens in the basal secretory test do not have any great significance. The total volume for the basal secretory hour will usually vary between about 10 and 100 ml; thus, Baron found a range of 10 to 80 ml with a mean of 36 ml for his 16 normal males and a range of 2 to 90 ml with a mean of 30 ml for the 15 normal females.[34] For the same 31 subjects, Baron reported a titratable acidity ranging from 0 to 71 meq/L.

Since the secretory response to pentagastrin stimulation is very similar to that of histamine, the data reported for histamine can be considered to be generally applicable to pentagastrin in the maximal stimulation test.[22] The study of Marks et al. of 20 healthy males and 15 healthy females revealed a maximal acid output—that is, the acid output for the entire 1 hour following histamine, ranging from 4.9 to 38.9 meq with a mean a 21.7 meq for males and from 0.1 to 29.2 meq with a mean of 15.0 meq for females.[33] As in the case of the basal-secretory study, these results are somewhat higher than those reported by Baron. Thus, the 16 healthy males in Baron's study had a maximal acid output ranging from 0.3 to 45 meq with a mean of 18.7, while the 15 healthy females had a range of 0.4 to 15.8 meq with a mean of 8.0 meq.[34] The volumes of secretion in the maximal stimulation test ranged from 38 to 360 ml/hour with a mean of 199 ml/hour for males and 24 to 212 ml/hour with a mean of 109 ml/hour for females in Baron's study. There was little difference in titratable acidity of gastric fluid between males and females with an aggregate range of 10 to 136 meq/L. In another study of the acid secretion of 20 healthy males and 20 healthy females, the peak acid output (expressed as two times the peak 30 minute value) was found to range from 0.3 to 50.2 meq/hour with a mean of 21.6 meq/hour for males and from 0.4 to 32.0 meq/hour with a mean of 12.3 meq/hour for females.[32]

When anacidity is defined as the failure of the pH of gastric fluid to fall below 6.0 in the maximal stimulation test, all adult patients with pernicious anemia will have anacidity. This does not hold true, however, for children with pernicious anemia, because they can have normal acid secretion. Anacidity occurs rather frequently in association with adenocarcinoma of the stomach but by no means in the majority of patients. Thus, in one series, only 16 of 52 patients with stomach carcinoma had anacidity.[33] Anacidity also occurs infrequently in patients with hypochromic anemia, rheumatoid arthritis, steatorrhea, and aplastic anemia, and in the healthy relatives of patients with pernicious anemia.[30]

Gastric peptic ulcers are associated with an essentially normal acid secretion.[33] There is evidence that pyloric or prepyloric gastric ulcers are associated with a somewhat greater than normal acid secretion in females but not in males.[34]

Duodenal peptic ulcers are associated with a significantly increased acid secretion in both the basal and maximal stimulation tests, but there is considerable overlap with healthy controls.[33,34] A maximal acid output greater than 40 meq is found in about 40% of males with duodenal ulcer but only rarely in healthy males.[35] Increased acid secretion also occurs in association with jejunal ulceration following partial gastrectomy with gastrojejunal anastomosis.[33]

The Zollinger-Ellison syndrome is characterized by an exceptionally high volume and acid output in the basal secretory test that ordinarily increase by a relatively small amount in the maximal stimulation test. In one series, the basal 1-hour acid output in 25 affected patients ranged from 11 to more than 80 meq.[36] In 21 of these patients, the acid output increased less than 25% from basal levels in the maximal stimulation test. The comparatively small increase above basal levels in the acid output of the maximal stimulation test is a reflection of the fact that the high circulating gastrin concentration in blood causes a near maximal stimulation of the gastric mucosa even in the resting state. The ratio of acid output in the basal secretory test to the maximal stimulation test is typically more than 60% in patients with the Zollinger-Ellison syndrome but rarely more than 40% in ordinary peptic ulceration whether of gastric or duodenal origin.[35]

The Insulin Hypoglycemia Test

The objective assessment of gastric function following vagotomy has been comprehensively reviewed by Read and Hall.[25] Guidelines for interpreting the data relating to acid output in the insulin hypoglycemia test have varied just as have the test protocols. In the Stempien modification of the Hollander procedure, complete vagotomy can be assumed if the acid output in the greater of the 2 postinsulin hours is less than that of the greater of the 2 basal hours or if the total acid output in the 2-hour postinsulin period does not exceed that of the 2-hour basal period by more than 0.5 meq.[26] The insulin hypoglycemia test is valid only if the blood-glucose concentration falls to 50 mg/dl or less during the test.

REFERENCES

1. Wallnöfer, H., and von Rottauscher, A.: Chinese Folk Medicine. New York, Crown, 1965, pp. 6 and 18.
2. Hollander, F., and Penner, A.: History and development of gastric analysis procedure. Am. J. Dig. Dis., 5:739, 1939.
3. Hollander, F., and Penner, A.: History and development of gastric analysis procedure. Am. J. Dig. Dis., 5:786, 1939.
4. Hollander, F., and Penner, A.: History and development of gastric analysis procedure. Am. J. Dig. Dis., 6:22, 1939.
5. Beaumont, W.: Experiments and Observations on the Gastric Juice and the Physiology of Digestion. Orig. pub. 1833. New York, Dover, 1959.
6. von Leube, W.: Diagnostik der magenkrankheiten. Deutsch. Arch. Klin. Med., *33*:1, 1883.
7. Rehfuss, M.: A new method of gastric testing with a description of a method for the fractional testing of the gastric juice. Am. J. Med. Sci., *147*:848, 1914.
8. Kay, A.: Effects of large doses of histamine on gastric secretion of HCl (an augmented histamine test). Br. Med. J., *2*:77, 1953.
9. Bock, O.: The concepts of "free acid" and "total acid" of the gastric juice. Lancet, *2*:1101, 1962.

10. Michaelis, L.: Some problems concerning the gastric juice. Harvey Lect., *22*:59, 1926.
11. Brown, J.: "Enterogastrone" and other new gut peptides. Med. Clin. N. Am., *58*:1347, 1974.
12. Jaffe, B.: Hormones of the gastrointestinal tract. *In* Endocrinology. Vol. 3. Edited by L. DeGroot, G. Cahill, L. Martini, D. Nelson, W. Odell, J. Potts, Jr., E. Steinberger, and A. Winegrad. New York, Grune & Stratton, 1979, pp. 1669–1698.
13. Hollander, F.: Gastric secretion of electrolytes. Fed. Proc., *11*:706, 1952.
14. Magee, D.: Pepsin. Med. Clin. N. Am., *58*:1277, 1974.
15. Piper, D., et al.: The diagnosis of gastric carcinoma by the estimation of enzyme activity in gastric juice. Gastroenterology, *45*:614, 1963.
16. Piper, D.: Tests of gastric function. Clin. Gastroenterol., *7*:247, 1978.
17. Rosenberg, J.: Present status of gastric analysis. Am. J. Gastroenterol., *42*:391, 1964.
18. Johnston, D., and McCraw, B.: Gastric analysis—evaluation of collection techniques. Gastroenterology, *32*:512, 1958.
19. Levin, E., Kirsner, J., and Palmer, W.: A simple measure of gastric secretion in man. Comparison of one hour basal secretion, histamine-secretion, and twelve hour nocturnal gastric secretion. Gastroenterology, *19*:88, 1951.
20. Lee, H., and Jones, R.: The histamine activity of some B-aminoethyl heterocyclic nitrogen compounds. J. Pharmacol. Exp. Ther., *95*:71, 1949.
21. Zaterka, S., and Neves, D.: Maximal gastric secretion in human subjects after Histalog stimulation. Comparison with augmented histamine test. Gastroenterology, *47*:251, 1964.
22. Khodadoost, J., Leitao, O., and Glass, G.: Comparison of pentagastrin and augmented histamine stimulation as tests of gastric acid secretion. Am. J. Gastroenterol., *57*:311, 1972.
23. Kay, A.: Memorial lecture: An evaluation of gastric acid secretion tests. Gastroenterology, *53*:834, 1967.
24. Hollander, F.: The insulin test for the presence of intact nerve fibers after vagal operations for peptic ulcer. Gastroenterology, *7*:607, 1946.
25. Read, R., and Hall, W.: Objective of gastric function after vagotomy. Curr. Probl. Surg. (July):1, 1974.
26. Stempien, S.: Insulin gastric analysis: Technic and interpretations. Am. J. Dig. Dis., *7*:138, 1962.
27. Segal, H., Miller, L., and Morton, J.: Determination of gastric acidity without intubation by use of cation exchange indicator compounds. Proc. Soc. Exp. Biol. Med., *74*:218, 1950.
28. Segal, H.: Clinical measurement of gastric secretion: Significance and limitations. Ann. Intern. Med., *53*:445, 1960.
29. Moore, E., and Scarlata, R.: The determination of gastric acidity by the glass electrode. Gastroenteroology, *49*:178, 1965.
30. Callender, S., Retief, F., and Witts, L.: The augmented histamine test with special reference to achlorhydria. Gut, *1*:326, 1960.
31. Card, W., and Marks, I.: The relationship between the acid output of the stomach following "maximal" histamine stimulation and the parietal cell mass. Clin. Sci., *19*:147, 1960.
32. Baron, J.: Studies of basal and peak acid output with an augmented histamine test. Gut, *4*:136, 1963.
33. Marks, I., Bank, S., Louw, J., and van Embden, B.: The augmented histamine test. An analysis of 672 consecutive tests. S. Afr. Med. J., *36*:807, 1962.
34. Baron, J.: An assessment of the augmented histamine test in the diagnosis of peptic ulcer. Gut, *4*:243, 1963.
35. Marks, I.: The augmented histamine test. Gastroenterology, *41*:599, 1961.
36. Ellison, E., and Wilson, S.: The Zollinger-Ellison syndrome: re-appraised and evaluation of 260 registered cases. Ann. Surg., *160*:513, 1964.

GASTRIC ANALYSIS PROCEDURES

The following are stimulants of gastric-acid secretion:

1. **Histalog** (3-beta-aminoethylpyrazole dihydrochloride). Inject 50

mg intramuscularly. If there is no acid secretion, repeat, using 100 mg dose. Some pathologists prefer 1.5 to 2.0 mg/kg of body weight. (Eli Lilly Co., Indianapolis, Ind. 46285. Supplied 50 mg/ml.)

2. **Histamine Phosphate.** Inject 0.04 mg/kg of body weight subcutaneously. (Eli Lilly Co., Indianapolis, Indiana, 46285. Supplied as histamine phosphate, 0.55 mg/ml.) Histamine administration must be preceded by intramuscular administration of a suitable antihistamine given 30 minutes previously, e.g., chlorpheniramine maleate (Chlor-Trimeton), 10 mg, or diphenhydramine hydrochloride (Benadryl), 50 mg. Antihistamine can be administered during the basal secretion test if desired. A suitable 1-ml syringe and vial of 1:1000 epinephrine hydrochloride should be immediately available if needed to counteract severe histamine reactions.
3. **Alcohol.** Instill 50 ml 7% (v/v) ethyl alcohol into stomach via intubation tube. This is useful in patients in whom Histalog is otherwise contraindicated.
4. **Ewald Meal.** Give one roll or two slices of dry toast (about 35 g) and 300 to 400 ml water or pure weak tea.
5. **Riegel Meal.** Give 200 ml beef broth, 150 to 200 g broiled beef steak, 100 g mashed potatoes.
6. **Caffeine.** Give caffeine sodium benzoate, 500 mg in 200 to 300 ml warm water, orally. This is used with the Diagnex Blue Azuresin tubeless analysis (E.R. Squibb & Sons, Inc., Princeton, N.J. 08540).
7. **Insulin.** Give 0.2 units regular zinc insulin per kg of body weight, intravenously (E.R. Squibb & Sons, Inc. Princeton, N.J. 08540).
8. **Peptavlon.** Inject 6 μg/kg of body weight subcutaneously. (Ayerst Laboratories, New York, N.Y. Supplied 0.25 mg/ml, 2 ml ampules.)

Special Medication for Provocative Tests

Insulin (U-40 regular zinc—40 units/ml; E.R. Squibb & Sons), a zinc-containing 51 amino acid polypeptide (M.W. 5,807)—produced by the pancreatic beta cells of the islets of Langerhans. It accelerates metabolism of glucose through all available pathways. Its fundamental action appears to involve facilitation of transport of glucose across the cell membrane and enhancement of the hexokinase reaction. Metabolism through the Embden-Meyerhof pathway, the pentose shunt, and the Krebs cycle is speeded up. Conversion of glucose to fat, and glycogen formation in liver are increased. Gluconeogenesis in liver, and ketogenesis are decreased. The net effect is a decrease in blood glucose within 30 minutes after subcutaneous injection, with maximal activity in 2 to 3 hours. An overdose produces *"insulin shock,"* characterized by weakness, profuse sweating, pallor, fatigue, emotional lability, and eventuating in coma. This shock can be counteracted with 5 to 20% (w/v) intravenous sterile glucose solutions, and glucagon—1 mg intravenously. This effect can be accentuated by 0.3 to 0.6 ml 1 in 1000

TABLE 3–2. Conversion of Pounds to Kilograms for Calculation of Medication Dosage for Provocative Tests.

lbs	kg	lbs	kg	lbs	kg
90	40.9	135	61.4	180	81.8
91	41.4	136	61.8	181	82.3
92	41.8	137	62.3	182	82.7
93	42.3	138	62.7	183	83.2
94	42.7	139	63.2	184	83.6
95	43.2	140	63.6	185	84.1
96	43.6	141	64.1	186	84.5
97	44.1	142	64.5	187	85.0
98	44.5	143	65.0	188	85.4
99	45.0	144	65.4	189	85.9
100	45.4	145	65.9	190	86.4
101	45.9	146	66.3	191	86.9
102	46.3	147	66.8	192	87.3
103	46.8	148	67.2	193	87.8
104	47.2	149	67.7	194	88.2
105	47.7	150	68.1	195	88.7
106	48.1	151	68.6	196	89.1
107	48.6	152	69.0	197	89.6
108	49.0	153	69.5	198	90.0
109	49.5	154	69.9	199	90.5
110	50.0	155	70.4	200	90.9
111	50.5	156	70.8	201	91.4
112	50.9	157	71.3	202	91.8
113	51.4	158	71.7	203	92.3
114	51.8	159	72.2	204	92.7
115	52.3	160	72.7	205	93.2
116	52.7	161	73.2	206	93.6
117	53.2	162	73.6	207	94.1
118	53.6	163	74.1	208	94.5
119	54.1	164	74.5	209	95.0
120	54.5	165	75.0	210	95.5
121	55.0	166	75.4	211	96.0
122	55.4	167	75.9	212	96.4
123	55.9	168	76.3	213	96.9
124	56.3	169	76.8	214	97.3
125	56.8	170	77.3	215	97.8
126	57.2	171	77.8	216	98.2
127	57.7	172	78.2	217	98.7
128	58.1	173	78.7	218	99.1
129	58.6	174	79.1	219	99.6
130	59.1	175	79.6	220	100.0
131	59.6	176	80.0	221	100.5
132	60.0	177	80.5	222	100.9
133	60.5	178	80.9	223	101.4
134	60.9	179	81.4	224	101.8

aqueous epinephrine, which will mobilize glucose from the liver by enhancement of phosphorylase activity. Preparations in use in the United States are extractions from hog (porcine) or cattle (bovine) pancreas. It can be stored for months at 2° to 10° C without loss of potency.

Glucagon (1 mg/ml; Eli Lilly Co.), a 29 amino acid straight-chain polypeptide (M.W. 3,485) produced by pancreatic alpha cells of the islets of Langerhans will increase blood glucose concentration by stimulation of hepatic glycogenolysis through activation of phosphorylase. Intravenous administration (0.5 to 1 mg) produces a gradual termination of insulin coma, usually within 20 minutes. Also, it may cause mild hypotension; a fall in blood nitrogen; an increase in renal electrolyte excretion; inhibition of gastric secretion and motility; and in large doses, nausea and vomiting. The drug should be administered concurrently with 50 ml of 50% (w/v) glucose intravenously (note— epinephrine will prolong its effect!). Local reactions have not been reported following intravenous administration. The dosage of 1 mg (1 ml) can be repeated once after 20 minutes (for a total of 2 doses). Since the drug is a protein, the possibility of hypersensitivity should be considered. Glucagon is soluble in water at pH ranges >3, <9.5. (It can be stored for 30 to 90 days at 2 to 10° C, without loss of potency.)

Basal Secretion Test

SPECIAL INSTRUCTIONS TO TECHNOLOGIST. Consult the pathologist if there is excessive difficulty in passing the tube, if food particles, blood, bile, or dark brown fluid are obtained by aspiration, or if more than 120 ml are obtained by aspiration.

METHOD. One-hour basal secretion test of Levin, Kirsner, and Palmer modified by Baron.

PRINCIPLE. The capacity of the gastric parietal cells to secrete hydrochloric acid is determined in the fasting state under basal conditions by intubation and analysis of acid content.

PROCEDURE

INTUBATION OF PATIENT

1. Patient must be in the fasting state with all food withheld for 12 hours and all fluid withheld for 8 hours. All medications that influence gastric secretion should be withheld for 48 hours. Explain the procedure to the patient with emphasis on the need for deep breathing by mouth and deliberate swallowing when instructed during passage of the tube. Instruct the patient to expectorate, not swallow, all saliva once the tube is in place and the test has begun.
2. Drape the patient appropriately with an apron or towel. Have the patient lean forward in the sitting position with the chin projected slightly forward and upward.
3. Lubricate the tip of the stomach tube with lubricating jelly or

glycerine and gently insert into one of the patient's nostrils, pointing the tube horizontally and eventually slightly downward. Gently pass the tube to a point above the glottis, have patient swallow to close the epiglottis, and gently pass the tube downward at intervals until the tube tip is positioned in the most dependent portion of the stomach as verified by fluoroscopic examination. Tape the free end of the tube to the cheek with surgical scotch tape. Attach a 50 ml syringe to the free end.

BASAL GASTRIC SECRETION

1. Following intubation, aspirate residual gastric contents, measure and record volume and appearance. If gastric content is red, brown, or bloody, contains food particles, or has a volume greater than 120 ml, notify the responsible physician promptly.
2. Aspirate and discard the first 15 or 30 minutes of secretion depending on the patient's degree of composure and apparent physiologic and psychologic adjustment to the intubation procedure.
3. With gentle, constant suction, aspirate gastric contents for 1 hour and deposit as 15-minute specimens in appropriately labeled containers.
4. For each 15-minute specimen, measure and record the volume in ml and the pH using a glass electrode.
5. Determine the titratable acidity of each specimen by titrating a suitable aliquot (5 to 10 ml) with 0.1 N NaOH to pH 7.0 (measured with a glass electrode).
6. Calculation:

$$\text{Titratable acidity (meq/L)} = \frac{100 \times \text{Volume (ml) of NaOH}}{\text{Volume (ml) of gastric fluid aliquot}}$$

$$\text{Acid output (meq)} = \frac{\begin{matrix}\text{Volume (ml)} \\ \text{of specimen}\end{matrix} \times \begin{matrix}\text{titratable} \\ \text{acidity}\end{matrix}}{1{,}000}$$

7. Report residual volume (ml), pH, volume (ml), titratable acidity, and acid output for each specimen; and aggregate volume and acid output for the entire 1-hour test (Fig. 3–3).

INTERPRETATION. Although data are inadequate to state a rigorous normal range, most patients will secrete 0 to 6 meq of acid in a volume of 10 to 100 ml in the 1-hour basal test. Residual volume will ordinarily be less than 75 ml. More than 100 ml is distinctly abnormal.

DISCUSSION AND CLINICAL SIGNIFICANCE. See pages 314 to 315.

MATERIALS AND REAGENTS

1. Levin tube, 14F or 16F, with radiopaque tip
2. 50 ml plastic syringe

GASTRIC ANALYSIS REPORT

Patient Jones, John
Unit No. 80-49875
Date 11/1/80

INITIAL ASPIRATE
Volume 22 ml
Appearance Clear, pale grey with mucus
Blood neg.
Bile neg.

BASAL SECRETION

	Sample	*pH*	*Volume (ml)*	*Titratable Acidity (meq/L)*	*Acid Output (meq)*
1.	15 min	1.59	16	38	.6
2.	15 min	1.56	10	40	.4
3.	15 min	1.52	12	42	.5
4.	15 min	1.60	11	36	.4
	60 min	—	49	—	1.9

STIMULATED SECRETION *Pentagastrin 6 μg/kg*

	Sample	*pH*	*Volume (ml)*	*Titratable Acidity (meq/L)*	*Acid Output (meq)*
1.	15 min	1.44	80	51	4.1
2.	15 min	1.28	103	77	7.9
3.	15 min	1.35	102	62	6.3
4.	15 min	1.43	66	44	2.9
	60 min	—	351	—	21.2

Technologist

Fig. 3–3. Sample report of basal and stimulated acid secretion tests that can be used in hospital and clinical laboratories.

3. Lubricating jelly or glycerin
4. Plastic urine containers with labels
5. pH meter and buffer standards for pH range 1 to 8
6. Burette, 25 ml
7. Beakers, 25 ml
8. NaOH, 0.1 N

REFERENCES

1. Baron, U.: Measurement and nomenclature of gastric acid. Gastroenterology, 45:118, 1961.
2. Levin, E., Kirsner, J., and Palmer, W.: A simple measure of gastric secretion in man. Comparison of one hour basal secretion, histamine-secretion, and twelve hour nocturnal gastric secretion. Gastroenterology, 19:88, 1951.

Maximal Stimulation Test

SPECIAL INSTRUCTIONS TO TECHNOLOGIST. If the patient has a history of asthma, hives, severe allergy, atropic eczema, or heart disease, consult the pathologist before the nurse gives the injection.

If no acid is obtained in 30- to 60-minute specimen, continue the test, collecting a 90-minute specimen.

METHOD. One-hour maximal pentagastrin stimulation test based on Kay and modified by Baron.

PRINCIPLE. The capacity of the gastric parietal cells to respond to a maximal stimulus is determined using pentagastrin as a stimulant.

PROCEDURE

1. Perform intubation and a basal secretion test as previously described.
2. Inject pentagastrin (Peptavlon) subcutaneously in a dose of 6 μg/kg body weight.
3. Immediately collect gastric fluid for 1-hour and deposit as 15-minute specimens in appropriately labeled containers.
4. Proceed to analyze specimens and report data as in the basal secretion test.

INTERPRETATION. As for the basal secretion test, data are inadequate to express a rigorous normal range. Most males will have an acid output of 1 to 40 meq in a volume of 40 to 350 ml in the entire hour. Lower values apply to females and older individuals.

DISCUSSION AND CLINICAL SIGNIFICANCE. See pages 315 to 316.

MATERIALS AND REAGENTS

1. See basal secretion test.
2. Pentagastrin (Peptavlon, Ayerst Laboratories, 685 Third Ave., New York, N.Y. 10017) 250 μg/ml, 2 ml ampuls.

REFERENCES

1. Baron, J.: Measurement and nomenclature of gastric acid. Gastroenterology, 45:118, 1961.
2. Kay, A.: Memorial lecture: an evaluation of gastric acid secretion tests. Gastroenterology, 53:834, 1967.
3. Kay, A.: Effect of large doses of histamine on gastric secretion of HCl (an augmented histamine test). Br. Med. J., 2:77, 1953.

Insulin Hypoglycemia Test

SPECIAL INSTRUCTIONS TO TECHNOLOGIST. Consult the pathologist before the test if the patient is older than 50 years of age or if he has had a gastrectomy of any type. Consult the pathologist before the nurse gives the injection if the patient is extremely thin, a diabetic, or is on any antiparasympathetic drugs (atropine, belladonna, Donnatol, Pamine, etc.). Only the nurse or physician should inject the insulin.

METHOD. Two-hour basal and 2-hour postinsulin test of Stempien based on Hollander.

PRINCIPLE. Hypoglycemia resulting from insulin administration stimulates the vagal nucleus in the brain from whence excitatory stimuli are transmitted via the vagus nerves to promote acid secretion by the parietal cells. Caution: this test should be performed only when a physician is readily available in the event of an adverse reaction. Caution must be exercised in requesting this test in patients over age 50, those with known arteriosclerotic cardiovascular disease, or those on antiparasympathetic drugs (atropine, belladonna, Pamine).

PROCEDURE

1. Perform intubation as in the basal secretion test.
2. Collect gastric contents for 2 hours as 15-minute specimens.
3. Collect a blood specimen for glucose determination.
4. Have a nurse or physician inject insulin (0.2 units crystalline insulin/kg body weight) intravenously. (Caution: have immediately available a 50 ml syringe filled with 50% (w/v) sterile glucose solution).
5. Continue to aspirate gastric fluid for 2 hours as 15-minute specimens.
6. Caution: Watch patient for complaints of severe hunger, irritability, paleness, fainting, palpitation, weakness, tremors, or any unusual emotional behavior, such as crying or laughing. If they develop, call physician immediately. At the conclusion of the test, the patient should be given a glass of orange juice.
7. Collect blood specimens for glucose determination at 30, 60, and 90 minutes after insulin injection.
8. For each gastric-fluid specimen in both the basal and postinsulin period, measure and record volume and pH using a glass electrode, determine the titratable acidity and calculate the acid output as in the basal secretion study.
9. Report the volume, pH, titratable acidity, and acid output for each specimen and the total volume and acid output for each of the 4 hours of the test.

INTERPRETATION. The test is valid only if the stomach is capable of secreting acid and if the blood glucose falls below 50 mg/dl at some point in the test, usually 30 minutes after insulin. Complete vagotomy can be assumed if the acid output in the greater of the 2 postinsulin hours is less than the greater of the 2 basal hours or if the total acid output in the 2 postinsulin hours does not exceed the total for the 2 basal hours by more than 0.5 meq. Incomplete vagotomy is also likely if the acid output in either basal hour is greater than 2 meq.

DISCUSSION AND CLINICAL SIGNIFICANCE. See pages 316 to 317.

MATERIALS AND REAGENTS

1. See basal secretion test.
2. Insulin injection (regular or crystalline insulin) U-40 (40 units/ml)
3. 5-ml syringes and stoppered tubes or vacuum tubes with hypodermic needles for blood collection.
4. 50 ml syringe with no. 20 needle
5. Glucose, 50% (w/v), sterile for injection

REFERENCES

1. Hollander, F.: The insulin test for the presence of intact nerve fibers after vagal operations for peptic ulcer. Gastroenterology, 7:607, 1946.
2. Stempien, S.: Insulin gastric analysis: technic and interpretations. Am. J. Dig. Dis., 7:138, 1962.

SPECIAL INSTRUCTIONS TO TECHNOLOGISTS FOR PATIENTS UNDERGOING GASTRIC ANALYSIS

Basal Test. If difficulty passing tube, consult pathologist.

If food particles, blood, bile, or dark brown fluid are obtained by aspiration, consult pathologist before continuing.

If more than 120 ml of gastric juices are obtained by aspiration, consult pathologist.

Histalog Test. If patient has history of asthma, hives, severe allergy, atopic eczema, or heart disease, consult pathologist before nurse gives injection.

If no acid is obtained in 30- and 60-minute specimen, continue test, collecting 90-minute specimen.

Insulin Test. If patient is older than 50 years of age, consult pathologist before test.

If patient has had gastrectomy of any type, consult pathologist before test.

If patient is on antiparasympathetic drugs (atropine, belladonna, Donnatol, Pamine, etc.), consult pathologist before nurse injects insulin.

If patient is extremely thin, consult pathologist before injection.

If patient is a diabetic, consult pathologist before injection.

Only nurse or physician is to inject insulin.

Insulin (U40–40 units/ml; Squibb Co.), a 50 amino acid polypeptide (M.W. 5,807-man) produced by pancreatic (islet of Langerhans) beta cells, accelerates a glucose oxidation (through hexokinase reaction); accelerates conversion of glucose to fat (through acetyl CoA reaction);

increases glycogen formation in liver (± inhibition of hormones producing hepatic glycogenolysis); inhibits gluconeogenesis in liver; and inhibits ketogenesis. The net effect is a decrease in blood glucose within 30 minutes after subcutaneous injection (but maximal action in 2 to 3 hours). Overdose produces "insulin shock" characterized by weakness, profuse sweating, pallor, fatigue, emotional lability, and coma. Counterreaction of this shock may be induced with 5 to 20% (w/v) IV sterile glucose solutions and glucagon-1 mg IV. This effect may be accentuated by 0.3 to 0.6 ml 1:1000 aqueous epinephrine, which will mobilize glucose from the liver. Human insulin is being synthesized in the laboratory by E. coli by gene splicing and genetic manipulation. It may be stored for months at 2 to 10° C without loss of potency.

REFERENCE

American Society of Hospital Pharmacists: American Hospital Formulary Service, *68*:20, 1976.

Glucagon (1 mg/ml; Eli Lilly Co.), a 29 amino acid straight chain polypeptide (M.W. 3,485) produced by pancreatic (islet of Langerhans) alpha cells, will increase blood glucose concentration by stimulation of hepatic glycogenolysis through activation of phosphorylase. Intravenous administration (0.5 to 1 mg) produces a gradual termination of insulin coma (≤ 20 minutes); mild hypotension; fall in blood nitrogen; increase in renal electrolyte excretion; inhibition of gastric secretion and mobility; and, in large doses, nausea and vomiting. The drug should be administered concurrently with 50 ml 50% (w/v) glucose intravenously (note: epinephrine will prolong effect!). Local reactions have not been reported with IV administration. Dosage of 1 mg (1 ml) may be repeated after 20 minutes (for two doses total). Since the drug is a protein, the possibility of hypersensitivity should be considered. Glucagon is soluble in HO at pH ranges 3 or 9.5. (It may be stored 30 to 90 days at 2 to 10°C without loss of potency.)

REFERENCE

American Society of Hospital Pharmacists: American Hospital Formulary Service, *68*:20, 1976.

Pentagastrin (Pentavalon 0.25 mg/ml in 2-ml vials; Ayerst Laboratories), is a polypeptide containing the same sequence of 4 amino acids formed in the C-terminal portion of the natural polypeptide, gastrin. This portion of the gastrin molecule is responsible for stimulation of gastric secretion. Pentagastrin is a colorless, crystalline solid, and is slightly soluble in water and in ethanol. The pH is 7 to 8. It should be stored at 4°C and has an expiration date of 2 years. The precise mechanism by which pentagastrin stimulates acid output is not known. The drug probably excites oxynitic cells of the stomach to secrete maximally.

The drug is only partially effective. Gastric secretion occurs within

10 minutes after subcutaneous administration, with peak activity in 20 to 30 minutes. The plasma half life is less than 1 minute. Pentagastrin metabolism is suspected to be by deamination to form pentagastrin acid, which is secreted in bile. About 40% is secreted unchanged, 40% as the acid, and 15 to 17% as unknown metabolites (experiments in dogs).

Side effects are infrequent and mild and include abdominal cramps, nausea, emesis, flushing, tachycardia, faintedness, dizziness, chills, and shortness of breath. Hypersensitivity reactions are rare. Adult dose: 6 μg/kg weight subcutaneously.

REFERENCE

American Society of Hospital Pharmacists: American Hospital Formulary Service, 68:36, 1976.

Chapter

4 Urinary Stone Analysis

ROBERT H. MORRISS
MYRTON F. BEELER
JAMES A. FREEMAN

Urinary stone is an ancient affliction, probably having plagued man from his very beginnings. A bladder stone, estimated to have been formed several centuries before the reign of Menes, the first Pharoah of Egypt (about 3200 B.C.), was found by Elliot Smith in the grave of a predynastic Egyptian at El Amara.[1] There is no mention of stone in the Papyrus (1871) discovered by George Ebers, the German Egyptologist. This Papyrus, mentioned in another chapter, is probably the oldest medical treatise in existence, dating from about 1,550 B.C. However, it is more a compendium of prescriptions and remedies than of descriptions of disease. Stone was probably uncommon amongst the ancient Egyptians, because Smith found only two in the more than 9,000 mummies he examined. Smith's second case was an interesting one, the stone having been found in the nasal fossa of a priest of the 21st Dynasty. The embalming custom dictated removal of intestines through an incision in the flank and removal of the brain by means of suction through the nasal passages. The stone was apparently removed from the urinary tract and then replaced in the enlarged nasal fossa, because it was a readily accessible area. Samuel Shattuck described a renal stone located near the second lumbar vertebra of a skeleton found in a tomb dating back to the 2nd Egyptian Dynasty (about 1,100 B.C.). Presumably, this was a urinary stone, although its composition has not been determined.[2] (One of the stones found by Smith was composed of uric acid, calcium oxalate, and ammonium magnesium phosphate—still common urinary stone constituents.) Stones were well known to American Indians. A urinary stone the size of a small pea was recovered from the pelvis of an American Indian mummy, estimated to date from about 1,000 B.C.

TABLE 4–3. Number of Calculi Containing Various Percentages of Each Crystalline Component, 464 Calculi.[7]

	100 %	90–99 %	80–89 %	70–79 %	60–69 %	50–59 %	40–49 %	30–39 %	20–29 %	10–19 %	0–9 %	Total Calculi	% of Total Calculi
Calcium oxalate monohydrate	51	25	14	19	18	10	16	20	40	35	15	275	59.3
Calcium oxalate dihydrate	11	12	33	21	17	18	13	15	20	30	10	200	43.2
Hydroxyl and carbonate-apatite	21	15	14	10	17	22	26	18	29	45	22	239	51.5
Magnesium ammonium phosphate hexahydrate	9	4	5	6	12	7	6	8	8	7	1	73	15.7
Calcium hydrogen phosphate dihydrate	2		2		1	1	2			1		9	1.9
Tricalcium phosphate	1	1	2						1	2		7	1.5
Calcium magnesium hydroxyl phosphate					1							1	0.2
Uric acid	16	11	8	6	3	3	1		3			51	11.1
Uric acid dihydrate	1				1	2		2	9	12	3	30	6.5
Ammonium acid urate	3		2			1					1	7	1.5
Sodium acid urate											1	1	0.2
Cystine	5			1								6	1.3

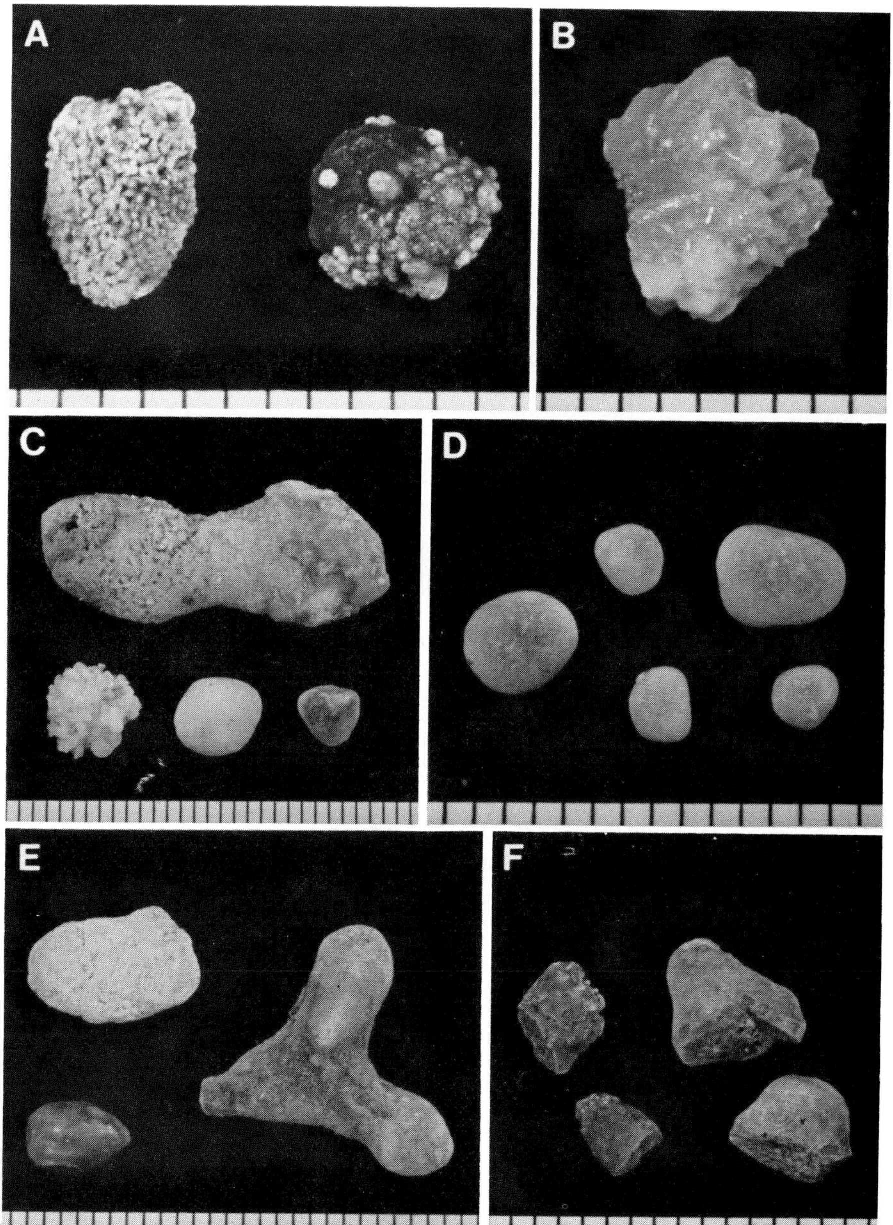

Fig. 4–1. Gross appearance of urinary stones of different composition. Scales are in millimeters. **A,** Calcium oxalate monohydrate stones of the mulberry type. **B,** Calcium oxalate dihydrate stone exhibiting large crystals. **C,** Variety of triple phosphate stones. **D,** Calcium hydrogen phosphate dihydrate multiple stones. **E,** Variety of apatite stones, including large stone of the staghorn type. **F,** Fragments of two uric acid stones.

to be much lighter in color than the monohydrate form of calcium oxalate. Figure 4–1C shows a variety of stones, each of which is composed of magnesium ammonium phosphate hexahydrate, commonly referred to as "triple phosphate." The large stone in the upper part of the figure occurred as a single stone in the kidney, whereas, the three smaller stones in the lower part of the figure are examples of multiple stones. The disparate forms demonstrate that composition alone does not determine the external appearance of urinary stones. Other factors, such as growth site and rate of growth, as well as all of the growth conditions, are important in determining the final form of a stone. The large, peanut-shaped stone is soft, porous, and uneven in surface texture. The stone in the lower left of the figure is a multiple bladder stone consisting of a loose aggregate of fairly large cystallites. The very light stone in the lower center is smooth and nearly spherical in shape. The medium brown stone in the lower right is a rounded tetrahedron, a form that sometimes results from friction when multiple stones are closely packed. The rare set of multiple stones shown in Figure 4–1D are pure calcium hydrogen phosphorus dihydrate. These stones are ellipsoidal in shape, have light smooth surfaces, and are very hard. A variety of pure apatite stones is illustrated in Figure 4–1E. The soft, chalky white stone in the upper left is fairly typical of pure apatite stones. Another common form is the staghorn stone shown on the right. These stones tend to be very large and can fill up the calyces and pelvis of the kidney. Staghorn stones occur as both single and multiple stones and often consist of a mixture of apatite and triple phosphate. Figure 4–1F shows uric acid stone fragments. Stones composed of pure uric acid tend to be irregular in shape, yellow ochre in color, and very hard. Pure uric acid stones are not very common; they usually occur as mixtures of the anhydrous and dihydrate forms of uric acid.

The appearance of stones on conventional diagnostic roentgenograms may also be helpful for differentiating stone composition (Fig. 4–2). Calcium oxalate stones sometimes have a stellate appearance, while triple phosphate stones often have dense concentric rings or layers upon x-ray examination. Cystine stones are purported to show a homogeneous dense shadow, but we have been unable to confirm this observation. Uric acid stones tend to give faint shadows, if any at all.

STRUCTURE OF STONES

Many stones exhibit considerable internal structure that can be revealed by cutting the stone in half. The cross sections of two commonly occurring mixed stones (apatite and calcium oxalates) reveal concentric laminations (Fig. 4–3). The upper stone (Fig. 4–3A) is a mixture of the two hydrates of calcium oxalate and apatite; it is characterized by concentric bands or lamellae, alternating light and dark, surrounding a central nucleus. The dark bands are calcium oxalate monohydrate, the

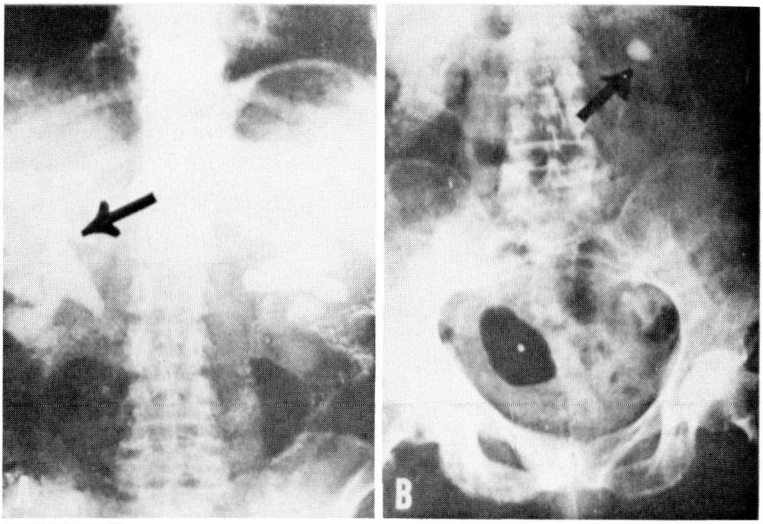

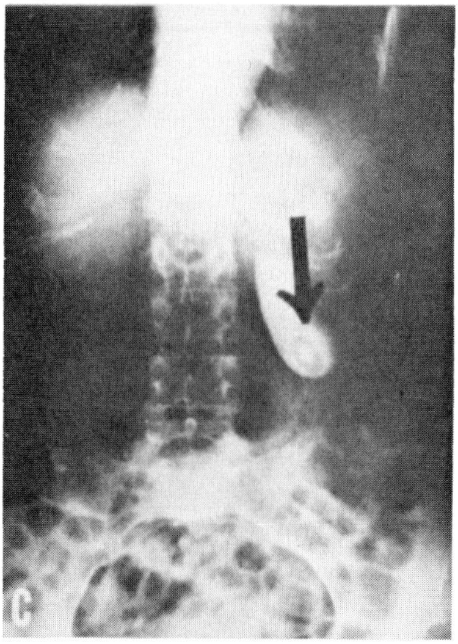

Fig. 4–2. X-ray appearance of kidney stones. **A,** Staghorn stones by abdominal upright x-ray examination. **B,** Apatite stones by abdominal upright x-ray examination. **C,** Cystine stones discovered during IV pyelogram x-ray. (Note the concentric laminations. The x-ray appearance of the dye and stones could be mistaken for gallbladder if found on the opposite side of the abdomen.)

light bands are primarily apatite, and the thick, outermost layer is calcium oxalate dihydrate. The lower stone (Fig. 4–3B) is a mixture of apatite and triple phosphate. The cross section is characterized by bands of different texture and an asymmetrical nucleus. The columnar structure (noticed particularly in the lower portion of the figure) is characteristic of triple phosphate. Much of the lighter material in the central region of the stone is apatite. The position of the nucleus suggests that the stone initiated its development from a calcium plaque on the surface of the renal papilla.

A wide variation of fine structure of urinary calculi is revealed by the scanning electron microscopy (Fig. 4–4). The calcium oxalate monohydrate stone shown in Figure 4–4A is characterized by preferred ori-

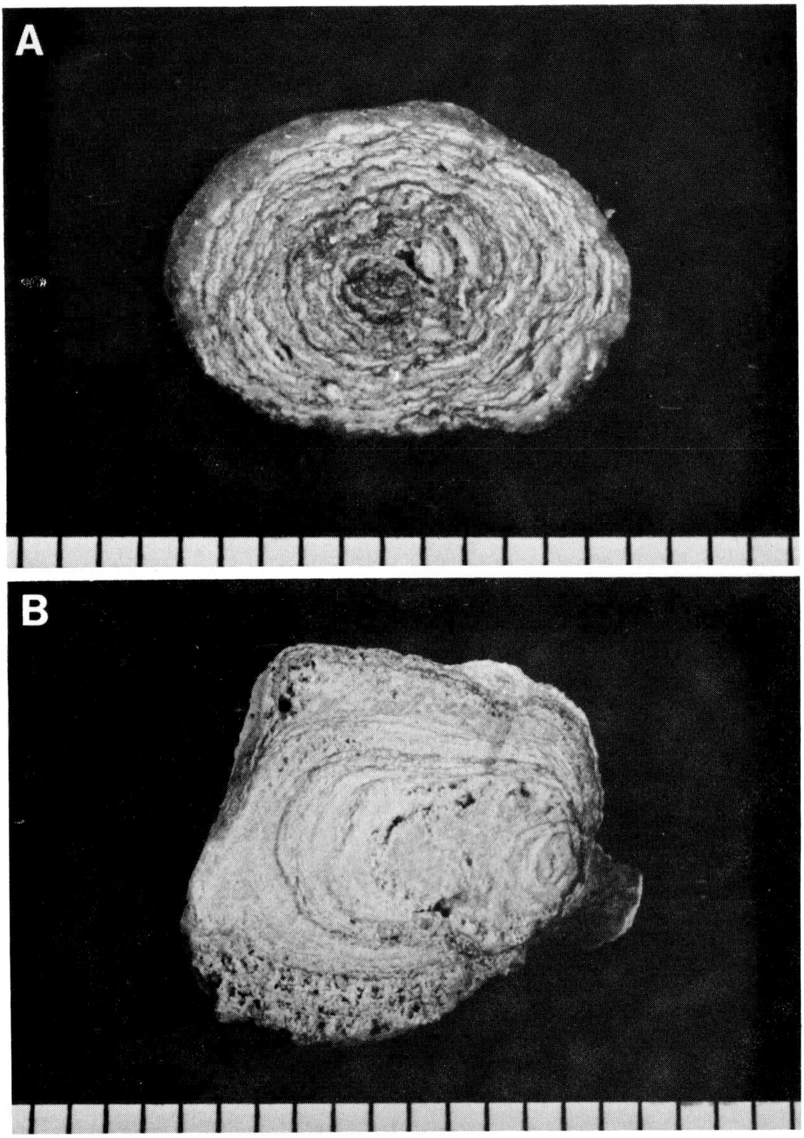

Fig. 4–3. Cross sections of two urinary stones. Scales are in mm. **A,** Mixed stone containing both hydrates of calcium oxalate and apatite, exhibiting concentric lamellae about a central nucleus. **B,** Mixed stone composed of apatite and triple phosphate, showing bands of different texture about an asymmetrical nucleus.

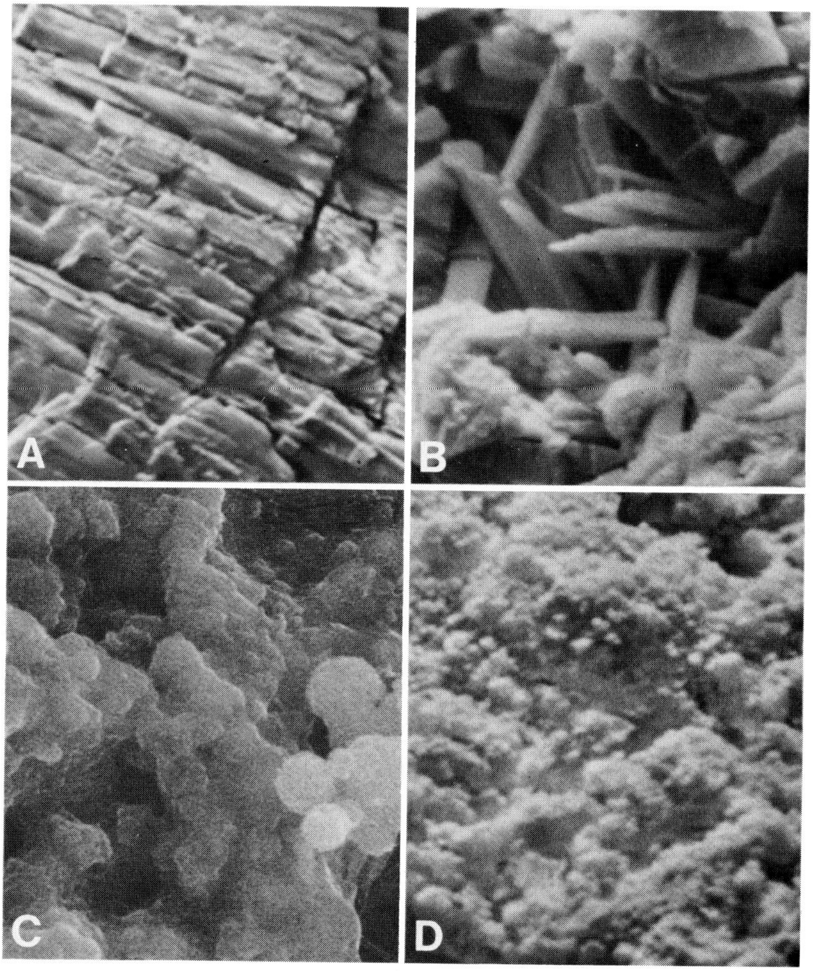

Fig. 4–4. Scanning electron micrographs of four types of urinary calculi revealing internal structure. Magnification ×1,000. **A,** Calcium oxalate monohydrate stone showing preferred orientation of crystallites. **B,** Calcium hydrogen phosphate dihydrate stone showing needle crystals randomly oriented. **C,** Triple phosphate stone composed of loose aggregate of platelets. **D,** Apatite stone composed of extremely fine grains.

entation—that is, a parallel alignment of neighboring crystallites. This is a fairly common texture observed in stones and is responsible for radial striations that often run perpendicular to concentric laminations. The calcium hydrogen phosphate dihydrate stone shown in Figure 4–4B is characterized by large, needle-shaped crystallites exhibiting little preferred orientation. The triple phosphate shown in Figure 4–4C appears to be a rather loose assemblage of platelets. Figure 4–4D shows apatite and is characterized by extremely fine grains that appear to be completely randomly oriented.

The external surface morphology of a calcium oxalate dihydrate stone as revealed by scanning electron microscopy is characteristic (Fig. 4–5). The upper micrograph (Fig. 4–5A) illustrates the well formed surface crystals in the shape of bitetrahedral pyramids that is a characteristic of this material. The higher magnification micrograph (Fig. 4–5B) of the same stone shows several intercrystal bridges. The morphology of the bridges suggest that they are noncrystalline and perhaps composed of organic matrix material. The surface crystals of calcium oxalate dihydrate shown in Figure 4–6 are encrusted with what appears to be apatite. There has been considerable speculation as to a possible role

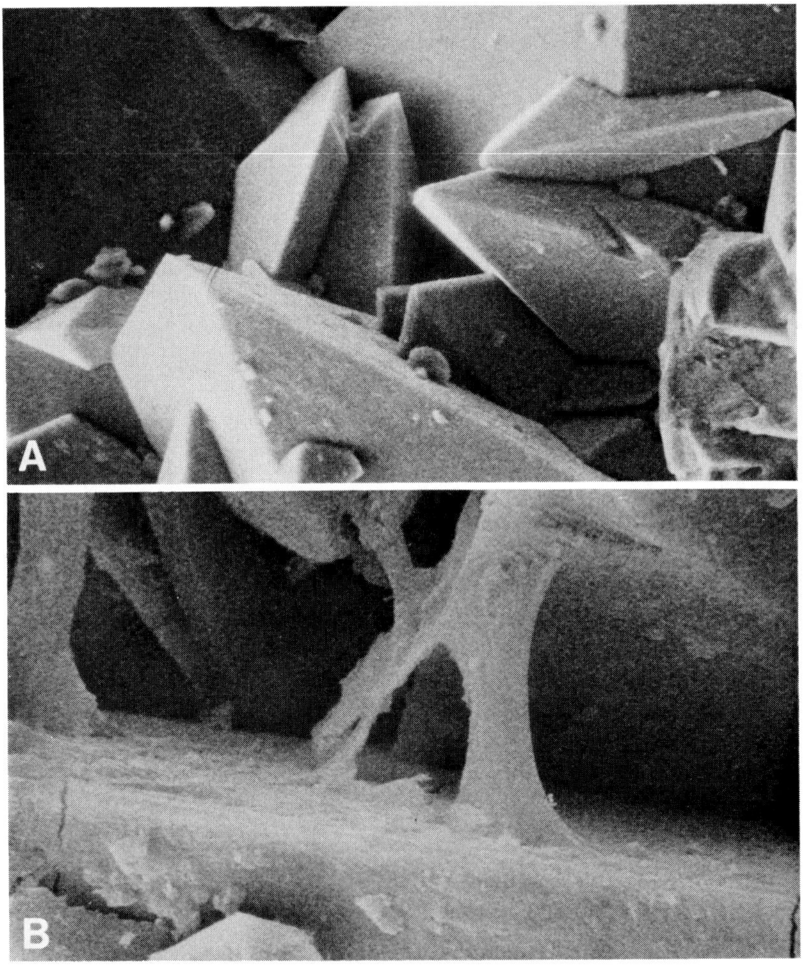

Fig. 4–5. Scanning electron micrographs of external surface of calcium oxalate dihydrate stone. **A,** Large well-formed crystals in shape of bitetrahedral pyramids (× 300). **B,** Several intercrystal bridges perhaps composed of amorphous organic matrix (× 1,000).

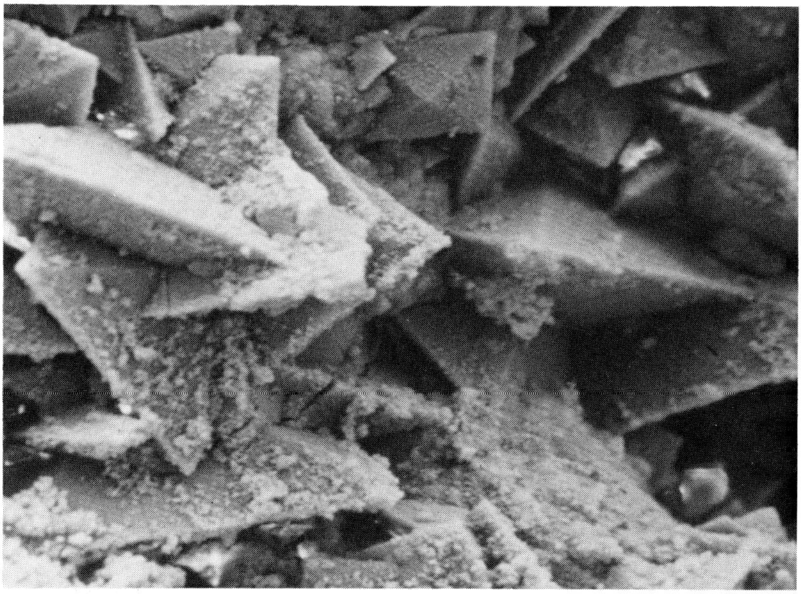

Fig. 4–6. Scanning electron micrograph of external surface of calcium oxalate dihydrate stone encrusted with very fine apatite particles (× 300).

played by both apatite and organic matrix material in the formation of urinary calculi; however, the definite influence of either has not been established.

Transmission electron microscopy gives an even closer look at the ultrastructure of urinary calculi (Fig. 4–7). Electron microscopy of calcium oxalate monohydrate reveals a foamy ultrastructure (Fig. 4–7A). A similar structure is exhibited by the dihydrate of calcium oxalate. Finlayson and Meyer have postulated that this structure results from the aggregation of spherulites 100 Å in diameter.[14] The electron microscopic appearances of tricalcium phosphate and triple phosphate also reveal a very fine grain structure (Fig. 4–7B and 4–7D). The individual crystallites of uric acid, on the other hand, appear to be much larger (Fig. 4–7C). The apatite stone (Fig. 4–7E) is characterized by extremely fine individual grains that are less than 100 Å in diameter. Apatite stones can thus be considered to exist in a colloidal state. Mineralogic apatite, on the other hand, shows much larger crystallites with electron microscopy (Fig. 4–7F). The fine-grain ultrastructure exhibited by so many urinary calculi suggests the possibility that the agglomeration of fine crystallites in urine plays a role in the growth of stones.

TECHNIQUES FOR ANALYZING STONES

Techniques for analyzing the crystalline constituents of urinary stones include:

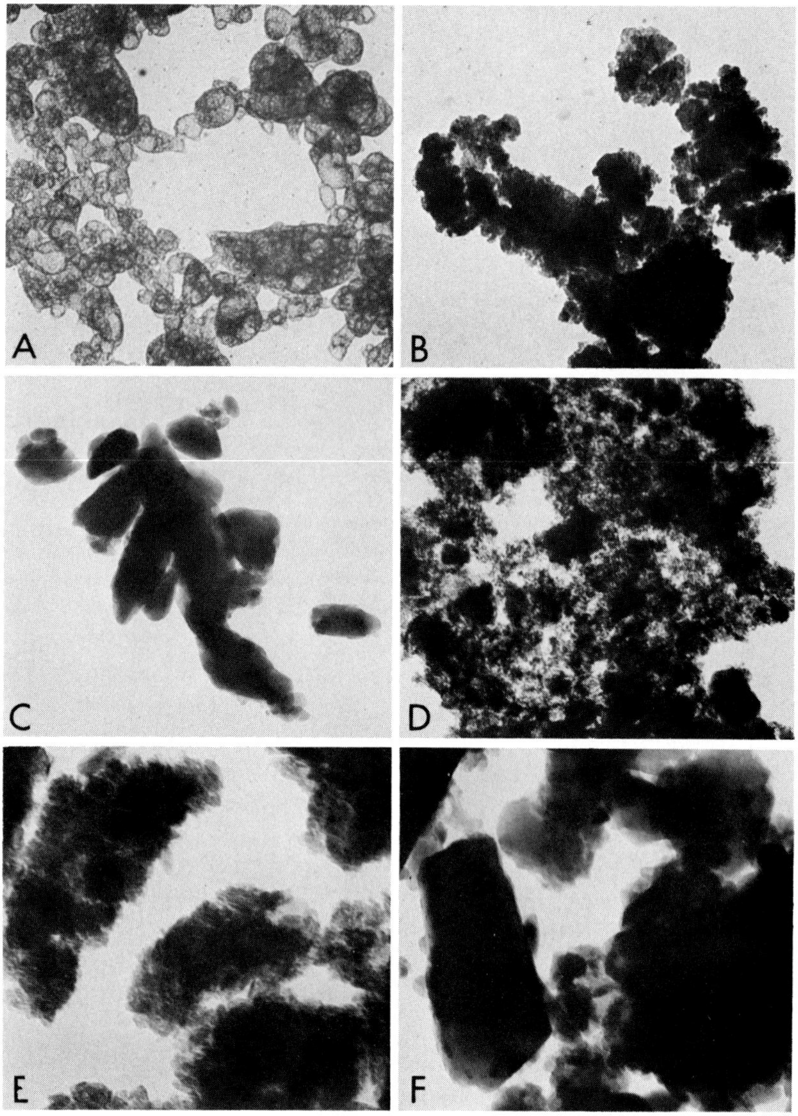

Fig. 4–7. Transmission electron micrographs of finely pulverized urinary stone showing ultrastructure. **A,** Calcium oxalate monohydrate stone exhibiting foam structure (× 15,000). **B,** Tricalcium phosphate stone revealing fine grain structure (× 15,000). **C,** Uric acid stone exhibiting large crystallites (× 25,000). **D,** Triple phosphate stone showing fine grain structure (× 25,000). **E,** Apatite stone showing extremely fine grains less than 100 Å in "diameter" (× 100,000). **F,** Mineralogical apatite showing much larger crystallites (× 100,000).

1. Chemical analysis
2. Polarizing (petrographic) microscopy
3. X-ray diffraction
4. Infrared spectroscopy
5. Electron microscopy

There is continuing debate about which method of analysis is the most accurate, the simplest, and the most useful. The organic matrix material has been much less carefully studied, and currently there are no practical, routine laboratory tests aimed at its analysis.

Edward Prien and Clifford Frondel, 1947, reported that the immersion optical method (petrographic microscopy with polarized light) was more satisfactory than either chemical or x-ray crystallographic analysis.[15] However, in 1964, Myrton Beeler, Daniel Veith, Robert Morriss, and Gerson Biskind concluded that chemical analysis was satisfactory for routine medical use in the clinical microscopy laboratory and was to be supplemented, on occasion, by x-ray diffraction or infrared spectroscopy.[16] Beeler and associates concluded that neither the immersion optical microscopic method nor the use of electron microscopy, electron diffraction, or thermoluminescence is suitable for routine use in the clinical laboratory. Although use of the petrographic microscope may appear simple to geologists and others familiar with crystallography, interpretation becomes difficult in the hands of those not primarily schooled in this technique.

In contrast to Prien and Frondel's condemnation of the chemical analysis, Beeler and associates found a high degree of correlation between chemical constituents (as determined by qualitative chemical study) and crystalline components (as determined by x-ray diffraction analysis). X-ray diffraction, because of the sophisticated, expensive instrumentation involved, is a technique generally available only in university or large reference laboratories. Chemical analysis, on the other hand, is rapid and can be performed in any laboratory, although it does require adequate attention to details of technique. There are, however, some serious objections to the sole use of chemical analysis. Although ions are reported by chemical analysis, a physician who gets a report of the presence of calcium and phosphate, for example, will not know whether the specimen is composed of hydroxyl apatite, calcium hydrogen phosphate dihydrate, or tricalcium phosphate. Also, chemical analysis does not differentiate between the two hydrates of oxalate, cannot distinguish the various forms of uric acid and the urates, and xanthine may be confused with uric acid. Oxalate may, on occasion, be missed when it is only a minor component.[10,16] The chemical method, on the other hand, is more sensitive than x-ray diffraction in detecting apatite and magnesium ammonium phosphate hexahydrate. Whereas the chemical method only provides qualitative analysis, x-ray diffraction provides semiquantitative results; however, this additional information is not especially useful for guiding treatment. Another limitation of the chemical method is that a minimum of about 4 to 5 mg of material is required for adequate analysis. The Reference Laboratory, Los Angeles, reported that about 10% of specimens were too small to be analyzed by chemical methods. Thus, when a stone is too small or if a small nucleus is distinguishable and a separate analysis is desired, the x-ray diffraction method should be applied. Infrared spectroscopy, like chemical analysis, detects chemical constituents from which one can predict the crystalline components.[12] The results are semiquantitative, and the method requires special, relatively expensive equipment, as does the method of x-ray diffraction.

PRINCIPLES OF CHEMICAL ANALYSIS

Julius Winer and Marjorie Mattice, in 1943, introduced a battery of simple qualitative chemical tests for analyses of the specific radical constituents of stones.[17] Reid Leonard and Arthur Butt shortly thereafter introduced a quantitative chemical method, but the technique was applicable to only a few of the possible constituents of calculi. Winer has subsequently advocated eight simple spot tests for identification of the constituents of stones. Another, somewhat similar battery of tests originating at the Stone Clinic of the Massachusetts General Hospital and described by Peter Maurice and Philip Henneman has been widely used.

The principles of the chemical analyses of urinary calculi are simple. The chemical tests are predominantly spot tests adapted to use in test tubes.

1. Calcium salts are dissolved in hydrochloric acid and subsequently detected by the cloudy flocculent of calcium hydroxide, which follows addition of sodium hydroxide.
2. Oxalate is detected by escaping bubbles of gaseous oxygen, which form when oxalate is oxidized by manganese dioxide in the presence of hydrochloric acid.
3. Phosphate is detected by appearance of the yellow color of ammonium phosphomolybdate, which forms in the presence of phosphate, ammonium molybdate, and nitric acid. The reaction is speeded by heat.
4. Carbonate is detected by bubbles of carbon dixoide, which are driven off by the action of hydrochloric acid on the carbonate ion.
5. Uric acid and urates are oxidized to allantoin in an alkaline solution, and a blue color is formed from reduction of phosphotungstic acid. Small traces of uric acid give a pale blue, while large amounts give a deep blue color.

6. Ammonium ions react with Nessler's reagent (potassium mercuric iodide) to form a yellow-brown compound.
7. Magnesium is detected by the purple color developed by p-nitrobenzeneazoresorcinol in the presence of magnesium. This appears to be a physical effect rather than a chemical reaction and is not well understood.
8. Cystine is detected by the reaction of sulfhydryl groups with nitroprusside following reduction of cystine by cyanide, with the resultant formation of beet-red compound.

The method of Winer and Mattice for the chemical analysis of urinary calculi is detailed at the end of the chapter.

PRINCIPLES OF POLARIZED LIGHT MICROSCOPY[18,19]

Optical characteristics result from the manner in which light behaves while passing through a substance. When an oblique beam of light passes from one medium (such as air) to another differing in optical density (such as liquid), the velocity and the direction of the beam are changed. Simply stated, the light is "refracted." A quantitative expression of this effect is given by Snell's law:

$$N_D = \frac{\sin i}{\sin r} = \frac{V}{V'},$$

where "N_D" is the ratio "n'/n" of the absolute refractive indices of the two media, "i" the angle of incidence, "r" the angle of light refraction, and "V" and "V′" are the velocities of light in the first and second media, respectively. Refractive index is also a function of wavelength. Substances show greater indices of refraction with violet light; lower with near-infrared light. (In practice a yellow filter is often used with a wavelength approximating the sodium D line [5,893 Å]. However, "daylight" substage or fluorescent "white light" illumination is satisfactory for most clinical work.)

The extent to which a beam of light is refracted depends on the number of atoms of substance in the light path, on the kind of atoms, and on the atomic arrangement of molecules. Crystalline substances can be powdered so finely that they become transparent or translucent, and when immersed in a liquid of appropriate refractive index, any single crystal will transmit or refract light to a characteristic degree, according to its molecular (crystalline) form and orientation in the light path. When they are viewed through a polarizing microscope, a halo of bright refracted light (called the Becke line) moves into or away from the crystal as the microscope is focused (Fig. 4–8). If the halo moves onto the crystal as the objective is lowered, the unknown crystal has a lower refractive index than the medium; if the halo moves into the medium, the unknown crystal has a higher index of refraction than the

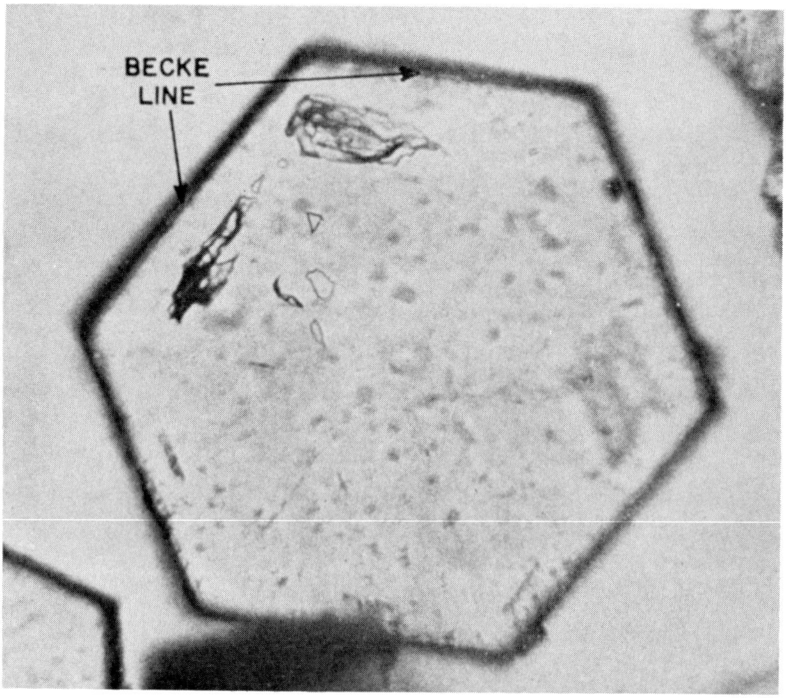

Fig. 4–8. Becke line or halo of refracted light around a crystal (the black image is due to photographic reversal of the image) as viewed through a polarizing microscope. (From Vieth, D.: Ph.D. thesis. New Orleans, Tulane University, 1964.)

medium. The reverse is the case when raising the objective. Through repeated trials, a mounting medium can be found that has nearly the same refractive index as the unknown. When a final match is approached, isotropic crystals will become nearly invisible, and in a perfect match, will actually disappear completely from sight. The refractive indices of uniaxial crystals can also be determined by observation at their "extinction" (blacking out) position. Since the refractive indices are characteristic for each crystal, this method may be used to establish identity (and purity) of crystals. The range of indices of practical value to the clinical pathologist extends from 1.40 to 2.00, which blankets the range seen in urinary stone constituents. R.P. Cargille Refractive Index Media are obtainable in complete sets covering the range of indices required for stone analysis (Fig. 4–9). (N_D25 1.41 to 1.78 in 0.01 increments, catalog no. C2655, Ward's Natural Science Establishment, P.O. Box 1712, Rochester, N.Y. 14603).

Identification of urinary calculi by refractometry requires at least a rudimentary knowledge of crystallography, optical physics, and microscopy; and a reasonably sophisticated polarizing microscope. In our

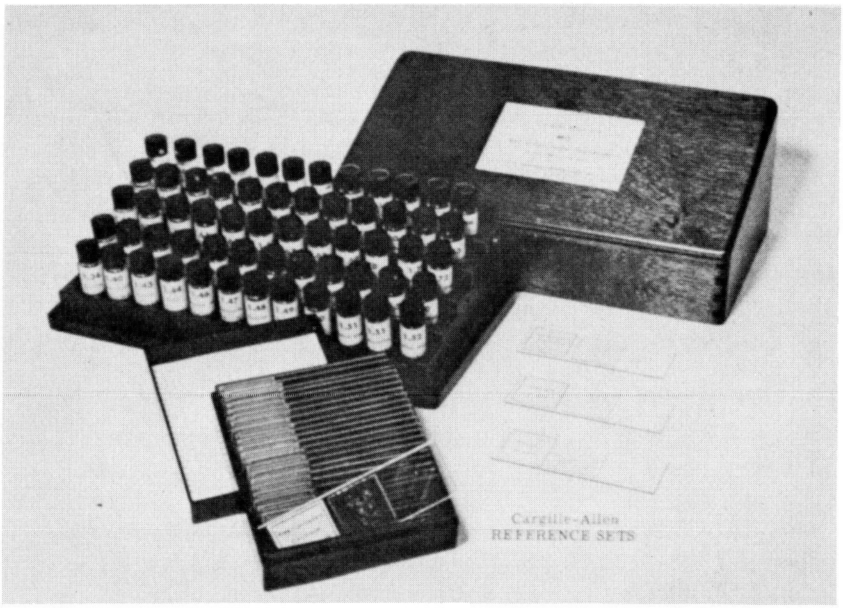

Fig. 4–9. Cargille-Allen M-1 Refractive Index Media Set. The usual range of indices of practical value to the clinical pathologist extends from 1.40 to 2.00, which blankets the range seen in urinary stone constituents. (Courtesy of Mr. John J. Cargille, R. P. Cargille Laboratories, Cedar Grove, N.J. 07009.)

hands, it has been found to be tedious, probably because of our relative inexperience and the limitations of our equipment. It is most useful when very little material is available for examination or as a supplement to the chemical examination; however, we prefer x-ray diffraction analysis for that purpose.

Crystals are solids naturally bounded by plane surfaces and having specific molecular patterns. The plane surfaces of a crystal are parallel to the plane of the atoms within the crystal. The combination of planes selected by the crystal is called its "habit." The cystallographic axes that are parallel to the principal edges of an ideal crystal form the basis of the usual classification of crystals into three groups and seven systems (that differ in length, width, depth, and the angle between their crystallographic axes). The first and simplest group is the isomeric or cubic system, with all axes of equal length and each at right angles to the others. The crystals of this system have a single refractive index (as do amorphous substances) and are said to be optically isotropic. Although none of the common constituents of urinary calculi belong to the cubic system, apatite is essentially isotropic due to its extremely fine-grained structure.

The second group are optically uniaxial systems and have two refractive indices, corresponding to the ω(omega) or O(ordinary) ray and the ϵ(epsilon) or E(extraordinary) ray. The birefringence of a uniaxial crystal is the difference between the two refractive indices. The optical sign of a uniaxial crystal is positive when n_ϵ is greater than n_ω, and the sign is negative when n_ω is greater than n_ϵ. This group includes the tetragonal system with three mutually perpendicular axes with the vertical (c) axis either larger or shorter than the other two. Calcium oxidate dihydrate belongs to this system. It is only slightly birefringent with $n_\omega = 1.523$ and $n_\epsilon = 1.544$; its optical sign is positive.[15] The second system of this group is the hexagonal system, similar to the tetragonal system, except that the three axes are at 60° angles to each other. Cystine, tricalcium phosphate, and apatite belong to this system; however, only cystine shows any appreciable birefringence. Cystine is optically negative since $n_\omega = 1.700$ and $n_\epsilon = 1.640$. The third system of this group is the rhombohedral system, which is similar to the hexagonal system.

The third group are optically biaxial systems that have three indices of refraction (α, β, γ or X, Y, Z). The birefringence of a biaxial crystal is the difference between α and γ, the smallest and largest indices, respectfully. The optical sign of a biaxial crystal is positive if $(\gamma - \beta)$ is greater than $(\beta - \alpha)$ and negative if $(\gamma - \beta)$ is less than $(\beta - \alpha)$. The first of these systems is the orthorhomic system, whose axes are mutually perpendicular but all of different length. Magnesium ammonium phosphate hexahydrate and uric acid belong to this system. Triple phosphate is only slightly birefringent and is optically positive, whereas, uric acid is highly birefringent. The monoclinic system is similar to the orthorhombic, except that one of the crystallographic axis angles is less than 90°. Calcium oxalate monohydrate and calcium hydrogen phosphate belong to this group. Calcium oxalate monohydrate exhibits a high degree of birefringence, whereas, calcium hydrogen phosphate is only slightly birefringent. Both have positive optical signs. The triclinic system has three axes of different lengths, all of different angles. Sodium acid urate belongs to either the triclinic or monoclinic system.

The interference figure is an optical characteristic of uniaxial and biaxial crystals useful in the determination of optical constants. It is a pattern seen under crossed prisms with a Bertrand lens (or when looking down the body of the microscope minus the eyepiece, if one has no Bertrand lens) when a properly oriented crystal is in the field. We have found it easy to demonstrate with reagent grade cystine crystals, but difficult to demonstrate with stone fragments, and so do not employ it. Interference figures do, however, provide an alternate method for calculating optical signs of uniaxial and biaxial crystals. The optical angle, 2v, is another characteristic of biaxial crystals that can be determined from interference figures, as well as from refractive indices.

When isotropic material is immersed in a fluid with a different index of refraction, it is surrounded by a black line whose intensity is a function of the difference. It also has a *halo (the Becke line)*, which behaves as already described. There are other methods of determining the index of refraction, known as the half shadow, oblique illumination, and double variation methods. The method for determining the refractive indices of uniaxial crystals is similar to that for isotropic material, except that the indices must be observed at their "extinction" (blacked-out) positions. One index will be due to the ordinary ray (ω); the other will approach the value for the extraordinary ray (ϵ), depending on the orientation of the crystal. In the case of biaxial crystals, the indices may be similarly determined for a crystal showing optimum birefringence. With other grains, the highest index noted will approach or be the $\gamma^{\omega}\beta$ index; the lowest the $\alpha^{\omega}\beta$. In the case of these crystals, only two, not three, indices will be found at any given orientation in their extinction positions.

The procedure for identifying the crystalline components of urinary calculi from refractive-index measurements using the polarizing microscope is outlined at the end of this chapter. We have included the table of optical characteristics of the crystalline components of urinary calculi given in Edward Prien's article.

PRINCIPLES OF X-RAY DIFFRACTION ANALYSIS[20–23]

X-rays were discovered in 1895 by Wilhelm Roentgen (for which he received the 1901 Nobel Prize in physics) and so named because their nature was not understood at the time. They were put to use almost immediately by physicians, since they were much more penetrating than light and could easily pass through the human body. In 1912 Max von Laue demonstrated that x-rays are electromagnetic waves of a very short wavelength by showing that x-rays are diffracted by the atoms of a crystalline substance in a manner similar to the diffraction of visible light by a finely ruled grating. Von Laue received the 1914 Nobel Prize in physics for this important work, which not only established the wave nature of x-rays but also proved the periodicity of the arrangement of atoms within a crystal. When a beam of x-rays impinges on a crystalline sample, the x-rays are diffracted in a specific manner depending on the atomic geometry of that particular crystal. The resulting diffraction pattern for each substance is unique, and in this lies its practicality for identifying the crystalline components of urinary calculi.

Crystalline materials are characterized by a periodic pattern of atoms in three dimensional space, a so-called crystalline lattice. This regular internal arrangement of atoms is often reflected in the external shape of the crystal, a fact that sometimes enables an immediate identification of large, single crystals. The unit cell is the smallest assemblage of atoms that can be repeated again and again to form the entire crystalline lattice. The size and shape of a unit cell can be described in terms of three vectors drawn from one corner of the cell taken as the origin. The lengths of these vectors (a,b,c) and the angles between them (α,β,γ) are referred to as the lattice constants of the unit cell. Figure 4–10 shows the unit cell for the cubic crystal KCl. The shape of this unit cell is a cube ($a = b = c$, $\alpha = \beta = \gamma = 90°$), and the dimension is twice the distance between neighboring K and Cl atoms.

A crystal can be thought of as a series of sets of parallel atomic planes, each set being characterized by an interplanar distance called a d-spacing. The orientation of each set of planes can be represented by three integers (h,k,l) referred to as Miller indices. Furthermore, each set of parallel planes within the crystal is like a grating, in that it is capable of diffracting x-rays if certain conditions are satisfied. Three equivalent sets of parallel planes, each characterized by the same d-spacing, are illustrated in Figure 4–10 for KCl. One can construct other sets of parallel atomic planes for this crystal, each represented by a different set of Miller indices and characterized by its own d-spacing. A three-dimensional crystal thus acts like a series of plane gratings of various orientations and spacings and is capable of diffracting x-rays to produce a pattern that is characteristic of its internal atomic arrangement.

Shortly after von Laue first demonstrated x-ray diffraction, Sir William H. Bragg and his son William L. Bragg expressed the conditions necessary for diffraction in a simple mathematical form (for which they shared the 1915 Nobel Prize in physics). The two essentials for x-ray diffraction are a wave motion capable of interference (x-rays) and a set

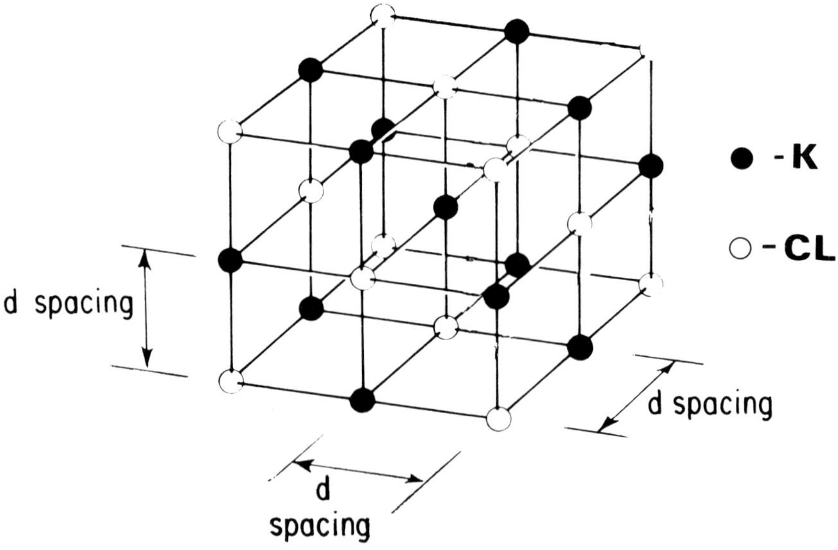

Fig. 4–10. Unit cell of cubic crystal of KCl. The d-spacings represent the interplanar spacing or grating space. (Modified and reproduced with permission from Richards, J., Sears, F., Wehr, M., and Zemansky, W.: Modern University Physics. Courtesy of Addison-Wesley, 1960.)

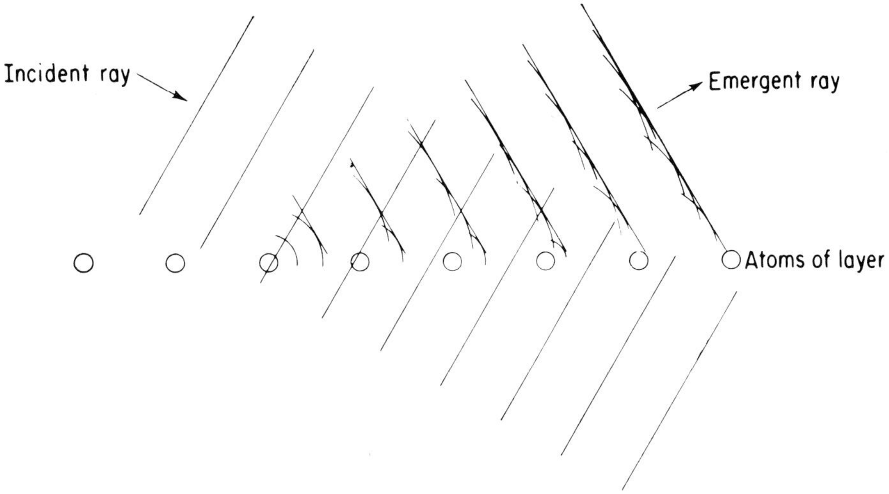

Fig. 4–11. When incident x-rays fall upon a crystal, the atoms of a crystal become the center of expanding wavelets that can combine constructively to produce a diffracted (emergent) beam. (Modified and reproduced with permission from Richards, J., Sears, F., Wehr, M., and Zemansky, W.: Modern University Physics. Courtesy of Addison-Wesley, 1960.)

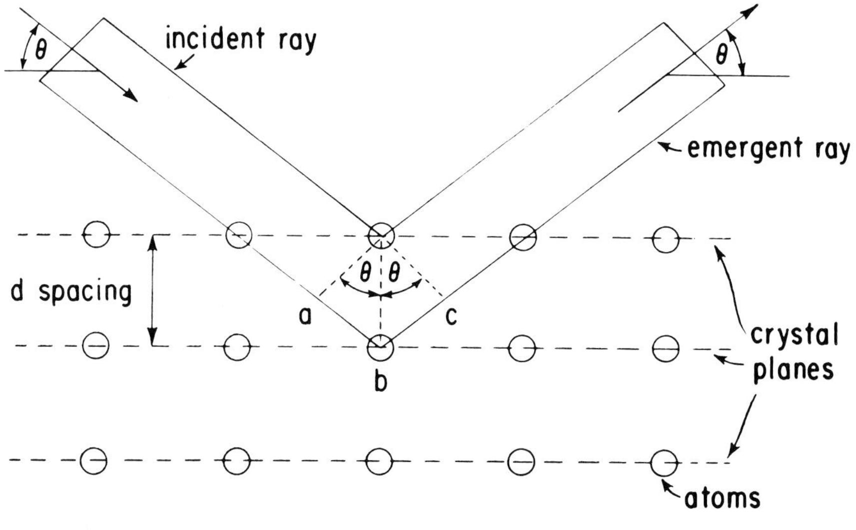

Fig. 4–12. Construction for deriving the Bragg relation that must be satisfied for diffraction, i.e., $n\lambda = 2d \sin \theta$ (Modified and reproduced with permission from Richards, J., Sears, F., Wehr, M., and Zemansky, W.: Modern University Physics. Courtesy of Addison-Wesley, 1960.)

of periodically arranged scattering centers (the atoms of a crystal). When an x-ray wavefront falls on the surface of a crystal, each atom scatters x-rays and, according to Huygen's principle, becomes the center of expanding wavelets (Fig. 4–11). The phase relations of the cooperative effect of scattering from large numbers of atoms are such that destructive interference occurs in most directions. However, in a few directions conditions are such that the secondary wavelets combine constructively to produce diffracted beams. One condition is that the emerging ray will always lie in the plane containing the incident ray and the normal to the crystal plane, and the emerging ray will make the same angle with the crystal plane as the incident ray. A second condition that must be met is that x-rays scattered by successive layers of a set of parallel crystal planes must be in phase so as to combine constructively. Figure 4–12 shows three layers of a crystal. It is noted that the ray scattered by the middle layer travels a greater distance than does the ray scattered by the upper layer. In order for these two rays to be in phase and hence, cause reinforcement, the path difference, $\overline{abc}$, must be an integral multiple of the x-ray wavelength, λ. Since the path difference is related to the interplanar spacing, d, and the angle of incidence, θ, by the relation, $\overline{abc} = 2d \sin \theta$, it follows that the condition for diffraction is given by Bragg's law in the form:

$$n\lambda = 2d \sin \theta,$$

in which n is the order of diffraction (1,2,3, etc.). It should be noted that the angle of diffraction—that is, the angle between incidence beam and the diffracted beam, is 2θ, and, it is this angle, rather than θ, which is usually measured experimentally.

A diffraction method commonly used to identify unknown materials is the Debye-Scherrer powder method. The sample is ground to a fine powder, placed in a narrow glass capillary tube, and positioned in a monochromatic beam of x-rays (Figs. 4–13 and 4–14). Since the tiny crystals are randomly oriented, some crystals will be oriented at the proper angle to satisfy the Bragg equation for each set of parallel lattice planes. The resulting diffraction pattern consists of a series of concentric cones with a common apex at the sample (Fig. 4–13). When recorded on a cylindrical strip of film in a Debye-Scherrer camera, these cones project as lines or arcs. An example of this type of diffraction pattern is illustrated in Figure 4–14. Each arc on the film is produced by diffraction from a particular set of parallel lattice planes (characterized by a d-spacing). From a knowledge of the camera diameter and by measuring the radius of the arc on the film, θ for that set of lattice planes can be easily calculated. The corresponding d-spacing can then be determined using Bragg's law, assuming that λ is known. A similar procedure for each diffraction line along with visual estimates of relative intensities will yield a set of diffraction data unique for that crystal. A

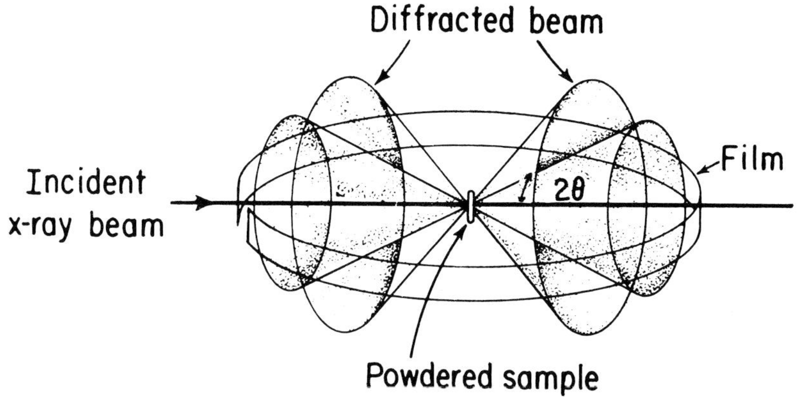

Fig. 4–13. Relation of incident and diffracted beams to sample and film in Debye-Scherrer powder diffraction method. Diffracted beams are in form of concentric cones of half-angle 2θ. (Modified and reproduced with permission from Richards, J., Sears, F., Wehr, M., and Zemansky, W.: Modern University Physics. Courtesy of Addison-Wesley, 1960.)

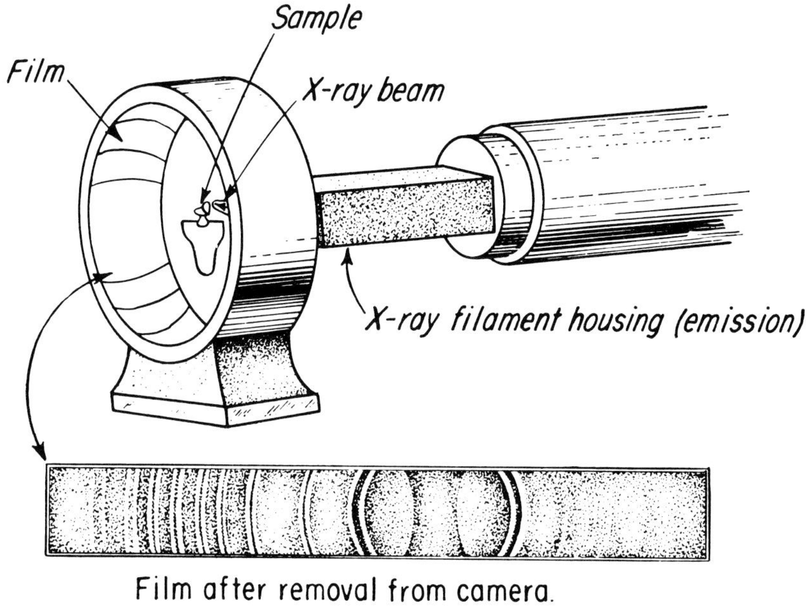

Fig. 4–14. Schematic of a Debye-Scherrer camera and a diffraction pattern produced on photographic film after processing of the film. (Modified and reproduced with permission from Harley, J., and Wilberley, S.: Instrumental Analysis. Courtesy of John Wiley & Sons, 1954.)

9-169

d	2.88	2.61	3.21	8.15	β-$Ca_3(PO_4)_2$
I/I_1	100	65	55	11	BETA CALCIUM ORTHO PHOSPHATE (WHITLOCKITE)

Rad. $CuK\alpha_1$ λ 1.5405 Filter Dia. 114.6MM
Cut off 50 I/I_1 PHOTOMETER
Ref. DEWOLFF, TECHN. PHYS. DIENST, DELFT, HOLLAND

Sys. HEXAGONAL S.G. D_{3D}^6 - $R\bar{3}c$
a_0 10.429 b_0 c_0 37.38 A C
α β γ Z 21 Dx 3.07
Ref. IBID. SPACE GROUP AND Z FROM ISOMORPH US WHITLOCKITE

εα nωβ εγ Sign
2V D mp Color
Ref.

SAMPLE OBTAINED BY HEATING COMMERCIAL SAMPLE

REPLACES 1-0941, 3-0690, 3-0713

d Å	I/I_1	hkl	d Å	I/I_1	hkl
8.15	11	102	2.607	65	220
6.49	15	104	2.562	5	1.0.14
6.22	5	006	2.553	7	223
5.21	20	110	2.520	11	2.1.10
4.90	1	113	2.499	5	311
4.39	7	202	2.407	9	2.1.11,226
4.15	3	108	2.375	5	315
4.06	15	204	2.263	9	1.0.16
4.00	3	116	2.249	3	1.1.15
3.45	25	1.0.10	2.241	1	402
3.40	3	211	2.195	13	404
3.36	9	212	2.165	11	3.0.12
3.25	7	119,208	2.103	3	2.1.14
3.21	55	214	2.076	7	2.0.16+
3.11	1	0.0.12,215	2.068	3	321
3.01	15	300	2.061	5	322
2.880	100	2.0.10,217	2.033	9	408
2.757	20	218	2.023	5	324
2.710	9	306	2.017	3	3.1.11
2.674	7	1.1.12	SEE FOLLOWING CARD		

Fig. 4–15. Typical reference file card for powder diffraction patterns compiled by the American Society for Testing Materials.

set of data for whitlockite as compiled by the American Society for Testing Materials is illustrated in Figure 4–15. Similar data for thousands of materials is contained in the X-ray Powder Data File along with a convenient index based on the d-spacings for the three most intense lines for each material. This provides a quick method for positively identifying unknown crystalline materials by the comparison of diffraction data with those of known materials.

Figure 4–16 shows some of the more common powder patterns observed in urinary calculi. These diffraction patterns were obtained using a Norelco x-ray generator equipped with a 114.59 mm Debye-Scherrer camera. Nickle-filtered copper Kα radiation produced at 35 kv and 20 ma was used with an exposure time of 2 to 4 hours. Lindemann glass capillary tubes of 0.3 to 0.5 mm inside diameter were used to hold the samples. Diffraction patterns for pure stones containing a single compound as well as mixed stones containing more than one compound are illustrated in the figure. It should be noted that when a stone contains more than one constituent, the resulting diffraction pattern is essentially the sum of the individual patterns. Relative porportions to within 5 to 10% can be estimated by visually comparing the most intense lines of the components. The pattern for pure apatite (Fig. 4–16C) is somewhat different from the others in that it contains relatively few, very broad diffraction peaks. This line-broadening results from the fact that the individual grains that make up apatite stones are extremely small (less than 100 Å in diameter). Figure 4–17 shows an x-ray diffractometer unit. This is a variation of the Debye-Scherrer camera technique in that it utilizes an ionization device to detect x-rays along with an automatic recording device.

PRINCIPLES OF INFRARED SPECTROSCOPY[11,12,22]

The atoms of any molecule not at absolute zero are constantly oscillating about their positions of equilibrium. The amplitudes (the vibrational-rotational spaces) of these interatomic motions are minute (10^{-9} to 10^{-10} cm), and the frequencies are high (10^{13} to 10^{14} cycles/second). When molecules are bombarded by infrared radiation (below 25 μ), the molecule absorbs some infrared energy and undergoes changes in the vibrational-rotational space of the molecule, with transmission of the remaining energy. When a molecule absorbs radiation of these short wavelengths, the energy changes are large and thus produce a pattern of spectral variations in the infrared region, characteristic for any given molecule, that can be graphically recorded with a spectrophotometer. An analysis of the transmitted infrared spectrum, therefore, constitutes an analysis of the mechanics of molecular motion of a compound.

The amount of radiation at one wavelength incident on a molecule (P_{-0}) can be related to the amount of energy transmitted by the molecule (P), to the length of the path of the radiation (b), and to the number or concentration of molecules (c) by the equation:

$$abc = -\ln \frac{P}{P_{-o}},$$

in which "a" is a constant for any given material at any given wavelength. This equation is merely another expression of the well-known Beer's law.

Each simple vibration producing an interatomic motion is referred to as a "fundamental" or "normal mode" of vibration. Any nonlinear molecule of "n" number (greater than 4) of atoms can be shown mathematically to possess 3n–6 normal modes, whereas a linear molecule possesses 3n–5 modes. Before a molecule can interact with any radiant energy with which it is bombarded and undergo a vibrational-rotational change, it is necessary that the molecule possess a dipole moment—that is, dissimilar atoms that can vibrate against each other and produce a change in electrical symmetry. For example, molecules composed of nitrogen and oxygen will not have a change of symmetry, and hence will not absorb in the infrared region, since the molecules are too similar in their atomic arrangement. In many of the normal modes of vibration of a molecule, the main participants are two dissimilar atoms held together by certain chemical bonds. Such modes of vibration have frequencies that depend not only on the masses of the two vibrating atoms, but also on the force constant on the bond joining them. Frequencies

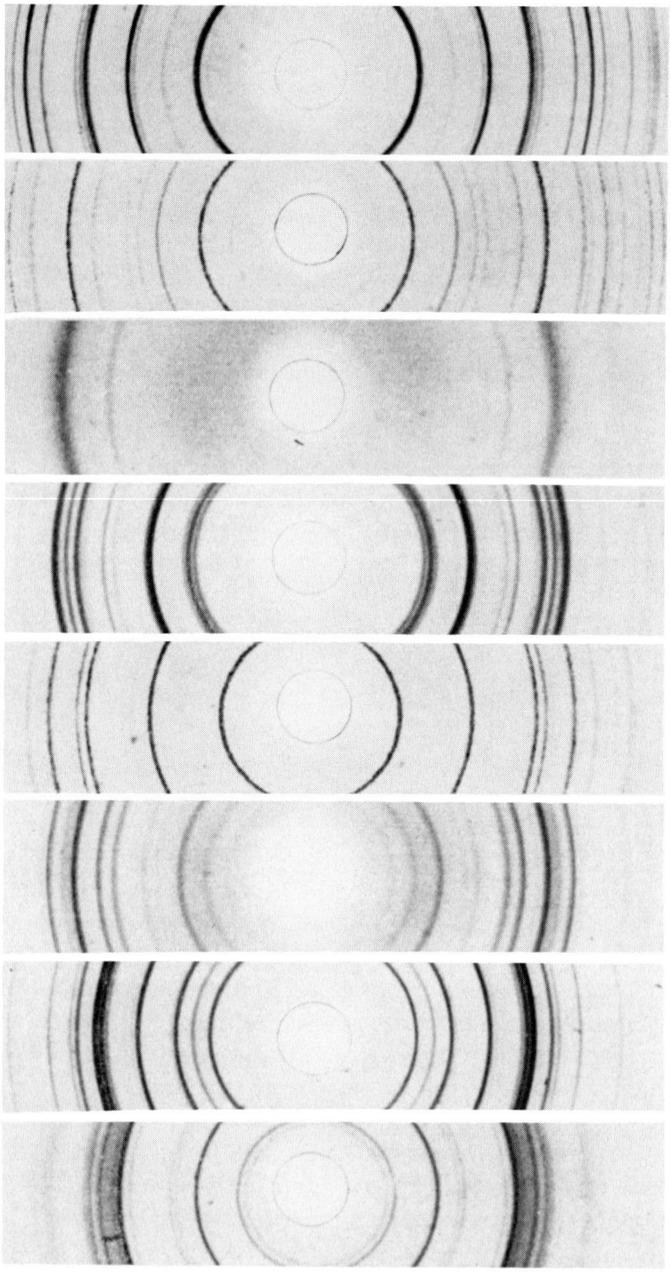

A. 100% calcium oxalate monohydrate

B. 100% calcium oxalate dihydrate

C. 100% apatite

D. 100% magnesium ammonium phosphate hexahydrate (triple phosphate)

E. 100% calcium hydrogen phosphate dihydrate

F. 100% tricalcium phosphate

G. 100% uric acid

H. 100% ammonium acid urate

Fig. 4–16. Reference x-ray diffraction patterns of the most common urinary stone constituents.

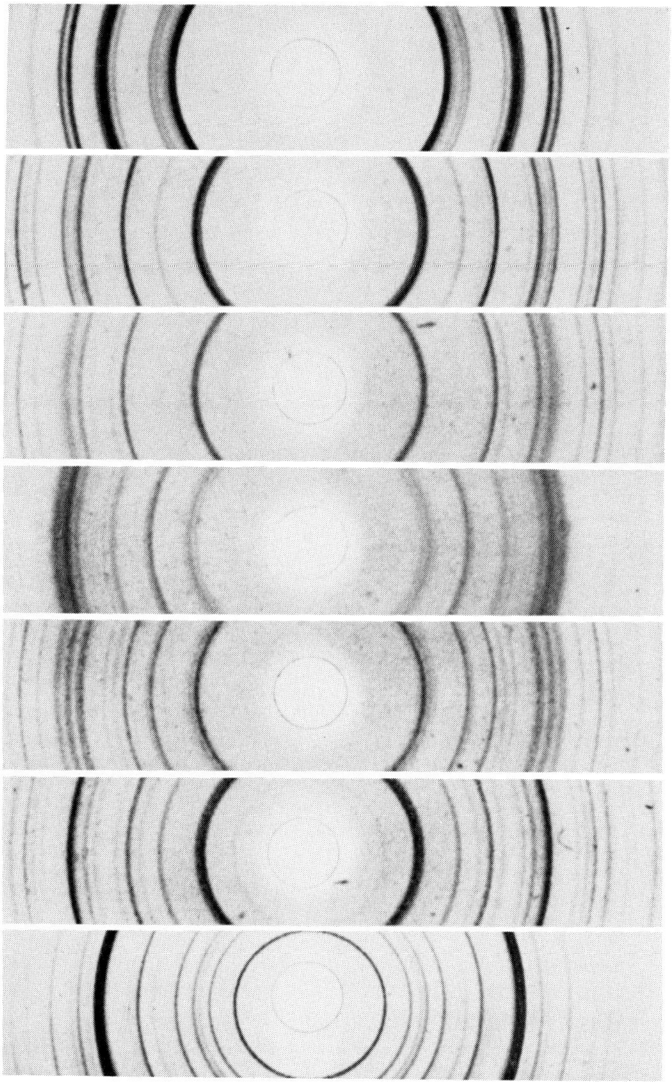

I. 100% cystine

J. 60% oxalate monohydrate
40% oxalate dihydrate

K. 50% oxalate monohydrate
50% apatite

L. 60% triple phosphate
40% apatite

M. 10% apatite
35% triple phosphate
55% oxalate monohydrate

N. 30% oxalate monohydrate
45% oxalate dihydrate
25% apatite

O. 70% uric acid
30% uric acid dihydrate

Fig. 4–16 (cont.)

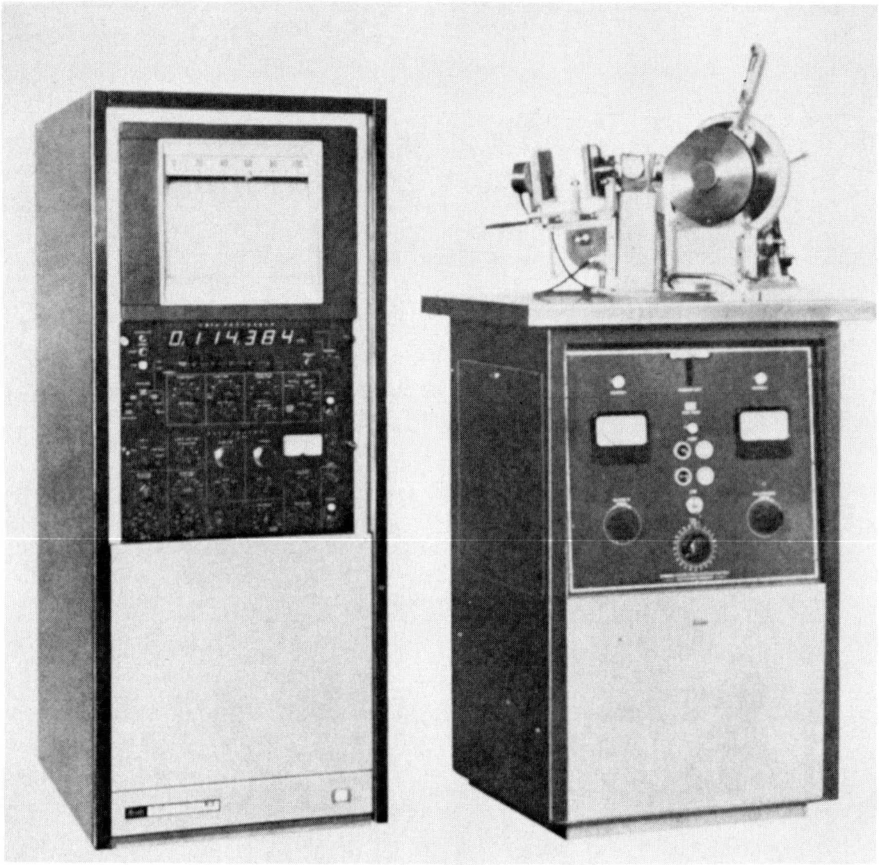

Fig. 4–17. Norelco x-ray diffractometer with recording device attached. (Courtesy of Phillips Electronics Instruments, Mount Vernon, N.Y. 10550.)

are only slightly affected by other atoms attached to the two atoms concerned; thus, these vibrational modes are characteristic of the specific groups in the molecule.

The infrared portion of the spectrum extends from the long wavelength limit of sensitivity of the human eye, about 0.75 μ, to the region of ultrashort radio waves, about 350 μ. The unit most often used by clinical pathologists for designating the spectrum is wavelength, mμ or Å units, the latter having one-tenth the magnitude of the former. But an alternate way of describing infrared radiation is in terms of its wave number ($\bar{v}$), which is defined as:

$$\bar{v}\ (\text{cm}^{-1}) = \frac{1}{\lambda}$$

in which "λ" is the wavelength. This description has been advocated as being preferable on certain theoretical grounds.

Infrared absorption spectra can be used for identification of pure substances or for detection and identification of impurities. Thus the infrared absorption spectrum of a compound can act as a "fingerprint" for the compound. For pure substances, it is necessary only to compare the spectrum of the substance with spectra of various known substances for identification. Fortunately, enough is usually known about the origin or nature of an unknown substance that a limited number of possibilities will be suggested. The spectrum of a mixture of compounds is essentially the sum of spectra of the individual components. Exceptions ocur in cases in which compound formation, association, disassociation, or polymerization takes place. But even shifts in the frequency of infrared bands from predicted values can be used as criteria for specimen identification. Since impurities will cause extra absorption bands to appear in the spectrum, they can be detected by comparison with the spectrum of the pure substance. Catalogs of infrared absorption spectra have been prepared by individuals (Barnes, Gore, Liddel, and Williams: Infrared Spectroscopy. New York, Reinhold, 1944), and in a series of punch cards by the American Society for Testing Materials (over 10,000 cards now on file).

William Herschel discovered the infrared spectrum in 1800, but the technique of identifying specific chemical compounds by infrared spectroscopy was not extensively utilized until early in the 20th century (William Coblens). Application of this technique to analysis of urinary stones has been recent, being fostered by Dietrich Beischer in 1955.

Spectrophotometers for the infrared range are composed of basic elements similar to instruments utilized for visible and ultraviolet spectrometry, but the optical detector system is more refined to eliminate stray radiation (Fig. 4–18). Transmittancy of most biologic samples necessitates use of a very thin aliquot (about 0.01 to 0.3 mm) for examination. Instruments employing the infrared range may have prism monochromators; but reflection gratings are utilized above 40μ, because transparent materials are not generally available in the latter range. Prisms can be constructed of glass, quartz, fluorite, rock salt (sodium chloride), lithium fluoride, potassium bromide, and thallium bromoiodide. These materials, in general, are very hydroscopic, and good control of the environmental humidity about the prisms of the infrared spectrophotometer is essential for obtaining good results.

In modern infrared spectrophotometers, double-beam systems are used whereby absorption by carbon dioxide and water in the atmosphere is compensated for by the reference beam. These two compounds are strong infrared absorbers and can reduce beam intensity at certain wavelengths to a point at which the spectrophotometer will not operate properly. Water vapor has the strongest absorption at 3 and 6 μ; and

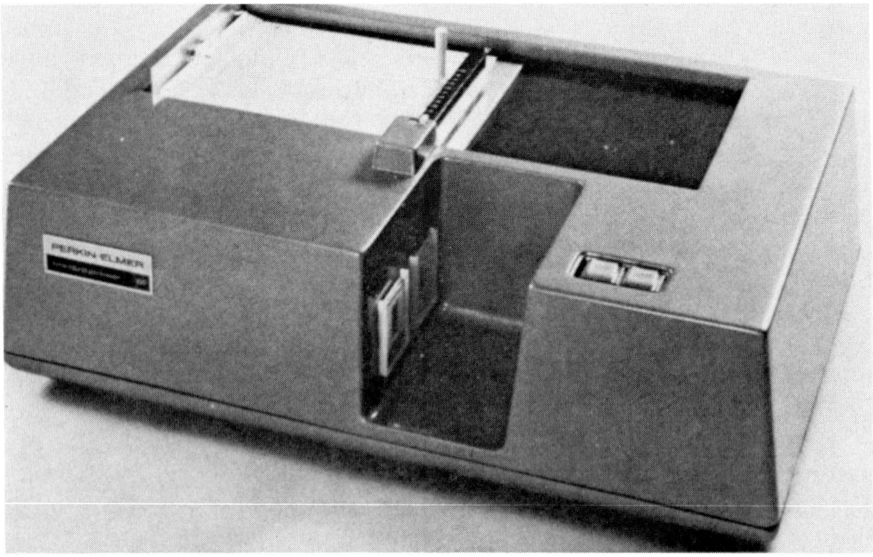

Fig. 4–18. Perkin-Elmer Model 700 Infrared Spectrophotometer with graphic spectral recording. (Courtesy of Perkin-Elmer Corporation, Norwalk. Conn. 06850.)

carbon dioxide at 4.2 and 14.5 μ. (The bands are fairly broad, so that the region extending 0.5 μ on each side of these wavelengths should be included in the absorption band of these compounds.) With commonly used instruments, such as the Perkin-Elmer, utilizing a sodium chloride prism in the monochromator, the infrared spectrum from about 2 to 15 μ can be scanned in 12 minutes, or in less time with special gears on the drum assembly. A good infrared spectrophotometer in sound operating condition does not in itself assure good results. As with all techniques, the validity of the results depends on sample handling techniques, selection of the proper instrument, and operating variables, as well as the specimen itself.

Stones can be prepared for analysis in numerous ways: solid, melted, powder, mull, and others. In the clinical microscopy laboratory, however, the mulling technique is most commonly used. Mulling, disbursing of a solid in a liquid background, is used to reduce the amount of light scattered from the solid, thus giving a spectrum with sharper absorption bands as well as preventing band shifting due to scattering effect. It should be ovious that addition of any substance to the stone to be analyzed will change or alter the peaks of the spectrum recorded in the graphic analysis. However, the reproducible artifact can be compensated for in the final analysis. Some mulls can be made with low-boiling-point organic solvents, and the solvent evaporated before the tracing is done. Mineral oil (*Nujol*) has only a few normal absorption bands in the infrared region (Fig. 4–19) and in general does not interfere with infrared bands produced by the common constituents of stones (Fig. 4–20). In the past few years, the potassium bromide (KBr) disc technique has become widely used. A few mg (less than 5 mg needed) of the stone are ground with about 0.25 to 1 g KBr and subjected to high pressure. A clear, nearly transparent disc results, which then can be supported in the infrared beam. Clearer discs are obtained if air is removed by applying a vacuum to the material before it is compressed under pressure (about 10,000 to 20,000 psi for 2 to 3 minutes). KBr has no absorption itself but sometimes with incomplete dehydration it shows weak absorption bands at 2.7 μ and 6 μ. Water cannot be used as a solvent for infrared analysis since water absorbs strongly beyond about 2.7 μ region (except for a region from 3.4 to 5.7 μ). Carbon tetrachloride is one of the best solvents, having only one region of very strong absorption from 12 to 14 μ.

INDICATIONS FOR URINARY STONE ANALYSIS[24,25]

Knowledge of the crystalloid or chemical composition of a stone suggests appropriate follow-up procedures aimed at identifying the underlying disease or derangement. Some conditions, such as hyperparathyroidism, can be cured. In other patients, appropriate attempts to prevent further stone formation may be initiated. Information from analysis may even obviate the need for more expensive and more difficult diagnostic techniques.

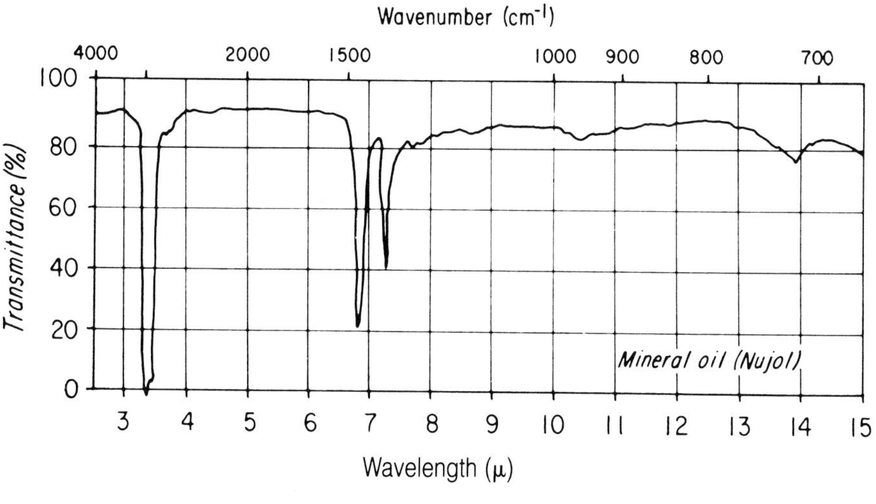

Fig. 4–19. Reference Infrared spectrophotometric pattern of mineral oil (Nujol). (Courtesy of Dr. D. James Lowell, Reference Laboratory, North Hollywood, Calif.)

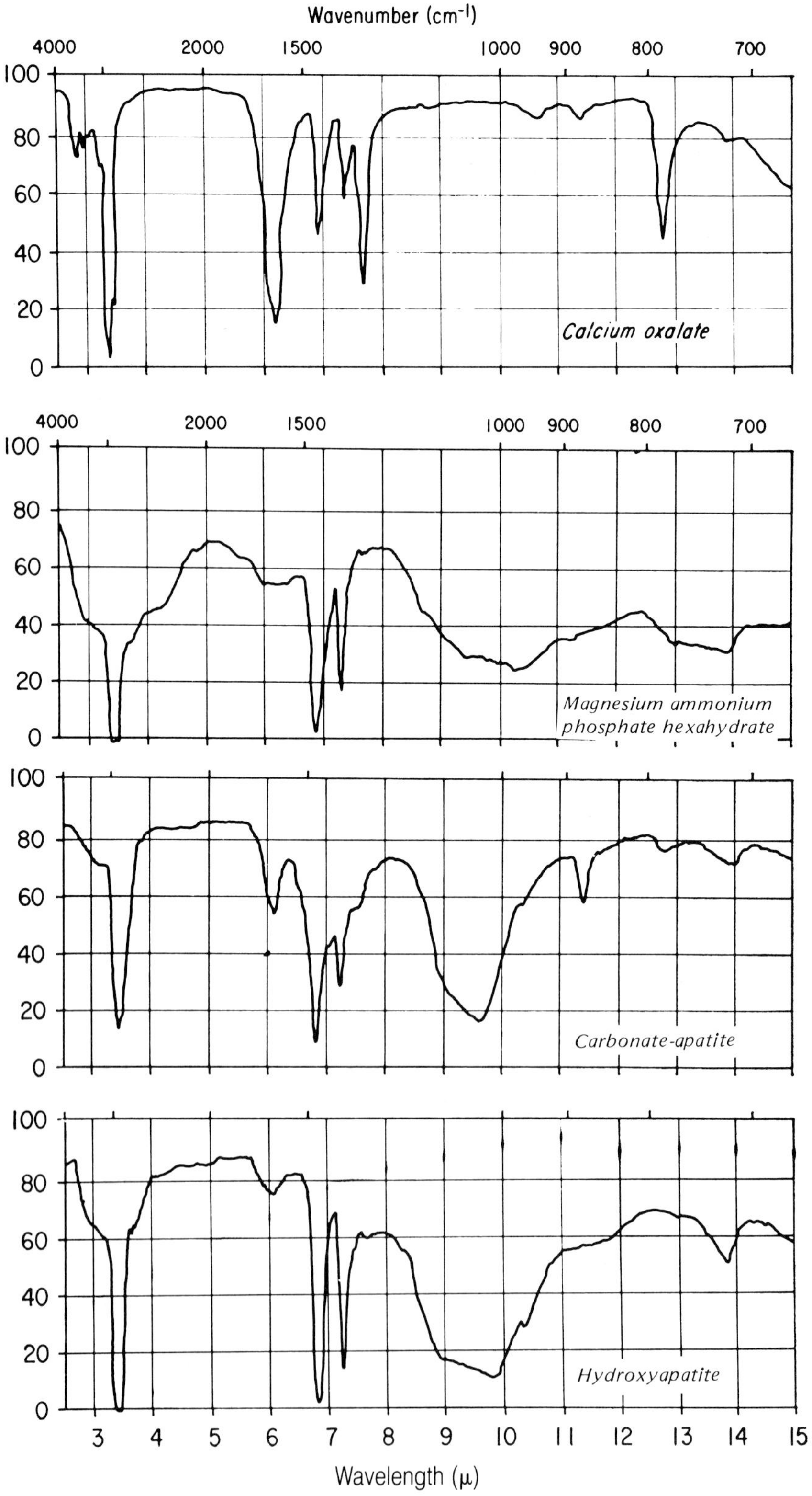
Wavenumber (cm^{-1})
4000
2000
1500
1000
900
800
700
100
80
60
40
20
0
Calcium oxalate
Magnesium ammonium phosphate hexahydrate
Carbonate-apatite
Hydroxyapatite
3
4
5
6
7
8
9
10
11
12
13
14
15
Wavelength (μ)

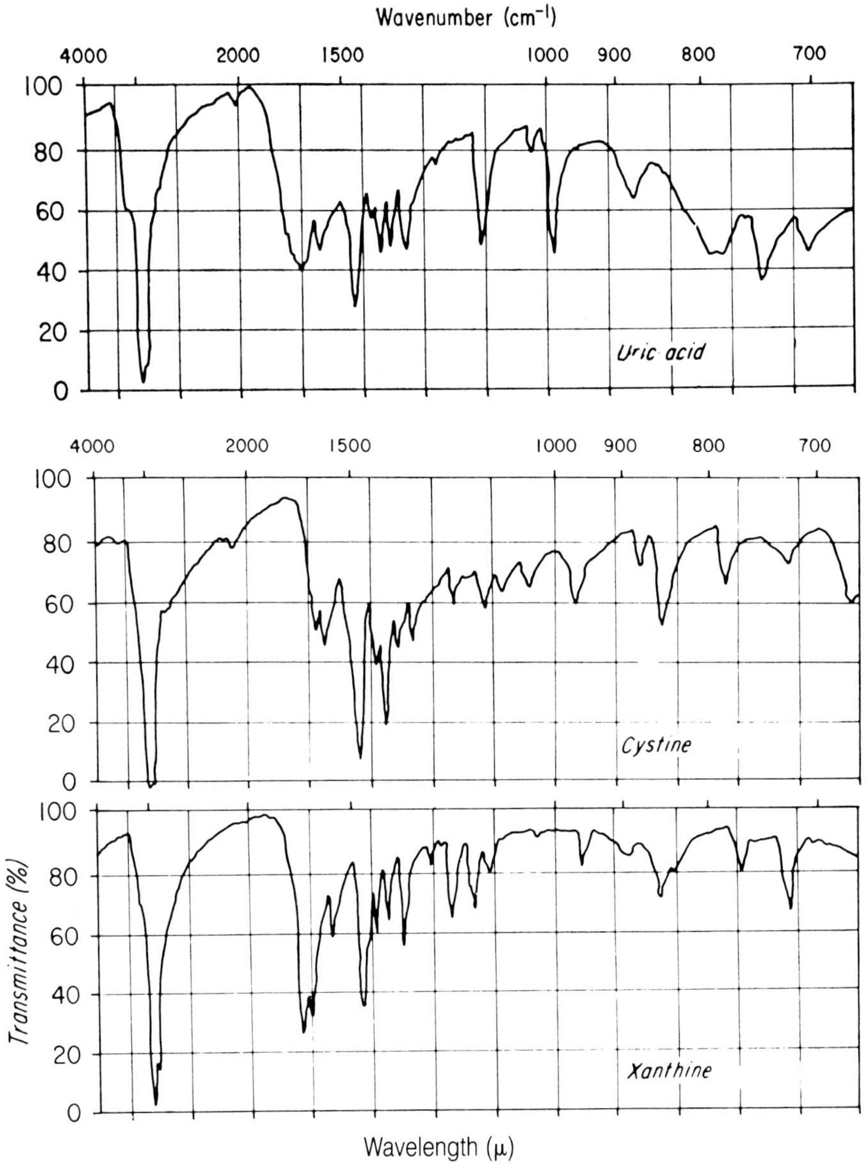

Fig. 4–20. Reference infrared spectrophotometric patterns of the most common urinary stone constituents after mulling in Nujol. (Courtesy of Dr. D. James Lowell, Reference Laboratory, North Hollywood, Calif. 91609.)

FACTORS INFLUENCING STONE FORMATION

Although there is constant dissolution and recrystallization of urinary crystalloids, disturbances of the normal equilibrium of the crystalloid colloid interface or disruptions of the urine-mucosal interface may initiate precipitation or conglomeration of mucopolysaccharides and mucoproteins, forming a nidus or matrix, and so preventing normal resolution of the precipitated crystalloids. Injury to renal tubular epithelial cells may have the same result. Several factors tend to disturb the normal urinary equilibrium, and thus predispose to stone formation:[24,25]

1. Metabolic, nutritional, and idiopathic disturbances (gout, polycythemia, oxaluria, cystinuria, hypophosphaturia, sarcoidosis, berylliosis, Cushing's disease, and some carcinomas)
2. Endocrinopathy (hyperparathyroidism, and others)
3. Urinary obstruction
4. Infection with urea-splitting organisms
5. Mucosal changes (avitaminosis A, dietary deficiency, and Randall's plaques)
6. Extrinsic and environmental factors (dehydration, alkali excess, purine drug excess, prolonged recumbency, chemotherapy)
7. Isohyduria with fixation of urinary pH and loss of normal acid and alkaline "tides"

Although any one of these disturbances may be present without concomitant calculi, there often are multiple associated factors that act synergistically in the formation of stones. Undoubtedly, all the causes and factors involved in kidney-stone formation are not yet well understood. The primary factor in all but oxalate-stone formation is probably precipitation from a supersaturated solution.

William Boyce and Stanton King have demonstrated that all renal stones have an organic matrix composed of a carbohydrate-protein conjugate termed "uromucoid."[26] They suggest that the molecules of uromucoid form a fibrillar or laminar gel, thus acting as an organic template for the decomposition of crystals during stone formation. According to this theory, the organic matrix is a prerequisite for stone formation, and crystal deposition is only a secondary phenomenon. Other organic masses can act as nidi, including blood clots, clumps of epithelial or pus cells, or even bacteria. Furthermore, necrotic ischemic tissue (neoplasm, ulceration) may favor precipitation of relatively insoluble substances.

The tip of nephrostomy or catheter tubes that have been in the urinary tract for more than a few days become encrusted with deposits of urinary phosphates. There is a great tendency for stones to form under such circumstances. This process is accentuated by the infection invariably induced by indwelling catheterization. There is a higher incidence of kidney-stone formation in areas of the country that are hot and dry in the summer than in those that are cool and wet. It seems almost certain that concentration of urine resulting from excessive perspiration and relative dehydration predisposes to stone formation. Some areas of the world, such as South China, have had "stone-forming" periods in the past. With regard to vesical calculi, a relatively uncommon disease of adult life (predominantly male) in the United States, pathologic changes in the bladder leading to development of urinary stasis serve as predisposing factors. These include:

1. Urethral strictures
2. Prostatic hyperplasia
3. Bladder diverticuli
4. Spinal cord injuries
5. Foreign bodies, such as sutures, catheters, or other objects introduced into the bladder through the urethra

The role of infection in the production of vesical calculi remains unsettled, although the association of bilharziasis with vesical calculi in Egypt is well recognized. In many parts of Asia, where it is primarily a disease of children, bladder stone is a major cause of illness.

OCCURRENCE OF STONE

It has been estimated that 9.47 persons per 10,000 population per year are admitted to hospitals with a diagnosis of renal stone.[27] Peter Maurice and Philip Henneman, in their review of the Medical Aspects of Renal Stones, record the incidence of stone as 1.12% in 25,000 autopsies cited.[28]

CALCIUM-CONTAINING STONES[16,27–29,32]

The great majority of urinary calculi in the United States (about 90%) contain calcium. Also, evidence indicates that all stones may contain some nuclear calcium. Urinary excretion of more than 250 mg calcium/24 hours (some authors report 200 mg/24 hours), by persons on a normal diet, may be considered hypercalciuria and a potential factor in stone formation. The incidence of hypercalciuria is great (60%) in patients with calcium oxalate, mixed calcium oxalate and apatite, and calcium phosphate (apatite) renal stones. Hypercalciuria and/or calcium-containing stone formation is known to be associated with at least seven major clinical syndromes:

1. Idiopathic hypercalciuria
2. Primary hyperparathyroidism
3. Bone disease (osteoporosis, Paget's disease and destructive diseases)

4. Excessive milk, alkali, or vitamin D intake
5. Renal tubular acidosis
6. Sarcoidosis
7. Berylliosis

Recently, R. McK. Chambers and Thomas Dormany have claimed that calcium/osmolarity ratios on 24-hour series of urines showed a clear diagnostic separation between recent and past renal stone formers and a number of different control groups. Some patients exhibited abnormally high urine calcium levels only relative to osmolarity.[30]

CALCIUM OXALATE STONES[24–25,28–29]

Approximately 30% of renal stones are composed of calcium oxalate. They are often found admixed with apatite. Mildly acid to near neutral urine (pH 5.5 to 6.0) favors calcium oxalate stone formation. Some patients with oxalate stones have hypercalciuria. Rare patients have oxalosis, with hyperoxaluria. Many patients with calcium oxalate stones have normal urinary calcium, oxalate, and pH, but are uninfected. These patients represent the largest unsolved etiologic puzzle in the area of urinary stone. Except in patients with oxalosis, there seems to be no correlation between the magnitude of urinary-oxalate excretion and the occurrence of calcium-oxalate stones. Increased oxalate excretion occurs, however, following ingestion of glycine and oxalates, in patients with liver disease, in patients with diabetes mellitus, following prolonged immobilization for fractures, in patients with poliomyelitis and spinal cord injuries. The great increase in the incidence of oxalate stone in central Europe following World War I has never been adequately explained, although many investigators feel that nutritional factors played a significant role. Pyridoxine deficiency produces calcium-oxalate stones in rats, but not in humans. Calcium oxalate calculi, in addition to the conditions listed for calcium-stone formers, have also been reported to occur in patients with:

1. Oxaluria (excretion of greater than 47 mg/day)
2. Incomplete catabolism of carbohydrates (diabetes mellitus)
3. Isohyduria at pH 5.5 to 6.0
4. Acetazolamide inhibition of carbonic anhydrase
5. Excess glycogen breakdown

The chemical test seems to be less sensitive than infrared analysis or x-ray diffraction for detecting oxalate. Experience is required to observe and interpret properly the result of the chemical test, and use of reagent grade manganese dioxide rather than native powder may cause false-negative results.

CALCIUM-PHOSPHATE STONES (APATITE, CALCIUM DIHYDROGEN PHOSPHATE DIHYDRATE, TRICALCIUM PHOSPHATE)[7,10]

The apatites are calcium-phosphate complexes in which other ions may replace some of the phosphates in the outer-absorption layers of the crystal. Although they are classified chemically as hydroxyl apatite or carbonate apatite, it is still a matter of controversy whether carbonate forms an integral part of the molecule or is merely adsorbed into the surface. Although the apatites have differing chemical compositions, their crystalline structures are very similar and are not distinguishable by x-ray diffraction analysis. Insofar as is known, in any case, differentiation of apatite into hydroxyl and carbonate forms has no clinical significance. Apatite occurs alone or in any degree of admixture with oxalate, and often has the same significance as calcium oxalate. Persistently alkaline urines and urinary infections with urea-splitting organisms also may be factors in the pathogenesis of apatite, as well as of triple-phosphate stones. Carbonate-apatite is a principal constituent of stones of the lachrymal duct, prostate gland, bronchi, and even in the calcified plaque of atherosclerosis. Pure apatite crystals are quite rare. Chemical analysis of calculi containing apatite usually detects calcium, phosphate, and on occasion, carbonate. The chemical tests are more sensitive for apatite than are x-ray diffraction techniques, because the characteristic small crystalline size of apatite in stones results in weak x-ray diffraction patterns. If apatite makes up less than 10% of the volume of the stone, it may be missed by x-ray diffraction. However, it can usually be detected chemically if it comprises as little as 1% of the stone.

MAGNESIUM AMMONIUM PHOSPHATE HEXAHYDRATE STONES[7,16]

Triple phosphate is found in approximately 15% of urinary calculi. It occurs alone or in any degree of admixture with apatite. Staghorn stones are often a mixture of triple phosphate and apatite. Chemical tests for magnesium and ammonium are extremely sensitive and often detect the presence of small amounts of triple phosphate not noticed by x-ray diffraction. Triple phosphate precipitates exclusively in alkaline urine and hence is the hallmark of alkaline (urea-splitting) infection.

URIC-ACID AND URATE STONES[28,29,31]

Uric-acid stones, usually pure, account for 5 to 10% of all kidney stones. They occur primarily in middle-aged and elderly individuals and, interestingly, are more common in Jews or persons of Italian extraction. Uric-acid stones are associated with:

1. Gout
2. Polycythemia

3. Leukemia
4. Lymphoma
5. Liver disease
6. Acid isohyduria
7. Theophylline and thiazide therapy
8. Conditions associated with rapid protein catabolism

Thirteen percent of patients with gout have uric-acid stones. However, there is often lack of correlation between serum uric-acid level, attacks of gouty arthritis, and urinary excretion of uric acid. Since the liver destroys 30 to 70% of endogenous uric acid, liver disease may, for this reason, be associated with hyperuricemia. Persistently acid pH of urine (less than pH 5.5) also favors formation of uric-acid stones and may be more common than hyperuricemia in uric-acid stone formers. At pH 5.0, even at normal levels of concentration, urine can become fourfold supersaturated with respect to uric acid. As urine becomes more alkaline, the solubility of uric acid increases, and urine is normally unsaturated with respect to uric acid at about pH 6.0. Even in patients with lymphomas and leukemias, in whom urinary uric acid excretion exceeds 2 g/day, the prime factor in formation of uric acid stones is acidity of urine. Prevention of stone recurrence is likely to be achieved by control of abnormal and persistent urinary acidity and maintenance of high urine volume.

In our study of 464 stones, anhydrous uric acid in the pure state was observed in 16 (or 3.2%) of the calculi. The most common associated material was the dihydrate of uric acid. Twenty-six (5.6%) calculi were found to be a mixture of the anhydrous and dihydrate forms. Ammonium-acid urate was observed in seven calculi, and sodium-acid urate was found as a minor constituent of a single calculus.[7]

CYSTINE STONES[28–29]

Cystine is relatively insoluble in urine, and cystine stones occur when more than 300 mg cystine per day are excreted. Cystinuria is found not only in patients with congenital cystinuria, but also in patients with:

1. Transient acute phases of chronic renal diseases, such as pyelonephritis
2. Heavy metal nephrotoxicity
3. Aminoaciduria (including Wilson's disease)
4. Renal tubular acidosis syndromes (hyperchloremic acidosis with nephrocalcinosis, Fanconi's syndrome, and Lowe's syndrome)

Cystinuria is almost always accompanied by other aminoacidurias, including ornithine, lysine, and arginine. These do not precipitate because of greater solubility. Cystine stone formers are relatively rare.

When there is greater than normal excretion of cystine, characteristic hexagonal cystine crystals may be seen in the urine sediment.

XANTHINE STONES[28–29]

Xanthine stone formers, who are extremely few, have an inborn error of metabolism, with congenital absence or decreased amount of xanthine oxidase; hence, stones usually appear in youngsters. These stones form primarily in persistently acid urine. Xanthinuria (excretion of greater than 25 mg/day) may also occur in renal disease when there is excessive clearance of xanthine from blood. It remains to be determined whether this is related only to a derangement of purine metabolism or also to excessive ingestion of xanthine and precursors. The pathogenesis of these stones cannot be defined due to insufficient data. (Xanthine stones may be misinterpreted as uric-acid stones; hence, xanthine may be missed by some methods of chemical analysis. They do not react with the method described and so may be missed, if pure.) Stones that leave no residue after microincineration or that yield a positive chemical test for uric acid from patients with low blood uric acids should be especially tested for xanthine. Xanthine is said to produce a yellow color, which turns orange after alkalinization with the murexide test. We have found differentiation from uric acid with the murexide test very difficult and so, recommend x-ray diffraction analysis.

The following list outlines the correlations between urinary pH and stone constituents:[32]

1. Acid pH (pH < 5.5): Uric acid, cystine, xanthine
2. Acid pH (pH 5.5–6.0): Calcium oxalate, apatite
3. Alkaline pH (pH > 7.0): Magnesium ammonium phosphate, calcium phosphates (apatite, calcium dihydrogen phosphate dihydrate, tricalcium phosphate)

REFERENCES

1. Joly, J.: Stone and Calculous Disease of the Urinary Organs. St. Louis, C.V. Mosby, 1929.
2. Barney, J.: Lithiasis. *In* History of Urology. Edited by B. Lewis. Baltimore, Williams & Wilkins, 1933.
3. Mathison, R.: The Shocking History of Drugs. New York, Ballantine Books, 1958.
4. Lonsdale, K.: Human Stones: Age, period, and world distribution. Science, *159*:1199, 1968.
5. Wells, C.: Bones, Bodies and Disease. New York, Praeger, 1964, p. 83.
6. Boyce, W.H.: Organic matrix of human urinary concretions. Am. J. Med., *45*:673, 1968.
7. Morriss, R., and Beeler, M.: X-ray diffraction analysis of 464 urinary calculi. Am. J. Clin. Path., *48*:413, 1967.
8. Prien, E.L.: Studies in urolithiasis II: Relationships between pathogenesis, structure and composition of calculi. J. Urol., *67*:821, 1949.
9. Parsons, J.: X-ray diffraction analysis of central Asian vesical calculi. Henry Ford Hosp. Med. Bull., *12*:187, 1964.
10. Herring, L.: Observations on the analysis of ten thousand urinary calculi. J. Urol., *88*:545, 1962.

11. Beischer, D.: Analysis of renal calculi by infrared spectroscopy. J. Urol., *73*:653, 1955.
12. Tsay, Y.: Applications of infrared spectroscopy to analysis of urinary calculi. J. Urol., *86*:838, 1961.
13. Lowell, D.J.: Personal communication, 1968.
14. Finlayson, B., and Meyer, A.S.: Stone ultrastructure. Proceedings of the National Resource Council Conference on Urolithiasis. Washington, D.C., 1971, p. 115.
15. Prien, E., and Frondel, C.: Studies in Urolithiasis: Composition of urinary calculi. J. Urol., *57*:949, 1947.
16. Beeler, M., Veith, D., Morriss, R., and Biskind, G.: Analysis of urinary calculus. Comparison of methods. Am. J. Clin. Path., *41*:553, 1964.
17. Winer, J.H., and Mattice, M.R.: Routine analysis of urinary calculi; rapid, simple method using spot tests. J. Lab. and Clin. Med., *28*:898, 1943.
18. West, P.: Chemical identification by means of polarized light microscopy. Chemist-Analyst, *43*, *46*, and *56*:77, 109, 1954.
19. Allen, R.: Practical Refractometry by Means of Microscope. 2nd Ed. Cedar Grove, N.J., R.P. Cargille Laboratories, 1962.
20. Parsons, J., and Eurs, F.: X-ray diffraction analysis of crystals in pathology. Am. J. Clin. Pathol., *32*:405, 1959.
21. Richards, J., Sears, F., Wehr, M., and Zemansky, W.: Modern University Physics. Reading, Mass., Addison-Wesley, 1960, p. 795.
22. Harley, J., and Wilberley, S.: Instrumental Analysis. New York, John Wiley & Sons, 1954, p. 310.
23. Cullity, B.: Elements of X-ray Diffraction. Reading, Mass., Addison-Wesley, 1956.
24. Winer, J.: Practical value of analysis of urinary calculi. J.A.M.A., *169*:1715, 1959.
25. Winer, J.: Value of analysis of urinary calculi. Mod. Med.:83, August 1, 1959.
26. Boyce, W., and King, J., Jr.: Present concepts concerning the origin of matrix and stones. Ann. N.Y. Acad. Sci., *104*:563, 1963.
27. Boyce, W., Garvey, F., and Strawcutter, H.: Incidence of urinary calculi among patients in general hospitals, 1948 to 1952. J.A.M.A., *161*:1437, 1956.
28. Maurice, P., and Henneman, P.: Medical aspects of renal stones. Med., *40*:315, 1961.
29. Melick, R., and Henneman, P.: Clinical and laboratory studies of 207 consecutive patients in a kidney stone clinic. N. Engl. J. Med., *259*:307, 1958.
30. Chambers, R., and Dormandy, T.: Measurement and interpretation of hypercalciuria on 24-hour urine series. Lancet, *2*:1378, 1967.
31. Krawcznski, J., Sagan, Z., Walajtys, E., and Ilowiecka, K.: Inborn enzymatic defect as the probable cause of the formation of renal stones containing uric acid. Am. J. Clin. Pathol., *18*:219, 1965.
32. Pak, C., et al.: Ambulatory evaluation of nephrolithiasis: Classification, clinical presentation and diagnostic criteria. Am. J. Med., *69*:19, 1980.

URINARY STONE-ANALYSIS PROCEDURES

Chemical Stone Analysis

METHOD. Winer and Mattice chemical analysis.*

PRINCIPLE. An aliquot of powdered calculus is submitted to simple qualitative chemical tests for uric acid, carbonate, oxalate, phosphate, calcium, magnesium, ammonium, and cystine.

SAMPLE. If stone is coated with extraneous matter, wash with distilled water and allow to dry.

PROCEDURE

1. Weigh on an analytical balance, measure diameters, and describe character.

---

*Complete kits with reagents and materials for chemical analysis can be obtained from:
1. C.W. Alban Co., 1645 South Grand Boulevard, St. Louis, Mo 63103
2. Oxford Laboratories, 1149 Chess Drive, Foster City, Calif. 94404

2. Fracture or cut with scalpel blade, jeweler's saw, or hack saw; describe cut surface.
3. Grind a representative aliquot (about 10 mg) in a small agate mortar.
4. Set up six test tubes in a rack and distribute 1 to 2 mg of powdered stone into each of the first five tubes by scraping off mortar bowl with scalpel blade.
5. To tube 1, add 1 drop of sodium carbonate and 2 drops of uric-acid reagent.
6. To tube 2, add 2 drops of hydrochloric acid (observe with hand lens several minutes).
7. Following cessation of bubble formation (if present), add a small amount of manganese dioxide to tube 2 and observe over a period of several minutes. (Microscopic bubbles may cause powder to rise to surface.)
8. To tube 3, add 3 drops of ammonium molybdate in nitric acid.
9. To tube 4, add 5 drops of hydrochloric acid. Mix by swirling, and divide by decanting half into another (empty) test tube (tube 6). To each of these, add 2 drops of sodium hydroxide. After addition of alkali to tube 4, compare clarity with that of tube 6 prior to addition of alkali.
10. To one of these tubes (tube 4), now add 2 drops of p-nitrobenzene-azoresorcinol. Observe over a period of 5 to 10 minutes (with reagent control if necessary).
11. To the other tube (tube 6), add 2 drops Nessler's solution.
12. To tube 5 (containing powdered stone), add a drop of ammonium hydroxide and a drop of sodium cyanide. Five minutes later, add 3 drops of sodium nitroprusside.

Interpretation

Tube No.	*Reagents Used*	*Color or Reaction*	*Results Reported*
1	Sodium carbonate and uric acid	deep blue pale blue	positive for uric acid trace uric acid
2	Hydrochloric acid, then manganese dioxide	(tiny) bubbles (tiny) bubbles	positive for carbonate positive for oxalate
3	Ammonium molybdate, then heating	strong yellow pale yellow	positive for phosphate trace phosphate
4	Hydrochloric acid and sodium hydroxide	cloudy or heavy precipitate	positive for calcium
6	→4-p-nitrobenzene-azoresorcinol →6-Nessler's reagent	blue orange pale yellow	positive for magnesium positive for ammonium trace ammonium
5	Sodium hydroxide, sodium cyanide, nitroprusside	beet red	positive cystine

DISCUSSION AND CLINICAL SIGNIFICANCE. In one series, 60% of stones were found to contain calcium oxalate monohydrate; 37% calcium oxalate dihydrate; 43% apatite; 15% magnesium ammonium phosphate hexahydrate; 8% uric acid; 4% ammonium acid urate; 5% cystine; 3% tricalcium phosphate; and 1% xanthine (Beeler, et al., Am. J. Clin. Path., *41*:553, 1964). Calcium stones suggest the possibility of hyperparathyroidism. They may also be found with idiopathic hypercalciuria and with hypercalciuria associated with excessive milk and alkali ingestion, hypervitaminosis D, bone disease, renal tubular acidosis and prolonged immobilization. Triple phosphate stones are found in patients with infected urinary tract. Oxalate stones may be found in patients with conditions associated with calcium-containing stones. They may also be found in oxalosis. Many are idiopathic. Uric acid stones may be found in association with constantly acid urine, gout, and with hyperuricemia of other causes (thiazide induced, etc.). Cystine stones are found in patients with cystinuria and complex aminoacidurias. In addition to metabolic disorders and infection, vitamin deficiency, foreign bodies, and physical chemical changes may play a role in stone formation. The importance of the mucoprotein matrix is still under active investigation (Boyce & King: Ann. N.Y. Acad. Sci., *104*:563, 1963).

It should be noted that one cannot distinguish, chemically, between apatite, calcium hydrogen phosphate dihydrate, and tricalcium phosphate. Also, the chemical method is less sensitive than x-ray diffraction for oxalate, but more sensitive for phosphate and ammonium. Most laboratories perform only chemical analyses. Chemical analysis is suitable for routine use, and x-ray diffraction is available by consultation in various parts of the country. Stones less than 5 mg should be analyzed by x-ray diffraction. So should stones weighing less than 3 to 5 mg, depending upon proficiency of the analyst.

MATERIALS AND REAGENTS

1. 20% (w/v) sodium carbonate
2. Uric-acid reagent (Folin): Place 100 g sodium tungstate (Na_2WO_4) (molybdate free) in 500 ml Florence flask. Add diluted phosphoric acid (33 ml of 86% [w/v] phosphoric acid added to 150 ml distilled water), and mix by shaking. Add a few glass beads and reflux gently for 1 hour (use a funnel holding a 200 ml flask of cold water) until solution is decolorized. Reheat on microburner until bromine fumes disappear. Dilute to 500 ml.
3. 10% (w/v) hydrochloric acid
4. Manganese dioxide (native powder). Reagent grade is unsatisfactory.
5. Ammonium molybdate: Dissolve 3.5 g ammonium molybdate $(NH_4)_6MO_7O_{24}\cdot 4H_2O$ in 75 ml distilled water. Add 25 ml concentrated nitric acid. Mix.

6. 20% (w/v) sodium hydroxide
7. Magnesium reagent: Dissolve 1 mg p-nitrobenzeneazoresorcinol (Eastman) in dl 1 N sodium hydroxide.
8. Nessler's reagent (Koch and McMeekin). Dissolve 30 g potassium iodide in 20 ml of water in a 500 ml Erlenmeyer flask. Add 22.5 g iodine. Mix until dissolved. Add 30 g metallic mercury. Shake well, cooling under running tap water, until supernatant has lost the yellow color of iodine. Pour off undissolved mercury. Test fluid for excess iodine by adding a few drops to 5 ml of 1% (w/v) starch solution in a test tube. If no blue color develops add iodine solution (3 g KI, 2.25 g I_2 and 10 ml H_2O) drop by drop to the decanted fluid until there is a slight excess of free iodine as determined by testing with starch. Dilute to 200 ml with water, mix, pour into 975 ml of 10% (w/v) NaOH (accurately prepared). Mix. (Store in dark for several days to permit precipitate to settle out, if present.)
9. 28% (w/v) (concentrated) ammonium hydroxide
10. Sodium cyanide: Transfer 500 g to 100 dl volumetric flask and dilute to mark with distilled water. Add 0.2 ml concentrated ammonium hydroxide. Mix. Use caution—very poisonous.
11. Sodium nitroprusside: Transfer 5 g to a dl volumetric flask and dilute to mark with distilled water. (Store in dark brown bottle; discard when it fades.)
12. Mortar and pestle
13. Dropping pipettes
14. Scalpel
15. Test tubes, 10 × 75 mm
16. Test tube rack

REFERENCES

1. Beeler, M., and Henry, J.: Pre-Workshop and Workshop Manuals on Urinalysis and Renal Function Studies. Chicago, Commission on Continuing Education, American Society of Clinical Pathologists, 1962.
2. Beeler, M., Veith, D., Morriss, R., and Biskind, G.: Analysis of urinary calculus. Comparison of methods. Am. J. Clin. Pathol., *41*:553, 1964.
3. Herring, L.: Observations on the analysis of ten thousand urinary calculi. J. Urol., *88*:545, 1962.
4. Maurice, P., and Henneman, P.: Medical aspects of renal stones. Med., *40*:315, 1961.
5. Winer, J., and Mattice, M: Routine analysis of urinary calculi; rapid, simple method using spot tests. J. Lab. Clin. Med., *28*:898, 1943.

Optical Stone Analysis

METHOD. Optical method of Prien, modified by Beeler.
PRINCIPLE. The birefringence of a powdered aliquot of the calculus

is noted, and the crystalline component(s) identified by means of their refractive indices.

PROCEDURE

1. Weigh stone on an analytical balance and describe character.
2. Fracture or cut with scalpel blade, jeweler's saw, or hack saw.
3. Grind a representative aliquot (about 10 mg) in a small agate mortar.
4. Spread a very small amount of powdered stone over a surface of a microscope slide.
5. Place on stage of polarizing microscope and examine for birefringence.
6. If highly birefringent crystals are present (calcium oxalate monohydrate and/or urates) place 2 drops of immersion fluid with index of refraction 1.65 on coverslip and invert over a portion of the stone powder. Focus. With analyzer in place, watch a small highly birefringent particle while the substage is rotated, until the particle disappears. Switch analyzer out, and observe behavior of Becke line (bright halo around fragment which moves in or out as objective is raised or lowered). On lowering focus, line moves in direction of medium with lower index of refraction; on raising, in direction of medium with higher index of refraction. Switch analyzer back in place and continue rotating substage in same direction while fragment reappears and disappears again. At the point of disappearance again, observe behavior of Becke line.
7. If refractive index is greater than 1.65, uric acid and/or sodium urates are present. If lower, probably calcium oxalate monohydrate is present.
8. To distinguish between the urates, repeat procedure, using fluid with index of refraction 1.83. Observe whether there is difference in behavior of Becke line when raising and lowering focus (to distinguish sodium acid urate and uric acid). See below.
9. If there is moderately birefringent material present (calcium oxalate dihydrate and cystine), try fluid with index of refraction 1.64. Observe Becke lines. Confirm impression by checking with fluid with index of refraction 1.54 (to distinguish cystine and calcium oxalate dihydrate). See below.
10. If there is material of very low or no birefringence present (apatite, magnesium ammonium phosphate, tricalcium phosphate and calcium hydrogen phosphate), immerse in fluid with index of refraction 1.26 (to distinguish tricalcium phosphate).
11. Immerse in fluid with index of refraction 1.50 (to distinguish apatite and magnesium ammonium phosphate). If some have higher indices than this, and no tricalcium phosphate is present, the material is probably apatite [isotropic and common] or, possibly calcium hydrogen phosphate [rare]. The indices of refraction

of apatite usually lie between 1.55 and 1.59, but may range from 1.52 to 1.61. The indices of refraction of calcium hydrogen phosphate are 1.54 and 1.55. Immerse in fluids with these indices and if none matches, the material is probably apatite. If some match, calcium hydrogen phosphate is probably present. The presence of apatite can be confirmed by checking other fluids within the known range of indices of this material.

Interpretation

Birefringence (Polarization):

None	*Moderate*	*High*
Magnesium ammonium phosphate	Cystine	Uric acid
Calcium hydrogen phosphate dihydrate	Calcium oxalate dihydrate	Urates
Apatites		Calcium oxalate monohydrate
Tricalcium phosphate		

Refractive Indices:

Highly Birefringent Crystals

$N_D > 1.65$: uric acid, sodium-acid urate
$N_D < 1.65$: calcium oxalate monohydrate
$N_D > 1.83$: sodium-acid urate
$N_D > 1.65$, but < 1.83: uric acid

Moderately Birefringent Crystals

$N_D < 1.64$ and $= 1.54$: calcium oxalate dihydrate
$N_D = 1.64$: cystine (rare)

Slightly Birefringent or Nonbirefringent Crystals

$N_D \geqslant 1.26$: tricalcium phosphate (rare)
$N_D \leqslant 1.50$: magnesium ammonium phosphate (common)
$N_D > 1.50$, and no tricalcium phosphate present:
apatite (common)
calcium hydrogen phosphate (rare)
(apatite N_D usually is 1.55 to 1.59, but may be 1.52 to 1.61)
($CaHPO_4$ usually is 1.54 to 1.55)

DISCUSSION AND CLINICAL SIGNIFICANCE. Refer to text discussion.

REAGENTS AND MATERIALS

1. Refractive Index Media (available as Professional Research Workers Set no. 1, series 1.41 to 1.78 in $^1/_4$ fluid ounce applicator vials, in steps of 0.01, catalog numbers C2655.1 from Ward's Natural Science Establishment, P.O. Box no. 1712, Rochester, N.Y. 14603).

2. Polarizing microscope
3. Microscope slides, 25 × 75 mm; coverslips.

REFERENCES

1. Allen, R.M.: Practical Refractometry by Means of the Microscope. 2nd Ed. Cedar Grove, N.J., R.P. Cargille Laboratories, 1962.
2. Gibb, T.R.P., Jr.: Optical Methods of Chemical Analysis. New York, McGraw-Hill, 1942.
3. Prien, E.L., and Frondel, C.: Studies in urolithiasis: Composition of urinary calculi. J. Urol., *57*:949, 1947.
4. West, P.W.: Chemical identification by means of polarized light microscopy. Chemist-Analyst, *43*:46, 56, 77, and 109, 1954.

Chapter

5 Pregnancy Testing

JAMES A. FREEMAN
MAXINE M. MARIONNEAUX

Since antiquity, man has desired to understand the mysteries of procreation and to detect the earliest moments of pregnancy. The oldest medical treatise in the Chinese language, the Pen Ts'ao Ching, records an abortifacient recipe attributed to Emperor Shen-Nung, who reigned about 2737 to 2696 B.C.[1] Hippocrates (460 to 377 B.C.) was interested in detecting and thwarting threatened abortions by prescribing parsley, which produced gaseous distention: a circumstance thought, at that time, to be good for maintenance of the pregnancy.[2] Aristotle stated "if it should happen among married people, that a woman, who already had a prescribed number of children, became pregnant, then before she felt life, the child should be driven from her."[2] Similar situations, involving medical, ethical, and moral questions, obviously still exist and are perhaps of even greater interest now than in Aristotle's time.

In an effort to understand the early stages of pregnancy, Aristotle visually studied the development of a chick embryo over 4,000 years ago. From what he could see of the chick, he mistakenly inferred that the human embryo developed out of "admixture of the male seminal fluid and the menstrual blood." He apparently thought that the substance of the embryo came solely from the female, while the male provided only the stimulus for growth. Five hundred years later, Galen of Pergamus added an authoritative (but incorrect) opinion, which persisted for more than 1,500 years: minute "prefabricated" embryos existed in the "female semen," and contact with the male merely brought about an unshelling of the embryo, permitting it to increase in size until birth. Every baby must, according to this theory, contain a preformed baby, one stacked inside the other, like Chinese boxes! Regnier deGraaf, a Dutch physician of the 17th century, really not understanding what he had seen, described something that broke like bubbles when he opened the reproductive tubes of a female rabbit.[3] The Estonian biologist, Karl Ernst von Baer, recorded his amazement when he recognized an ovarian follicle under the microscope. In 1827, writing in his treatise, de Ovi Mammalium et Hominis Genesi, he stated:

> I saw plainly. . . a yellowish-white point. . . led by curiosity. . . I opened one of the follicles and took up the minute object on the point of my knife, finding that I could see it very distinctly. When I placed it under the microscope, I was utterly astonished for I saw an ovule and so clearly that a blind man could hardly deny it.[3]

Anton von Leeuwenhoek's visualization of sperm led to more scientific controversy, if not to absolute confusion. Man's descent was said to be matrilineal; the sperm merely serving to incite expansion of the mother's ready-made baby. The relative simplicity of structure of the early sperm, ovum, and embryo led some people to equate human structure with animal structure, a problem accentuated by Charles Darwin's Origin of Species, published November 24, 1859 (all 1,250 copies of the first edition sold out in 1 day!).[3] What was to Darwin a harmo-

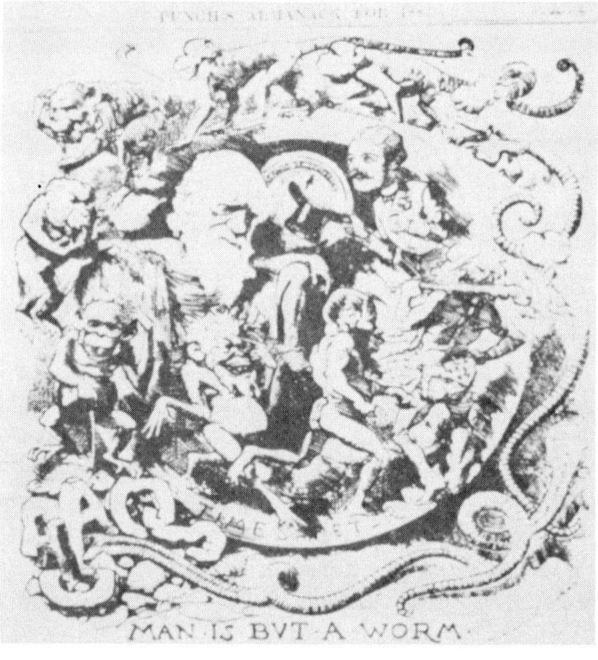

Fig. 5–1. Cartoon that appeared in Punch's Almanac, 1882, ridiculing Charles Darwin's theories on evolution of man. The worm at the bottom is shown (clockwise) developing into a monkey, a human dwarf, a cave man, then a "dandy." The bearded man is a depiction of Charles Darwin.

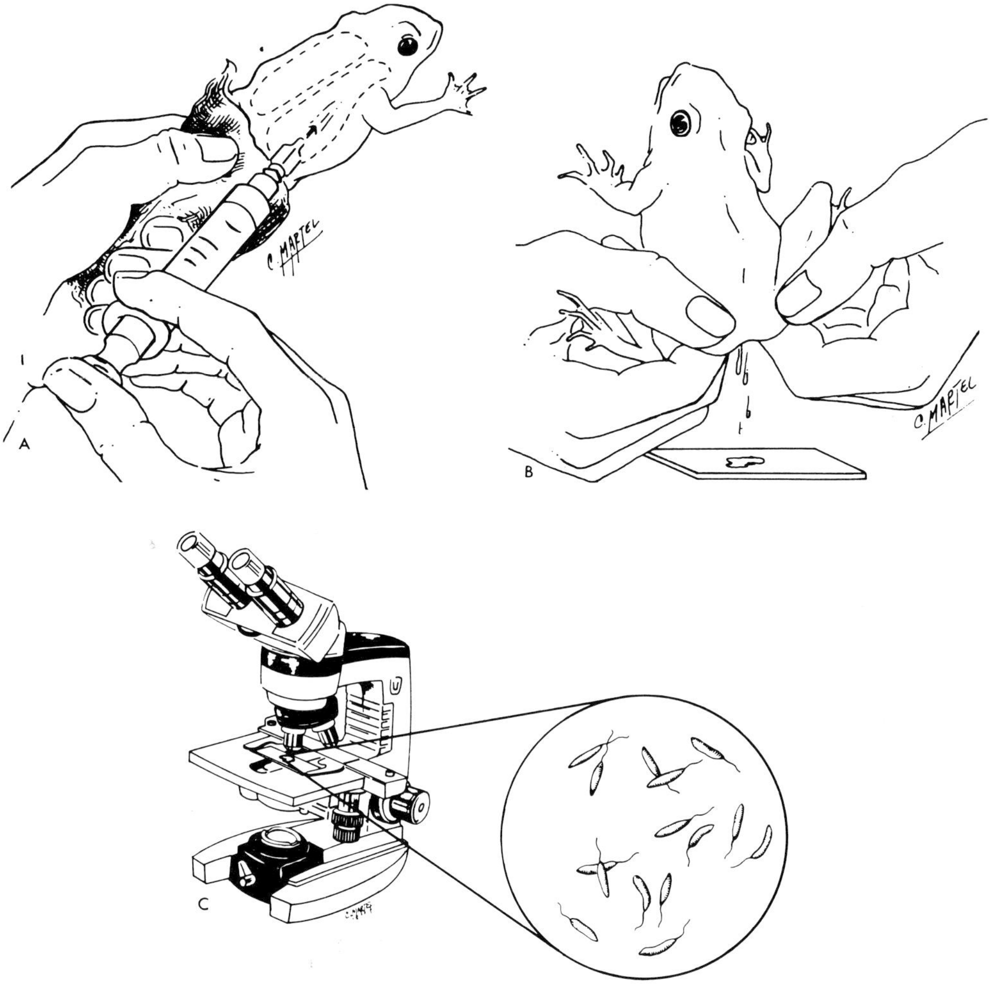

Fig. 5–2. Diagrammatic representation of frog bioassay procedure. **A,** Human urine is injected into the dorsal sac; **B,** urine is expressed from the amphibian; and **C,** microscopic appearance of sperm.

nious unity in nature obviously did not look the same to all men (Fig. 5–1).

Many investigators, both medical and lay, had tried rather unsuccessfully to develop reliable methods for diagnosing the pregnant state until Selmar Aschheim and Bernhard Zondek, in 1928, developed a bioassay system for measuring chorionic gonadotropin hormone.[4,5] Their methods, although difficult, laid the scientific basis for assay of human chorionic gonadotropin, which, in essence, is still the basis of pregnancy testing (Figs. 5–2 and 5–3). Aschheim and Zondek's procedure

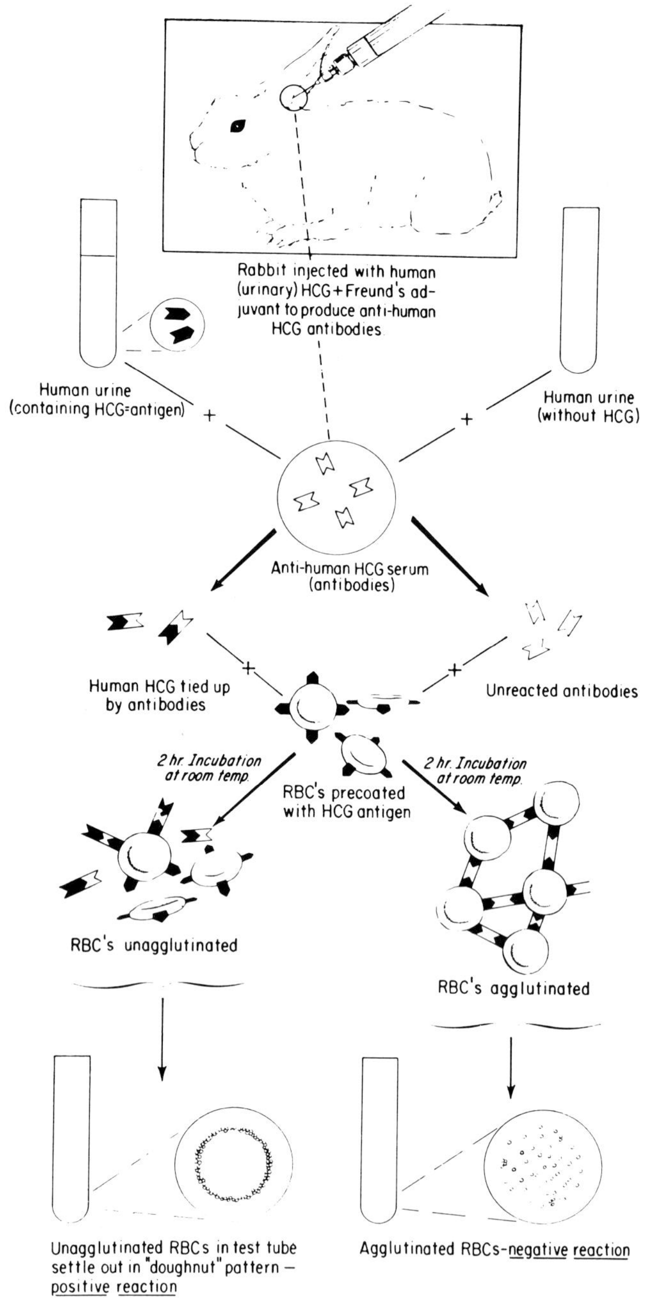

Fig. 5–3. Diagrammatic representation of procedures of latex-inhibition immunoassay and of hemagglutination-inhibition assay.

was laborious, requiring examination for hemorrhagic follicles and corpora lutea in five to six immature female mice 96 hours after injection of test urine. A year after the method was published, Maurice Friedman (1929) found that urine containing hCG caused ovulation in mature female rabbits 24 to 48 hours following injection, and he made this the basis of a pregnancy test.[6,7] Numerous modifications of the Aschheim-Zondek and Friedman tests have appeared subsequently, but all have as their basic principle hCG stimulation of ovarian follicle maturity or uterine hypertrophy. So many modifications have been made that the tests referred to as "A-Z Tests" currently may have little resemblance to Aschheim and Zondek's original procedure.

Other test animals also have been used, including rats. In 1930, Lancelot Hogben discovered that the mature female South African clawed toad (Xenopus laevis) would extrude eggs 4 or more hours after injection of human urine containing hCG.[8] David Miller and his students adapted the male frog (Rana pipiens) to hCG bioassay in 1948, using spermation from ½ to 2 hours after injection of test urine as the biologic endpoint (Fig. 5–2).[9] Although amphibians are less sensitive to stimulation than mice, rats, or rabbits, concentration of hCG by kaolin absorption in urine (Hon-Morris procedure) permits almost any desired degree of sensitivity.[10,11]

Attempts at detection of hCG by means of antibody tests were first made shortly after James Collip described "anti-hormones" (antibodies to hCG) in 1934. Specific antisera became commercially available only recently, however; subsequently, several immunologic tests (immunoassay systems) for detection and quantitation of hCG have been developed.[12,13] Kaolin concentration and alcohol precipitation methods have been used widely for concentration of hCG for bioassay techniques,[6,10] but it was not until Freund's adjuvant was added to hCG for injection into laboratory animals that enough hCG antibody was produced to make clinical use of immunoassay techniques practical.

CHORIONIC GONADOTROPIN

Human chorionic gonadotropin is a mucoprotein with an approximate weight of 80,000 daltons. hCG consists of two noncovalently bound dissimilar polypeptide subunits: α subunit (molecular weight about 15,000 to 20,000 daltons) and β subunit (molecular weight about 25,000 to 30,000 daltons). The α subunit is nearly identical to the α subunits of human luteinizing hormone (LH) and that of the α subunit of human follicle-stimulating hormone (FSH). It is also molecularly similar to the subunit of thyroid stimulating hormone (TSH). The biologic activity of hCG, therefore, may cross react with LH in bioassay systems (thus producing false-positive tests) (see Table 5–2). Such a problem also occurs in immunoassay systems, but to a lesser degree when the antigenic substance is directed against only the β subunits. The β subunit seems to determine the biologic and immunologic specificity of hCG, while the carboxyl terminal end of the β subunit is immunologically specific.

Physiology of Chorionic Gonadotropin

Human chorionic gonadotropin is produced from the cytotrophoblastic cells of the forming placenta after nidation. Usually, the exact time of initial hormone production cannot be detected with scientific certainty, inasmuch as knowledge of conception in most fertile women is, at best, a guess! Using available radionuclide technique, hCG has been detected as early as 1 week after conception or, in other words, 1 week before the expected missed mensis. To the reader is left the intellectual (or even social) problem of determining such an occurrence (as conception) with exact certainty! With the new horizons provided by in vitro human fertilization, a greater understanding of the date, or even moment, of production of chorionic gonadotropin should be forthcoming.

There is some evidence for the existence of a threshold level for excretion of human chorionic gonadotropin, but excretion is not related to renal clearance rates. This has not been defined with certainty. If it exists, however, one would expect elevated serum levels of hCG in the earliest stages of pregnancy to be more readily detectable in blood than in urine. Some investigators report that serum concentrations early in pregnancy are about 1.5 times higher than urine values in the same patients.

STANDARDIZATION OF HUMAN CHORIONIC GONADOTROPIN FOR PREGNANCY TESTING[14]

The original International Standard for LH activity, also used for hCG activity, was at the National Institute of Medical Research at Mill Hill, London, England. Human chorionic gonadotropin (hCG) values, expressed as IU/ml, represent the specific amount of gonadotropic activity contained in 0.0013 mg of dried hCG standard distributed by the Institute. The International Reference Preparation of human menopausal gonadotropin (hMG 24), a kaolin extract of human menopausal urine, contains both LH and FSH activity. Other materials have been produced by the National Institutes of Health of the United States, the United States Public Health Service Department of Health, Education and Welfare, the Armour Company in the United States, the National Institute for Biologic Standards and Control in London, England, and others. Data are not available, however, in terms that permit ready comparison of all international standards. Including these standards, there simply is no known pure hCG. Most synthetic proteins have relatively poor purity; hence, synthetic hCG may not be the answer. Until the complete chemical structure of "purified" hCG is known, in reality, we cannot know if "purified" hCG is truly pure![6,15,16]

The second International Standard of Human Chorionic Gonadotrophin for Bioassay, established in 1964, has been widely used for bioassays and immunoassays of hCG. Because of its heterogeneity, however, this international standard was not suitable for use in all immunoassay systems; it is about 20% (w/w) pure on the basis of its biologic potency and contains quantities of glycoprotein subunits as well as other substances.

The World Health Organization (WHO) Expert Committee on Biological Standardisation, in 1974, established a separate International Reference Preparation (IRP) of hCG for immunoassay, which consists of a highly purified preparation of hCG and contains insignificant amounts of subunits. WHO also established international reference preparations of the α and β subunits of hCG for immunoassay. These subunit preparations were derived from the same batch of highly purified hCG used for the International Reference Preparation of hCG, and each is substantially pure.

The International Reference Preparation of hCG was assayed in terms of the international standard in an extensive international collaborative study, in which the International Reference Preparations of the α and β subunits were included as well as coded samples of serum and urine of early and later pregnancy, by a wide variety of bioassay and immunoassay procedures. The in vivo and in vitro bioassays, which estimate intact hCG, as well as receptor binding assays, gave results that were homogeneous with a mean value of 650 IU per ampule. In contrast, several immunoassay systems (which included several that were shown to cross react with other glycoproteins and subunits as well as hCG) gave lower and heterogeneous values; those that were more specific for hCG appeared to give estimates of hCG closest to those obtained by bioassay. In accordance with the policy stated in its twenty-first report, the WHO expert committee assigned a unit of 650 IU per ampule to the Intenational Reference Preparation of hCG on the basis of the bioassay results.

A hormone preparation selected for use as a standard for immunoassay should consist of the naturally occurring form of the hormone with a high potency in a classic in vivo bioassay recognized by the scientific community as definitive for that hormone.

As may be expected from the transition between an impure standard and a standard of pure material, the use of the International Reference Preparation of hCG may cause a change in the numerical values of estimates made with any assay system that is not specific for intact hCG. For this reason, the WHO expert committee also recommended that the sensitivity and ranges of normal values of pregnancy test kits should, for an interim period, be stated in terms of units defined both by the new International Reference Preparation of hCG and by those of the international standard; the committee emphasized that this step would not necessarily involve a change in the reagents themselves.

Certain pregnancy test kits are designed to detect any molecules resembling hCG (or its β subunit), but not to be specific for hCG itself (or the β subunit) and would be particularly affected in this way. The explanation of the new calibration units for such assay systems could be confusing for medical and public test kit users.

It has also been suggested that a working standard consisting of freeze-dried urine of early pregnancy could be useful for manufacturers of pregnancy test kits. It is difficult to reproduce exactly a complex mixture of several components unless the amount of each component is known. This suggestion would lead to more confusion.

The international collaborative study showed that the new International Reference Preparation of hCG is entirely suitable for immunoassays of hCG in blood and urine, and this International Reference Preparation should be used to calibrate such assay systems. Similarly, the newly established International Reference Preparation of the α subunit of hCG and the International Reference Preparation of the β subunit should be used to calibrate immunoassay systems for these respective substances. Moreover, the IRPs can be used to evaluate the specificity of such kits, as recommended in the recently published WHO requirements for immunoassay kits.

Thus, in summary, a standard consisting of a mixture containing substances A(hCG), B(hCG-α), and C(hCG-β) has been replaced by separate standards, one for A, one for B, and one for C. Assay systems intended to estimate A should be specific for A and should use the standards for A; similarly, assays for B should use the standard for B. Assays designed to be nonspecific and detect A and B and other undefined substances should now have their sensitivity calibrated at least in terms of each identified component, i.e., the standards A, B, and C.

Confusion is worsened by some manufacturers who label their kits "β hCG kits" (because they use an antiserum raised to the β subunit of hCG) when such kits are designed to assay hCG and not the β subunit of hCG. WHO recommends that an assay kit be labeled unambiguously, to describe the analyte that the assay system is intended to estimate, and that a statement of the results of an assay should record the assay method used and the standard and its units.

ACCURACY, SPECIFICITY, AND SENSITIVITY OF PREGNANCY TESTING

The usefulness of any diagnostic test, especially a screening test, depends in part upon the incidence of the disease it detects in the population tested, as well as on the diagnostic specificity and sensitivity of the test (taken together, its diagnostic accuracy). Diagnostic specificity can be defined as the ability of the test to yield a negative result for patients without the disease. The less specific the test, the greater the percentage of positive test results in patients without the disease. Diagnostic specificity can be expressed quantitatively as follows:

$$\text{Specificity} = \frac{\text{number of negative test results in patients without the disease}}{\text{number of people tested without the disease}} \times 100$$

Thus, if there are no "false-positive" test results, the test is 100% specific.

Sensitivity is defined as the ability of the test to yield a positive result for patients with the disease. It can be expressed quantitatively as follows:

$$\text{Sensitivity} = \frac{\text{number of positive test results in patients with the disease}}{\text{number of people tested with the disease}} \times 100$$

If there are no "false-negative" test results, the test is 100% sensitive.

Diagnostic accuracy can be defined as the ability of the test to correctly classify the entire population tested for the disease in question. Because most diseases have a low incidence in the population at large, accuracy depends more on specificity than on sensitivity.

Thus, the usefulness of a test depends on the incidence of the disease in the population screened, as well as on its sensitivity and specificity. The greater the incidence of the disease, the lower the specificity that can be economically accepted; the lower the incidence, the greater the specificity required. Specificity may sometimes be sacrificed for greater sensitivity (the two often tend to be reciprocal) in screening tests, when the penalties for missing the diagnosis are greater than those of falsely suspecting the diagnosis.

In testing for pregnancy, we shall use the terms "sensitivity," "specificity," and "diagnostic accuracy" in their general clinical diagnostic use. By "sensitivity" we shall generally mean the percentage of pregnant women who yield a positive test, unless by context it is clear that we refer to the ability of the test to detect small concentrations of human chorionic gonadotropin. By "specificity" we shall generally refer to the percentage of "negative" results found in urine from women demonstrated not to be pregnant. By "diagnostic accuracy" we shall refer to both pregnant and nonpregnant patients correctly characterized by the test results.

Obviously, estimates of diagnostic accuracy will differ with the incidence of pregnancy in the population tested, with the normality and duration of the pregnancies, and with the certainty with which the diagnosis of pregnancy can be made (as well as with sensitivity and specificity of the test system). Some pregnancies may terminate in undiagnosed abortions, and positive results may incorrectly be interpreted as false-positive results. It should be noted that chemical diagnostic accuracy and clinical accuracy are two different concepts. To repeat, for our purposes, we will define "diagnostic accuracy" as the percentage of "correct" diagnoses.

It should now be clear that it is not possible to set a single titer for hCG above which all positive test results indicate pregnancy and below which no nonpregnant patient is included. For this reason, sensitivities of immunoassay test systems have been arbitrarily set by the manufacturers in an effort to achieve a reasonable balance between excessive sensitivity with low specificity on the one hand and high specificity with low sensitivity on the other hand. Exact sensitivities vary from lot to lot, and manufacturers usually include this information in their brochures.

It would be good practice either to use one test of high and one of low sensitivity for each patient, or to set up two tests with the more sensitive methods for each patient: one with undiluted urine; one with urine diluted 1:1 or 1:2. If both tests are negative, they can be so reported; if both are positive, they can be so reported. Such immunoassay systems of tests might include a latex technique and a hemagglutination-inhibition technique. If the hemagglutination-inhibition technique is positive and the latex technique is negative, results may be regarded as equivocal and another urine specimen may be requested. Continued discrepancies might merit more sophisticated laboratory and clinical investigation. Regardless of test sensitivity used for detection of pregnancy in the young female, results will depend in part on the duration of gestation (calculated from the first day of last known menses). The greater the number of days from the last menses, the higher the usual hCG activity (during the first trimester).

In general, immunoassay systems have been reported to be nearly 100% sensitive 41 days after the last menses; 96% to 100% sensitive between 30 and 40 days after the last menses.[17–24] Results are variable before 30 days after the last menses. Since the last menses may bear no constant relationship to the time of ovulation, this method of calculation of course cannot be related absolutely to duration of pregnancy in many cases. In many women, estimation of the dates of last menses is a guess at best!

Although sensitivity of immunoassay systems has been determined by comparison with international reference standard material, this material was developed for bioassay systems as noted previously (see

Standardization of Human Chorionic Gonadotropin in Pregnancy Testing). The biologically active portion of the hCG molecule does not correspond exactly to the immunologically active portion. Therefore, the two systems seem to measure different variables and this can differ independently.[18] This difference is seen during pregnancy and increases as pregnancy progresses. After the beginning of the second trimester, bioassay values for hCG drop, while immunoassay values increase.[24] Many authors have used the earliest detection of pregnancy to determine the relative merit of immunoassay systems as opposed to bioassay systems. Although this may roughly parallel sensitivity, as we have seen, there is no absolute standard, since the exact date of conception in these pregnancies cannot be known, and for the other reasons already discussed, these comparisons are not necessarily helpful. Diagnostic accuracy may be the more meaningful parameter.

Precision (reproducibility), however, can be calculated following repeated performance of tests on the same specimen or by the method of blind duplicates. Adequate estimates require consideration of day-to-day variability between specimens, technologists and reagent lots. Twenty daily determinations would be a minimum desirable number on which to base estimates.

False-Positive and False-Negative Pregnancy Tests

The findings of false-positive and false-negative results are basically different problems.[22,23] In one sense, it is incorrect to consider the test result to be false positive, if, as in menopausal women, elevated gonadotropins secreted by the pituitary, rather than pregnancy, are the cause (inasmuch as the α subunits of chorionic and pituitary gonadotropins cross react in some immunoassay systems).[21] If we are applying the test for early detection of pregnancy, however, then early detection (or confirmation) of pregnancy (diagnostic accuracy) should be one of the guidelines for determining clinical usefulness of immunoassay systems. For this purpose, also, we may wish to consider false-negative results to be negative results in patients with viable pregnancies. From psychosocial as well as legal points of view, false-positive test results in young single girls are highly undesirable. Therefore, it may be desirable to employ test systems set at different sensitivities for various situations, as noted previously. In general, the hemmaglutination-inhibition procedures are manufactured to be more sensitive than the latex-inhibition procedures; radioimmunoassay and radioreceptor assay procedures are the most sensitive (Table 5–1).

TECHNIQUES FOR ASSAY OF CHORIONIC GONADOTROPIN

In general, techniques for chorionic gonadotropin assay can be divided into: bioassay systems and immunoassay systems (Figs. 5–2 and 5–3). Bioassay systems include:

1. Aschheim-Zondek mouse follicle assay
2. Friedman rabbit test
3. Rat ventral prostate test
4. Rat ovarian hyperemia test
5. Rat ovarian weight test
6. Rat uterine weight test
7. Amphibian spermation (Rana pipiens, Buffo americanus, and Buffo marinus) and ovulation (Xenopus laevis)

TABLE 5–1. Comparison of Bioassay and Immunoassay Systems in Pregnancy Testing

	Approximate Sensitivity for hCG (IU/ml)	Time Required for Assay	Test Specimen	Type of Test*
Bioassay System				
Aschheim-Zondek (mouse follicle)	1.5 to 6	96 hours		
Friedman (rabbit corpora lutea)	10 to 15	48 hours		
Rat ovarian (hyperemia)	1.2 to 20	6 to 24 hours		
X. laevis (ovulation)	75	18 hours		
R. pipiens (spermation)	22 to 45	4 hours		
B. americanus (spermation)	12 to 45	4 hours		
B. marinus (spermation)	35 to 50	5 hours		
Immunoassay System				
Pregnosticon	0.75 to 1.5	2 hours	Urine	HAI
Wampole UCG (titration)	0.3	2 hours	Urine	HAI
(undiluted urine)	0.75 to 1.0	16 hours	Urine	HAI
Perpuerin	0.75 to 1.5	2 minutes	Urine	HAI
Immunoplate	6.0	2 minutes	Urine	HAI
Pregnosis	1.5 to 2.5	2 minutes	Urine	HAI
DAP test	2 to 3	2 minutes	Urine	HAI
Placentex	1.0	1½ hours	Urine	HAI
Sensi-Tex	0.25	1½ hours	Urine	HAI
Gest ♀ State	2.0 to 4.0	2 minutes	Urine	HAI
Neocept	0.2	2.1 hours	Urine	HAI
Posta-Tec	0.03	1 hour	Serum	RIA
HCG-B (Preg/STAT)	0.015	1 hour	Serum	RIA
UCG-slide	2.0	3 minutes	Urine	HAI
UCG-tube	1.0	2.2 hours	Urine	HAI
Biocept-G	0.2	0.2 hour	Serum	RRA
Tandem HCG	any	2.5 hours	Serum	IMRA

(Compiled from Venning: Obstet. Gynecol., *25*:110, 1965; Henry and Freig: CP Bull., State University of New York, Syracuse, 1966; and Hon: Pregnancy Testing Manual, Yale, 1955; Chung: South. Med. J., *74*:1387, 1981, and manufacturer's brochures)[11,22,23,26]

*HAI = hemagglutination-inhibition; RAI = radioimmunoassay; RRA = radioreceptor assay; IMRA = immunoradiometric (monoclonal antibody) assay

Commercially available immunoassay systems, at the time of writing, include:

1. **Pregnosticon** (Organon, Inc., Div. of Azkona, Inc., West Orange, N.J. 07052), includes H-I tube and L-I slide

2. **Prepuerin** (Burroughs Wellcome Co., Research Triangle Park, N.C. 27709), includes H-I tube test
3. **Wampole UCG** and **β-hCG slide** (Wampole Laboratories, Div. Carter-Wallace, Inc., Cranbury, N.J. 08512), includes H-I tube and LI slide
4. **Neocept** (Organon, Inc., Div. of Akzona, Inc., West Orange, N.J. 07052), H-I tube test
5. **Immunoplate** (Hyland Labs, Div. Travenol Labs., Inc., Costa Mesa, Calif. 92626), includes direct latex slide
6. **Natatel** (Pfizer Laboratories, Div. of Pfizer, Inc., New York, N.Y. 10017), includes direct latex slide
7. **Gonadex** (Leo Pharm. Prod., Copenhagen, Denmark), includes H-I tube test
8. **Pregnosis** (Roche Labs., Div. Hoffman-LaRoche, Inc., Nutley, N.J. 07110), includes L-I slide
9. **DAP Test** (Organon, Inc., Div. of Akzona, Inc., West Orange, N.J. 07052), includes direct latex slide
10. **Pregnosticon** Dri-Dot (Organon, Inc., Div. of Akzona, Inc., West Orange, N.J. 07052), include L-I slide
11. **Gest ♀ State** (Lederle Laboratories, Div. of American Cyanamid, Pearl River, N.Y. 10965), includes L-I tube
12. **Sensi-Tex** (Roche Labs., Div. Hoffman-LaRoche, Inc., Nutley, N.J. 07110), includes L-I slide
13. **Placentex** (Roche Labs., Div. Hoffman-LaRoche, Inc., Nutley, N.J. 07110), includes L-I slide
14. **E.P.T.** (Warner/Chilcott Laboratories, Morris Plaines, N.J. 07950), includes H-I tube
15. **Tandem HCG** (Hybritech, Inc., San Diego, Calif. 92121), IRMA tube test, IEMA tube test
16. **HCG-BETA** (Serono Laboratories, Braintree, Maine 02184), RIA tube test
17. **Biocept G** (Wampole Laboratories, Cranbury, N.J. 08512), RRA tube test
18. **Gamma Dab** (Clinical Assays, Division of Travenol Laboratories, Cambridge, MA 02139), RID tube test

Bioassay Systems

The bioassays at best are crude methods for hormonal assay. It is difficult to standardize bioassay systems, primarily because of variation among test animals. Bioassays have been standardized against an international reference preparation of hCG, which is crude. Its biologic activity is the result of synergistic reaction with pituitary (gonadotropic) follicle-stimulating hormone (FSH). The bioassay technique for the detection of chorionic gonadotropin developed by Aschheim and Zondek was based on observation of development of "blood points" or corpora lutea in ovarian follicles, with urine from pregnant women, the effect being secondary to both luteinizing hormone (LH) and FSH. hCG predominantly has LH activity (from the α subunit detection).

Although some authors have indicated the order of accuracy of bioassay tests in the (widely used) rat as follows: (1) vaginal estrus in the uncastrated rat, (2) uterine hypertrophy, (3) blood points or corpora lutea, and (4) ovarian hypertrophy, there is no conclusive evidence that any one bioassay system is more accurate than any other.

Some authors have felt that the bioassay system commonly used clinically (and referred to), the Friedman rabbit test, is not desirable since it is expensive, gives no differentiation of gonadotropin activities, and lacks specificity and sensitivity.[6] Furthermore, the ratio of biologically inactive to immunologic activity of hCG, as it is excreted in the urine, varies.[15]

There are also other disadvantages of using biologic specimens in

TABLE 5–2. Some Causes of False-Positive Results in Pregnancy Testing

A. Cross Reaction Between Pituitary Gonadotropin (LH, FSH) and Chorionic Gonadotropin (hCG)
- Amenorrhea
- Menstrual irregularities
- Menopause
- Postclimacteric (postmenopause)

B. Systemic Diseases
- Urinary tract infection
- Proteinuria
- Hematuria
- Chronic active hepatitis
- Tubo-ovarian abscess
- hCG-producing tumors (choriocarcinoma, hydatidiform mole, other malignant diseases)

C. Medications
- Phenothiazines
- Barbiturates
- Chlorpromazine
- Thioridazine
- Methadone
- Penicillin

Some Causes of False-Negative Results in Pregnancy Testing

A. Specimen
- Dilute urine (specific gravity <1.010 or osmolality <500 mmol/Kg)
- Low concentrations of hCG in early pregnancy

B. Technical
- Inexperienced personnel testing
- Reagent outdating

(Compiled from Chung: South. Med. J., *74*:1387, 1981; Wide and Gemzell: Acta Endocrinol., *39*:539, 1962; Doraisey: Can. Med. Assoc. J., *102*:975, 1970; Marks and Shackcloth: Br. Med. J., *1*:517, 1966; Ravel et al.: Am. J. Obstet. Gynecol., *105*:1222, 1969; Arkin and Noto: Am. J. Clin. Pathol., *58*:314, 1972.)

hCG assay. Quinine and aspirin derivatives, so frequently found in urine specimens, are both toxic to rabbits, and so may kill test animals in bioassay systems (Table 5–2). The rat hyperemia test is difficult to interpret, and sensitivity to hCG varies markedly. Chlorpromazine and allied drugs may produce false-positive results in male frogs (but not in rabbits or mice).[25,26] Frogs may develop often fatal "red leg" disease. It is necessary to "refrigerate" amphibians to simulate hibernation to suppress spontaneous ovulation or spermation. Both frogs and toads have seasonal variation in responsiveness and may give false-positive reactions in the spring. Furthermore, there is seasonal difficulty in obtaining amphibians. Refrigeration and air conditioning have not overcome the latter two problems. When frogs are removed from refrigeration to warmer room temperature, they may spontaneously spermate, as though it were springtime, producing a false-positive test result. Xenopus toads should not be fed 24 or more hours before the test, since injection of urine causes regurgitation of partially digested food, which may interfere with visualization of the eggs.

All these problems militate against use of bioassay systems in laboratory testing for the pregnant state. *We do not recommend any of these test systems.*

Immunoassay Systems

Most currently available immunoassays for testing of urine are either hemagglutination-inhibition or latex particle-inhibition procedures.[26] hCG is the antigen. The antibody, prepared by injection of hCG and Freund's adjuvant into rabbits, is adsorbed onto red blood cells or latex particles, which serve as visible carriers for the agglutination reaction. While some of these tests are based on hemagglutination-inhibition and others on latex-inhibition, the principal underlying test is similar (Fig. 5–3). Antibody is incubated with test specimen (urine), followed by addition of particles (red blood cells or latex balls) coated with antigen. Visible agglutination in this system indicates that antigen was not present in the test specimen in sufficient amounts to bind all antibody; this test result is therefore negative. Absence of agglutination indicates that the antibody reacted with the antigen (hCG) in the test specimen prior to addition of the hCG-coated particles; hence, the test is positive.

Latex agglutination-inhibition tests have the advantage of rapidity (about 2 minutes), and so have been extensively used in clinical office practice. Hemagglutination-inhibition tests have greater sensitivity but yield more false-positive test results.

The latex procedures are rapid, simple to perform, and can be useful in emergency situations; they should not be discarded! Furthermore, some latex procedures, such as Neocept, are almost as accurate as the β subunit radioimmunoassay testing.[26] Regardless of the type of testing procedure, a positive result in the hands of a physician who can exercise good clinical judgment is a valuable piece of laboratory information. If a false-negative procedure is suspected, in clinical office practice, a beta subunit radioimmunoassay procedure, or a repeat immunoassay procedure on a first morning urine obtained 7 days later, is considered standard practice (Table 5–2).[26,27] In the pregnant patient with elevated prolactin levels, the immunoassay tests may be negative.

With currently available techniques for producing high levels of antibodies to hCG, immunoassay system sensitivity can be set as high as desired. Difficulty arises in deciding what level of sensitivity is most desirable. It should be high enough to detect hCG in early pregnancy, but low enough not to detect small functional increases of pituitary gonadotropin that occur during the menstrual cycle.[8] The excretion of pituitary LH reaches a peak of 0.2 to 0.4 IU/L in urine at time of ovulation.[20,26] LH levels are 0.1 to 0.4 IU/ml urine in postmenopausal women. Also, there is an even more marked increase in secretion of pituitary gonadotropins during the climacteric. Therefore, the level of test sensitivity for detection of pregnancy in women in or nearing the climacteric perhaps should be set higher than the level for detection of pregnancy in young women. (The problem is the same whether using bioassay or immunoassay systems.)

Radioassay Procedures[28–30]

Radioimmunoassay systems use antibodies directed against the antigenic sites of the beta subunit of hCG. The antibodies are usually produced by immunizing rabbits. The procedures depend upon binding of the antibodies competitively with unlabeled antigens, and radionuclide-labeled antigens. Radioreceptor (RRA) procedures differ from radioimmunoassay (RIA) procedures in that they are based on specific binding of antigenic sites, without the competitive aspect. Procedures that depend on β-hCG subunit binding are more specific for hCG, inasmuch as they will not cross react with α subunits of LH and FSH. Consequently, radioimmunoassay and radioreceptor assays are more sensitive than hemagglutination-inhibition or latex inhibition procedures.

Proteinuria and phenothiazine-type drugs have been known to produce false-positive latex agglutination reactions with most immunoassay test systems using urine, but not in the Gest ♀ State™ system (Table 5–2).[26] Few, if any, pregnant women have urine that is totally protein free. Other substances in urine may nonspecifically "bind" the hCG antibody and produce false-positive reactions, in bioassay and non-β-subunit specific assay systems (Table 5–2). Dilute urine (with specific gravity less than 1.010 or osmolality less than 500 mmol/kg) and low hCG concentration early in pregnancy may produce false-negative results in many commercially available test systems (Table 5–2).

Immunoradiometric and Immunoenzymatic Procedures

Two-site immunoradiometric assays (IRMA) and immunoenzymatic assays (IEMA) have recently been introduced citing an advantage over the RIA and RRA. Two antibodies, each directed against a distinct site, must bind before quantitation can occur. One of the antibodies is radiolabeled or enzyme-labeled and the second antibody immobilized on a solid base: the concentration of the analyte is directly proportional to the bound radioactivity or antibody-enzyme, conjugate. These techniques effectively using two monoclonal antibodies, obviates interference from free α and β subunit, LH, FSH, TSH, and only native hCG molecules are measured. The IRMA or IEMA technique contrasts with β-subunit-specific RIA and RRA techniques, in which free radicals of β subunits, that may not be structurally intact within the hCG molecule, can react in the RIA and RRA systems.

INDICATIONS FOR PREGNANCY TESTING

While man had been prompted by his social if not intellectual curiosity for many centuries to detect the earliest moments of conception, the medical significance of pregnancy testing lies in:

1. Recognition of pregnancy in patients with disease that could increase mortality or morbidity in the pregnant state;
2. Differential diagnosis of ruptured ectopic pregnancies (in fallopian tubes, intra-abdominal cavity, and elsewhere) in a patient presenting with an acute surgical emergency;
3. Avoidance of unintentional abortion during medical and surgical procedures;
4. Desire of induced abortion (medically indicated or otherwise);
5. Differential diagnosis of complete versus incomplete spontaneous abortion;
6. Avoidance of fetal irradiation during roentgenographic or radionuclide procedures;
7. Differential diagnosis of hCG-secreting tumors, in both male and female;
8. Following results of hCG-secreting tumor therapy; and
9. Medicolegal problems.

SPECIMEN COLLECTION

Dilute urine (specific gravity < 1.010 or osmolality < 500 mmol/kg) may contain too small a quantity of hCG per unit volume of urine to be detectable with immunoassay systems as noted. Therefore, it is more desirable to obtain a concentrated first morning urine specimen.[6] In the office practice of medicine, it is more often necessary to use an isolated urine collection at varying hours of the day; for the reasons stated, a negative "pregnancy test" with such a random urine specimen should be repeated with a more concentrated first morning urine.

Of course, in patients presenting with suspected ectopic pregnancy or, worse yet, with ruptured ectopic pregnancy, the physician cannot wait for an opportune time to collect urine and must rely on a catheterized urine specimen obtained immediately. Catheterization will eliminate the possibility of blood contamination and a false-positive immunoassay test. Serum RIA and IRMA procedures, being more specific for β subunit hCG, have been more valuable in evaluating patients with suspected ectopic pregnancies, but these suffer the disadvantage of not being emergency procedures. More often than not, the physician must rely on a "quickie test" (2-minute latex agglutination procedure) using urine to evaluate patients in the emergency room, relying on a RIA, RRA, or IRMA procedure to confirm diagnosis. Unfortunately this confirmation is usually made after surgical procedures have been performed, and the emergency has abated, at such time when there is no longer clinical need (which makes the test not as clinically useful).

It is better to collect a 24-hour urine specimen rather than a random specimen in order to minimize the many variables that may alter apparent hormone secretion. It is good practice to dehydrate the patient, starting 8 hours before actual urine collection, by restricting fluids sufficiently so that the total urine volume will be 1 L or less in 24 hours. Collection of an accurately timed 24-hour urine specimen is difficult to achieve even under the best of circumstances in a hospital, and it seems that interested patients do better than uninterested nurse's aides. Some nurse's aides, nurses, and even physicians fail to recognize the crucial importance of instructing patients to discard urine voided at the start of a 24-hour collection so that one starts collection with an empty bladder and empties the bladder at the end of the collection period. Many nurse's aides and patients also appear to believe that the collection must be exactly for 24 hours and that this is more important than accurate recording of the time.

Urine should be refrigerated to minimize loss of hormone activity. Because of the problems of aesthetics, home refrigeration, specimen transport, and patient inconvenience, most physicians have used first voided morning urine samples. Some authors record similar results from morning specimens and 24-hour specimens, but this has also been challenged scientifically.[6,20]

PREGNANCY

It must be emphasized that *assaying gonadotropic hormones is not testing for pregnancy per se* (when pregnancy is defined as a state existing after conception—a relative association of sperm and ovum with subsequent orderly development). The same assay system may also be employed to detect hCG secretion of hormones by trophoblastic neoplasms: chorionepithelioma, hydatidiform mole, and male testicular tumors and, depending on the level of test sensitivity, α subunits of pituitary LH and FSH. Since hCG is not secreted until after development of cytotrophoblastic cells, as noted previously, *chorionic go-*

nadotropin assay does not detect the earliest moments of pregnancy. Accurate estimation of the day of conception is nearly impossible. "Days from last menses" is the formula most commonly used for estimating gestational age.

Nevertheless, partially because of patient curiosity and partially because of potential medical usefulness, continuing attempts are made to develop laboratory tests that will detect the pregnant state even earlier (greater sensitivity). Tests such as the two-site immunoradiometric monoclonal antibody (IRMA) or the immunoenzymatic (IEMA) assays have been developed. Levels of chorionic gonadotropin during the earliest moments of pregnancy are clinically relevant, although not measurable. Workers, however, have achieved very early detection of appearance of the hormone, but it is probable that a level of chorionic gonadotropin detectable by bioassay methods usually is not reached until about the tenth day after implantation. Detectability by RIA and RRA methods, however, may reduce the detection time to under 7 days postimplantation. Methods more sensitive than this, such as IMRA, may lower this time but, as pointed out, would be liable to yield false-positive results from detection of pituitary gonadotropins (less specificity).

In the United States, several pregnancy tests, one such being the EPT In-Home Pregnancy Test™, are marketed for "in-home" use by patients whose curiosity or psychosocial instability induces them to attempt to determine privately if they are pregnant. The EPT test is alleged by the manufacturer to be 97% "accurate" when implantation has occurred at least 9 days previously. Is this diagnostic accuracy or chemical accuracy? Is this nonsense in untrained persons? Can observation be considered equally valid from one individual to another?

In cases of "subfertile" patients, in which the knowledge of implantation date is critical to prevention of recurrent early spontaneous abortion, the detection of pregnancy-specific β subunit of hCG is now in widespread use by radioimmunoassay technology. The use of the β-subunit assay does not totally avoid cross reactivity with endogenous luteinizing hormone (LH) and exogenous pituitary and/or chorionic gonadotropins used therapeutically. This is especially a problem when the sensitivity of the test is set by the manufacturer to detect less than half the amount of hCG usually detected by HI and LI techniques (about 0.6 IU hCG/ml urine in HI technique). hCG is detectable in urine by the toad bioassay 20 to 30 days after the last known menses. By 40 to 50 days in the average pregnancy, a level of about 5000 IU hCG/24 hours is reached. By days 50 to 90 (usually 60 to 70), levels of up to 500,000 IU/24 hours are reached, but these levels rarely exceed 10 days' duration (Fig. 5–4).

For the remainder of pregnancy, urinary hCG usually ranges between 4000 to 11,000 IU/24 hours (athough sometimes it may go as low as 2000 IU/ml) (Fig. 5–4). Leif Wide and Bruce Gemzell have demonstrated, using hemagglutination-inhibition techniques, rises in urinary

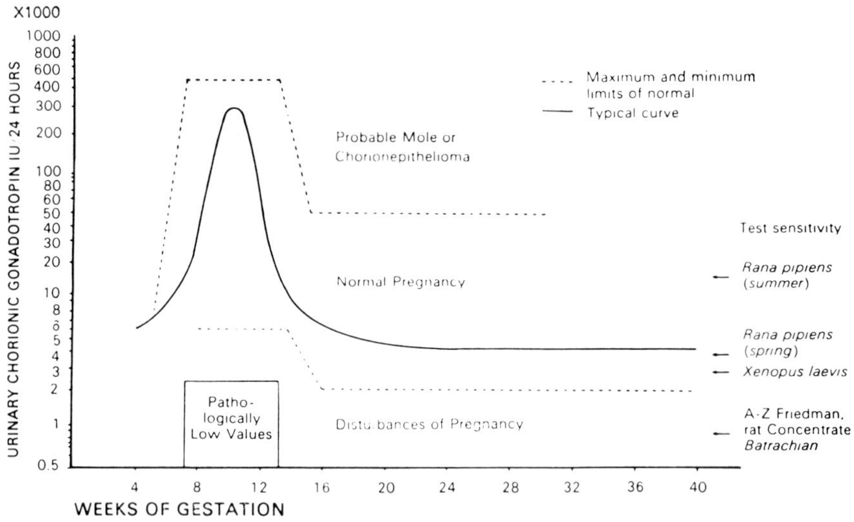

Fig. 5–4. Limits of urinary chorionic gonadotropin excretion during pregnancy as determined by various bioassay systems. The relative test sensitivity is noted on the right of the diagram. (Reproduced with permission from Hon, E.: A Manual of Pregnancy Testing. Courtesy of Little, Brown, 1961.)

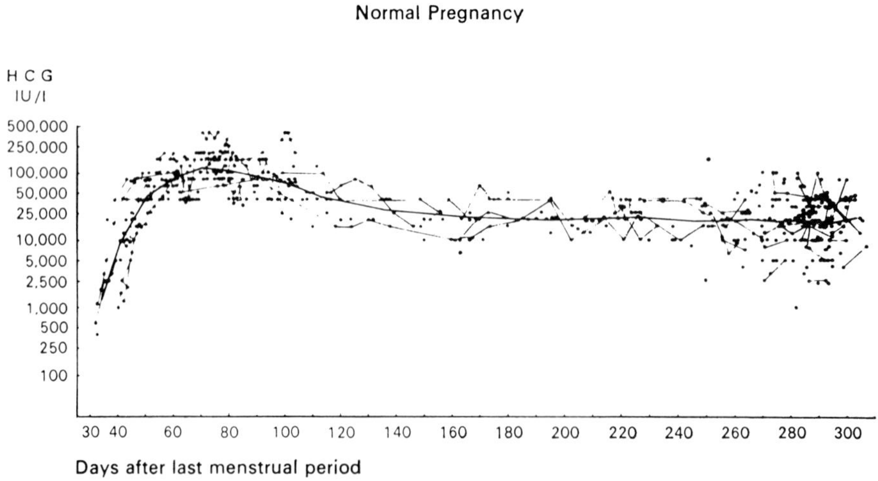

Fig. 5–5. Range of chorionic gonadotropin levels during pregnancy determined by hemagglutination-inhibition assays in 522 first morning urines collected from 240 women with normal pregnancies. The heavy line represents the mean values. (Reproduced with permission from Wide, L., and Gemzell, C.: Determinations of gonadotropins in urine by a hemagglutination-inhibition reaction. *In* Ciba Foundation Colloquia on Endocrinology. Immunoassay of Hormones. Vol. 14. Edited by G. Wolstenholme and M. Cameron. Courtesy of Little, Brown & Co., 1962.)

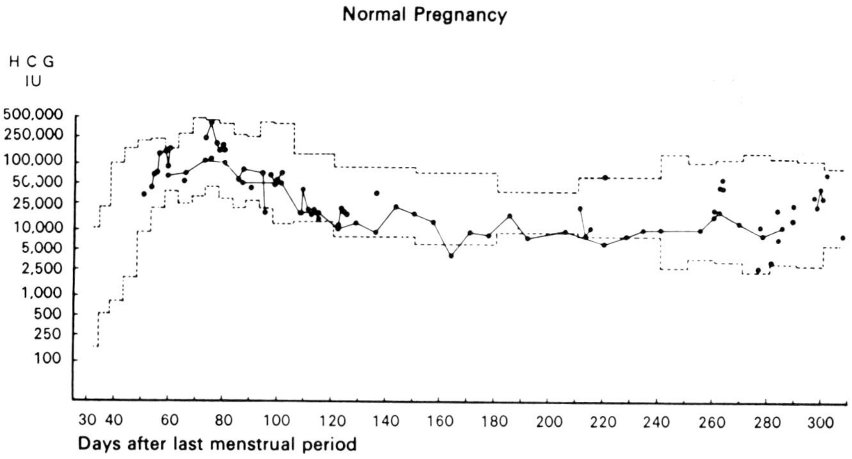

Fig. 5–6. Range of chorionic gonadotropin levels during pregnancy as determined by hemagglutination-inhibition assays in 87 24-hour urines collected from 29 women with normal pregnancies. The dots represent individual determination; the broken lines, the limits of error of the immunologic hCG activity. (Reproduced with permission from Wide, L.: An immunological method for the assay of human chorionic gonadotropin. Acta Endocrinol., *41* (Suppl. 70):84, 1962.)

TABLE 5–3. Comparative Sensitivity of Some Pregnancy Tests

	Number of Patients	Sensitivity (Positive) Results		Specificity (Negative) Results	
		Correct	"False"	Correct	"False"
Frog	145	47(96%)	2(4%)	76(79%)	20(21%)
Pregnosticon	130	51(96%)	2(4%)	69(90%)	8(10%)
Immunoplate	139	30(86%)	5(14%)	71(68%)	33(32%)
Wampole UCG	137	44(86%)	7(14%)	66(77%)	22(23%)
Gravindex	138	45(86%)	6(14%)	67(78%)	20(22%)

Table 5–3 lists comparative results of tests (in patients with viable pregnancies). According to the authors, this series does not provide evidence of a significant difference among tests as regards false-positive results (sensitivity) judged by the chi square test. The durations of pregnancy were not recorded by the authors. (Reproduced with modifications with permission from Thompson, R., Mayo, R., and Bell, W.: A critical evaluation of pregnancy tests. Am. J. Clin. Pathol., *35*:585, 1965.)

hCG levels about 30 to 40 days after the last menses, reaching a peak of 50,000 to 250,000 IU/L by 60 to 80 days, then slowly decreasing to 25,000 to 50,000 IU/L by 100 days. The latter values are usually sustained throughout the remainder of pregnancy (Figs. 5–5 and 5–6).

Quantitative urinary assays in the second and third trimesters have little value in normal pregnancy. Bioassays demonstrate a fall in activity, while with immunoassays, there is a second peak (0.75 to 96 IU/ml; mean, 18 IU/ml) in the third trimester, suspected to be partly the result of hormonal secretion by female fetuses and partly due to un-

TABLE 5–4. Comparative Studies of Immunoassay and Frog Bioassay Tests on Pregnant and Nonpregnant Patients

Studies on Pregnant Patients

Cases proven to be pregnant by (subsequent) delivery	Number of Cases		Days from first day of last menstrual period: < 36 days (pts)		36–49 days (25 pts)		> 49 days (25 pts)	
	Pos.	Neg.	Pos.	Neg.	Pos.	Neg.	Pos.	Neg.
Frog (R. pipiens)	38	18	11	5	15	10	22	3
Pregnosticon	50	6	4	2	23	2	23	2
Immunoplate	28	28	2	4	13	12	13	12
Wampole UCG	39	17	4	2	16	9	19	6
Gravindex	28	18	3	3	17	8	18	7

Studies on Nonpregnant Patients

	Number of Cases		Days from first day of last menstrual period: < 36 days		36–44 days		> 49 days	
	Pos.	Neg.	Pos.	Neg.	Pos.	Neg.	Pos.	Neg.
Frog	0	53	0	19	0	20	0	14
Pregnosticon	1	52	1	18	0	20	0	14
Immunoplate	2	51	2	17	0	20	0	14
Wampole UCG	5	48	2	17	2	18	1	13
Gravindex	4	49	3	17	3	17	1	13

(Reproduced with permission from Thompson, R., Mayo, R., and Bell, W.: A critical evaluation of pregnancy tests. Am. J. Clin. Pathol., *35*:585, 1965.)

known reasons. The urinary immunoassay peak of the first trimester, as we have seen, is usually from 12 to 192 IU/ml (mean, 60 IU/ml).[15] The higher level of hCG near term in patients with female fetuses (as opposed to those with male fetuses) does not have diagnostic application at present.

Tables 5–3 and 5–4 list comparative results of various urinary immunoassay tests in pregnant and nonpregnant patients with calculated gestational duration.[31] In the 36-day group, there was no significant difference between tests. In the over-49-day group, the Immunoplate™ yielded fewer positive results ($p = 0.01$ by the chi square test).

Inasmuch as we are not testing for pregnancy per se, but for the existence of hCG, there is no level below which all tests will be negative, or above which all tests will be positive.[34] In The College of American Pathologist Comprehensive Survey (1982-Set H-B) 1364 participants found a negative result, 692 participants a positive result, and 63 participants an inconclusive result when dealing with an hCG level that was assayed at 0.28 IU/ml. The difference in the results was ascribable to the level of sensitivities of the different testing systems that were used by the participants, who were all pathologists, medical technologists, laboratory specialists, and technicians. Confusion arose as to whether the specimen should have been negative or positive, as expressed in letters to the Clinical Microscopy Resource Committee of The College of American Pathologists. If such confusion existed in the minds of trained technical specialists, just think of the confusion that would exist in the minds of untrained women using these test systems at home. Variance of the test systems to detect pregnancy is not understood by the untrained women using the "do-it-yourself" kits. Many such patients end up in abortion clinics after a deceiving "do-it-yourself-kit" positive test. Such women should be first forgiven; secondly, admonished; and next, educated regarding these problems.

Manufacturers rely on the same principle of manufacturing these substances as they do for testing in hospitals and medical laboratories, i.e., test systems that set a specific sensitivity. These systems should require the same concern and technical expertise as that necessary in medical laboratories!

Ovulation

Maximum estrogen effect, from increase in luteinizing hormone elaborated immediately before ovulation, can be detected by daily immunoassay determinations using procedures that detect the α subunit hCG. The excretion of LH into urine peaks at 0.2 to 0.4 IU/L at the time of ovulation. In most instances, the increase is detected before the temperature shift noted in ovulatory cycles and also correlates with vaginal cytologic examination by the maturation index count, and the "fern test."

Abortion

The value of quantitative assay of hCG by immunologic methods in pathologic pregnancies has been widely debated.[17] In general, results are thought to be less reliable than in normal pregnancies. Levels less than 3000 IU/24 hour urine with frog spermation bioassay in the first 50 to 90 days of gestation frequently are associated with inevitable abortion. Levels less than 19 IU/ml in a first voided morning urine by hemagglutination-inhibition immunoassay also have been associated with nonviable gestation (Fig. 5–7). Although patients with inevitable abortion may initially present with normal hCG levels, immunoassay methods usually demonstrate a fall to 5 to 10 IU/ml about 1 to 2 days prior to abortion. Hence, quantitative daily assays may have real prognostic value.[15] Only rarely will low levels of hCG be encountered in a pregnant patient who will proceed uninterrupted to term.[35] Serum-free estriol levels performed daily have more clinical usefulness in this regard, but are laborious and expensive.

In the United States and Europe there has been a proliferation of independent agencies, medical, paramedical, and otherwise, that pro-

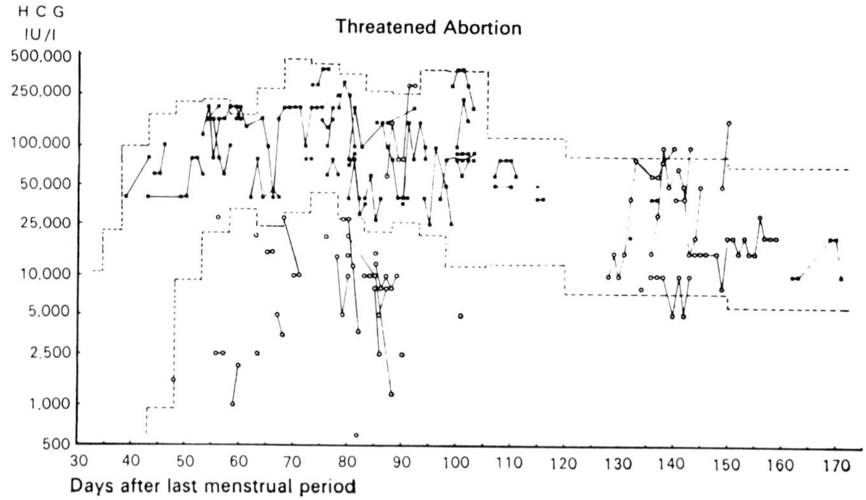

Fig. 5–7. Immunologic hCG activity in 229 morning urines from 72 women hospitalized for threatened abortion. The open circles represent 33 patients who aborted spontaneously; in the other 39 patients, represented by solid squares, pregnancy went to term. The dotted lines represent the limits of error of the immunologic hCG activity. (Reproduced with permission from Wide, L.: An immunological method for the assay of human chorionic gonadotropin. Acta Endocrinol., *41*(Suppl. 70):88, 1962.)

vide "on-call" abortion service, many times without prior pregnancy testing. Women's magazines carry "do-it-yourself" test information, and entire shelves in pharmacies or apothecaries are lined with the test kits. During the course of clinical medical practice, one of the authors (JAF) has had several experiences with women who have paid for "abortions" on the basis of a "do-it-yourself" pregnancy test, ultimately the test being proven to have had a false-positive result!

Chorionic Gonadotropin Secreting Tumors

Marked elevation of hCG above normal extremes or persisting elevation during the second trimester has been associated with hydatidiform mole, trophoblastic neoplasms, and chorionepithelioma.[36] Lack of detectable hCG, however, may not rule out choriocarcinoma or hydatidiform mole in all suspected cases, because some of these tumors may not secrete hCG.[18]

The radioimmunoassay techniques for β-subunit hCG are currently recommended for postoperative or postirradiation follow-up of these patients. Male testicular tumors (seminoma, teratoma, embryonal carcinoma) may secrete hCG, and so may be detectable and suitable for postsurgical or postirradiation follow-up by quantitative hCG determinations. Urinary hCG should fall to undetectable levels 5 to 10 days after complete removal of tumors. The hCG level should fall to normal levels within 6 to 12 weeks after removal of a hydatidiform mole. Elevated values also have been seen in patients with polyhydramnios, twin pregnancies, and those culminating in fetal death from erythroblastosis fetalis, but values may overlap normal levels, making clinical interpretation difficult in these cases.

Leif Wide and Bruce Hobson have studied the radio of biologic to immunologic activity (B/I) utilizing the ventral prostate of rat bioassay and the hemagglutination-inhibition reaction. In the first trimester of normal pregnancy, the ratio was less than unity and averaged 0.40. In urine of patients with hydatidiform mole, the ratio was greater than 1.[19] This approach may be useful for detecting abnormalities early in the pregnancy state.

Ectopic Pregnancy

hCG levels are usually, but not invariably, below 10 IU/ml by bioassay in urine of patients with ectopic pregnancy (Fig. 5–8).[11]

The test system of choice for detection of ectopic pregnancy are radioassay procedures: RIA, RRA, or IMRA. Since most patients suspected of having an ectopic pregnancy, in fact, do not have an ectopic pregnancy, the major advantage of using radioassay procedures is to rule out a pregnancy. (Keep in mind that patients with abdominal pain and elevated hCG levels may not have ectopic pregnancy, but instead, may have intrauterine pregnancy.) An intrauterine pregnancy can be suspected if hCG is above 6 IU/ml and enlargement of the uterus is identified by other technology (such as ultrasonographic techniques). In the event that an intrauterine sac is demonstrated by ultrasonogram, and the hCG is above 10 IU/ml, this can be taken as positive evidence of pregnancy. In emergency situations, these findings should militate

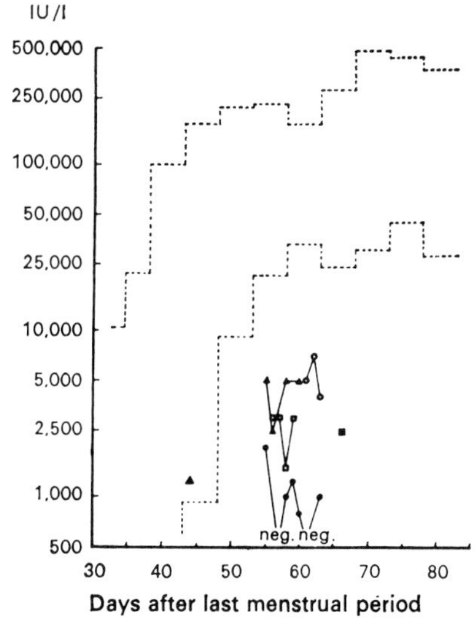

Fig. 5–8. Immunologic hCG activity in 20 morning urines from 6 women with ectopic pregnancies. The dotted lines represent limits of error of immunologic hCG activity in morning urines of women with normal pregnancies. (Reproduced with permission from Wide, L.: An immunological method for the assay of human chorionic gonadotropin. Acta Endocrinol., *41* (Suppl. 70):89, 1962.)

against operative intervention for ectopic pregnancy. The level of sensitivity of test systems used for this purpose needs to be low enough to detect small amounts of hCG (usually less than 1 IU/ml). The possibility of encountering false-positive results from pituitary gonadotropins, however, must also be considered when using tests set at this level of sensitivity.[38]

Nicholas Kadar and Roberto Romero have suggested that increase of hCG in two specimens over 48 hours time can help distinguish between normal intrauterine pregnancies and ectopic pregnancies.[37] The percent increase in hCG should be 66% or greater in normal pregnancies for the time interval. Of course, the clinical diagnosis should not depend solely on this laboratory parameter, inasmuch as 15% normal pregnancies could be termed abnormal by this parameter. The rate of increase of hCG was below this level in 87% of patients with ectopic pregnancy. *A sensitive hCG determination can provide the physician with a basic information only and cannot substitute for good clinical judgment.* Again, it is most important for the physician to exclude the diagnosis when considering an acute pelvic surgical catastrophe.[38]

PELVIC SURGERY

We believe that a pregnancy test should be performed (and its results negative) before hysterectomy and elective pelvic surgery! In some laboratories, performance of dual test systems is necessary prior to such a procedure.

Women who have had intrauterine devices (IUD) inserted into the uterus as a contraceptive device have become pregnant. In such cases the IUD may become intimately entwined into the protoplasm of the developing fetus. We have examined aborted fetuses with IUDs through the neck, head, and limbs. The presence of an IUD does not eliminate the possibility of pregnancy, which may need to be ruled out or confirmed with hCG test systems. Several studies have shown that ectopic pregnancy is more apt to occur in women who have had an IUD than in women who have not had an IUD. An increased risk of pelvic or intrauterine infections (endometritis) with IUD use is also known to increase the possibility of ectopic pregnancy, even after removal of the IUD.

Ectopic pregnancy in young fertile women who have had excision or cauterization of fallopian tubes, when presenting with acute lower abdominal pain or evidence of an acute surgical abdomen, usually can be ruled out or confirmed with radioassay procedures. This is especially important because the number of tubal fulguration (cauterization) procedures, via laparoscopic technique, are increasing annually in the United States. Tubal ligation procedures are being performed in ambulatory surgical clinics, in hospitals, and other less regulated institutions, without having prior demonstration of a negative hCG test.

REFERENCES

1. Wallnöfer, H., and von Rottanscher, A.: Chinese Folk Medicine, New York, Cron, 1965, p. 18.
2. Taussig, F.: Abortion Spontaneous and Induced: Medical and Social Aspects. St. Louis, C.V. Mosby, 1963, p. 31.
3. Flanagan, G.: The First Nine Months of Life. New York, Simon and Schuster, 1962, p. 8.
4. Aschheim, S.: Early diagnosis of pregnancy, chorionepithelioma, and hydatidiform mole by Aschheim-Zondek test. Am. J. Obstet. Gynecol., *19*:335, 1930.
5. Aschheim, S.: Pregnancy test. J.A.M.A., *104*:1324, 1935.
6. Segaloff, A.: The gonadotropins. *In* Methods in Hormone Research. Volume 2. Edited by R. Dorfman. New York, Academic Press, 1962.
7. Friedman, M.: Mechanisms of ovulation in rabbit; ovulation by injection of urine from pregnant women. Am. J. Physiol., *90*:617, 1929.
8. Schneider, P.: A hormone test for the diagnosis of early pregnancy. Surg. Gynecol. Obstet., *52*:56, 1931.
9. Hogben, L.: Zenopus test for pregnancy (letter to editor). Br. Med. J., *2*:38, 1939.
10. Wiltberger, P., and Miller, D.: The male frog, Rana pipiens, as a new test animal for early pregnancy. Science, *107*:198, 1948.
11. Hon, E.: A system of pregnancy testing using male toads and frogs (Laboratory manual). New Haven, Yale University School of Medicine, 1955.
12. Wide, L., and Gemzell, C.: An immunologic pregnancy test. Acta Endocrinol., *35*:261, 1960.
13. Islami, Z., Fisher L., and Kupfer, H.: Rapid slide test for pregnancy. Am. J. Obstet. Gynecol., *89*:586, 1964.
14. Baughman, D., and Starring, P.: Standardisation of human chorionic gonadotropin testing for pregnancy. Lancet, *1*:390, 1982.
15. Brody, S., and Carlstrom, G.: Problems associated with the quantitative immunoassay of human chorionic gonadotropin. *In* Gonadotropins: Physico-chemical and Immunological Properties. Ciba Foundation Study Group no. 22. Edited by G. Wolstenholme and J. Knight. London, J. & A. Churchill, 1965, p. 46.
16. Wilde, C., and Bagshavoe, K.: The purification of chorionic gonadotropin. *In* Gonadotropins: Physiochemical and Immunological Properties. Ciba Foundation Study Group No. 32. Edited by G. Wolstenholme and J. Knight. London, J. & A. Churchill, 1965, p. 46.
17. Gots, P., and Mighorst, J.: Comparative examinations of serologic pregnancy test and the frog test. Am. J. Obstet. Gynecol., *89*:590, 1964.
18. Wide, L, and Hobson, B.: Immunological and biological activity of human chorionic gonadotropin in urine and serum of pregnant women and women with a hydatidiform mole. Acta Endocrinol., *54*:105, 1967.
19. Sato, T., and Greeblat, R.: Detection of early pregnancy. Immunologic tests versus the rat hyperemia test. Am. J. Obstet. Gynecol., *91*:31, 1965.
20. Wide, L., and Gemzell, C.: Determination of gonadotropins in urine by a hemagglutination-inhibition reaction. *In* Immunoassay Endocrinology. Volume 14. Edited by G. Wolstenholme and M. Cameron. Boston, Little, Brown, 1962, p. 296.
21. Evans, J., and Simpson, M.: Physiology of the gonadotropins. *In* The Hormones. Volume 2. Edited by G. Pincus and K. Thimann. New York, Academic Press, 1950.
22. Henry, J., and Krieg, A.: Critique-Clinical Chemistry "Check Sample" No. CC-35: Human Chorionic Gonadotropin. Chicago, Commission on Continuing Education, American Society of Clinical Pathologists, 1965.
23. Venning, E.: Pregnancy tests. Obstet. Gynecol., *26*:110, 1965.
24. Thompson, R., Mayo, R., and Bell, W.: A critical evaluation of pregnancy tests. Am. J. Clin. Pathol., *35*:585, 1965.
25. Hilbert, G.: False positive pregnancy tests caused by Sparine and Thorazine (letter to editor). Am. J. Clin. Pathol., *31*:466, 1959.
26. Chung, S.: Review of pregnancy test. South. Med. J., *74*:1387, 1981.
27. Das, S.: Pregnancy in a patient with the negative pregnancy tests and hyperprolactinemia. Am. J. Obstet. Gynecol., *138*:590, 1980.
28. Elkins, R.: Merits and disadvantages of different labels and methods of immunoassay.

In Immunoassays for the 80's. Edited by A. Voller, A. Bartlet, and D. Bidwel. Baltimore, University Park Press, p. 5, 1981.
29. Shimizu, S., Present, W., Sevier, E., Wang, R., and Sanders, R.: Choriogonadotropin measures by use of monoclonal antibodies in a two-site immunoradiometric assay. Clin. Chem., *28*:546, 1982.
30. Hirsh, J.: Routine pregnancy testing: Is it a standard of care? South. Med. J., *73*:1365, 1980.
31. Thompson, R., Mayo, R., and Bell, W.: A critical evaluation of pregnancy tests. Am. J. Clin. Pathol., *35*:585, 1965.
32. Derman, R., Corson, S., Horwitz, C., Lau, H., and Soderstrom, R.: Early diagnosis of pregnancy. J. Reprod. Med., *26*:149, 1981.
33. Horwitz, C., and Lee, C.: Pregnancy testing. Postgrad. Med., *63*:145, 193, 1978.
34. Biesecker, J., and Rippey, J.: Performances of urine pregnancy tests on College of American Pathologists survey specimens. Am. J. Clin. Pathol., *76*(supplement):543, 1981.
35. Morrow, C., et al.: Clinical laboratory correlates of pregnancy and trophoblastic disease. Am. J. Obstet. Gynecol., *128*:424, 1977.
36. BiPietro, D.: Ectopic pregnancy: Interpreting hCG levels. Lab Management, Nov., 1981.
37. Kadar, N., Caldwell, B., and Romero, R.: A method of screening for ectopic pregnancy and its indications. Obstet. Gynecol., *58*:162, 1981.
38. Lindstedt, G., Janson, O., and Thorburn, J.: Sensitivity of serum chorionic gonadotropin assay for ectopic pregnancy. Lancet, *1*:781, 1981.

CHORIONIC GONADOTROPIN

METHOD. Wampole latex-inhibition β-hCG slide test, qualitative and quantitative.

PRINCIPLE. The test is based on the lack of agglutination of chorionic gonadotropin (hCG antigen)-coated white latex particles by anti-hCG when hCG is present in the test urine; when no hCG is present in urine, there is agglutination.

SAMPLE. For the quantitative procedure, collect an accurately timed and measured 24-hour urine sample. For the qualitative procedure, collect first morning urine and save 10 ml. (Specific gravity of the specimen should be greater than 1.010, or osmolality should be over 500 mmol/kg.) Specimens should be tested within 12 hours of collection, and they should be refrigerated in the meantime.

PROCEDURE. Test a negative control, using normal male urine, and a positive control, using urine from patients known to be pregnant, preferably those whose duration of pregnancy is between 50 and 90 days, with each group of unknowns.

Qualitative Procedure

1. Place 1 drop of urine in the circle on the test slide (well cleaned) with a disposable pipette.
2. Add 1 drop of UCG antiserum (antibody).
3. Mix well with applicator stick and rock slide gently for 30 seconds.
4. Add 1 drop of thoroughly shaken UCG slide test latex-coated antigen.
5. Mix well with applicator stick, spreading over an area about 1¼ inches in diameter.

6. Rock slide gently and slowly so the urine-antiserum-antigen mixture barely moves on the slide.
7. Observe for agglutination under fluorescent lighting for no longer than 2 minutes after mixing.

QUANTITATIVE TEST (NOT OFTEN USED)

1. Record volume of 24-hour urine.
2. Withdraw 2 ml sample and make the following dilutions with saline: 1:2, 1:8, 1:16, 1:32, 1:64, 1:128, 1:256, 1:512.
3. Test 1 drop of each dilution on the slide as in the qualitative method.
4. The endpoint is the reciprocal of the highest dilution in which there is no agglutination (for example, no agglutination at 1:8, and agglutination at 1:16, indicates an endpoint of 8).
5. Calculation:
   IU/24 hours = (Volume urine (ml) × (Dilution endpoint) × Sensitivity listed on brochure with each lot; IU/ml)

INTERPRETATION

QUALITATIVE TEST. Positive test—no agglutination within 2 minutes.

QUANTITATIVE TEST. First trimester pregnancy (35 to 100 days)—agglutination in dilutions 1:8 to 1:16, but may be as high as 1:64.

DISCUSSION AND CLINICAL SIGNIFICANCE. The assay is set by manufacturer to detect as little as 0.5 IU hCG/ml of urine. This level of hCG is usually reached by > 10 days after the first missed menses (or about 40 days after onset of last menstrual period). Negative tests prior to 40 days after the last menstrual period should be repeated in 1 week before being interpreted as ruling out pregnancy. Hydatidiform mole and chorionepithelioma (uterine and testicular) usually yield positive test results. Titers greater than 1:64 suggest a pathologic condition. Tests yielding a titer of 1:128 between 60 and 120 days following the onset of the LMP should be repeated 20 days later. A continued high titer suggests hyperpituitarism, chorionepithelioma, or hydatidiform mole. A titer higher than 1:64 prior to 60 days or after 120 days also suggests pathologic conditions, such as toxemia of pregnancy, diabetes, or Rh sensitization of female.

Warning: The kit contains sodium azide, which can be explosive in lead, copper or metallic plumbing! When disposing of reagents, flush with large volumes of water.

MATERIALS.

1. Wampole UCG Slide Test Kit (Wampole Laboratories, Cranbury, N.J. 08512).

REFERENCES

1. Hutcheson, W., Schwartz, H., and Bates, H.: A simple slide pregnancy test with the use of an immunological technique. Am. J. Obstet. Gynecol., 89:70, 1964.

2. Thompson, R., Mayo, R., and Bell, W.: A critical evaluation of pregnancy tests. Am. J. Clin. Pathol., *35*:585, 1965.
3. Wampole Brochure on test.

CHORIONIC GONADOTROPIN

METHOD. Pregnosticon Wide-Gemzell hemagglutination-inhibition procedure, slightly modified by Organon.

PRINCIPLE. The test is based on an antigen-antibody reaction between human gonadotropin and rabbit antiserum. When the antiserum is mixed with erythrocytes sensitized with hCG, the erythrocytes agglutinate. If hCG-containing urine is mixed with the antiserum in a previous step, the antibody is bound to antigen, agglutination of erythrocytes fails to occur, and the erythrocytes settle to the bottom of a test tube in a characteristic ring-shaped pattern.

SAMPLE. For the quantitative procedure, collect an accurately timed and measured 24-hour urine sample. For the qualitative procedure, collect at least 50 ml of a first voided morning urine.

PROCEDURE. Test negative controls using normal male urine and the positive controls using urine from patients known to be pregnant, preferably those whose duration of pregnancy is between 50 and 90 days.

Qualitative Test

1. Filter sample of urine to be tested. Discard the first few milliliters of filtrate and retain the following 25 to 50 ml for testing.
2. Pipette 4.0 ml of buffer into vial of erythrocytes and shake.
3. Break off neck of ampul containing dried serum (scoring is not necessary) and place ampul in mirrored rack.
4. Pipette 0.1 ml of filtered urine into ampul of dried serum and mix by flicking with finger.
5. Within 5 minutes, pipette 0.4 ml erythrocyte suspension into ampul containing serum and urine.
6. Shake rack gently to achieve thorough mixing and place where it will not be disturbed by vibration or heat.
7. Read endpoint 2 hours later.

Quantitative Test.

1. Collect accurately timed 24-hour urine and record volume.
2. Filter about a 50-ml aliquot of urine into a clean, dry container.
3. Make serial dilutions of 1:10, 1::100, and 1:500 by mixing 1 ml filtered urine with 9 ml diluent (1:10). Then mix 1 ml of this dilution with 9 ml diluent (1:100). Finally, mix 2 ml of this dilution with 8 ml of diluent (1:500).
4. Perform procedure as a qualitative test (steps 2 though 5).

INTERPRETATION.

Qualitative Test. If the test is positive, a clearcut brown ring will appear on the bottom of the ampul; if negative, a diffuse yellow-brown sediment will appear.

An ill-defined, unbroken brown ring indicates that sedimentation has been disturbed and the test should be repeated. The density of the color of the ring is roughly proportional to the amount of hCG present.

QUANTITATIVE TEST. Report quantitative hCG content as the value of the range between greatest positive dilution and next negative dilution multiplied by the sensitivity factor printed on the test package (usually about 750 IU/L). For example:

Greatest possible dilution factor (1 in 10 dils, factor = 10)
Next negative dilution factor (1 in 100 dils, factor = 100)

CALCULATION.

$$IU/L = 10 \times 75 = 750 \text{ AND}$$
$$100 \times 75 = 7500$$

So, hCG range = 750 to 7500 IU/L. (Other dilutions between 1:10 and 1:100 could be used to determine the range more precisely if desired.)

DISCUSSION AND CLINICAL SIGNIFICANCE. This immunologic test is very sensitive and is able to detect about 0.7 IU/ml chorionic gonadotropin or pituitary gonadotropin, including some biologically inactive gonadotropins. (A positive test thus occurs when the hCG titer is 700 to 1400 IU/24-hour specimen (assuming a 24-hour volume of 1000 to 2000 ml). A positive test result caused by pituitary gonadotropin may occur in menopausal women and in certain normal males or after injury to or removal of gonads. Positive tests caused by hCG also occur in patients with choriocarcinoma (male and female) and hydatidiform mole. The test may remain positive after delivery or abortion for about a week. Because of its sensitivity, the test is potentially useful in detecting ectopic pregnancy.

Dirty pipettes, detergent, sunlight, heat (100° C for 1 hour may inactivate hCG, but Pregnosticon test usually still yields positive results), bacterial growth in urine, extreme pH shifts, adsorption of hCG to filter paper (Whatman No. 4, least absorptive), and adsorption of dilute hormone to glass all may result in negative test results.

MATERIALS.

1. Pregnosticon Test Kit (Organon, Inc., Div. of Akzona Inc., West Orange, N.J. 07052).
2. Whatman No. 4 filter paper
3. Filter funnel
4. Volumetric pipette, 1 ml
5. Volumetric pipette, 5 ml
6. Volumetric pipette, 10 ml

REFERENCES

1. Organon brochure on test.
2. Rag, G., et al.: Two-hour immunodiagnostic pregnancy test. Curr. Ther. Res., 5:273, 1963.

3. Wide, L., and Gemzell, C.: An immunologic pregnancy test. Acta Endocrinol., *35*:261, 1960.

CHORIONIC GONADOTROPIN

METHOD. Wampole hemagglutination-inhibition β-hCG tube test, qualitative and quantitative.

PRINCIPLE. In the presence of human chorionic gonadotropin (hCG) antiserum, red blood cells coated with hCG will agglutinate and settle out to form a mat of cells on the bottom of a test tube. When hCG in the urine of pregnant women is added to this system, inhibition of the combination of coated cells and antibody takes place. A visual endpoint of a "doughnut" pattern of cells, equivalent to that seen in the control, is a positive pregnancy test. The urine of nonpregnant women, containing no hCG, does not inhibit the hemagglutination reaction, and a mat of cells with or without a faint ring then develops in a negative pregnancy test.

PROCEDURE.

QUALITATIVE TEST

1. Remove and discard cap from the UCG-BETA STAT REAGENT test tube and place the tube into test tube holder.
2. Pipet 0.1 ml of urine specimen into UCG-BETA STAT REAGENT tube.
3. Using dropper supplied, expel two (2) drops of diluent into UCG-BETA STAT REAGENT tube.
4. Tap or vortex the tube until the freeze-dried reagent is completely mixed with the liquid. DO NOT MIX BY INVERSION OF TUBE.
5. Place test tube back into test tube holder and leave undisturbed at room temperature for 60 minutes. *Test results must be read no later than 75 minutes.* Positive urine is often readable within 35 to 40 minutes. Do not report a test as negative until 60 minutes have elapsed.

QUANTITATIVE TEST

1. A quantitative estimate of the concentration of hCG in a specimen can be determined if serial doubling dilutions of urine are made using isotonic saline or distilled water. Test each dilution according to the "Qualitative Procedure."
2. The quantitative estimate of the concentration of hCG is obtained by noting the highest dilution of the specimen that gives a positive result and then taking into consideration the dilution factor and UCG-BETA STAT REAGENT sensitivity.

   Example: If last dilution to produce a positive result is 1:32, and UCG-BETA STAT REAGENT sensitivity is 0.2 IU hCG/ml, then hCG = 32 × 0.2 = 6.4 IU hCG/ml.
3. For routine quantitation of hCG levels in urine, the use of a kit

offered for this purpose, Wampole's UCG-TITRATION SET, is recommended.

On rare occasions (less than 1%), interfering factors in the urine may inhibit the formation of a ring in the control tube. It is therefore recommended that the urine be tested for pregnancy (by the qualitative test procedure), before quantitation is attempted. When found to be present, these interfering factors may be removed by dialysis or the following procedure:

1. Mix the contents of one capsule of reagent powder into approximately 5 ml of filtered, undiluted urine in a clean vial.
2. Allow to stand for 5 minutes. Clarify by filtration using a hard, retentive filter paper (S&S 576 and Whatman N. 50, for example).
3. Use this clear urine filtrate to prepare the dilutions described previously.

INTERPRETATION. After 1 hour at room temperature, the cell patterns at the bottom of the tubes are interpreted and recorded. The best way to view the cell pattern is through the bottom of the test tube. Do this by carefully lifting up the rack, then reading from the bottom, or by using the mirror under the UCG test rack holder. Results are positive when the pattern in both the control and patient tubes are comparable. Positive—"doughnut" or ring pattern; Negative—no specific or mat pattern.

DISCUSSION AND CLINICAL SIGNIFICANCE. The assay is set by the manufacturer to detect as little as 0.2 IU hCG/ml of urine. This level of hCG is usually reached by 7 to 10 days after the first missed menses (or about 40 days after onset of last menstrual period). Negative tests prior to 40 days after the last menstrual period should be repeated in 1 week before being interpreted as ruling out pregnancy. Hydatidiform mole and chorionepithelioma (uterine and testicular) usually yield positive test results. Titers greater than 1 in 64 suggest a pathologic condition. Tests yielding a titer of 1 in 128 between 60 and 120 days following the onset of the LMP should be repeated 20 days later. A continued high titer suggests hyperpituitarism, chorionepithelioma, or hydatidiform mole. A titer higher than 1 in 64 prior to 60 days or after 120 days also suggests pathologic conditions, such as toxemia of pregnancy, diabetes, or Rh sensitization of the female.

Warning: The kit contains sodium azide, which can be explosive in lead, copper, or metallic plumbing! When disposing of reagents, flush with large volumes of water.

MATERIALS AND REAGENTS

1. 0.85% (w/v) saline
2. Small funnel and filter paper (or centrifuge, if preferred)
3. Clean, detergent-free, tuberculin-type syringe (clean pipettes or calibrated droppers for delivery of ¼ ml may be used instead)

4. Test tubes, 10 × 75 mm
5. Wampole UCG BETA-STAT Kit (Wampole Laboratories, Cranbury, N.J. 08512).

REFERENCES

1. Southam, A., et al.: Evaluation of a rapid immunologic test for pregnancy. Am. J. Obstet Gynecol., 85:495, 1963.
2. Wampole UCG-BETA STAT brochure on test.

CHORIONIC GONADOTROPIN

METHOD. GammaDab β-hCG quantitative radioimmunoassay.

PRINCIPLE. The β-hCG procedure is competitive radioimmunoassay binding technique, which utilizes antibody-bound radionuclide antigen and unbound radionuclide antigen to compete for binding sites on the β-hCG antibody. The amount of radionuclide hCG "tracer" that will bind to the antibody is inversely proportional to the amount of nonradioactive hCG present in the assay system. The precipitating antiserum reagent containing the second antibody in a polymer solution is used to separate the antibody-bound radioactive hCG from unbound radioactive hCG by immunoprecipitation. The antibody-bound radioactive hCG in the precipitate is counted by a gamma radiation detector. The relative hCG values in controls and unknown samples are assessed by comparison with a calibrator.

SPECIMEN. Collect a venous blood sample by red top tube (without additives) and allow to coagulate at room temperature; separate the serum by centrifugation. Patient samples are stable 48 hours at 2° to 8° C and may be stored frozen for up to 3 months. (EDTA or heparinized plasma samples are known to depress hCG values; hemolyzed, lipemic, or icteric samples may interfere with the assay. Remove any visible particles by centrifugation before assay.) If the specimen has been frozen, be sure to completely thaw and mix before performing the assay.

PROCEDURE.

1. Allow all reagents to reach room temperature, 22° to 25° C, and mix well by vortexing without foaming.
2. Label polypropylene test tubes in duplicate according to the following scheme.
   1&2—hCG calibrator, 25 mIU/ml
   3&4—Positive control, which is your third level serum control
   5&6—Negative control
   The remainder of the tubes are your patient unknowns in duplicate.
3. Add to the appropriate tubes in duplicate using Oxford pipette:
   a. 200 μL of the 25 mIU/ml calibrator.
   b. 200 μL of each control and sample.
4. Add 100 μL of blue radioactive hCG tracer to all tubes.

5. Add 100 μL of red rabbit anti-β-hCG serum to all tubes. Mix reagents by vortexing each tube at a low speed.
6. Incubate tubes 45 minutes at room temperature.
7. Add 1 ml of precipitating antiserum to all tubes.
8. Mix by vortexing at low speed. To ensure a homogeneous mixture, stir the precipitating antiserum reagent continuously or hand swirl every 10 to 15 pipettings.
9. Incubate tubes 5 minutes at room temperature.
10. Centrifuge all tubes at 22° to 25° C for 15 minutes at full speed of centrifuge.
11. Decant by gently inverting all tubes once, preferably at the same time, discarding the supernatants into a radioactive waste container or down the drain. Keeping the tubes inverted, place them on absorbent paper for blotting. To facilitate removal of remaining droplets, tap the rims of the tubes on the paper gently. Allow tubes to drain for about 30 seconds.
12. Count all tubes for 1 minute in a gamma counter with the window suitably adjusted for ^{125}Iodine.
13. Compare results.
14. Record the counts per minute (CPM).
15. Average the CPM bound for the calibrator tubes. Calculate the indeterminate range from 95% to 105% of the calibrator average CPM.
16. Compare the CPM bound for each sample with the range calculated previously.

INTERPRETATION

For samples with CPM less than 95% of the calibrator CPM, the test is positive for pregnancy (after other conditions are excluded).

For samples with CPM greater than 105% of the calibrator CPM, the test is negative for pregnancy.

Samples with CPM between 95% and 105% of the calibrator CPM are indeterminate with respect to pregnancy. hCG values found in this range are typically 15 to 35 mIU/ml and may result from early stages of pregnancy or abnormal elevations of hCG. (A retest done on a second serum sample obtained 48 hours later is recommended in the latter case.)

LIMITATIONS OF PROCEDURE

1. The components supplied in the kit are intended for use as an integral plot. Do not mix lot numbers, and do not use beyond expiration date.
2. Reagents should be stored at 2° to 6° C. After removing reagents from the refrigerator, they should be allowed to equilibrate to room temperature before pipetting.
3. Mix all standards and controls before pipetting. Mix reagents in the assay tubes by carefully vortexing each tube. Also, be sure to

stir precipitating antiserum continuously or by hand every 10 to 15 pipettings.
4. Patients samples are stable 48 hours at 2° to 6° C and may be frozen for up to 3 months. Thaw samples at room temperature and mix well before pipetting. Do not thaw samples in a 37° C waterbath.
5. Do not use samples that have anticoagulants in them, such as EDTA or heparin. These anticoagulants are known to depress hCG values. Hemolyzed, lipemic, or icteric samples may interfere with the assay.
6. Be sure to blot tubes adequately following decantation. Improper blotting may cause poor replication and spurious values.
7. Sensitivity of this test is calculated to be at 2 mIU/ml.

DISCUSSION AND CLINICAL SIGNIFICANCE. In pregnant women, an increase in serum hCG levels occurs approximately 21 days after the last menstrual period (LMP), hCG levels reach a peak 8 weeks post LMP, and decline to lower values for the remainder of the pregnancy.

Healthy men and nonpregnant women have nondetectable or barely detectable levels of hCG in serum. Tests have shown approximately 90% of normal men, 80% of nonpregnant women, have hCG levels below 5 mIU/ml. Elevated levels of β-hCG are sometimes seen in patients with malignant disease.

Human chorionic gonadotropin (hCG) is a glycoprotein produced by the placenta shortly after implantation of the embryo into the uterine wall. The level of hCG in maternal serum increases nearly exponentially, and then drops to a plateau for the remainder of pregnancy. Normal variation of hCG levels in the third trimester is considerable, making other hormones such as estriol more useful for monitoring late pregnancy. hCG is detectable by radioimmunoassay prior to the onset of clinical symptoms of pregnancy. Radioimmunoassay provides a sensitive and specific technique allowing early detection of pregnancy about 7 days after the first missed menses.

Because of structural similarities among the subunits of human hormones, hCG, luteinizing hormone (LH), follicle stimulating hormone (FSH), and thyroid stimulating hormone (TSH), the primary antiserum used in the hCG radioimmunoassay should demonstrate low cross reactivity to these subunits.

If the qualitative assay is negative, pregnancy should not be ruled out. Either drawing and testing a second serum sample at least 48 hours later or repeat testing of the same sample in a quantitative test may aid in the detection of early pregnancy. The quantitative assay may also aid in the detection of ectopic pregnancy, threatened abortion, or other conditions associated with low but detectable hCG levels.

MATERIAL AND REAGENTS

1. GammaDab (^{125}I) hCG Radioimmunoassay Kit. hCG standards and

control are calibrated to the World Health Organization's immunoassay standard, the First International Reference Preparation (1975) and labeled in milli-International units per ml. One hCG control is provided in the kit. The nomimal value is 60 ± 12.0 mIU/ml (Clinical Assays, Division of Travenol Laboratories, Cambridge, Mass. 02139).

The following is a list of other reagents contained in the kit:
One vial of radioactive hCG tracer, 8 mc at calibration; 13 ml.
One vial rabbit anti-β-hCG serum; 13 ml
One vial β-hCG nonspecific binding reagent; 1 ml
One bottle precipitating antiserum reagent; 65 ml
One vial hCG control, 60 mIU/ml; 10 ml
One vial hCG blank, 0 mIU/ml; 10 ml
Five vials hCG standard, calibrated at 5, 10, 50, 100, 200 mIU/ml; 2 ml of each
One vial hCG calibrator/standard, calibrated at 25 mIU/ml; 6 ml

All these reagents are stored at 2° to 6° C until used. Kit must be warmed to room temperature before using. Do not use after expiration date.

2. Test tube rack
3. Polypropylene test tubes, disposable, 12 × 75 mm
4. Precision pipette, 100, 200, and 1000 ml
5. Vortex mixer
6. Magnetic mixer
7. Spin bar (optional)
8. Gamma counter for ^{125}I gamma radiation detector
9. Plastic-backed absorbent paper

REFERENCES

1. Henry, J.: Clinical Diagnosis and Management by Laboratory Methods. 16th Edition. Philadelphia, W.B. Saunders, p. 680, 1979.
2. Tietz, N.W.: *Fundamentals of Clinical Chemistry*. 2nd Edition. Philadelphia, W.B. Saunders, p. 707, 1976.
3. Human Chorionic Gonadotropin (hCG), in Rx: RIA for Physicians, 2, August 1977.
4. Hunt, W.B.: Population Report, J, J-109, 1975.
5. GammaDab brochure.

Chapter 6 Synovial-Fluid Analysis

DONALD C. CANNON
ALVIN J. MATHEWS

In paleopathology (a term popularized by Sir Marc Armand Ruffin in the 19th century), diseases of the joints are probably the oldest of all human diseases studied. Fossils of the "Ape Man" of the Pliocene Period (some 2 million years ago), of the Java Man, the Lansing Man (500,000 years ago), the Egyptian mummies, and the pre-Columbian Indians have all revealed some pathologic changes of chronic joint diseases.[1] Physicians in antiquity recorded observations and theories related to joint diseases.[2] Hippocrates (460 to 377 B.C.) penned references to gout, but he did not distinguish the multiple etiologies and clinical syndromes of joint diseases. Also, Hippocrates had probably unknowingly observed gonococcal arthritis, as evidenced by this statement in Aphorisms: "A young man does not take gout until he indulges in coition."[3] The Babylonian Talmud, written from the second to the sixth century B.C., discusses reduction of joint dislocation by the uman (professional surgeon). In the first century A.D., Cornelius Celsus unknowingly described rheumatic fever when he associated nosebleeds, headaches, and joint pains. Celsus, a medical, military, and agricultural genius, was best noted for his description of inflammation (rubor et tumor cum calor et dolor [redness and swelling with heat and pain]), which is still taught in medical curricula today! A callus has been found in an arm bone of a reptile of the Paleozoic Permian period. Arthritis in dinosaurs and prehistoric animals was so common that early scholars coined the term "cave gout." Even the Neanderthal Man of 40,000 to 70,000 years ago, had evidence of advanced arthritis, apparently accounting for the bended knees and rounded spine in the skeleton of this earliest Homo sapiens, discovered in 1856.

Judging by the tenets of the present, we have been able to understand these diseases; although this precept may have led to erroneous concepts about early man's "cults of healing," not all beneficial acts were "good medicine." Included among Celsus' recommended therapies for arthritis were the application of heat, skin cautery, and an ointment composed of the rinds of poppy seeds boiled in oil and mixed with wax salve made of rose oil.[2] Guillaume de Baillou first applied the name of rheumatism to acute arthritis, in 1570. Thomas Sydenham (1624–1689) was the first physician known to have distinguished gout from other types of acute and chronic arthritides. In 1782, William Heberden described the arthritic nodules of degenerative joint disease, which were observed arising from bone-spur formation at the articular margins of the distal interphalangeal joints of the fingers.

Theophrastus Bombastus von Hohenheim, who, as noted in Chapter 2, renamed himself Phillipus Aureolus Paracelsus, after the master Celsus, actually coined the term synovial fluid (etymologically derived from the Greek "syn" meaning "with" or "associated with" and the Latin ovum meaning "egg"). This derivation was prompted by the resemblance of joint fluid to uncoagulated egg albumin.

In spite of the medical interest in joint afflictions over the course of many centuries, relatively little attention was devoted to synovial-fluid analysis until the mid-20th century. In 1930, Walter Bauer and coworkers reported the first of many studies on synovial fluid, initially using young cattle, and later human beings.[4] Their work culminated in the classic monograph of Marian Ropes and Walter Bauer in 1953, Synovial Fluid Changes in Joint Disease, which firmly established the value of synovial fluid analysis in medical diagnosis and thus led to general acceptance of the laboratory analysis of joint fluid.[5] Although Alfred Baring Garrod in 1848 had suggested that uric-acid crystals could be responsible for the acute inflammation of gout, it was not until 1961 that Daniel McCarty and Joseph Hollander first conclusively identified uric-acid crystals in the synovial fluid of gouty arthritis.[6,7] In the following year, positive identification of calcium pyrophosphate crystals in the synovial fluid of some arthritic patients allowed recognition of the pseudogout syndrome, clearly distinguishing the syndrome from gout.[8] This report is of even greater significance in that it emphasized the importance of polarizing microscopy in crystal identification. Synovial-fluid analysis continues to have an expanding role in the diagnosis of joint diseases.

STRUCTURAL-FUNCTIONAL RELATIONSHIPS OF JOINTS

There are basically two types of joints: *synarthroses* and *diarthroses*. Synarthroses are characterized by little or no movement, the articulating bones being directly connected with other bone (synostosis), cartilage (synchondrosis), or fibrous tissue (syndesmosis).

Diarthroses permit considerably freer movement of the articulating bones because of the presence of a joint cavity (a schematic illustration of a diarthrodial joint is shown in Fig. 6–1). The joint cavity is enclosed by a dense, fibrous-tissue investment, which is lined on its inner surface by synovial membrane. The synovial membrane is reflected from the joint capsule to cover the otherwise exposed bone within the joint cavity and meshes with the perichondrium of the articular cartilage. Numerous folds can be present in the synovial membrane to accommodate joint movement. The articulating bone surfaces of diarthrodial joints are covered with hyaline cartilage. The outer surface of the articular cartilages is free of synovial covering but continuous with the synovium at the cartilagenous margins. To provide greater strength and stability, most diarthrodial joints contain an assortment of ligaments, which are covered by synovial membrane, menisci, and intra-articular disks (the latter of which are free of synovial investment except at their peripheral surfaces).

In contrast to articular cartilage, which is free of both blood vessels and lymphatics, the synovial membrane is highly vascular, as would be expected from its primary functions of secretion and waste removal. In addition to lining joints and the associated intra-articular structures, synovial membrane also lines bursae and synovial tendon sheaths. The synovial membrane consists of a cellular layer facing the joint space and a connective-tissue backing layer that merges with the joint capsule.

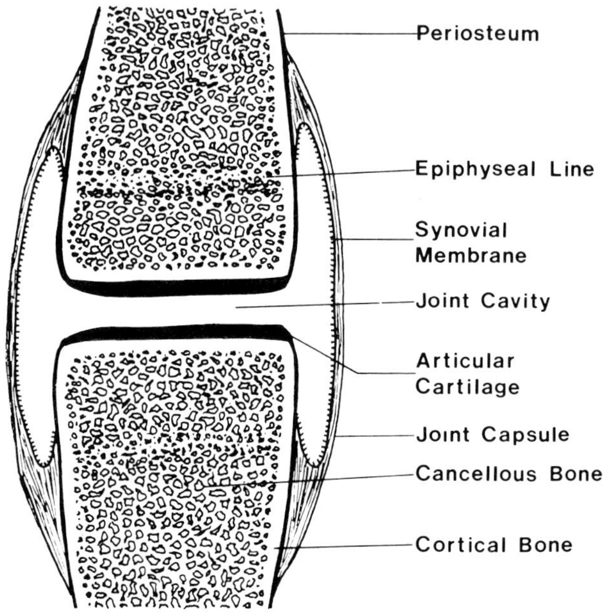

Fig. 6–1. Structure of a diarthrodial joint.

The cellular layer is composed of three morphologic types of cells: type A, type B, and intermediate type cells.[9,10]

One atypical characteristic of synovial cells is that they lack a true basement membrane, or basal lamina, such as exists for most other epithelial cell layers in the body. Type A cells have prominent Golgi complexes and many vesicles and vacuoles but minimal rough endoplasmic reticulum. Their function has been considered to be primarily phagocytic; hence, they are sometimes designated as "M cells" for macrophage activity. Recent evidence suggests, however, that the A cells also have the important function of synthesizing and secreting hyaluronic acid. Type B cells are ordinarily the most common cell type. They have abundant rough endoplasmic reticulum, a feature that is consistent with the elaboration and secretion of proteins. B cells are encased in microfibrils and thus, are sometimes referred to as "F cells," because of their resemblance to fibroblasts. Intermediate cells are aptly named because they have a rough endoplasmic reticulum and a Golgi complex. It is probable that all three cell types have both secretory and phagocytic functions and that they are functional variants of a common cell type.

CHEMICAL COMPOSITION OF SYNOVIAL FLUID

Synovial fluid is a dialysate of blood plasma altered by the addition of hyaluronic acid from the active secretion of the synovial cells. The result is a clear, pale-yellow viscous fluid, which has three major functions:

1. Lubrication of the joint surfaces
2. Nutrition of the intra-articular joint structures
3. Removal of waste material, both metabolic waste and detritus, which is carried to the synovial membrane for phagocytosis.

Electrolytes are distributed between blood plasma and synovial fluid essentially in accord with the Donnan equilibrium, while nonelectrolytes have basically equal concentrations in the two fluids, except for those that are readily metabolized by cells and tissues (glucose, for example). The chemical composition of synovial fluid has been the subject of recent comprehensive reviews.[10–11]

Hyaluronic acid is a nonsulfated polysaccharide polymer composed largely of 2-acetamido-2-deoxy-3-0-β-D-glucopyranosyluronic acid-D-glucose linked by 1,4 β-glycosidic linkages.[11] Approximately equal amounts of D-glucuronic acid and N-acetyl-D-glucosamine are obtained by hydrolysis. The viscosity of hyaluronic acid is a consequence of both the high molecular weight of up to 10^7 daltons and its ability to form complexes of polysaccharide chains with tertiary and quaternary structures that involve interaction with adjacent chains and possibly other constituents of synovial fluid. The concentration of hyaluronic acid in joint fluid is about 0.3 g/dl.[10] In addition to hyaluronic acid, a glycoprotein that has been isolated from synovial fluid appears to play an important role in lubrication of the articular cartilage.[11] This glycoprotein has been named *LGP-1* (lubricating glycoprotein fraction 1).

The total protein concentration of synovial fluid is about 1.8 g/dl and thus, is about one-fourth that of blood serum.[10] Compared with serum, however, there are differences in the relative amounts of various proteins, which can be explained in part on the basis of differences in molecular size. This would be expected in the case of a dialysate, because it is unlikely that cells of the synovial membrane synthesize proteins in any significant amount, except for the immunoglobulins secreted by antibody-forming lymphoid and plasma cells in the various inflammatory diseases. Thus, on a relative basis, albumin is increased, as is alpha-acid glycoprotein; transferrin is present in about the same relative amount; γ- and β-2-macroglobulin, haptoglobin, ceruloplasmin, IgG, and IgM are decreased; and fibrinogen is essentially absent.[10–11] These relative amounts of proteins are greatly altered in inflammatory diseases that disrupt the semipermeable character of the synovial membrane so that large molecules can more or less freely enter the synovial fluid.

The glucose concentration of synovial fluid closely approximates that of plasma but is ordinarily less than that of plasma by no more than 10 mg/dl. This small difference in concentration probably reflects metabolic consumption of glucose by the various joint tissues. The entrance of glucose into the synovial fluid does not, however, follow the expected behavior for a freely diffusible substance.[12] Changes in the glucose concentration of normal synovial fluid lag behind those of plasma by an hour or more.

Data relating to the acid-base, lactate, and oxygen status of normal synovial fluid are not adequate to state normal ranges; a few generalizations are possible, however. The pH of normal synovial fluid appears to be about 7.3 to 7.4, and thus, is only slightly lower than that of plasma.[13] As might be expected from metabolic considerations, the lactate and pCO_2 of synovial fluid are higher than those of plasma, while the pO_2 is lower. These differences are accentuated by inflammatory diseases of the joints, which cause increased cellular metabolism.[14]

CLASSIFICATION OF JOINT DISEASES

Following the precedent set by other authors, there is some advantage to classifying joint diseases according to synovial-fluid changes.[5,12–16] These classifications are basically the same. The classification scheme shown in Table 6–1 is based on that of Frank Schmid and Roger Ogata.[12] There is considerable overlap, particularly between the group-1 (noninflammatory) and group-2 (inflammatory) diseases. Lupus erythematosus, for example, can be associated with either a noninflammatory synovial fluid transudate or a true inflammatory exudate. Rheumatoid

TABLE 6–1. Classification of Diseases with Synovial-Fluid Manifestations.*

Group 1 (noninflammatory)	Group 2 (inflammatory)	Group 3 (septic)	Group 4 (hemorrhagic)
Osteoarthritis	Rheumatoid arthritis	Pyrogenic bacteria	Trauma
Trauma	Rheumatic fever	Mycobacteria	Neuroarthropathy
Rheumatoid arthritis (early stages)	Acute gout	Fungi	Neoplasms
Gout and pseudogout (quiescent stages)	Acute pseudogout		Pigmented villo-nodular synovitis
Osteochondromatosis	Psoriatic arthritis		Scurvy
Osteochondritis dissecans	Viral arthritis		Hemophilia
Rheumatic fever	Reiter's syndrome		
Articular amyloidosis	Systemic lupus erythematosus		
Hypertrophic pulmonary osteoarthropathy	Hypertrophic pulmonary osteoarthropathy		
Systemic lupus erythematosus			
Neuroarthropathy			

*Based on Schmid and Ogata.[12]

arthritis typically causes an inflammatory involvement of the synovial fluid, but in very early stages or in the quiescent phase of chronic disease, the synovial fluid can more closely resemble a transudate.

The various categories of joint diseases can be represented by characteristic synovial-fluid manifestations.[5,12–16] There is considerable variation among the various diseases within a given category in terms of the synovial-fluid changes and also in the manifestations of a given disease based on such factors as stage and severity of the disease, superimposed diseases, and host factors. Table 6–2, therefore, represents only typical synovial-fluid changes and must not be rigidly interpreted.

SPECIMEN COLLECTION AND PREPARATION

Although some have stated that there is no absolute contraindication to diagnostic aspiration of joint fluid (arthrocentesis),[12] it is prudent not to attempt the procedure when it would necessitate passing a needle through infected skin or subcutaneous tissues.[12] In addition, great caution must be exercised in attempting arthrocentesis on any patient with a serious coagulation disorder, such as hemophilia A.

The risks of arthrocentesis are otherwise relatively slight. Minimal bleeding virtually always occurs and is seldom of any consequence. Infection is rare. Daniel McCarty, for example, states that he has never

TABLE 6–2. Typical Synovial-Fluid Findings in Joint Diseases.*

	Normal	Noninflammatory	Inflammatory	Septic	Hemorrhagic
Color	pale yellow	yellow	yellow, green, or white	grey, brown-green, bloody	bloody or xanthochromic
Turbidity	clear	clear	turbid	turbid to opaque	turbid to opaque
Viscosity	high	moderate to high	low	low to absent	variable
Fibrin clot	none	usually none	yes	yes	usually none
Mucin clot	good	fair to good	fair to good	poor	variable
Total nucleated cells (per μL)	<200	<1,000	2,000–50,000	20,000–150,000	<5,000
Polymorphonuclear leukocytes (%)	<25	<25	>50	>80	<50
Plasma-synovial fluid glucose difference (mg/dl)	<10	<10	>25	>25, often >50	<10
Microbiologic culture	negative	negative	negative	positive	negative

*Based on Schmid and Ogata.[12]

experienced an iatrogenic joint infection from percutaneous arthrocentesis in 20 years of experience with the procedure.[13]

Arthrocentesis is most frequently performed on the knee, but this merely reflects the frequency of disease involvement of this joint. Other large joints are readily accessible, however, and are frequently aspirated (hips, ankles, shoulders, elbows, and wrists, for example). Even the joints of the hands and feet can usually be aspirated without great difficulty. Arthrocentesis should be performed by a physician familiar with the technique. The conduct of the procedure in relation to anatomic features is described in detail elsewhere.[17–18]

Except for a frank explanation of the procedure, no special preparation of the patient is necessary. If glucose is to be analyzed, however, it is essential that the patient be fasting for at least 6 hours immediately prior to specimen collection.

Although basic sterile precautions are obviously necessary, sterile drapes and gloves are not essential.[13] The skin over the area of entry should be washed thoroughly with green surgical soap and shaved if necessary. Disinfection should proceed with tincture of iodine followed by 70% (v/v) alcohol, or use of a Frepp/Sepp skin preparation. The skin and subcutaneous tissues down to the joint capsule can be infiltrated with 2% (w/v) lidocaine (Xylocaine) using a 5-ml syringe with 25-gauge × $^1/_2$-inch needle. Usually 1 or 2 ml of lidocaine will suffice. The size of the syringe and needle will vary with the joint to be aspirated, the anticipated volume of the joint fluid, and individual preference. For the knee joint, a 10- or 20-ml plastic disposable syringe with 20-gauge × $1^1/_2$-inch or larger disposable needle will suffice.

Failure to aspirate fluid is common if the amount of fluid is not pathologically increased. Even the knee joint normally contains only about 1 ml of synovial fluid that can be aspirated.[19] Ideally, at least 10 ml of synovial fluid should be obtained. The fluid should be distributed in specimen tubes as follows:

1. Sterile heparin tube (prepared to contain 200 units of heparin, which is sufficient to anticoagulate at least 7 ml of synovial fluid). Aliquot 2 to 4 ml of synovial fluid into this tube for microbiologic cultures.
2. EDTA tube (prepared to contain 5 mg of disodium ethylenediamine tetracetate; commercially available tubes for blood collection are satisfactory). Aliquot 3 to 4 ml of synovial fluid for cell enumerations, differential cell counts, wet mounts for crystal examination and identification and for exfoliative cytology.
3. Plain tube. Aliquot 3 to 4 ml of synovial fluid for viscosity evaluation, mucin-clot test, fibrin clot test, and, if desired, complement assays.
4. Oxalate-fluoride tube (commercially available tubes for blood col-

lection are satisfactory). Aliquot 1 to 2 ml of synovial fluid for glucose determination. Glucose analytic procedures in some laboratories require other specimen preservatives because of interference of methodology by fluoride.

These recommended volumes can be scaled down in the event that only a small amount of synovial fluid is available. Protocol in various clinical laboratories varies considerably. For example, it is not only acceptable, but desirable, to inoculate microbiologic culture media directly from the aspirating syringe if it can be done immediately after aspiration so that coagulation, which frequently occurs in association with the infectious arthritides, can be avoided. The use of oxalate as an anticoagulant should be avoided (except when it is used for glucose measurement), because calcium-oxalate crystals may form, which in time, can be phagocytized by leukocytes and perhaps be confused with the crystal-deposition diseases.

INDICATIONS FOR SYNOVIAL-FLUID ANALYSIS

As with most other clinical laboratory analyses, synovial-fluid analysis usually does not provide pathognomonic information. Notable exceptions to this generalization are the bacterial arthritides that yield positive microbiologic cultures and the two major crystal deposition diseases of joints. In most cases, the results of synovial-fluid analysis must be interpreted from the perspective of a wealth of clinical information. Investigation of joint diseases often requires various radiologic studies, histopathologic interpretations of synovial biopsies or related connective tissue lesions, rheumatoid factor and antinuclear antibody studies, LE cell tests, streptococcal antibody determinations, assays of total hemolytic complement and complement factors, evaluations of erythrocyte sedimentation rates, determinations of serum uric acid and C-reactive protein, and a variety of other tests.

In general, there are four indications for performing synovial fluid analysis:

1. To diagnose joint disease, especially bacterial arthritides or diseases that are not characteristic of any of the clinical syndromes
2. To assess the degree of inflammatory activity
3. For direct therapeutic benefit, either to remove transudate, blood, or exudate from a swollen and painful joint
4. To administer medication into the joint space

ROUTINE SYNOVIAL FLUID ANALYSIS

The routine analysis of synovial fluid has never been defined, and it is not a diagnostic-test battery that has been considered in most laboratories. Many laboratories, however, have come to the conclusion that there are several procedures that are usually considered when a synovial-fluid analysis is requested by the physician. In our laboratories, we have found that most clinically relevant information can be obtained by the following procedures:

1. Color and turbidity
2. Fibrin-clot formation
3. Viscosity
4. Volume
5. Mucin-clot test
6. Microscopic evaluation of synovial fluid cells and differential cell counts
7. Morphologic description of cells
8. Crystal detection and identification

Microbiologic studies are ordered when it is suspected that infectious processes exist in the joint. In these cases, the joint fluid is aspirated with a syringe and needle and transferred directly to culture plates. The miscellaneous tests on synovial fluid occupy a special place in diagnostic testing and are not considered routine.

Color and Turbidity

Normal synovial fluid is completely transparent, pale yellow, and highly viscous. Clarity or turbidity is classically evaluated by attempting to read print through the test tube containing the unaltered specimen. In the event that spontaneous coagulation has occurred, this feature can be evaluated on the aliquot anticoagulated with EDTA. Turbidity is evaluated on a 0-to-4 + scale, with 0 being the normal state of total transparency and 4 + turbidity being such that prominent print cannot be seen at all through the specimen. The most common cause for markedly turbid specimens is increased leukocytes, whether they are associated with septic or aseptic inflammation. Crystals and bacteria also contribute to turbidity but are ordinarily accompanied by numerous leukocytes. The loss of selective permeability of the synovial membrane in inflammation results in fibrinogen exudation, so fibrin strands can occur in vivo and be evident on gross inspection. Erythrocytes will also cause turbidity but will impart a red color to the fluid unless they are present in only small numbers.

Blood in synovial fluid can vary from flecks of blood resulting from the arthrocentesis itself to gross hemorrhage. Bleeding incidental to the arthrocentesis can often be identified by observing that the blood, usually of slight amount, is unevenly distributed throughout the specimen, that the amount of blood decreases as the fluid is aspirated, or less commonly, that the blood increases as aspiration progresses because of trauma from manipulating the needle.[10] Gross hemorrhage into a joint (hemarthrosis) is most commonly a consequence of trauma but also occurs as a result of blood-coagulation disorders, particularly hemophilia A (classical hemophilia), pigmented villonodular synovitis, and neoplasms involving the joint space, which are usually metastatic.

Like cerebrospinal fluid, synovial fluid will exhibit xanthochromia after blood has been in the joint space for a number of hours. Xanthochromia is difficult to evaluate in synovial fluid, however, because of its intrinsic pale-yellow color. Conjugated bilirubin from the blood plasma appears to enter the synovial fluid freely and can cause a distinct yellow color in patients with hyperbilirubinemia.

Joint effusions associated with tuberculous arthritis can appear as xanthochromic exudates or can assume a yellow-white gelatinous appearance depending, presumably, on the duration and severity of involvement.[20] Acute gout often causes the synovial fluid to appear milky. A cloudy to frankly turbid fluid with a green hue occurs in various inflammatory diseases including rheumatoid arthritis, pseudogout, and gout.[21–22] Pyogenic arthritis typically results in a highly turbid synovial fluid that is grey-to-brown, green, or even frankly bloody.[23]

Droplets of free-floating fat frequently occur in association with bone fractures that communicate with the joint space. Fat droplets are also commonly detected in trauma that does not cause fractures, and in these cases, they presumably originate from the fat pads of the joints. In one large series, free fat was found in 85% of all hemarthroses.[24] Osteoarthritis can cause cartilaginous debris to be suspended in the synovial fluid. The finding of marrow particles in joint fluid by microscopic examination is suggestive of fracture through the articular surface.[24]

Rice bodies are aptly named because of their similarity, in terms of size, shape, and color, to grains of polished rice. They have been found in various types of arthritides, including juvenile and adult rheumatoid arthritis as well as tuberculous and pyogenic infections.[25] Rice bodies represent a nonspecific response to inflammation and probably arise from microinfarction of the synovium. They are predominantly composed of fibrin with smaller amounts of collagen, but blood vessels can be detected.[26]

Fibrin-Clot Formation

Because fibrinogen is excluded by the semipermeable nature of the intact synovial membrane, normal synovial fluid will not coagulate either spontaneously or upon the addition of thrombin. Increased permeability of the synovial membrane is related to the severity of inflammatory involvement and thus to the amount of fibrinogen exudation. Fibrin clots can be evaluated on a 0-to-4+ scale on which

1. 0 represents normal fluid without any fibrin.
2. 1+ represents the specimen with fibrin strands.
3. 2+ represents the presence of a definite but small fibrin clot comprising less than 10% (v/v) of the specimen volume.

4. 3+ represents a larger clot comprising 10 to 50% (v/v) of the specimen volume.
5. 4+ represents a clot comprising 50 to 100% (v/v) of the volume.

It may be trite to remind the reader that observation for fibrin-clot formation must be conducted on a specimen without added anticoagulant, but we have seen this happen more than once. In general, the larger the eventual clot, the sooner coagulation will occur. A specimen with other findings of inflammation, such as decreased viscosity, turbidity, and increased cell count, should be observed for at least 4 hours at room temperature before being designated as negative for fibrin-clot formation.

Viscosity

Viscosity is dependent upon both the concentration and physicochemical state of hyaluronic acid. It can be readily evaluated by expelling drops of synovial fluid from a Pasteur pipette. Normal viscosity is such that the fluid will create a string that is at least 4 cm and often up to 10 cm or more, in length. Virtual loss of viscosity is reflected in a specimen that readily allows discrete drops to form. Although viscosity can be precisely measured with instruments such as an Ostwald viscometer, this is not warranted for routine diagnostic purposes.

Decreased viscosity typically accompanies joint inflammation and thus is a characteristic of many joint afflictions from rheumatoid arthritis and gout to septic arthritis.

Volume

Measurement of specimen volume, even when the joint space is maximally evacuated, has no diagnostic significance. It is common for experienced physicians to obtain only a few drops of synovial fluid or even none at all from arthrocentesis of a joint. Marian Ropes, Elsie Rossmeisl, and Walter Bauer studied the knee joints of 124 normal human volunteers and were able to aspirate an average volume of only 1.1 ml with a range of 0.13 to 3.5 ml.[19]

Mucin-Clot Test

The mucin-clot test is frequently referred to by the eponym, "Ropes test," after Marian Ropes, who described a "ropey" precipitate of mucin when normal synovial fluid was added to dilute acetic acid.[27] The coagulum that forms is not, however, mucin, but it does have a mucinous appearance. This observation was not original with Marian Ropes and co-workers, who indeed noted that Frerichs had described the phenomenon in 1846.

As with synovial-fluid viscosity, the mucin-clot test is a reflection of the concentration and physicochemical state of hyaluronic acid, particularly its degree of polymerization. Results of the two tests almost always parallel each other, and some investigators feel that the mucin-clot test is superfluous.[22] One situation in which a discrepancy can occur between the results of the mucin clot test and viscosity determination is acute noninflammatory serous effusion of the joint, which causes dilution of the synovial fluid so that viscosity is reduced but mucin-clot formation is qualitatively unaltered albeit quantitatively reduced.

Various procedures have been described for the mucin-clot test. Recommended acetic-acid concentrations have ranged from 2% to 5% (v/v) and the amount of specimen from a few drops to 1.0 ml. As a matter of fact neither the strength of acetic acid nor the volume ratio between the specimen and acetic acid is critical. The quality of mucin clot is evaluated descriptively—that is, good, fair, poor—or semiquantitatively on a 0 to 4+ scale. With the latter, a 4+ clot represents a tight ropey or mucinous coagulum (Fig. 6–2A) while 0 represents a turbid white suspension of small granular particles (Fig. 6–2B).

As with viscosity determination, diminished mucin-clot formation occurs as a result of inflammatory joint diseases. The test is nonspecific.

Microscopic Examination of Synovial-Fluid Cell Counts

Cells in synovial fluid can be readily enumerated in much the same manner as in blood. The usual red and white-blood-cell diluting fluids cannot be used, however, because they contain acetic acid, which will precipitate hyaluronic acid. A suitable diluent is physiologic saline to which methylene blue dye is added to a concentration of 0.1% (w/v). This stains cell nuclei and thus facilitates cell identification. The erythrocytes in specimens containing abundant blood can be readily lysed by using either a hypotonic diluent such as 0.3% (w/v) saline or the 1% (w/v) saponin solution used in hematologic studies.[28] Care must be taken to mix the specimen thoroughly with a suitable mechanical mixer prior to aliquoting because the viscosity of synovial fluid can cause an uneven distribution of cells. (The EDTA-anticoagulated specimen is drawn to the 0.5 mark in a white-blood-cell pipette and diluted to the 11 mark for a 1:20 dilution. Both chambers of a hemacytometer, preferably one with improved Neubauer ruling, are filled. The leukocytes in the four large corner squares of each chamber (a total of 8 mm^2) are then counted. The total number of cells is then multiplied by 25 to determine the cell concentration per μL.)

There is little if anything to be gained from counting the erythrocytes. In some cases, it is desirable to perform a microhematocrit to estimate the amount of blood. In the event that exceptionally high leukocyte counts are anticipated, the specimen can be initially diluted 1:10 to

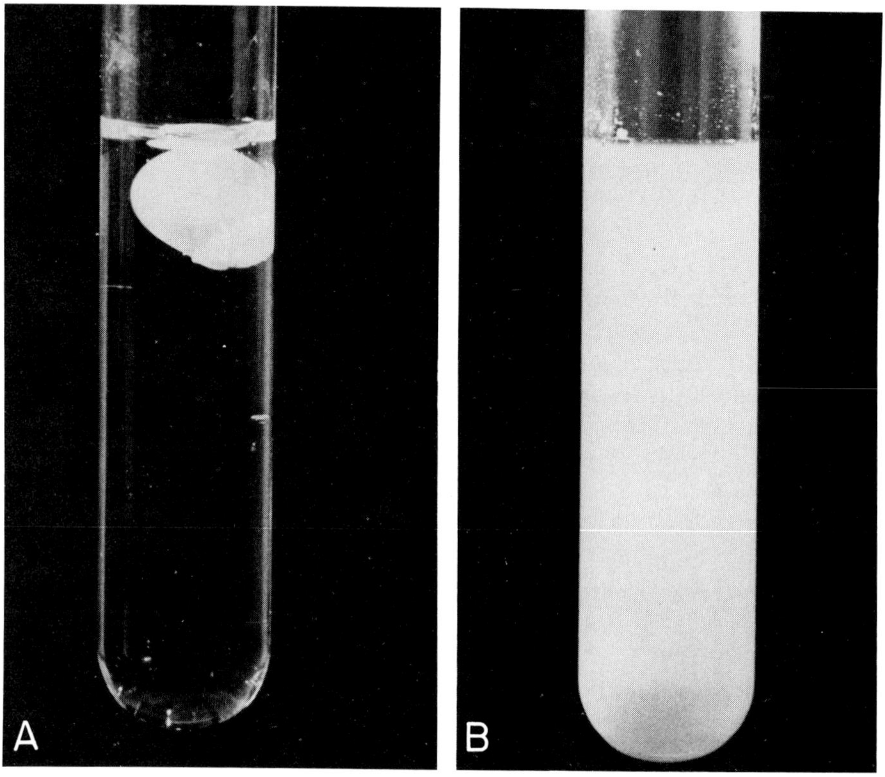

Fig. 6–2. Mucin-clot test. **A,** Normal result showing a tight mucinous clot. **B,** Markedly abnormal result consisting of granular particles suspended in a turbid medium.

1:100 with physiologic saline prior to filling the white-blood-cell pipette.

Data related to cell counts are relatively sparse. The normal total nucleated cell count is frequently stated to be less than 200/μL, but this appears to be more an approximation than a rigorous interpretation of data. Howard Coggeshall, Charles Warren, and Walter Bauer in 1940 reported the nucleated cell counts of 29 normal humans and found a range of 13 to 180/μL with a mean of 63/μL.[29] Although some investigators have characterized the various categories of joint diseases as if rigid distinctions can be made on the basis of nucleated cell counts, others have correctly indicated the considerable overlap that exists, particularly between aseptic inflammatory diseases such as rheumatoid arthritis, gout, pseudogout, and the infectious arthritides.[10,12–14] Probably the most extensive study of synovial-fluid leukocytosis is that of Phoebe Krey and David Bailen, who studied 378 specimens from 310 patients.[30] In 50 patients with culture-proven bacterial arthritis, they found a range of 6,100 to 284,000/μL with a mean of 87,000/μL. There were no appreciable differences in numbers of leukocytes with various bacterial etiologies—that is, Neisseria gonorrhoeae, staphylococcus species, streptococcus species, and gram-negative bacilli. This same study included 124 specimens from 76 patients with rheumatoid arthritis, 67% of which had cell counts between 2,500 and 25,000/μL while only 4% had cell counts between 50,000 and 100,000/μL. Furthermore, of 126 specimens from 113 patients with gout, 44% had cell counts between 2,500 to 25,000/μL. Although the leukocyte count varies considerably in tuberculous arthritis, it is usually in the range of 10,000 to 20,000/μL.[20] Data are very sparse regarding the synovial fluid manifestations of arthritis associated with various viral diseases, such as rubella, varicella, and hepatitis B. Apparently, leukocyte counts are usually in the range of 1,000 to 10,000/μL.[10] The cell counts in noninflammatory joint effusions are usually less than 1,000/μL and virtually never exceed 5,000/μL.[10]

Differential Cell Counts

The differential count of leukocytes can be performed in much the same manner as for blood. The EDTA-anticoagulated specimen that remains after the total cell count should be centrifuged, and the sediment resuspended in the few drops of synovial fluid remaining in the tube after the supernatant fluid is decanted. A drop is then placed on a microscope slide and smeared as in the preparation of a peripheral blood smear. The smear should be relatively thin, because not only will hyaluronic acid interfere with optimal staining, it can also cause artifactual distortion of the cells as drying occurs. The smear can be stained with Wright's stain or Wright-Giemsa stain.

In normal synovial fluids, polymorphonuclear leukocytes will constitute fewer than 25% of the nucleated cells with the remainder being composed of lymphocytes, monocytes, and macrophages. Synovial cells that either have been sloughed into the fluid as a consequence of cell senescence or dislocated by the unavoidable trauma of arthrocentesis will also occur. Clumps of synovial cells are often seen (Fig. 6–3). As is characteristic of the inflammatory reaction in other tissues and body fluids, polymorphonuclear leukocytes increase more or less proportionally to both the acuteness and severity of the inflammatory stimulus. Consequently, pyogenic bacterial infections of the joint are usually associated with an increase in polymorphonuclear leukocytes so that they constitute more than 90% of all nucleated cells. Partly as a reflection of its slower onset and more chronic nature, tuberculous arthritis is associated with a preponderance of polymorphonuclear leukocytes, but they uncommonly exceed 90% of the total nucleated cells.[20] Polymorphonuclear leukocytes usually predominate in rheumatoid arthritis and in the arthritides of rheumatic fever, gout, pseudogout, and Reiter's syndrome.[10] Even large effusions of a noninflammatory nature

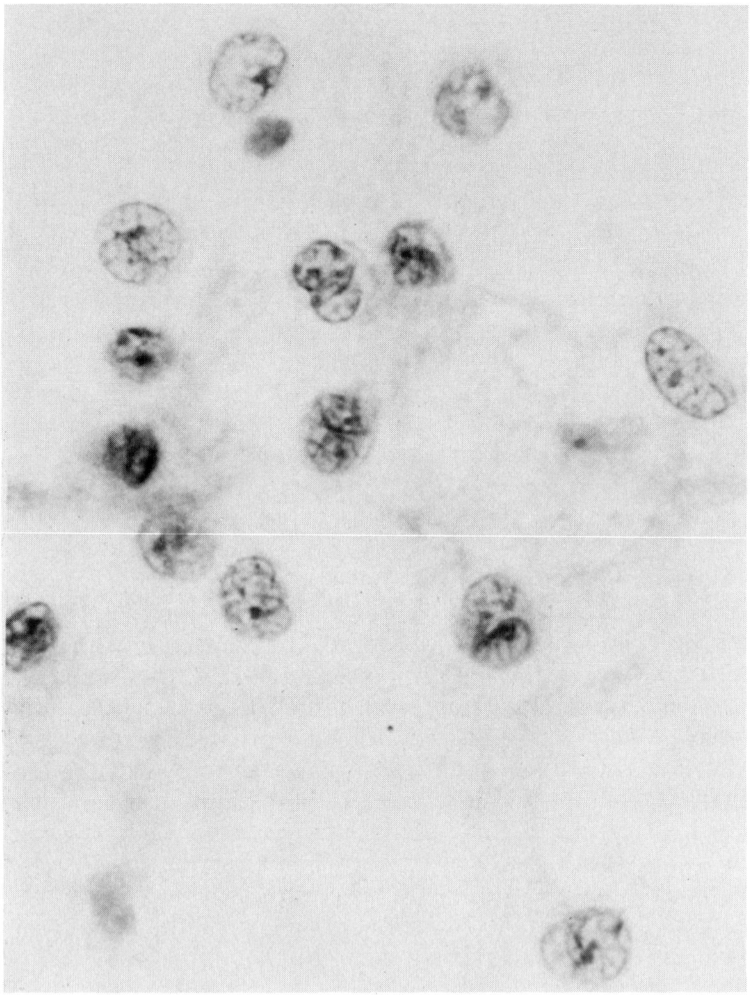

Fig. 6–3. Synovial cells stained by Papanicolaou stain have vesicular nuclei with prominent nuclear membranes and distinct nucleoli. × 500.

are usually associated with fewer than 30% or at most 40% polymorphonuclear leukocytes.

Recently, a disease syndrome, acute monocytic arthritis, has been described which consists of fever, skin rash, and acute polyarthritis.[31] The disease is similar to some other viral arthritides. The synovial-fluid nucleated cell count varied from 1,000 to 13,000/μL with at least 80% monocytes in the five cases reported.

Qualitative Cell Morphology

Occasionally, it is desirable to study cell morphology in greater detail than is ordinarily rendered by the routine stained smear. Actually, the basic Wright-stained or Wright-Giemsa stained smear can often be significantly improved by depolymerizing the hyaluronic acid with hyaluronidase.[13] Hyaluronidase is available in pharmacies as a preparation for human administration under the trade name Wydase (Wyeth Laboratories, Div. American Home Products, P.O. Box 8299, Philadelphia, Pa. 19101). Approximately one part of the prepared enzyme solution, which contains 150 N.F. units/ml in physiologic saline, can be added to 3 parts of synovial fluid and the mixture incubated at about 30°C for 1 hour. After centrifugation, smears are prepared from the sediment as previously described, and abnormal cell types can be evaluated:

1. Malignant cells
2. RA cells (ragocytes)
3. Reiter's cells
4. Mononuclear cells in villonodular synovitis
5. LE cells

MALIGNANT CELLS

In the event that neoplastic involvement of the joint cavity is suspected, an ample specimen of synovial fluid should be submitted for exfoliative cytologic examination. The EDTA-anticoagulated specimen is desirable and should be refrigerated as soon as possible. Excellent morphologic detail can be achieved by either filtration or centrifugation followed by Papanicolaou staining.[32,33] (See procedure described in Chapter 8—Cerebrospinal Fluid Analysis.) The differential cell count can also be conducted on these preparations.

RA CELLS

Rheumatoid, or RA, cells were originally named because, in a study of more than 600 patients with rheumatoid arthritis, those cells were found to comprise from 3 to 97% of all nucleated cells in approximately 95% of synovial-fluid specimens.[55] They have also been referred to as ragocytes, inclusion body cells, and raisin cells. RA cells are polymorphonuclear leukocytes that contain 1 to 20 dark granules varying from about 0.5 to 1.5 μ in diameter and are located principally at the cell periphery. Phase microscopy reveals that these granules are actually vacuoles containing granular material and are phagosomes. Similar extracellular particles have been described in the synovial fluid of many patients with rheumatoid arthritis.[56] The granules are aggregated precipitates of IgM (rheumatoid factor), IgG, and complement. RA cells are not, however, specific for rheumatoid arthritis, and similar cells have been observed in other conditions, including gout and pyogenic arthritis.[21]

REITER'S CELLS

Large macrophages with ingested polymorphonuclear leukocytes have been described in Reiter's syndrome (urethritis, uveitis, and polyarthritis) and termed "Reiter's cells."[48] This designation is also not entirely appropriate, because such cells can be identified in other joint diseases.[13] Synovial cells in Reiter's syndrome are often swollen and exhibit appreciable variation in size.[32] Although chlamydial organisms have been described as inclusions in the synovial cells, Reiter's syndrome is associated with various other infectious diseases including salmonella, shigella, and campylobacter.[32]

MONONUCLEAR CELLS IN PIGMENTED VILLONODULAR SYNOVITIS

Pigmented villonodular synovitis is characterized by a preponderance of mononuclear cells; papillary aggregates of synovial cells, and multinucleated foreign body giant cells.[32,33] Golden-brown, granular deposits of hemosiderin are usually readily apparent both in histiocytes and synovial cells. Hemosiderin can be verified, if necessary, by its blue-green staining reaction with Prussian blue.

LE CELLS

Autoantibodies to deoxyribonucleoprotein regularly occur in lupus erythematosus and are the basis for the LE-cell phenomenon. LE cells are phagocytes, usually polymorphonuclear leukocytes, that have engulfed into the cytoplasm the homogeneous product resulting from the reaction of the deoxyribonucleoprotein antibody with the nuclear material of other cells. LE cells were found in the synovial fluid of 7 of 10 selected patients in one series, and in one of these cases, the LE cells were present in synovial fluid but not in blood preparations.[34,56] It is thus well established that LE cells can form in vivo in synovial fluid.

TRAUMATIC JOINT DISEASE AND OSTEOARTHRITIS

Aseptic traumatic-joint disease is associated with nonspecific synovial-fluid findings. In addition to marked hemorrhage and usually only slightly increased numbers of polymorphonuclear leukocytes, sheets of synovial cells, clumps of degenerated cartilage cells, and various tissue fragments can often be identified. Hemosiderin deposits are frequently found in synovial cells and histiocytes when the hemarthrosis has been present for more than 1 or 2 days.

Cellular features of osteoarthritis include sheets of synovial cells, multinucleated cartilage cells, other multinucleated cells that have been identified as osteoclasts, and minimal or absent inflammatory cells.[32,33]

Crystal Identification

JOINT CRYSTALS AND DISEASE

Examination of the sediment for crystals is a critical part of the synovial-fluid examination. Identification of monosodium urate or calcium pyrophosphate dihydrate crystals is tantamount to the diagnosis of gout or pseudogout, which are the prototypes of crystal deposition joint diseases (Fig. 6–4). A third crystal type, calcium hydroxyapatite (apatite), has recently been described in both acute undiagnosed arthritis and osteoarthritis.[35–36] Apatite has not been conclusively established as a crystal deposition disease, but it appears to be of some pathogenetic importance in various conditions.[6]

The fact that even corticosteroid crystals can induce synovitis when administered into the joint cavity for therapeutic purposes suggests that the crystalline structure of a particular substance rather than its chemical composition is the key factor in initiating an inflammatory response in the joint cavity.[12,37] The pathogenesis and clinical aspects of crystal-induced inflammation of the joint cavity have been recently reviewed.[38] The pathogenesis of crystal-induced inflammation appears to be as follows:

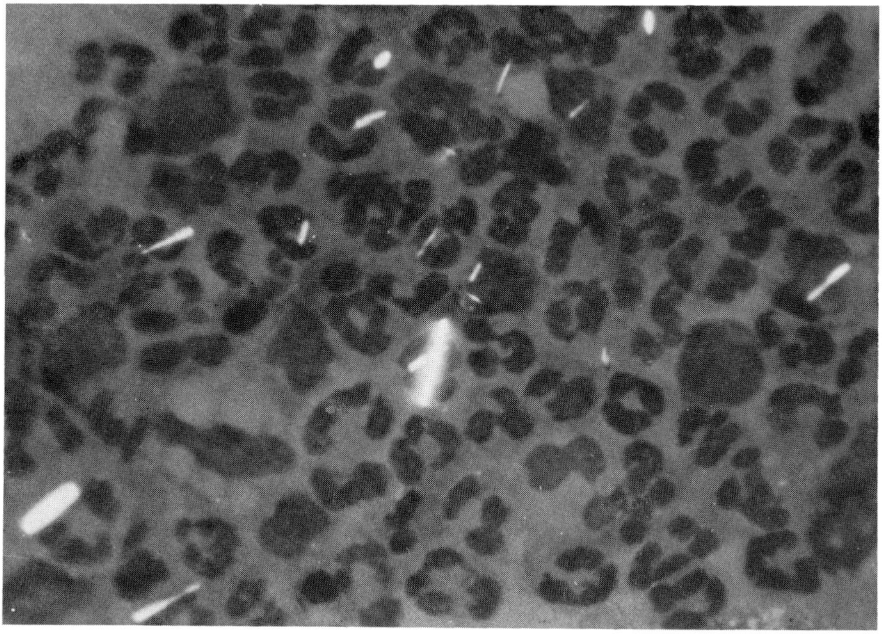

Fig. 6–4. Urate crystals in acute gout. The crystals are located both extracellularly and within polymorphonuclear neutrophils. The field is partially polarized to allow observation of cell outlines. × 756. Courtesy of Dr. Kirtikant V. Sheth, Portland, Ore.

1. Crystal formation
2. Phagocytosis of crystals by both polymorphonuclear leukocytes and monocytes
3. Rupture of the phagolysosomes so that proteolytic enzymes and chemotactic factors are released
4. Attraction of additional polymorphonuclear leukocytes by chemotactic factors

The inflammatory response is augmented by activation of the kinin system, which occurs, in part, from direct interaction of the Hageman factor with crystals.

MICROSCOPIC EXAMINATION

The microscopic examination to detect and identify crystals is usually performed on a wet-mount preparation. A drop of sediment from the EDTA anticoagulated specimen is placed on a microscope slide and covered with a coverslip, which can be rimmed with petrolatum or clear fingernail lacquer to prevent drying. It is important that an oxalated specimen not be used for crystal examination because of the possible formation of calcium oxalate crystals. It is also essential that the microscope slide and coverslip be scrupulously free of dust and other particles that might polarize light and be mistaken for intrinsic crystals. Dried smears have also been recommended for crystal examination because they can be stained for the differential cell count, examined at leisure, and filed for future reference.[39]

The disadvantage of staining dried smears is that crystals can be dissolved or washed away during the procedure. The slide preparation should be scanned by ordinary-light microscopy using a low power (10 ×) objective to determine fields that are particularly worthy of more critical examination. The slide should then be examined with polarized light—that is, with the planes of the polarizer and analyzer at right angles to each other (the "crossed polar" relationship)—using the high-dry (40 or 44 ×) objective. Birefringent (optically anisotropic or "doubly refractile") crystals, which might otherwise be missed by examination with ordinary-light microscopy, will be readily apparent as bright structures on a dark background (Fig. 6–5). All of the crystals of known importance in joint disease are at least weakly birefringent.

For practical purposes, the crystals of major importance in synovial fluid can be identified on the basis of crystal morphology and birefringent characteristics. The birefringent characteristics of each crystal type can be determined by using a polarizing microscope fitted with a first-order red compensator, which will be located in the optical pathway between the microscope objective lens and the analyzer.[40] A compensator separates light into its fast and slow vibration components and is inserted into the optical path so that the direction of its slow component is at an angle of 45% with the planes of the polarizer and analyzer. The

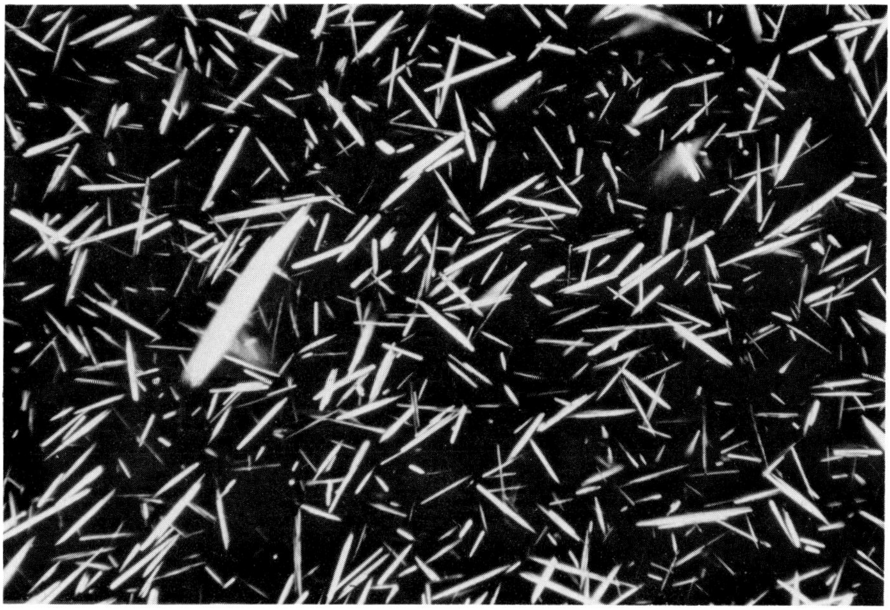

Fig. 6–5. Urate crystals from a gouty tophus that had ruptured into a joint. ×100.

direction of the slow component is ordinarily indicated on the compensator by a single arrow, the shorter of two arrows, or an arrow designated by a gamma (γ) symbol. The red compensator retards red light so that the field appears red instead of black with crossed polars. The mechanical stage of the microscope is rotated so that the long axis of the particular crystal is parallel to the slow component of the red compensator. A crystal that appears blue in this orientation is designated as positively birefringent, while crystals that appear yellow are negatively birefringent. Turning the microscope stage another 90° so that the crystal axis is now at right angles to the slow component of the compensator will cause positively birefringent crystals to be yellow and negatively birefringent crystals to be blue. Actually, as the mechanical stage of the microscope is rotated through 360°, all birefringent crystals will have, in addition to the two orientations in which they appear blue and the two in which they appear yellow, four intermediate positions, one in each quadrant, in which the crystals assume the red color of the background.[22] The particular orientation in relation to the planes of the polars at which the crystals appear red is determined by the angle of extinction of the particular crystal type. (See Chap. 9 for a more detailed discussion of the microscope and microscopy.)

In the event that a polarizing microscope is not available, kits can be purchased to add this capability to ordinary microscopes. The result is of lower quality but nevetheless acceptable for most purposes in diagnostic microscopy. Since the compensator can be placed anywhere in the optical path between the polarizer and analyzer, various substitutes have been devised for the optically ground quartz plate that constitutes the red compensator in high-quality polarizing microscopes. Layers of cellophane between two glass slides or two thicknesses of cellophane tape (some brands of cellophane tape are not adequate, but Mystik tape gives good results) applied to a glass slide or directly to the ocular side of the polarizer have been substituted for a red compensator.[41] In these cases, the cellophane or tape must be empirically oriented to render a red background when the polars are crossed—that is, the field is otherwise black.

As previously noted, the relationship of these crystals to disease is uncertain.[6] Cholesterol crystals are rarely encountered in synovial fluids, and when present, they are usually associated with chronic inflammatory diseases, especially rheumatoid arthritis.[42] The typical crystals are large plates usually shaped as rhomboids or parallelograms with notched corners and are strongly birefringent. The sign of birefringence cannot be meaningfully expressed because the plates do not have definable longitudinal axes.

Corticosteroids that have recently been injected into the joint space can be detected in the synovial fluid. The various types of corticosteroids have crystal structures varying from needles to pleomorphic aggregates and birefringence that is positive in some types and negative in others.[37] When corticosteroids have been recently administered intra-articularly, no diagnostic conclusions can be drawn from crystals that are found in the synovial fluid examination.

MICROBIOLOGIC STUDIES

Microbiologic studies of synovial fluid can frequently provide unique diagnostic information and should be pursued in depth on any case even remotely suggesting bacterial arthritis. In 90% of cases, bacterial arthritis is mono-articular and most often involves the knee joint. In children younger than 2 years, Hemophilus influenzae type B is the most common causative organism, while in young adults, Neisseria gonorrhoeae is the most common etiology.[43] In older children and older adults, Staphylococcus aureus is the predominate causative agent. Gram-stained smears of the synovial-fluid sediment will reveal the bacterial organisms in more than 50% of cases (Fig. 6–6).[44] Cultures should include chocolate agar for incubation in 10% carbon dioxide, sheep agar, and an appropriate anaerobic fluid, such as chopped-meat medium or thioglycollate broth.

Mycobacterial infection of the joints is very uncommon in the United States. About 20% of the cases of tuberculous arthritis will have a synovial-fluid smear that is positive for acid-fast organisms.[20] The smear and culture for mycobacteria should be performed in any suspected

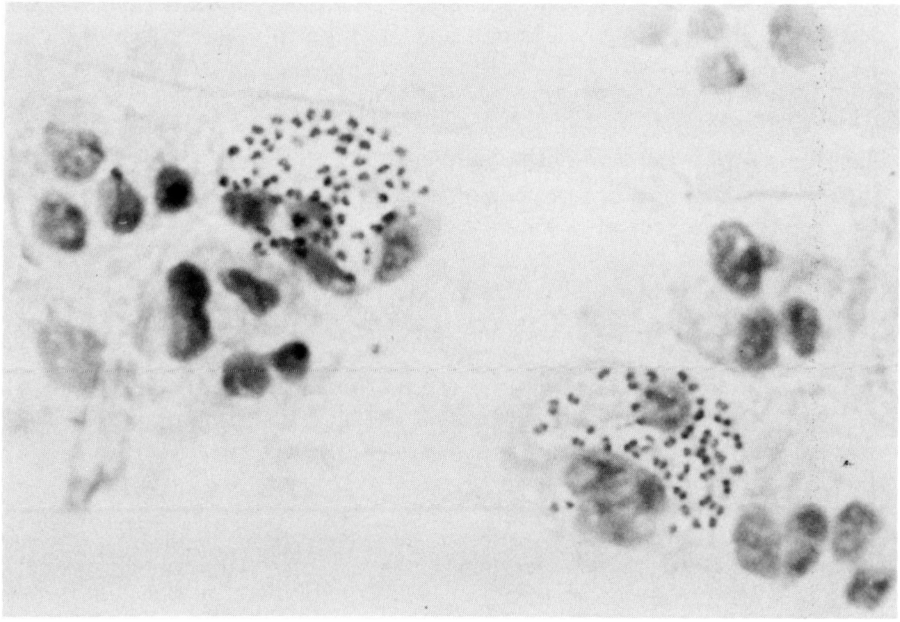

Fig. 6–6. Acute gonococcal arthritis. Polymorphonuclear neutrophils containing organisms of Neisseria gonorrhoeae. × 100. Gram stain.

case. Mycobacterium kansasii and M. intracellulare are the most common of the atypical mycobacteria to cause arthritis.[43]

Sporothrix schenkii is the most common cause of fungal arthritis.[43] Other fungal agents include Coccidioides immitis, Candida albicans, and Cryptococcus neoformans among others.

Various viruses can cause arthritis as a manifestation of systemic disease. Parasitic arthritis is virtually unknown in the United States.

CHEMICAL TESTS OF SYNOVIAL FLUID

Glucose

Analysis of glucose in synovial fluid is of only limited value in clinical diagnosis and management. One situation in which synovial-fluid glucose can be of some value is in substantiating the clinical diagnosis of pyogenic arthritis in the absence of demonstrable organisms on stained smears and prior to the availability of bacterial-culture results. Under normal physiologic conditions, the synovial-fluid glucose concentration is only slightly less than that of plasma and usually well within a difference of 10 mg/dl. An increased synovial fluid-plasma glucose difference reflects increased metabolic activity within the joint cavity, which for practical purposes, relates to increased numbers of inflammatory cells, chiefly polymorphonuclear leukocytes but also monocytes, or to the presence of bacteria. Inflammation of any etiology can thus increase the metabolism of glucose and thereby increase the synovial fluid-plasma glucose differential. Furthermore, the severity of the acute inflammation is roughly proportional to the magnitude of the glucose differential. As would be expected, the lowest synovial-fluid glucose concentrations can occur in acute pyogenic arthritis, in which the glucose differential is frequently more than 50 mg/dl, and in rare cases, glucose is undetectable in the synovial fluid. There is considerable overlap, however, in the glucose differentials of pyogenic arthritis and those of other acute inflammatory diseases including gout, rheumatoid arthritis, and tuberculosis.

As previously discussed, glucose apparently does not enter the synovial fluid from the blood plasma by a process of simple ultrafiltration. A significant delay of an hour or more is required for glucose in synovial fluid to equilibrate with that in blood. For this reason, patients should be fasting for at least 6 hours before the synovial fluid and blood specimens are obtained.

Hemolytic Complement (CH50)

Complement is normally present in synovial fluid, and numerous studies have been made of the diagnostic value of measuring total hemolytic complement (CH50) or individual complement components, such as C2 or C3. CH50 activity in synovial fluid is usually about one-third to one-half that of plasma. The unique importance of synovial fluid CH50 to clinical diagnosis is not, however, in measuring its absolute activity levels, but in relative changes in concentration to values expected with increased synovial permeability. This can best be done by relating complement activity to total protein.

The synovial fluid CH50 is regularly decreased in rheumatoid arthritis and probably reflects the antigen-antibody reaction and immune-complex formation in this disease.[45,46] There is a reasonable correlation between the extent of CH50 suppression and the activity and severity of the disease.[47] Hemolytic complement activity is also frequently decreased in bacterial arthritis (especially gonococcal and staphylococcal arthritis), systemic lupus erythematosus, and, occasionally, in gout and pseudogout.[45,46] Increased synovial fluid CH50 occurs in Reiter's syndrome.[48]

Enzymes

Enzymes are normally present in very low levels in synovial fluid.[22] Increased enzyme concentrations in disease basically reflect the increased metabolism associated with cellular exudation. No specific enzyme has yet been shown to have any specific relationship to a particular disease entity.[10]

Hyaluronic Acid

Hyaluronic acid can be assayed by measuring the uronic acid released by hyaluronidase digestion.[10] There is little if any clinical indication for this assay. Indeed, the quantity and degree of polymerization of hyaluronic acid can be evaluated by the simple viscosity test and mucin-clot test.

Protein

The total protein of normal synovial fluid varies from about 1.3 to 2.7 g/dl, which is about one-fourth to one-third the concentration in plasma.[10] The total protein of synovial fluid increases as the selective permeability of the synovial membrane deteriorates because of inflammation or trauma. By itself, the total protein concentration does not render any uniquely useful information. Indeed, estimates of the integrity of the synovial membrane and the degree of inflammatory activity are available from other tests, such as tests for turbidity, viscosity, fibrin clot, mucin clot, total cell count, and differential cell count. Probably the unique indication for determining the total protein of synovial fluid is to provide a relative index for the hemolytic complement assay. Analytic methods for total-plasma proteins are generally applicable to the synovial fluid.

Rheumatoid Factor

Detection of rheumatoid factor in serum is important in confirming the clinical diagnosis of rheumatoid arthritis. Many patients with obvious clinical disease, however, frequently or persistently exhibit negative test results for rheumatoid factor. In one series of 100 patients with rheumatoid arthritis, the sera of 30% were negative with the Waller-Rose test (sheep red blood cells coated with anti-sheep red-blood-cell antibodies), 19% were negative with the latex test (latex particles coated with human gamma globulin), and 13% were negative with both tests.[49] In the hope of detecting rheumatoid factor in patients who are seronegative, the various tests have been performed on synovial fluid. Although there is a good correlation between rheumatoid-factor test results on serum and those on synovial fluid, the additional detection rate is insufficient to justify their routine performance on synovial fluid.[49–50]

Other Immunologic Markers

Immunoglobulin quantitation in synovial fluid in the form of ratios to serum immunoglobulins generally reveal ratios less than 1.0 and roughly equivalent distribution of IgG, IgA, and IgM. These measurements do not seem to offer useful criteria for distinguishing the various types of arthritis with the exception of Reiter's syndrome, in which the ratio is often greater than 1 with prominent IgM elevation.

Immune complexes, usually containing IgG and IgM along with complement components, can be detected in most patients with rheumatoid arthritis. Such assays appear to have little clinical value to date.[51,52] These correlate with intracellular aggregates (ragocytes), seropositivity, lowered synovial fluid C3 complements, and other parameters of active inflammation.[53]

Oligoclonal immunoglobulins have been identified in the synovial fluid of many patients with arthritis, particularly the seronegative types.[51] This phenomenon is analogous to findings in the cerebrospinal fluid in patients with multiple sclerosis and may represent a localized, nonspecific stimulation of B-cell clones. The clinical application of this observation is not clear at this point.[54]

Cryoprecipitates have been found in the synovial fluid of various types of arthritis. In patients with rheumatoid arthritis, these usually represent IgG-IgM complexes or IgG alone. Similar precipitates have been found in nonimmune mediated arthritis and may therefore represent a nonspecific phenomenon related to the degree of inflammation. Various auto-antibodies have likewise been studied including antinuclear antibody, antismooth muscle antibody and antithyroid antibody, but the clinical utility of these measurements is unclear at this point.

REFERENCES

1. Osgood, R.: The medical and social approaches to the problem of chronic rheumatism. Am. J. Med. Sci., *200*:429, 1940.
2. Hormell, R.: Notes on the history of rheumatism and gout. N. Engl. J. Med., *223*:754, 1940.
3. Hippocrates: Aphorisms. *In* The Genuine Works of Hippocrates. Vol. 2. Edited by F. Adams. New York, William Wood and Company, 1929, p. 255.
4. Bauer, W., Bennett, G., Marble, A., and Claflin, D.: Observations on normal synovial fluid of cattle: The cellular constituents and nitrogen content. J. Exp. Med., *52*:835, 1930.
5. Ropes, M., and Bauer, W.: Synovial Fluid Changes in Joint Disease. Cambridge, Harvard University Press, 1953.
6. Dieppe, P., et al.: Synovial fluid crystals. Q. J. Med., *48*:533, 1979.
7. McCarty, D., and Hollander, J.: Identification of urate crystals in gouty synovial fluid. Ann. Intern. Med., *54*:452, 1961.
8. McCarty, D., Kohn, N., and Faires, J.: The significance of calcium phosphate crystals in the synovial fluid of arthritic patients: The pseudogout syndrome. Ann. Intern. Med., *56*:711, 1962.
9. Ghadially, F.: Fine structure of joints. *In* The Joints and Synovial Fluid. Vol. 1. Edited by L. Sokoloff. New York, Academic Press, 1978, pp. 105–176.
10. Cohen, A., Brandt, K., and Krey, P.: Synovial fluid. *In* Laboratory Diagnostic Procedures in the Rheumatic Diseases. 2nd Ed. Edited by A. Cohen. Boston, Little, Brown, 1975, pp. 1–64.
11. Swann, D.: Macromolecules of synovial fluid. *In* The Joints and Synovial Fluid. Vol. 1. Edited by L. Sokoloff. New York, Academic Press, 1978, pp. 407–435.
12. Schmid, F., and Ogata, R.: Synovial fluid evaluation in joint disease. Med. Clin. North Am., *49*:165, 1965.
13. McCarty, D.: Synovial Fluid. *In* Arthritis and Allied Conditions. 9th Ed. Edited by D. McCarty. Philadelphia, Lea & Febiger, 1979, pp. 51–69.

14. Godkhindi, K., Tilve, G., and Nair, K.: Synovianalysis. Postgrad. Med. J., *24*:63, 1978.
15. Teloh, H.: Clinical pathology of synovial fluid. Ann. Clin. Lab. Sci., *5*:282, 1975.
16. Wolf, A., et al.: Current concepts in synovial fluid analysis. Clin. Orthop., *134*:261, 1978.
17. Miller, J.: Joint paracentesis from an anatomic point of view: Shoulder, elbow, wrist, and hand. Surgery, *40*:993, 1956.
18. Miller, J.: Joint paracentesis from an anatomic point of view: Hip, knee, ankle, and foot. Surgery, *41*:999, 1957.
19. Ropes, M., Rossmeisl, E., and Bauer, W.: The origin and nature of normal human synovial fluid. J. Clin. Invest., *19*:795, 1940.
20. Wallace, R., and Cohen, A.: Tuberculous arthritis. A report of two cases with review of biopsy and synovial fluid findings. Am. J. Med., *61*:277, 1976.
21. Yehia, S., and Duncan, H.: Synovial fluid analysis. Clin. Orthop., *107*:11, 1975.
22. Currey, J., and Veron-Roberts, B.: Examination of synovial fluid. Clin. Rheum. Dis., *2*:149, 1976.
23. Gregg, J., Nixon, J., and DiStefano, V.: Neutral fat globules in traumatized knee. Clin. Orthop., *132*:219, 1978.
24. Lawrence, L., and Seil, B.: Bone marrow in joint fluid: A clue to fracture. Ann. Intern. Med., *74*:740, 1971.
25. Cheung, J., Ryan, L., Kozin, F., and McCarty, D.: Synovial origins of rice bodies in joint fluid. Arthritis Rheum., *23*:72, 1980.
26. Berg, E., et al.: On the nature of rheumatoid rice bodies: An immunologic, histochemical, and electron microscope study. Arthritis Rheum., *20*:1343, 1977.
27. Ropes, M., et al.: Synovial fluid mucin. Acta Med. Scand., *196*:700, 1947.
28. Donaldson, L.: Technique for performing white cell counts in joint fluids. Med. Lab. Tech., *29*:1, 1972.
29. Coggeshall, H., Warren, C., and Bauer, W.: The cytology of normal human synovial fluid. Anat. Rec., *77*:129, 1940.
30. Krey, P., and Bailen, D.: Synovial fluid leukocytosis. A study of extremes. Am. J. Med., *67*:436, 1979.
31. Brawer, A., and Cathcart, E.: Acute monocytic arthritis. Arthritis Rheum., *22*:294, 1979.
32. Naib, Z.: Cytology of synovial fluids. Acta Cytol., *17*:299, 1973.
33. Broderick, P., et al.: Exfoliative cytology interpretation of synovial fluid in joint disease. J. Bone Joint Surg., *58A*:396, 1976.
34. Hunder, G., and Pierre, R.: In vivo LE cell formation in synovial fluid. Arthritis Rheum., *13*:448, 1970.
35. Dieppe, P., Crocker, P., Huskisson, E., and Willoughby, D.: Apatite deposition disease: A new arthropathy. Lancet, *1*:266, 1976.
36. Schumacker, H., Smolyo, A., Tse, R., and Maurer, K.: Arthritis associated with apatite crystals. Ann. Intern. Med., *87*:411, 1977.
37. Kahn, C., Hollander, V., and Schumacher, H.: Corticosteroid crystals in synovial fluid. J.A.M.A., *211*:807, 1970.
38. McCarty, D.: Pathogenesis and treatment of crystal-induced inflammation. *In* Arthritis and Allied Conditions. 9th Ed. Edited by D. McCarty. Philadelphia, Lea & Febiger, 1976, pp. 1245–1261.
39. Good, A., and Frishette, W.: Crystals in dried smears of synovial fluid. J.A.M.A., *198*:80, 1966.
40. Phelps, P., Steele, A., and McCarty, D.: Compensated polarized light microscopy: Identification of crystals in synovial fluids from gout and pseudogout. J.A.M.A., *203*:508, 1968.
41. Wild, J., and Zvaifler, N.: On office technique for identifying crystals in synovial fluid. Am. Fam. Physician, *12*:72, 1975.
42. Ettlinger, R., and Hunder, G.: Synovial effusions containing cholesterol crystals: Report of 12 patients and review. Mayo Clinic Proceedings, *54*:366, 1979.
43. Smith, J.: Infectious arthritis. *In* Principles and Practice of Infectious Diseases. Vol. 1. Edited by G. Mandell, R. Douglas, and J. Bennett. New York, John Wiley & Sons, 1979, pp. 933–945.
44. Ward, J., and Atcheson, S.: Infectious arthritis. Med. Clin. North Am., *61*:313, 1977.

45. Bunch, T., et al.: Synovial fluid complement determination as a diagnostic aid in inflammatory joint disease. Mayo Clinic Proceedings, *49*:715, 1974.
46. Townes, A., and Sowa, J.: Complement in synovial fluid. Johns Hopkins Med. J., *127*:23, 1970.
47. Bunch, T., Hunder, G., Offord, K., and McDuffie, F.: Synovial fluid complement: Usefulness in diagnosis and classification of rheumatoid arthritis. Ann. Intern. Med., *81*:32, 1974.
48. Pekin T., Malinin, T., and Zvaifler, N.: Unusual synovial fluid findings in Reiter's syndrome. Ann. Intern. Med., *66*:677, 1967.
49. Huskisson, E., Hart, F., and Lacey, B.: Synovial fluid Waller-Rose and latex tests. Ann. Rheum. Dis., *30*:67, 1971.
50. MacSween, R., Dalakos, T., Jasani, M., and Buchanan, W.: Rheumatoid factor in serum and synovial fluid. Scand. J. Rheumatol., *1*:177, 1972.
51. Halla, J., et al.: Immune complexes in rheumatoid arthritis seen in synovial fluid. Arthritis Rheum., *22*:440, 1979.
52. Male, D., Roitt, I., and Hay, F.: Analysis of immune complexes in synovial effusions of patients with rheumatoid arthritis. Clin. Exp. Immunol., *39*:297, 1980.
53. Hasselbacher, P.: Extracellular aggregates of immunoglobulin in synovial fluids from rheumatoid arthritis. J. Rheumatol., *6*:374, 1979.
54. Mellbye, O., Syrand, O., Brath, J., and Olsen, E.: Oligoclonal immunoglobulins and smooth muscle antibodies in arthritis joints. Clin. Exp. Immunol., *40*:103, 1980.
55. Hollander, J., McCarty, D., Gonzalo, A., and Castro-Murillo, E.: Studies on the pathogenesis of rheumatoid joint inflammation: The "R.A. cell" and a working hypothesis. Ann. Intern. Med., *62*:271, 1965.
56. Hasselbacher, P.: Extracellular aggregates of immunoglobulin in synovial fluid from rheumatoid arthritis. J. Rheumatol., *6*:374, 1979.

COLOR AND TURBIDITY

METHOD. Visual physical evaluation.

PRINCIPLE. Color, turbidity, fibrin-clot formation, viscosity, and mucin-clot formation are all physical observations that can be made visually on joint fluid. Although these observations are qualitative or semiquantitative estimations, they are reproducible enough to compare specimen to specimen, and disease to disease, and are characteristic enough to confirm some diagnoses in the study of joint diseases.

PROCEDURE

1. Visually observe and record synovial fluid in the test tube.
2. Record color and turbidity.

INTERPRETATION

COLOR. Fluid should be clear and transparent (with the consistency of uncooked egg albumin).

TURBIDITY

0 = Transparent, clear
1+ = Slightly hazy
2+ = Distinctly cloudy; difficulty reading small print from newspaper through the tube
3+ = Very turbid. Only large print can be read through the tube.
4+ = Opaque

DISCUSSION. The most common cause for markedly turbid specimens is polymorphonuclear leukocytes. Although crystals and bacteria cause some turbidity, they are almost always accompanied by leukocytes. Erythrocytes will also cause red discoloration of the fluid, which should be fairly obvious to the naked eye. In patients with tuberculous arthritis, the fluid may assume a yellow-white gelatinous appearance or become xanthochromic. Acute gouty arthritis is often accompanied by milky synovial fluid. Patients with rheumatoid arthritis or pseudogout can have frankly turbid (4+) synovial fluid, which is of a somewhat green hue. Pyogenic arthritis produces a grey-brown or green, and sometimes bloody, synovial fluid. Even fat droplets, in cases of trauma, can cause some turbidity; however, they will usually float on the surface of the specimen.

MATERIALS AND REAGENTS. Test tube, 10 × 100 mm.

REFERENCE

1. Hollander, J., Jessar, R., and McCarty, D.: Synovianalysis: An aid in arthritis. Bull. Rheum. Dis., *12*:263, 1961.

FIBRIN-CLOT FORMATION

METHOD. Visual physical evaluation.

PRINCIPLE. Normally, synovial fluid does not clot; in disease processes, especially inflammation, there is increased permeability of the synovial membrane permitting fibrin to be present and thus producing clotting. This can be observed visually.

SPECIMEN. Synovial fluid without anticoagulant should be examined within 4 hours of collection.

PROCEDURE

1. Observe and record fluid for fibrin strand or clot formation in a test tube.
2. Record observations.

INTERPRETATION. The results can be observed visually and the amount of fibrin can be estimated:

0 = Absence of fibrin
1+ = Strands of fibrin
2+ = Definite but small clot comprising less than 10% of the total volume
3+ = Clot comprising 10 to 50% of the specimen volume
4+ = Clot comprising 50 to 100% of the specimen volume

DISCUSSION AND CLINICAL SIGNIFICANCE. Synovial fluid does not coagulate spontaneously or upon the addition of thrombin. With fibrin exudation as the result of inflammatory processes, there is an increase in the tendency to clot formation that is proportional to the severity of the inflammation. This is a nonspecific finding and can be produced in any inflammatory arthritis.

MATERIALS AND METHODS. Test tube, 10 × 100 mm.

REFERENCE

1. Hollander, J., Jessar, R., and McCarty, D.: Synovianalysis: An aid in arthritis. Bull. Rheum. Dis., *12*:263, 1961.

VISCOSITY

METHOD. Viscosity of synovial fluid is dependent upon the concentration and physicochemical state of hyaluronic acid. It can be evaluated by visually observing drops of synovial fluid expelled through a Pasteur pipette.

PROCEDURE

1. Pipette 4 to 10 ml synovial fluid using the Pasteur pipette.
2. Observe the stringiness as the fluid courses through the narrow end of the pipette.
3. Record observation.

INTERPRETATION. Viscosity can be estimated as follows:

0 = Droplets have the character of water or milk and are not stringy.
1+ = Barely detectable distension of the droplet
2+ = Obvious strand less than 1 cm length
3+ = Strands of 1 to 4 cm
4+ = Strands formed that are longer than 4 cm

DISCUSSION AND CLINICAL SIGNIFICANCE. There are more technically precise ways of determining viscosity, including the Ostwald viscometer, but this precision is not necessary in clinical medical practice. Decreased viscosity occurs with any joint inflammation. Although this is a nonspecific finding, it helps confirm that a disease process is present.

MATERIALS AND REAGENTS

1. Test tubes, 10 × 100 mm
2. Pasteur pipette

REFERENCES

1. McCarty, D.: The physiology of the normal synovium. *In* The Joints and Synovial Fluid. Vol. 2. Edited by L. Sokoloff. New York, Academic Press, 1980, p. 293.
2. Schmid, F., and Ogata, R.: Synovial fluid evaluation of joint disease. Med. Clin. North Am., *49*:165, 1965.

MUCIN-CLOT TEST

METHOD. Ropes test.

PRINCIPLE. When diluted acid is added to synovial fluid, a "ropey" precipitate is produced that can be observed visually.

SPECIMEN. Specimen should be collected without anticoagulant.

PROCEDURE

1. Slowly layer about 1 ml of synovial fluid (without added anticoagulant) to 4 ml of 5% (v/v) acetic acid in a test tube.
2. Gently agitate tube at 30 second intervals for 3 minutes.
3. Evaluate and record the coagulum.

INTERPRETATION. The coagulum can be recorded as follows:

0 = Turbid white suspension with small granular particles of coagulum
1+ = Threads and large granules in a turbid solution
2+ = Large and small clumps of stringy precipitate in a slightly turbid solution
3+ = Loose coagulum that may break up into several pieces in a clear solution upon agitation
4+ = Tight ropey or mucinous coagulum

DISCUSSION AND CLINICAL SIGNIFICANCE. The coagulum that forms when acetic acid is added to synovial fluid is not mucin but does have a mucinous appearance. The mucin-clot test is a reflection of the polymerization and concentration of hyaluronic acid; consequently, it is similar in clinical relevance to the viscosity measurement. In cases of acute noninflammatory serous effusions, the viscosity may be reduced but the mucin-clot formation unaltered. Diminished clot formation occurs in most inflammatory disease. The test was popularized by Marion Ropes, although the phenomenon has been known since 1846.

The volume and strength of acetic acid and the ratio of acetic acid to specimen is critical.

MATERIALS AND METHODS

1. Test tubes, 10 × 100 mm.
2. Acetic acid, 5% (v/v)
3. Volumetric pipettes, 1.0 ml.

REFERENCE

1. Ropes, M., and Bauer, W.: Synovial Changes in Joint Disease. Cambridge, Harvard University Press, 1953.

CYTOLOGIC AND HISTOLOGIC EVALUATION

PRINCIPLE. Normally, synovial fluid contains only desquamated cells of the synovial lining, but in disease processes, other cells (leukocytes) can be recognized, counted, and their morphology identified. These cells may be characteristic of the type of inflammatory process.

SPECIMEN. Use an EDTA anticoagulated specimen of synovial fluid.

PROCEDURE

1. Mix the specimen thoroughly using a vortex mixer.
2. Draw the specimen into a white-blood-cell pipette to the 0.5 mark and dilute with 0.85% (w/v) saline diluent to the 11 mark. (If the specimen contains many erythrocytes, it should be diluted with 0.3% (w/v) saline diluent to lyse the erythrocytes.)
3. Mix the fluid in the pipette by gentle rotation for 5 minutes.
4. Charge both chambers of a hemacytometer with the diluted specimen after discarding the first two drops.

5. Count the leukocytes in the four large corner squares of each chamber (total of 8 mm^2). If the leukocytes are increased (>5,000/μL) or greatly increased (>50,000/μL), the specimen can be prediluted 1:10 or 1:100, respectively, with 0.85% (w/v) saline.
6. Multiply the number of counted leukocytes by 25 to determine the concentration in terms of cells/μL. Record the results as leukocytes/μL.
7. Centrifuge the remaining EDTA anticoagulated specimen. Decant the supernate (it can be used for other tests).
8. Resuspend the sediment in the small amount of residual fluid.
9. Prepare smears on microscope slides and stain with Wright or Wright-Giemsa stain in the same manner as for a peripheral blood smear.
10. Perform a differential leukocyte count in the same manner as a peripheral blood smear; count 200 cells.
11. Note any morphologically abnormal cells and the presence of synovial cells.
12. Record the percentages of the various leukocytes, including polymorphonuclear leukocytes, monocytes, lymphocytes, and eosinophils.

MICROSCOPIC EXAMINATION

1. Place a drop of the resuspended sediment from the EDTA anticoagulated specimen on a microscope slide and cover with a coverslip rimmed with petrolatum.
2. Scan with ordinary bright-field microscopy using the 10× objective to determine crystals and debris.
3. Examine for crystals with the polarizing microscope using the 40× objective and crossed polarizers.
4. If crystals are detected, determine the type of birefringence by inserting the red compensator into the optical path.
5. Align the long axis of the crystal with the direction of the slow component of the compensator.
6. Record the type of birefringence. (If the crystal appears blue, it is positively birefringent; if the crystal is yellow, it is negatively birefringent.)
7. Report the type and number of crystal, and whether the crystals are intracellular or extracellular—that is, few or many uric-acid crystals.

INTERPRETATION. Cells can be counted in synovial fluid much the same as they are in blood and enumerated appropriately. The total number of nucleated cells should be less than 200/μL; a range of 13 to 180/μL (mean 63/μL) is considered "normal." Polymorphonuclear leukocytes constitute less than 25% of nucleated cells in normal synovial fluid.

DISCUSSION AND CLINICAL SIGNIFICANCE. Qualitative cell morphology permits the identification of malignant cells when there is joint cavity involvement in either metastatic or primary neoplastic disease. It also permits the detection of RA cells (ragocytes), Reiter cells, LE lupus erythematosus cells, and the mononuclear cells seen in pigmented villonodular synovitis. The fluid is usually free of crystal and tissue particles except for clusters of synovial cells.

Most of the cells of interest are leukocytes. There are no appreciable differences in the number of the leukocytes with bacterial diseases; nevertheless, their identification does identify an arthritic disease. Cell counts are less than 1,000/μL in noninflammatory joint effusions. Cell counts in inflammatory arthritides can range to 284,000/μL (mean 87,000/μL).

Red and white blood cell diluting fluids cannot be used because the acetic acid will precipitate hyaluronic acid on the counting chamber.

There is no clinical value to counting erythrocytes.

MATERIALS AND METHODS

1. Counting chamber with Neubauer ruling
2. White-cell pipette
3. Methylene blue, 0.1% (w/v)
4. Saline, 0.85% (w/v)
5. Saponin solution or saline, 0.3% (w/v)
6. Microscope, bright field and polarizing

REFERENCES

1. Cohen, A., Brandt, K., and Krey, B.: Synovial fluid. *In* Laboratory Diagnostic Procedures in Rheumatic Diseases. 2nd Ed. Boston, Little, Brown, 1975, p. 1.
2. Hollander, J., McCarty, D., Gonzalo, A., Castro-Murillo, E.: Studies on the pathogenesis of rheumatoid joint inflammation: The "RA cell" and a working hypothesis. Ann. Intern. Med., *62*:271, 1965.
3. Hunder, G., and Pierre, R.: In vivo LE cell formation in synovial fluid. Arthritis Rheum., *13*:448, 1970.
4. McCarty, D.: Synovial fluid. *In* Arthritis in Allied Conditions. 9th Ed. Philadelphia, Lea & Febiger, 1979, p. 51.
5. Perkins, T., Malinin, T., and Zvaifler, N.: Unusual synovial fluid findings in Reiter's syndrome. Ann. Intern. Med., *66*:667, 1967.

CRYSTAL IDENTIFICATION

METHOD. Polarization microscopy.

PRINCIPLE. Under the microscope using crossed polarizers, crystals can be localized because of the birefringence and identified because of their characteristic physical appearance.

SPECIMEN. Fresh specimen of noncoagulated synovial fluid should be used shortly after collection of the EDTA anticoagulated specimen.

PROCEDURE

1. Aspirate a drop of synovial fluid into Pasteur pipette.
2. Place on microscope slide and coverslip.

3. Rim the coverslip with lacquer or petroleum jelly to prevent drying.
4. Examine under microscope with polarization capability.
5. Observe crystal morphology and birefringent characteristics and record.
6. Examine by polarized light with a polarizer and analyzer at right angles to each other (crossed-polarizer relationship).
7. Anisotrophic (doubly refractile) crystals will be birefringent.

INTERPRETATION. Crystals will appear as bright-colored structures on a dark background. All of the crystals that occur in joint disease are birefringent to some extent. If crystals appear blue, they are positively birefringent; if crystals appear yellow, they are negatively birefringent.

Crystal	*Morphology*	*Birefringence*
Monosodium urate crystals	slender rod 2 to 20 mm	strong negative
Calcium pyrophosphate dihydrate crystals	less than 10 mm	weak positive
Hydroxyapatite crystals	0.1–1 mm needle shape	weak positive
Cholesterol crystals	rhomboid plates with notched corner	positive or negative
Corticosteroid crystals	nondescript	positive, negative, or none

DISCUSSION AND CLINICAL SIGNIFICANCE. The crystals within joints are all birefringent and can be identified by polarization microscopy. Monosodium urate crystals occur in gout; calcium pyrophosphate dihydrate crystals occur in pseudogout; and hydroxyapatite crystals are seen in osteoarthritis and other nonspecific arthritides.

MATERIALS AND METHODS

1. Neubauer counting chamber
2. White-cell pipette
3. Methylene blue, 0.1% (w/v)
4. Saline, 0.85% (w/v)
5. Saponin solution or saline, 0.3% (w/v)
6. Polarizing microscope with first-order red compensator

REFERENCES

1. Ettlinger, R., and Hunder, G.: Synovial effusions contained in cholesterol crystals: Reported 12 cases in review. Mayo Clinic Proceedings, *54*:336, 1979.
2. Good, A., and Frishete, W.: Crystals and dried smears in synovial fluid. J.A.M.A., *198*:80, 1966.
3. Phelps, P., Steele, A., and McCarty, D.: Compensated polarized light microscopy: Identification of crystals in synovial fluid for gout and pseudogout. J.A.M.A., *203*:508, 1968.

Chapter

7 Seminal-Fluid Analysis

DONALD C. CANNON
JAMES A. FREEMAN

In 1677, Antoni van Leeuwenhoek credited Mr. Ham, a medical student at Leiden, with the actual discovery of "living animalcules" (male spermatozoa) in semen. Leeuwenhoek, who was neither a physician nor a scientist, but rather a linen merchant from Delft, Holland, had a consuming interest in optical lenses and simple microscopes, which he constructed to study such diverse subjects as skeletal muscle, red blood cells, bacteria, and the microcirculation in frogs and eels. Although a crude compound microscope had been constructed by Hans and Zacharias Jansen about 1590, Leeuwenhoek used only simple, minute lenses that he had ground so carefully that magnifications of about 270 times could be achieved. Being untrained in science, Leeuwenhoek did not publish his findings as formal scientific reports; rather, he wrote letters to scientists and addressed symposia of men of distinction. In a letter to the president of the Royal Society in November, 1677, he initially described spermatozoa:

> These animalcules were smaller than the corpuscles, which impart a red colour to the blood, so that I judge a million of them would not equal in size a large grain of sand. Their bodies, which are round, were blunt in front and ran to a point behind. They were furnished with a thin tail, about 5 or 6 times as long as the body, and very transparent and with the thickness about one twenty-fifth that of the body. . . . They moved forward owing to the motion of their tails like that of a snake or an eel swimming in water.[1]

Leeuwenhoek and his contemporaries had no concept of the ovum or the process of fertilization, and the belief was prevalent that the spermatozoon was, in fact, a miniature human being, or homunculus, which simply grew in size, without the need for structural differentiation, to become a fetus. Niklaas Hartsoeker (1656–1725), one of Leeuwenhoek's contemporaries, published pictures showing tiny, preformed men (the homunculi) in the spermatozoa he examined through a microscope. By the end of the 17th century and throughout much of the Renaissance period, there were two opposing views on how the embryo formed. *Preformation*, the dominant theory, was the doctrine of embodiment, which had adherents from ancient times. According to this doctrine, each individual and those of succeeding generations lay encapsulated in a miniature, but fully differentiated form within their mothers. This doctrine was challenged in the early 17th century by William Harvey. Expressing the doctrine of *epigenesis*, which explained the organism as a primitive substance that expanded and changed through a series of stages, in which the mature embryo was achieved—a maturation of sorts. (Harvey's reports, however, contained many factual errors; but this did not alter the meritorious recognition of Harvey's brilliance in delineating the continuous circulation of the blood.) The latter discovery was probably the most significant achievement of medicine in the 17th century, although this idea had been recorded in the ancient Chinese Nei Ching (Canon of Medicine) by Yi Hsiung, ca. 2600 B.C. The Preformative theory was not decisively discredited until 1759 when Caspar Friedrich Wolff published his treatise, Theoria Generationis, based on his observations of anatomic differentiation in developing chick embryos. Interestingly, mammalian ova were not discovered until the investigations of Karl Ernst van Baer in 1827 (this was mentioned in Chap. 5).

Fertility was a favorite subject of ancient sculpturers, as evidenced by the statuary and carvings of menhirs and fertility goddesses, such as the female seated figure (ca. 6500–5700 B.C.) found during the excavations of Catal Huyuk in Turkey (the figurine is now exhibited in the Archeological Museum of Ankara). The ancient Mexican god, Quetzacoatal, was considered a god of fertility and life. The Mesopotamians (ca. 1400–1200 B.C.) were known to create gold figurines as fertility images (Norbert Schimmel Collection, New York, N.Y.), The ancient Egyptians must have had some knowledge of the role of semen in fecundation, because a bas-relief from Saggara (exhibited in the Louvre, Paris) shows a bull and cow in the position of insemination. The Amerindian medicine man, the Congo witch doctor, and the old world shaman were all concerned with reproduction. One of the eight monumental gates to the Babylonia of Nebuchadnezzar II (ca. 575 B.C.) was dedicated to the fertility deity Ishtas.

By the early 20th century, methods for the investigation and treatment of infertility had become firmly established within medical practice, albeit in a superficial form. Although Max Hühner published a book, Sterility in the Male and Female and Its Treatment (1913), the concern of early investigations was preponderately directed to the female as the cause of infertility in barren marriages.[2] Indeed, it was not until 1929 that a precise technique was reported for enumerating spermatozoa in seminal fluid.[3]

The art forms of our more permissive society have not escaped preoccupation with sperm and ova, genetics and breeding, or fertility and sterility; witness the book, The Führer Seed (Gus Weill, 1979).

The scope of infertility investigations has been expanded as a result of advances in biogenetics and the general availability of endocrine tests in hospital and clinical laboratories since the late 1970s. A more balanced approach to the study of fertility and sterility reflects the recognition that the male is the major contributor to infertility problems in 30 to 50% of barren marriages.

PHYSIOLOGY OF SEMINAL FLUID

In one respect, seminal fluid is analogous to blood in that it consists of cells (spermatozoa) suspended in a complex solution of proteins and enzymes (seminal plasma). Another similarity is that both of these body fluids are capable of coagulation and spontaneous clot lysis. Here the similarity ends. Seminal fluid should not be considered a transudate or a modified ultrafiltrate of blood plasma as are urine, cerebrospinal fluid, and body-cavity fluids.

The functions of seminal plasma include:

1. Activation of spermatozoal motility
2. Provision of nutritive substances
3. Conveyance of spermatozoa to the endocervical mucus and coagulation (the latter of which is probably an evolutionary mechanism to help avoid loss of semen from the vagina immediately after coitus).

The role of seminal plasma is transitory, because spermatozoa must penetrate the endocervical mucus within at most a few hours after ejaculation or be inactivated by the low pH of vaginal secretions. Indeed, motile spermatozoa can be detected in the fallopian tubes within 5 to 15 minutes from the time the liquified seminal fluid is deposited in the vagina. Fertilization ordinarily occurs in the distal third of the fallopian tubes but probably not for at least 4 or 5 hours, during which time capacitation occurs. Capacitation involves disintegration of the acrosome, a membrane-lined cell organelle that envelops the anterior two-thirds of the sperm head, with the resultant release of hydrolytic enzymes that assist the spermatozoon in penetrating the cumulus oophorus, corona radiata, and zona pellicuda of the ovum. (Penetration of the ovum, however, by another ovum without spermatozoa, has been achieved in vitro, with development of only an XX zygote— an experiment with somber moral and genetic implications!)

Spermatozoa constitute less than 5% of the seminal-fluid volume. Seminal plasma is derived from secretions of the prostate, seminal vesicles, epididymides, vasa deferentia, bulbourethral (Cowper's) glands, and urethral (Littre) glands. In the process of tumescence, a few drops of clear viscid secretion from the bulbourethral and urethral glands enter the urethra and frequently appear at the urethral meatus. This fluid is thought to lubricate the urethra for passage of the ejaculated seminal substance. Although this secretion is sometimes considered to be the first of three secretory fractions in the ejaculatory process, this notion is not entirely correct, because this initial secretion can occur whether or not ejaculation follows. The first true ejaculatory fraction comprises about 30% of the total seminal-fluid volume and consists largely of prostatic secretion, small amounts of secretion from the vasa deferentia and epididymides, and most of the spermatozoa. The final fraction consists largely of mucoid secretion from the seminal vesicles.

TESTES

Subsequent to the onset of puberty, spermatozoa are produced from germ cells (spermatogonia) of the testicular tubules by maturation (spermatogenesis): the spermatogonia develop into primary and secondary spermatocytes, then into spermatids, and finally, into mature spermatozoa.

In the formation of spermatids, meiotic division results in a haploid complement of chromosomes. Spermatogenesis is strongly endocrine-dependent, but the relative importance of the various hormones has not been conclusively established.[4] Follicle-stimulating hormone (FSH) appears to be necessary, at least for the initiation of spermatogenesis in the immature testis. Subsequently, spermatogenesis seems to proceed provided that testosterone is present in adequate amounts. Testosterone is produced in males largely by the interstitial (Leydig) cells of the testes under the influence of luteinizing hormone (LH). Both FSH and LH are produced by the adenohypophysis in response to a gonadotropin-releasing hormone secreted by the hypothalamus and modulated through a negative-feedback mechanism that involves androgens (chiefly testosterone) and, to a lesser extent, estrogens and progesterone.

Spermatozoa are not actively motile until ejaculation. They are passively transported from the testes through the epididymides and vasa deferentia largely by peristaltic action to the ampullae (expanded terminal portions of the vasa deferentia), where they are stored until ejaculation. The ampullae are connected to the urethra by the short (2 cm) ejaculatory ducts. Spermatozoa can apparently survive in a relatively quiescent state of low metabolic activity in the ampullae for a month or more, although prolonged storage does result in progressive loss of subsequent motility.

PROSTATE

The prostate completely surrounds the urethra immediately below the bladder neck and is composed of a dense, fibromuscular stroma that surrounds 30 to 50 compound tubuloalveolar glands, which empty into the urethra by as many as 32 separate excretory ducts. Prostatic secretion is an opalescent fluid with a pH of about 6.5; it contains a high concentration of citric acid, zinc, "acid phosphatase," and numerous other enzymes, including diastase, beta glucuronidase, and several proteolytic enzymes that are responsible for both the clotting and liquefaction of semen. Although acid phosphatase can cleave phosphorylcholine, which is present in high concentrations in seminal-vesicle secretion, its biochemical significance is otherwise not clear. Prostatic secretion also frequently contains small concretions, corpora amylacea, which form from inspissated secretion in the glandular alveoli. Corpora amylacea are usually 100 to 500 μ in diameter, but they may reach several millimeters. They are readily identified under the microscope by their concentric laminations.

SEMINAL VESICLES

The seminal vesicles are hollow, tortuous organs about 5 to 8 cm long and are closely apposed to the posterior aspect of the urinary bladder. They empty into the urethra via the ejaculatory ducts. Seminal-vesicle secretion constitutes about 60% of the entire seminal-fluid volume. The secretion is viscid, neutral to slightly alkaline, and pale to deep yellow-brown as a consequence of its high flavin content. This secretion provides the substrate responsible for coagulation of semen. Seminal-vesicle secretion is also rich in fructose and phosphorylcholine.

INDICATIONS FOR SEMINAL-FLUID ANALYSIS

Seminal-fluid examination is usually performed as part of a comprehensive investigation of infertile marriages. In view of its high potential for providing diagnostic information, its low cost, and technical simplicity, the seminal-fluid examination should be one of the first tests performed in the infertility investigation.

Most cases of infertility have anatomic abnormalities in semen; some cases, however, involve physiologic (functional) problems.

Functional infertility in the male is a result of:

1. Impotence
2. Inadequate spermatogenesis
3. Obstruction to the delivery of spermatozoa into the urethra during ejaculation, caused by postinfectious strictures of the ejaculatory ducts of vasa deferentia and surgical ligation of the vasa deferentia, for example
4. Anatomic anomalies that prevent seminal fluid from entering the vagina during ejaculation (retrograde ejaculation into the urinary bladder or via hypospadias, for example)

Other reasons for seminal-fluid analysis include:

1. Qualification of donors for artificial insemination programs
2. Documentation of the completeness of vasectomy
3. Evaluation of semen quality for semen banking
4. Examination of vaginal or oral washings, rectal swabs, or clothing and fabric stains for the presence of semen in alleged or suspected rape or in association with other crimes
5. Forensic indication for seminal-fluid examination in the investigation of a denial of paternity allegation based on a claim of absolute sterility, albeit rare.

Preservation of spermatozoa by freezing also has therapeutic applications in that it allows concentration of oligospermic semen and multiple inseminations into a woman who ovulates irregularly. (Except for artificial-insemination programs, semen banking has only limited applications—for storage of semen prior to vasectomy or to the institution of surgical, radiation, or chemotherapeutic treatment for malignancies, for example).[5]

At the present time, only a minority of the conditions producing inadequate spermatogenesis can be treated adequately.

The following outline lists the causes of inadequate spermatogenesis[6,7]:

A. Primary testicular dysfunction
    1. Anatomic
        a. Testicular agenesis
        b. Testicular ectopia (cryptorchism)
    2. Circulatory
        a. Testicular torsion
        b. Varicocele
        c. Atherosclerosis
    3. Physical agents
        a. Ionizing radiation
        b. Heat
    4. Pharmacologic/toxic agents
        a. Alkylating agents (nitrogen mustard, chlorambucil, triethylenemelamine, cyclophosphamide, etc.)
        b. Chemotherapeutic agents (vincristine, methotrexate, mercaptopurine, etc.)
        c. Various industrial chemicals (pesticides, fungicides, solvents, etc.)
    5. Infectious
        a. Viral infections (mumps)
        b. Granulomatous disease (tuberculosis, leprosy, tertiary syphilis, autoimmune orchitis, etc.)
    6. Chromosomal/hereditary enzyme defects
        a. Klinefelter's syndrome (XXY)

b. XX syndrome
c. XYY syndrome (some cases)
d. Congenital adrenal hyperplasia types IV, V, VI (inability of both adrenals and testes to form androgens)
7. Miscellaneous
a. Myotonic dystrophy
b. Noonan's syndrome ("male Turner syndrome")
c. Reinfenstein's syndrome
d. Sertoli only syndrome
e. Severe malnutrition
f. Idiopathic conditions

B. Secondary testicular dysfunction
1. Hypothalamic insufficiency (craniopharyngioma, metastatic neoplasm, trauma, etc.)
2. Adenohypophyseal insufficiency (panhypopituitarism, pituitary adenoma, metastatic carcinoma, trauma, surgical excision, etc.)
3. Excessive sex steroids
a. Androgen or estrogen-producing neoplasms of the adrenals
b. Congenital adrenal hyperplasia Types I, II, III
c. Exogenous (therapeutic or toxic exposure)

Nevertheless, maximum information is essential to the husband and wife of an infertile marriage so that reproductive alternatives—adoption or artificial insemination—can be considered.

SPECIMEN COLLECTION AND PRESERVATION

No advance preparation of the patient is required. A frank discussion of the importance of the seminal-fluid examination to the overall investigation of the infertility problem is, of course, useful. Although many physicians prescribe a 3- or 4-day period of abstinence from sexual intercourse or ejaculatory activity prior to collection of the seminal-fluid specimen, a more convincing argument can be made for collecting the specimen after a period of abstinence consistent with the usual frequency of coitus for the couple. Since it is purported by sex therapists that most couples have sexual intercourse twice weekly, additional abstinence is not necessary.

The best seminal-fluid specimen is collected by masturbation in the immediate vicinity of the clinical laboratory, so that the entire process of coagulation and liquefaction can be observed and the risk of accidental exposure to extreme heat or cold can be avoided.

Do not believe that all males understand the term "masturbation." It may be necessary to explain the process in more earthy terms, or at last resort, to gesticulate!

It is desirable for the patient to urinate immediately prior to collection in order to cleanse the urethra as much as possible. Care must be taken to deposit the specimen in a chemically clean container. Disposable plastic or polyethylene containers used for urine or sputum specimens are cheap, readily available, and ordinarily free of any toxic residues (see Chap. 1). Glass jars are not always satisfactory collection containers, because they frequently contain undetectable soap or detergent residues, which can rapidly inactivate spermatozoa. If the specimen is to be transported to the laboratory from a distant location, it should be submitted within 2 hours of collection and must not be subjected to temperature extremes. It appears that avoidance of cold exposure is particularly important until liquefaction is complete, about 20 to 30 minutes after collection.[8]

Whether for psychologic, religious, moral, or aesthetic reasons, some patients cannot or will not collect seminal fluid by masturbation. Some patients, however, will permit their spouses to masturbate them, while others will refuse any form of masturbation. In such patients, collection with special containers during intercourse or coitus interrruptus may be necessary. The first portion of the ejaculate, which contains most of the spermatozoa, is frequently lost with collection by coitus interruptus; if this occurrence can be avoided, the specimen is satisfactory. Collection in ordinary latex condoms is usually unacceptable, because condoms frequently contain toxic residues and are often precoated with spermicidal lubricants. Efforts to wash condoms with soap and water are not entirely satisfactory, because soap or detergent residue can inhibit sperm motility. A recently introduced silastic device (Dow Corning, P.O. Box 1-M, Midland, Mich. 48640) resembling an ordinary condom has been reported to yield excellent preservation of sperm motility.[9] The Milex Seminal Pouch (Milex Products, 5915 Northwest Highway, Chicago, Ill. 60631) is another plastic collection device that maintains good preservation of sperm motility.

ROUTINE SEMINAL-FLUID ANALYSIS

There are no specific parameters or laboratory procedures that have been considered "routine" in seminal-fluid analysis. Because seminal fluid, like urine, is a complex mixture of fluid, cells, spermatozoa, enzymes, and other substances, analysis of this substance is truly a composite examination. Therefore, it has become customary, if not totally appropriate, to perform a battery of tests on seminal fluid. A clinically relevant battery of testing has yet to be developed; but hopefully, the laboratories with which we are associated perform the following procedures:

1. Color and clarity
2. pH
3. Viscosity
4. Volume

5. Coagulation and liquefaction
6. Motility
7. Sperm count (concentration)
8. Morphologic evaluation/microscopic examination for abnormal spermatozoa
9. Postcoital testing

Studies for detection of seminal fluid and investigation of alleged rape and sexual assault have been more commonly performed in the United States over the past few years, because some 51,000 rape cases are reported yearly (about 900 weekly, 140 daily, or 1 every 10 minutes). It is believed that more than twice this many cases are unreported. Without laboratory corroboration of the presence of seminal fluid (detection of spermatozoa and high levels of acid phosphatase) in such cases, the investigating authorities would have no recourse. Justice and public demand require conclusive scientific evidence in rape cases, to adjudicate more fairly and actively the rights of all parties. This has placed a burden on the clinical laboratory.

Color and Clarity

Subsequent to liquefaction of the initial coagulum, seminal fluid is a somewhat viscous, translucent, grey-white fluid with a distinct, somewhat pungent, odor. This odor is considered to be the result of oxidation of spermine, which is secreted by the prostate.[10] Prolonged abstinence prior to specimen collection can cause a yellow color as a consequence of increased flavin content from the seminal vesicles. A dense, white, turbid appearance can be caused by large numbers of leukocytes associated with inflammation in the urethra or in one of the accessory ejaculatory glands. A red color is suggestive of blood, the presence of which can be verified by microscopic examination.

pH

The pH of fresh seminal fluid is usually in the range of 7.3 to 7.9.[11] The pH eventually increases slightly, probably as a result of carbon-dioxide loss. The presence of numerous leukocytes can cause a progressive decrease in pH because of metabolic-acid accumulation. Vasectomy also causes a significant decrease in seminal-fluid pH.[12] A pH of less than 7.0 suggests that the seminal fluid consists mainly of prostatic fluid because of either blockage of the ejaculatory ducts from acute inflammation or because of inflammatory stricture or congenital absence of the seminal vesicles.

Viscosity

Viscosity is readily evaluated by pouring the liquefied specimen from its container into a graduated cylinder for measurement of volume. A specimen of normal viscosity can be poured in small discrete droplets. Alternatively, viscosity can be evaluated by aspirating an aliquot of the specimen into a Pasteur pipette and observing the character of the expressed droplets. Viscosity is commonly evaluated on a scale of 0 to 4+, 0 representing normal viscosity and 4+ being a gelatinous mass that cannot be poured and only gradually conforms to the container in which it is placed.[13] Viscosity decreases significantly following bilateral vasectomy.[12] Excessive viscosity can interfere with sperm motility.

Volume

Volume can be measured to the nearest 0.1 ml in a suitable graduated cylinder. In a 1975 study of 1300 men who had fathered two or more children, a mean seminal-fluid volume of 3.2 ml with a range of 0.1 to 11.0 ml was reported.[14] This is significantly more than the mean of 2.8 ml reported in a 1974 study of 386 males who had fathered at least one child.[15] A 1951 study revealed a mean volume of 3.4 ml for 1000 fertile males compared with 3.6 ml for 800 males of infertile marriages, a difference that is statistically significant.[16] The 1974 study included sufficient data to allow nonparametric analysis, which indicates a normal range of approximately 0.7 to 6.5 ml. Small volumes of seminal fluid can be associated with infertility because of inadequate seminal plasma to convey spermatozoa to the endocervix and to counteract the strong acidity of vaginal secretions. Abstinence causes an increase in volume at least for a week or so.[17] One study indicated an incremental increase in volume of 0.4 ml/day for periods of up to 7 days.[18] As might be expected, vasectomy does not significantly change the seminal-fluid volume.[12] Infertile males can have a volume greater than 10 ml for reasons yet unknown.

Coagulation and Liquefaction

Semen normally coagulates within a few seconds following ejaculation to form a thick, grey-white coagulum, which spontaneously liquefies within 15 to 20 minutes. The event that triggers the coagulation process is the mixing of clotting substrate from the seminal vesicles with clotting enzymes from the prostate. The semen of males with bilateral agenesis of the seminal vesicles or bilateral obstruction of the ejaculatory ducts does not coagulate.[10]

Motility

Motility of sperm is considered synonymous with anatomic integrity and fertility. Actually motility is a function of energy expenditure and of the mitochondrial production of ATP. Motility is readily evaluated by placing a drop of seminal fluid on a microscope slide and covering the drop with a coverslip; the drop should be large enough to cover the underside of the coverslip but not so excessive that spermatozoa can move vertically out of the plane of focus. Ideally, the slide should be prewarmed and maintained at 37° C until the evaluation is completed. Cold does inhibit sperm motility. The high dry objective should be used to evaluate 200 spermatozoa in at least 10 different fields in order to compensate for the marked differences in sperm motility that can be observed from field to field in many specimens. The entire depth of the field should be examined in order to include dead or otherwise nonmotile sperm that may gravitate to the bottom of the field of focus. Spermatozoa should be considered motile if they exhibit definite forward progression. Some investigators recommend a semiquantitative estimation of sperm motility using a 0 to 4+ scale.[13]

0 = No motion
1 = Sperm movement without forward progression
2 = Sperm movement with slow forward progression
3 = Sperm moving in an almost straight line with moderate speed
4 = Sperm moving in a straight line with high speed

In view of the wide range of percentages of motile sperm from fertile males and the significant effect of both temperature and the time interval between ejaculation and examination, it can be reasonably questioned whether a motility subclassification such as this is clinically relevant.

In a study of 1300 males of proven fertility, a range of motile spermatozoa from 5 to 95% with a mean of 65% was found.[14] Nonparametric analysis of these data indicates a normal range of about 20 to 90%. This is similar to the mean motility reported by MacLeod and Gold of 61% for 732 fertile males, which contrasted with 54% for 869 males associated with infertile marriages.[19] An upper limit for the normal range of motility has no known pathophysiologic importance and can be ignored. Although infertile males as a group have lower sperm motility than do fertile males, there is a broad overlap between the two groups. In comparing the 732 fertile males with 869 infertility-associated males, MacLeod and Gold found that fertile males were underrepresented in the categories below 40% motility and overrepresented above 60% (these data emphasize the distinction between normal range and prevalent range). It would appear appropriate to consider a sperm motility of less than 40% as abnormal but by no means synonymous with infertility. Sperm motility is significantly less in semen with sperm counts of less than 20 million/ml.[19] There is a slight decrease in the percentage of motile sperm after the age of 40.[16] In one study, a significant decrease in the percentages of motile sperm was noted as the period of abstinence increased from 3 to 10 days.

Historically, many investigators have recommended continuing evaluation of motility over a 24-hour period. This should be abandoned, because it has no physiologic basis. (Spermatozoa must either penetrate the endocervical mucus within a short time after ejaculation or be inactivated by vaginal secretions.)

Sperm-Count Concentration

Spermatozoa can be enumerated in much the same way as blood cells are counted. The diluting fluid usually contains either formalin or phenol to inactivate the spermatozoa. Ordinarily, the semen can be conveniently diluted 1:20 in an ordinary white-blood-cell pipette and the spermatozoa enumerated in a standard hemacytometer, e.g., one with improved Neubauer ruling. Difficulty can be encountered in attempting to perform sperm counts in seminal fluid with significantly increased viscosity. In such a situation, the seminal fluid can be diluted with equal parts of suitable mucolytic agents such as Alevaire (Breon Laboratories Inc., 90 Park Avenue, New York, N.Y. 10016).

All hemacytometer enumerations of spermatozoa are relatively imprecise at best. Thus, in one study, duplicate sperm counts by the same technologist had a mean difference of 20%.[20] Even more striking was the finding that counts performed by three technicians, each of whom used duplicate pipettings on the same sample, had a coefficient of variation of 26%.

The sperm counts found in four studies involving 5,229 fertile males and 800 males associated with infertile marriages are summarized in Table 7–1. Of interest in Table 7–1 is the significant decrease in sperm counts over the 27-year period. Also, there is considerable overlap between fertile males and those associated with infertile marriages. MacLeod did find a preponderance of males associated with infertile marriages when sperm counts were less than 20 million/ml.[16] It would seem advisable, therefore, to consider sperm counts of less than 20 million/ml as suspect, although this is not synonymous with a desig-

TABLE 7–1. Comparison of Sperm Counts in Four Large Studies.

Investigators	MacLeod[16] (1951)	MacLeod[16] (1951)	Nelson, Bunge[15] (1974)	Rehan, Sobrero, Fertig[14] (1975)	Smith, Stultz, Jackson, Steinberger[21] (1978)
Type of subjects	fertile	infertile marriages	fertile	fertile	fertile
Number of subjects	1,000	800	386	1,300	2,543
Mean sperm count ($\times 10^6$/ml)	107	90	48	79	70
% of subjects with sperm counts:					
Less than 20×10^6/ml	5	14	20	7	19
Greater than 100×10^6/ml	44	38	7	24	23

nation of infertility, a prevalent or referent range, or a normal range in the traditional sense of the term. Sperm counts increase with abstinence at least up to a 10-day period.[17] The incremental increase in one study was 13 million/ml per day of abstinence.[18] Changes in the public sex habits in our more permissive society could explain the decreased sperm counts noted over the period 1951 through 1978. Sperm counts do not change appreciably with age.[14] There is a suggestion that polyzoospermy, a sperm count of greater than 250 million/ml, is associated with an increased incidence of abortion.

Morphologic Evaluation/Microscopic Examination

Examination of an appropriately stained smear of seminal fluid allows evaluation of sperm morphology as well as the detection of inflammatory cells, microorganisms, blood, and miscellaneous structures such as calculi. Smears are prepared in essentially the same manner as peripheral blood smears and stained after fixation. Georges Papanicolaou's staining technique or the Kernechtrot stain give excellent morphologic rendition. These staining techniques are recommended for exfoliative cytology in those clinical laboratories that use these techniques routinely. The only requirement for preparing the smear is that it be fixed immediately in either 95% (v/v) ethanol or 50% (v/v) ethanol-ether. A laboratory that does only occasional seminal-fluid examinations and does not use the Papanicolaou procedure for exfoliative cytology or for other applications should consider the Kernechtrot or other staining procedure for the occasional seminal-fluid examination.

Morphologic categorization ordinarily presents no problem, although occasionally it is difficult to distinguish macrophages, epithelial cells from the accessory sex glands, and germinal epithelial cells, particularly in the presence of inflammatory disease. One detailed study of 100 males who had previously fathered two or more children and whose wives were currently pregnant, indicated a mean of 73% morphologically mature and normal spermatozoa with a range from 21 to 90%.[22] Nonparametric analysis of the data from this study indicates a normal range of approximately 40 to 90%. Another study of 386 fertile males reported a mean of 74% morphologic forms.[15] In a comparative study of the sperm morphology of 989 fertile males and 969 males associated with infertile marriages, MacLeod and Gold found a considerable overlap in the percentages of morphologically normal forms in the two groups.[23] There was, however, a significant underrepresentation of fertile males with more than 40% abnormal forms. It would seem reasonable, therefore, to establish the criterion of normalcy as over 60% morphologically normal forms. As with sperm motility and sperm counts, this criterion does not distinguish fertile from infertile males; also, it is not the lower limit of a normal range, in the classic sense of the term, either by parametric or nonparametric estimation. What it does imply is that, with fewer than 60% morphologically normal spermatozoa, a male has a significantly increased chance of having a fertility problem.

The percentage of morphologically normal spermatozoa does not change with increased periods of abstinence.[17] The percentage of abnormal forms does tend to increase significantly with decreasing sperm counts.[23]

Hematoxylin staining of an air-dried smear permits observation of morphologic detail; it is simple and recommended. The Kernechtrot stain is advocated by forensic scientists. Other stains that can be used effectively include Giemsa, basic fushsin, and crystal violet stains.

At least 200 spermatozoa should be evaluated. The percentage of normal and abnormal forms should be recorded in similar fashion:

1. Percentage of normal spermatozoa
2. Percentage of immature forms
3. Percentage of abnormal forms (Figs. 7–1 – 7–3)

Various abnormal shapes occur, including giant head or pin head, amorphous heads, double heads or tails (Fig. 7–4).

In the course of the morphologic evaluation, one should notice inflammatory cells, blood, crystals, and foreign material. Corpora amylacea have been discussed previously. Smears from specimens that have had a prolonged interval between collection and examination can contain colorless, needle-shaped crystals of spermine phosphate.

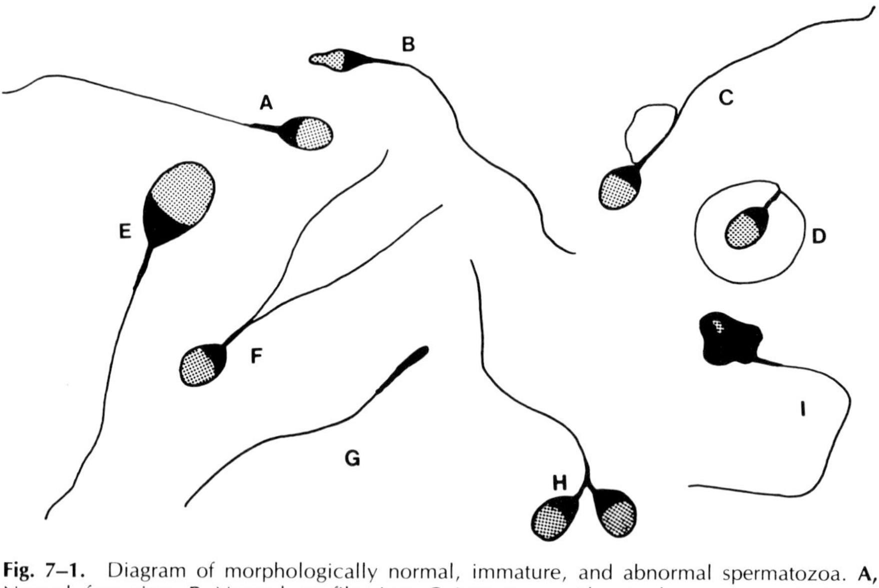

Fig. 7–1. Diagram of morphologically normal, immature, and abnormal spermatozoa. **A,** Normal, face view. **B,** Normal, profile view. **C,** Immature, with cytoplasmic remnant at neck region. **D,** Immature, with tail coiled in cytoplasm. **E,** Giant head. **F,** Double tail. **G,** Pin head. **H,** Double head. **I,** Amorphous head.

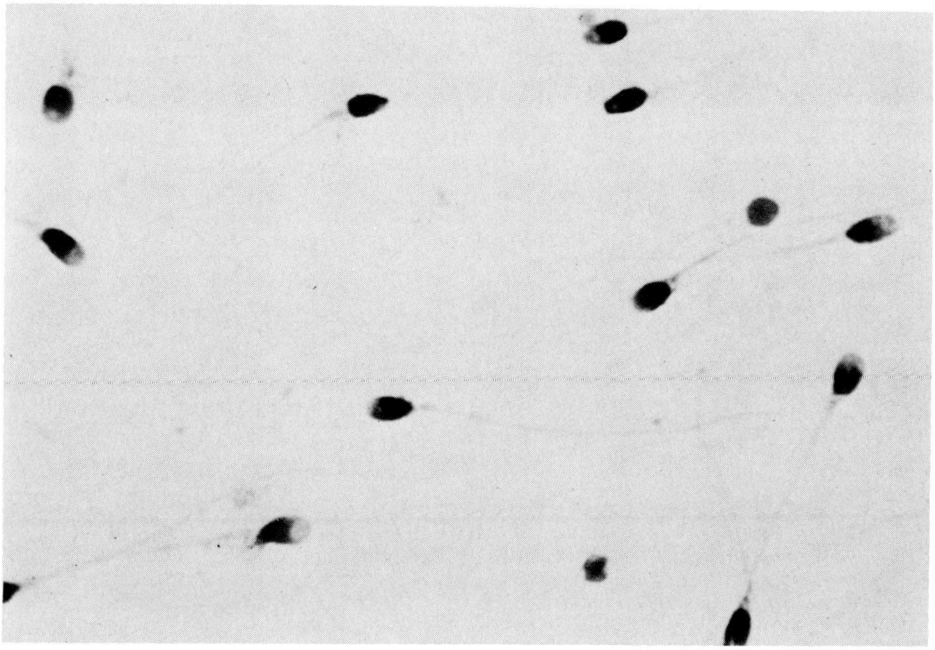

Fig. 7–2. Morphologically normal, mature spermatozoa. × 400. Papanicolaou stain.

POSTCOITAL TEST

Examination of the cervical mucus following coitus was first recommended as an approach to infertility investigation by Marion Sims in Uterine Surgery, published in 1866.[24] The study was later endorsed by Max Hühner in his 1914 book, Sterility in the Male and Female and Its Treatment.[2] Consequently, the postcoital test is frequently referred to as the Sims-Hühner test. The test is now commonly utilized in infertility investigations, because it is a direct measure of the receptivity of endocervical mucus to spermatozoa. The interaction between endocervical mucus and spermatozoa has recently gained increased attention because of the possibility that antispermatozoal antibodies exert their untoward effects at this site. It has been suggested that functional abnormalities of the cervix and its secretions may be responsible for as many as 5 to 10% of all cases of infertility.[25]

Cervical mucus is rich in carbohydrates and glycoproteins. Its character changes markedly throughout the menstrual cycle as a consequence of hormonal regulation. Estrogen stimulates copious amounts of watery mucus, while progesterone causes a viscous mucus that is virtually impenetrable to spermatozoa. Cervical mucus achieves the optimal status for sperm penetration in the period immediately prior to ovulation.

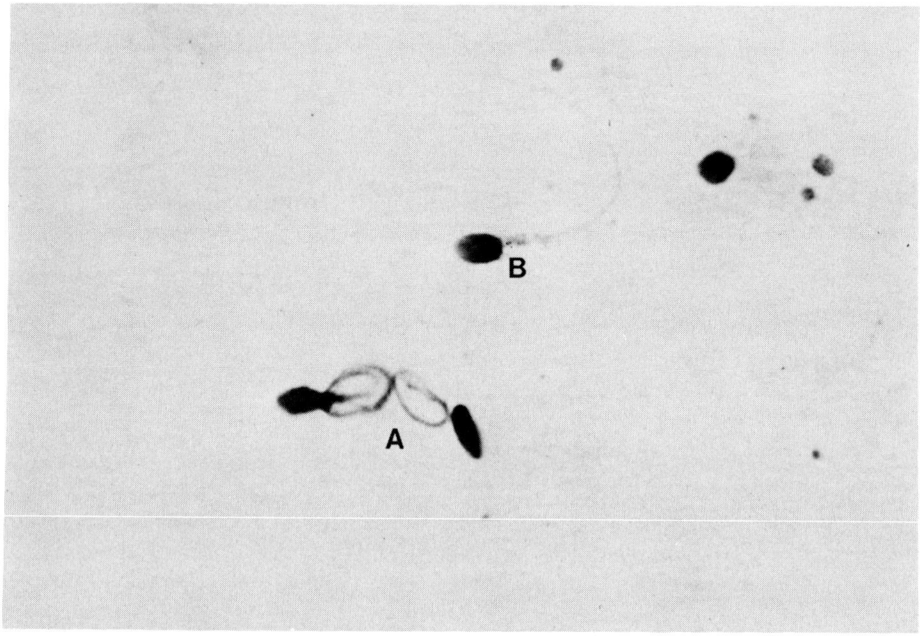

Fig. 7–3. Immature spermatozoa. **A,** Two spermatozoa have their tails coiled in a cytoplasmic remnant of the spermatid. **B,** This spermatozoon is almost mature but has a small cytoplasmic remnant on the neck piece. × 400. Papanicolaou stain.

The female should report to her physician for the examination within several hours after coitus, as close as possible to the time of ovulation as determined by basal temperature records. Although motile spermatozoa can persist in the endocervical mucus for as long as 36 or even 48 hours, the test should be performed within 8 hours of coitus because the number of spermatozoa seems to decrease rapidly after this time period.[26] This vaginal speculum can be moistened with water or saline but not with petrolatum, lubricating jellies, or other oils commonly used by physicians in office practice. The external os is wiped clear of mucus. The endocervical mucus can be aspirated with either a tuberculin syringe or a glass cannula attached by a rubber hose to a 10-cc Luer syringe. The syringe may be a convenient container for transporting the aspirated specimen to the clinical laboratory.

Upon receipt in the laboratory, the volume of the specimen should be measured, whereupon it can be expelled from the syringe container into a Petri dish for observation. At midcycle, the mucus should be clear, copious, and watery. The viscosity and tenacity of the mucus are evaluated by a feature known as spinnbarkeit, which is tested by grasping a portion of the mucus with forceps and observing the distance to which it can be pulled from the initial mass without breaking. At mid-

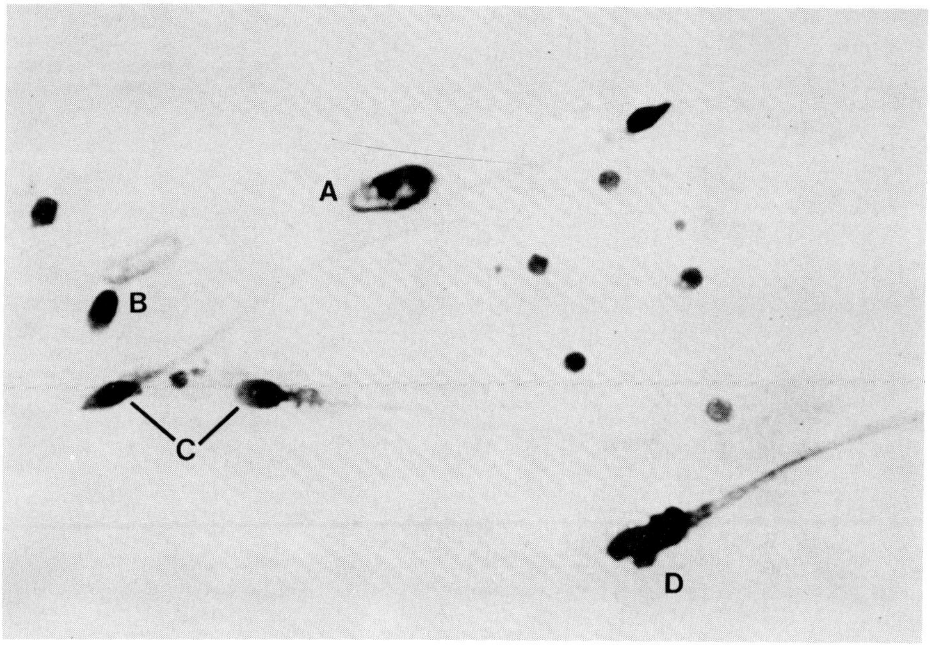

Fig. 7–4. Immature and abnormal spermatozoa. **A,** This spermatid has an amorphous nucleus. **B,** Immature spermatozoon with tail coiled in cytoplasmic remnant. **C,** Two immature spermatozoa with cytoplasmic tags at the neck pieces. **D,** A grossly amorphous giant-head spermatozoon. × 400. Papanicolaou stain.

cycle, an acceptable spinnbarkeit is at least 10 cm. A representative drop of mucus is then placed on a microscope slide, covered with a coverslip, and examined with the 40 × (high dry) objective for the number and motility of spermatozoa. The number of spermatozoa reach a peak about 2 to 3 hours after coitus, after which their numbers remain relatively constant for at least 6 to 8 hours. During this period, the number of motile sperm should be at least 10/high-power microscopic field.[25]

ANTIBODIES TO SPERMATOZOA

During the past 2 decades, considerable interest and investigational effort have focused on the immunogenicity of spermatozoa and the relationship of spermatozoal antibodies to male and female infertility and to other immune diseases. It is now firmly established that spermatozoa possess tissue-specific antigens and that antispermatozoal antibodies can occur in both males and females in the serum and in other body fluids (seminal plasma, vaginal secretion, and endocervical mucus, for example). Furthermore, significant levels of antibodies are more common in both males and females who are associated with infertile marriages.[27] Antibodies to spermatozoa occur in most males following vasectomy, but there is no known association of this postvasectomy immune response with other autoimmune disease or with immune-complex formation.[28]

Various techniques have been developed for the detection and quantitation of antibodies to spermatozoa, including immunofluorescent, cytotoxic, complement fixation and agglutination tests.[29] Agglutination tests have received the most attention and various protocols have been recommended: gelatin (Kibrick), slide, tray (Friberg), and tube-slide (Franklin-Dukes).[29] The tube-slide test has been somewhat controversial and current evidence suggests that the agglutination in this test may be the reaction of either a steroid-protein complex or a beta-agglutinin that is not an immunoglobulin. All of these tests are technically demanding and should be performed only by qualified laboratories.

DETECTION OF SEMINAL FLUID FOR MEDICOLEGAL PURPOSES

The clinical laboratory may be requested to examine secretions or washings from the vagina; stains on clothing, skin, or hair; or other sources for the presence of seminal fluid. When such examinations are requested for medicolegal purposes, care must be taken to maintain a chain of evidence; this requires a routing format, or sheet, to record who had possession of the specimen at what times. Each person who had possession of the specimen should verify the identification of the specimen, the steps taken to maintain its physical security, and information about its biochemical preservation, if appropriate. This information should be recorded on the routing sheet with dates, times, and signatures appended.

Material from the vagina can be obtained by direct aspiration of secretions or by saline lavage performed by a physician. Seminal fluid typically exhibits a green-white fluorescence under ultraviolet light, and this may be helpful in identifying stains that deserve further investigation. If the fabric can be sacrified, a 1-cm piece can be cut out and soaked in several milliliters of physiologic saline in a test tube. It is desirable to obtain a similar piece of material remote from the stain to serve as a control. Stains on skin or hair can be removed with a small pledget of gauze moistened in saline and then deposited in a test tube containing a small amount of saline.

Stained smears should be prepared for microscopic examination from the direct aspirate of vaginal contents or from the centrifuged sediment of lavage fluid or washings. Under such circumstances, spermatozoa are exceptionally fragile, so their tails are frequently broken away. Such smears should be kept secure as permanent evidence or should be photographed for demonstration. Spermatozoa can be detected in the vagina as long as 72 hours after coitus.[30] Spermatozoa can be identified in dried smears after a much longer period of time, however.

Acid phosphatase can also be assayed on the direct aspirates, lavages, or washings. Acid phosphatase is present in seminal fluid at a concentration exceeding 3500 King-Armstrong units, or 100,000 IU/L, while its concentration in other body fluids does not exceed about .08 IU/L. Although acid phosphatase usually disappears from vaginally deposited semen within 18 hours, it can be detected, albeit in much lesser concentrations, in dried stains after longer periods of time (7 days in one study).[31] Determination of acid phosphatase does not significantly improve the sensitivity of semen detection above and beyond the identification of spermatozoa.[31]

A, B, and H blood group substances occur in the seminal fluid of the 80% of males who are secretors, but of course, they also occur in the vaginal secretions of female secretors. Detection of blood-group substances in seminal fluid, secretions, lavage, or washings is based on the ability of the test solution to neutralize the agglutinating ability of a specific anti-A, B, or H reagent serum. The identification of a specific blood-group substance is potentially valuable for medicolegal purposes.

OTHER TESTS OF SEMINAL FLUID

Fructose is produced by the seminal vesicles. It has been recommended that a qualitative test for fructose be performed on all azoospermic seminal-fluid specimens in order to detect bilateral aplasia of the vasa deferentia and seminal vesicles, which have a common embryologic origin, or bilateral obstruction of the ejaculatory ducts.[13] This would seem to be superfluous in view of the fact that the same information can be gained by simply observing the seminal fluid for adequate clot formation, which is evidence that seminal vesicle secretion is entering the ejaculate.

The Florence test was formerly used as a screening test for the detection of seminal fluid, but it is of historical interest only. The test was based on the identification of a rhombic or needle-like crystal of choline periodide formed from the reaction of choline in semen with Lugol's iodine solution. The test is relatively insensitive and subject to false-positive results with other tissue fluid.

REFERENCES

1. Leeuwenhoek, A.: The Collected Letters of Antoni van Leeuwenhoek. Vol. 2. Amsterdam, Swets and Zeitlinger, 1941.
2. Hühner, M.: Sterility in the Male and Female and Its Treatment. New York, Rebman, 1913.
3. Macomber, D., and Sanders, M.: The spermatozoa count: Its value in the diagnosis, prognosis, and treatment of sterility. N. Engl. J. Med., *200*:981, 1929.
4. Steinberger, E.: Hormonal control of spermatogenesis. *In* Endocrinology. Vol. 3. Edited by L. DeGroot, et al. New York, Grune and Stratton, 1979, pp. 1535–1538.
5. Beck, W.: Artificial insemination and preservation of semen. Urol. Clin. North Am., 5:593, 1978.
6. Snyder, P.: Endocrine evaluation of the infertile male. Urol. Clin. North Am., 5:593, 1978.
7. Steinberger, E.: Disorders of testicular function (male hypogonadism). *In* Endocri-

nology. Vol. 3. Edited by L. DeGroot, et al. New York, Grune and Stratton, 1979, pp. 1549–1565.
8. Watson, A., and Robertson, C.: Male infertility: A reappraisal of semen analysis. J. Med. Lab. Tech., *23*:1, 1966.
9. Schoenfeld, C., Amelar, R., Dubin, L., and Skwerer, R.: Evaluation of a new sialastic seminal fluid collection device. Fertil. Steril., *30*:319, 1979.
10. Parrish, R., Polakoski, K., and Zaneveld, L.: Standards of analysis and clinical biochemistry of semen. Prog. Reprod. Biol., *3*:12, 1978.
11. Raboch, J., and Skachova, J.: The pH of human ejaculate. Fertil. Steril., *16*:252, 1965.
12. Nikkanen, V.: The effects of vasectomy on viscosity, pH, and volume of semen in man. Andrologia, *11*:123, 1979.
13. Amelar, R., and Dubin, L.: Semen analysis. *In* Male Infertility. Edited by R. Amelar, L. Dubin, and P. Walsh. Philadelphia, W.B. Saunders, 1977, pp. 105–140.
14. Rehan, N., Sobrero, A., and Fertig, J.: The semen of fertile men: Statistical analysis of 1300 men. Fertil. Steril., *26*:492, 1975.
15. Nelson, C., and Bunge, R.: Semen analysis: Evidence for changing parameters of male fertility potential. Fertil. Steril., *25*:503, 1974.
16. MacLeod, J.: Semen quality in one thousand men of known fertility and in eight hundred cases of infertile marriage. Fertil. Steril., *2*:115, 1951.
17. MacLeod, J., and Gold, R.: The male factor in fertility and infertility: Effect of continence on semen quality. Fertil. Steril., *3*:297, 1952.
18. Schwartz, D., Laplanche, A., Jouannet, P., and David, G.: Within subject variability of human semen in regard to sperm count, volume, total number of spermatozoa and length of abstinence. J. Reprod. Fertil., *57*:391, 1979.
19. MacLeod, J., and Gold, R.: The male factor in fertility and infertility: An analysis of motile activity in the spermatozoa of 1000 fertile men and 1000 men in infertile marriage. Fertil. Steril., *2*:187, 1951.
20. Freund, M., and Carol, B.: Factors affecting haemocytometer counts of sperm concentration in human semen. J. Reprod. Fertil., *8*:149, 1964.
21. Smith, K., Stultz, D., Jackson, J., and Steinberger, E.: Evaluation of sperm counts and total sperm counts in 2543 men requesting vasectomy. Andrologia, *10*:362, 1978.
22. Sobrero, A., and Rehan, N.: The semen of fertile men: Semen characteristics of 100 fertile men. Fertil. Steril., *26*:1048, 1975.
23. MacLeod, J., and Gold, R.: The male factor in fertility and infertility. IV. Sperm morphology in fertile and infertile marriages. Fertil. Steril., *2*:394, 1951.
24. Sims, M.: Uterine Surgery. New York, William Woods Co., 1866.
25. Moghissi, K.: Postcoital test: Physiologic basis, technique, and interpretation. Fertil. Steril., *27*:117, 1976.
26. Danezis, J., Sujan, S., and Sobrero, A.: Evaluation of the postcoital test. Fertil. Steril., *13*:559, 1962.
27. Menge, A.: Clinical immunologic infertility: diagnostic measures, incidence of antisperm antibodies, fertility and mechanisms. *In* Immunological Aspects of Infertility and Fertility Regulation. Edited by D. Dhindsa and G. Schumacher. Amsterdam, Elsevier North Holland, 1980, pp. 205–224.
28. Rümke, P.: Autoantibodies against spermatozoa. *In* Spermatozoa, Antibodies and Infertility. Edited by J. Cohen and W. Hendry. London, Blackwell Scientific Publications, 1978, pp. 67–79.
29. Boettcher, B.: Immunity to spermatozoa. Clin. Obstet. Gynecol., *6*:385, 1979.
30. Soules, M., Pollard, A., Brown, K., and Verma, M.: The forensic laboratory evaluation of evidence in alleged rape. Am. J. Obstet. Gynecol., *130*:142, 1978.
31. Dahlke, M., et al.: Identification of semen in 500 patients seen because of rape. Am. J. Clin. Pathol., *68*:740, 1977.

COLOR AND CLARITY EVALUATION

METHOD. Visual physical evaluation.

PRINCIPLE. Visual examination of seminal fluid can be used to separate obvious pathologic specimens from the usual normal fluid.

SPECIMEN COLLECTION. Specimen should be submitted within

2 hours of collection in a dry, clean test tube and should be permitted to sit for at least 30 minutes after collection to ensure liquefaction.

PROCEDURE

1. Examine the color and clarity (turbidity) of the seminal fluid in a test tube.
2. Record color and clarity.

INTERPRETATION. Normal seminal fluid, after liquefaction, is translucent, viscid, grey-white, and has a mildly pungent odor.

DISCUSSION AND CLINICAL SIGNIFICANCE. A dense, white, turbid appearance is usually associated with inflammation caused by polymorphonuclear leukocytes. A red color is suggestive of blood. Confirmation in either circumstance can be achieved by microscopic examination.

MATERIAL AND METHODS. Test tube, 10 × 100 mm.

REFERENCES

1. Amelar, P., and Dubin, L.: Semen analysis. *In* Male Infertility. Edited by R. Amelar, L. Dubin, and P. Walsh. Philadelphia, W.B. Saunders, 1977, p. 105.
2. Hepler, O.: Manual of Clinical Laboratory Methods. Springfield, Ill., Charles C Thomas, 1961, p. 160.

PH

METHOD. pH indicator paper visual examination.

PRINCIPLE. The H+ in the specimen reacts with mixed-color indicators (usually sodium dinitrophenolazo-naphthol disulfonate) to produce a variety of color that is proportioned to hydrogen-ion activity.

PROCEDURE

1. Dip paper into seminal fluid in suitable container and shake off excess.
2. Immediately compare color with reference chart.

INTERPRETATION. pH range of seminal fluid is 7.3 to 7.9.

DISCUSSION AND CLINICAL SIGNIFICANCE. Normally, the pH is a ratio of the buffer system in the specimen and will increase on standing as a result of carbon-dioxide loss. pH decreases in postvasectomy specimens. A pH of <7.0 indicates predominately prostatic secretion. Leukocyte presence in seminal fluid will also decrease pH.

MATERIALS AND REAGENTS

1. Nitrazine paper (E.R. Squibb & Sons, Princeton, N.J. 08540), pHydrion paper (MicroEssential Lab Laboratory, Brooklyn, N.Y. 11200) or Labstix (Ames Company, Elkhart, Ind. 46514).
2. Seminal fluid container

REFERENCE

1. Hepler, O.: Manual of Clinical Laboratory Methods. Springfield, Ill., Charles C Thomas, 1961, p. 160.

VISCOSITY

METHOD. Visual physical evaluation.

PRINCIPLE. The viscosity of seminal fluid is a reflection of the contents of the substances that comprise seminal fluid, and when abnormal viscosity is decreased. Although an Ostwald viscometer can be utilized, simple visual observation of the specimen is adequate enough for clinical purposes.

SPECIMEN COLLECTION. Specimen should be submitted within 2 hours of collection in a dry, clean test tube and should be permitted to sit for at least 30 minutes after collection to ensure liquefaction.

PROCEDURE

1. After liquefaction occurs in the specimen, mix by swirling in test tube.
2. Pour specimen from test tube into graduated cylinder.
3. Record viscosity on the scale of 0 to 4+.
4. Place a drop of seminal fluid on a microscopic slide and cover with a clean coverslip (the drop should be large enough to fill the entire area).

INTERPRETATION

0 = Watery specimen that can be poured
1+ = Slight viscosity that is somewhat stringy
2+ = Progressive stringiness
3+ = Slight coagulum that drops in a jelly-like manner
4+ = Gelatinous mass that cannot be poured

MATERIALS AND METHODS

1. Test tube, 10 × 100 mm.
2. Microscope slide, 1 × 3 mm.
3. Graduated cylinder, 50 ml.
4. Microscope coverslips

REFERENCES

1. Amelar, P., and Dubin, L.: Semen analysis. *In* Male Infertility. Edited by R. Amelar, L. Dubin, and P. Walsh. Philadelphia, W.B. Saunders, 1977, p. 105.
2. Hepler, O.: Manual of Clinical Laboratory Methods. Springfield, Ill., Charles C Thomas, 1961, p. 160.

SPERM MOTILITY, CONCENTRATION, AND MORPHOLOGY

METHOD. Visual observation.

SPECIMEN. Seminal fluid should be obtained in a dry, clean container, preferably by masturbation.

PRINCIPLE. Liquefaction can be observed visually. Motility can be estimated on a wet mount; pH is determined by pHydrion or Nitrazine paper; viscosity can be determined by visual observation; and volume can be measured in a small graduated cylinder—all on the same specimen. The concentration of spermatozoa is determined by enumeration in a hemacytometer. Morphologic evaluation is performed on slide mount.

PROCEDURE

DETERMINATION OF MOTILITY

1. Place a large drop of seminal fluid on a chemically clean microscope slide (prepare a wet mount) and cover with a chemically clean coverslip (the drop should be large enough to fill under the entire area of the coverslip but not so large as to cause free floating of the coverslip).
2. Using the high-dry microscope 40 × objective, evaluate the motility of 200 spermatozoa present in at least 10 fields. (The entire depth of each field must be examined so that immobile spermatozoa that have gravitated to the bottom of the field will be included.)
3. Consider any spermatozoon as motile if it exhibits definite forward progression.
4. Record the number of motile spermatozoa out of the 200 examined.
5. Report the percentage of motile spermatozoa by dividing the number in the 200 count by 2.

DETERMINATION OF SPERM CONCENTRATION

1. Mix the seminal fluid specimen thoroughly and draw an aliquot to the 0.5 mark in a white-blood-cell pipette.
2. Dilute the aliquot 1 in 20 by drawing formalin diluting fluid into the pipette until the volume reaches the 11 mark. (In the event that the specimen is exceptionally viscous, make a preliminary 1 to 1 dilution of a small aliquot with Alevaire. In this event, the final count will have to be multiplied by 2.)
3. Mix the fluid in the pipette by gently rotating for 5 minutes.
4. Fill both chambers of hemacytometer with the diluted specimen.
5. Count the spermatozoa in two large (1 sq mm) squares, one in each chamber of the hemacytometer.
6. Calculate and report the concentration of spermatozoa/mm by multiplying the total spermatozoa in two large squares by 100,000.

MICROSCOPIC EVALUATION OF SPERM MORPHOLOGY

1. Prepare a smear of seminal fluid on a microscope slide in the same manner as a peripheral blood smear.
2. If the Papanicolaou or Kernechtrot techniques are available in the laboratory, immediately fix the smear in ethanol; otherwise, air dry the smear and stain as follows in Coplin jars:
   a. Neutral formalin (1 minute)
   b. Water rinse (5 dips)
   c. Harris's hematoxylin (2 minutes)
   d. Water rinse (5 dips)
   e. Air dry

3. Evaluate 200 spermatozoa and categorize as normal, immature, or abnormal morphology (also note the presence of blood, inflammatory cells, or crystals).
4. Report the percentages of normal, immature, and abnormal spermatozoa by dividing the number in each of the categories in the 200 cell enumeration by 2.

Morphologic evaluation of the stained smear should include abnormalities of the head (too small, too large, pointed, ragged edges, atypical, distributor of chromatin, vacuoles, double head); middle piece (absent, bifurcated, swollen); and tail (double, curled, rudimentary, absent).

INTERPRETATION. Normal seminal fluid is grey-white and translucent and has a water viscosity that allows dropwise pouring (viscosity of 0 on a 0 to 4+ scale, whereas 4+ is a gelatinous mass that will not pour). Liquefaction should be complete within 30 minutes. Volume should be in the range of 0.7 to 6.5 ml with a mean of about 3.0 ml. The mean sperm concentration in fertile males is about 70 million/ml.

DISCUSSION AND CLINICAL SIGNIFICANCE. Decreased fertility is associated with a sperm motility of less than 40% (see text for evaluation of motility) although the mean motility in fertile males is about 65%. Decreased fertility is associated with sperm concentrations below 20 million/ml, and normal counts can go up to 150 million/ml. The mean percentage of morphologically normal and mature spermatozoa is about 75%. Fewer than 60% morphologically normal and mature spermatozoa are associated with decreased fertility.

MATERIALS AND REAGENTS

1. Formalin diluting fluid. To a 100 ml volumetric flask, add 1 ml 37% (w/v) formaldehyde and 5 g sodium bicarbonate. Dilute to 100 ml with distilled water.
2. Alevaire (Breon Laboratories Inc., 90 Park Ave., New York, N.Y. 10016).
3. Ethanol, 95% (v/v)
4. Neutral formalin, 10% (v/v). To a 100 ml volumetric flask, add 0.4 g monobasic sodium phosphate, 0.65 g diabasic sodium phosphate, and 10 ml 37% (w/v) formaldehyde. Dilute to 100 ml with distilled water.
5. Harris's hematoxylin. Dissolve 0.5 g hematoxylin in 5 ml of absolute ethanol. Dissolve 10 g potassium alum in 100 ml distilled water with heating as needed. Mix the two solutions in a beaker and rapidly bring to a boil. Remove the solution from heat and add 0.25 g red mercuric oxide. Reheat the solution until it becomes dark purple (approximately 1 minute). Immediately cool the solution by placing the beaker in cold water. Add 0.4 ml glacial acetic acid.
6. Disposable plastic urine or sputum containers for specimen collection

7. 10 ml graduated cylinder. Clean in 20% (v/v) acetone and polish interior dry with gauze.
8. Microscope slides and coverslips. Clean in 20% (v/v) acetone and polish with clean gauze.
9. Microscope with high-dry objective (40 ×)
10. White-blood-cell pipettes
11. Hemacytometer with improved Neubauer ruling

REFERENCES

1. Amelar, R., and Dubin, L.: Semen analysis. *In* Male Infertility. Edited by R. Amelar, L. Dubin, and P. Walsh. Philadelphia, W.B. Saunders, 1977, p. 105.
2. Hepler, O.: Manual of Clinical Laboratory Methods. Springfield, Ill., Charles C Thomas, 1961, p. 160.

POSTCOITAL TEST OF ENDOCERVICAL MUCUS

METHOD. The Sims-Hühner test as described by Danezis, Sujan, and Sobrero.

PRINCIPLE. The test is a measure of the penetration of spermatozoa into the endocervical mucus. The mucus achieves an optimal state of receptivity for penetration by sperm immediately prior to ovulation (presumably due to estrogen, carbohydrate, glycoproteins, and other factors in the mucus). Therefore, measure of spermatozoa activity can reflect the receptivity of mucus, or the converse, by the presence of hostile factors (such as antispermatozoa antibodies).

SPECIMEN COLLECTION. During the ovulatory phase of the menstrual cycle as determined by basal temperature records, the female reports to the physician within 2 to 8 hours after coitus. Endocervical mucus is aspirated with syringe and long needle from the os and submitted as the specimen.

PROCEDURE

1. Measure the volume of mucus in a syringe (if this served as the specimen container) or in a graduated cylinder.
2. Pour the specimen into a petri dish and evaluate its color, consistency, and clarity.
3. Determine the spinnbarkeit by grasping a portion of the mucus with forceps and noting the distance it can be pulled without breaking.
4. Place a drop of mucus on a chemically clean microscope slide and cover with a coverslip. Examine microscopically with a high-dry objective (40 ×).
5. Determine the average number of motile spermatozoa in 10 high-power fields.
6. Report the appearance, spinnbarkeit, and average number of motile spermatozoa/HPF.

INTERPRETATION. At the ovulatory phase of the menstrual cycle, endocervical mucus should be clear and watery and have a spinnbarkeit of at least 10 cm. The number of motile spermatozoa reach a peak in endocervical mucus about 2 or 3 hours after coitus. At that time, their numbers remain relatively constant for 6 to 8 hours, after which the number of motile spermatozoa decreases. The number of motile spermatozoa should be at least 10/HPF.

DISCUSSION AND CLINICAL SIGNIFICANCE. When a patient has sperm counts of less than 20 million/ml, he is suspected of being sterile. Infertile males have a lower sperm motility than fertile males; however, there is too much overlap for this type of parameter to be diagnostic. In general, normal average motility of sperm is about 65% (but can range from 9 to 95%). Motility is significantly lower in males with sperm counts less than 20 million/ml.

MATERIALS AND REAGENTS

1. Graduated cylinder, 10 to 20 ml. Clean in 20% (v/v) acetone and polish interior with gauze.
2. Plastic, disposable petri dish
3. Forceps
4. Microscope slides and coverslips. Clean in 20% (v/v) acetone and polish with clean gauze.
5. Microscope with high-dry objective

REFERENCE

1. Danezis, J., Sujan, S., and Sobrero, A.: Evaluation of the postcoital test. Fertil. Steril., *13*:559, 1962.

SPERMATOZOA STAINS

METHOD. Papanicolaou technique.

PRINCIPLE. The Papanicolaou staining procedure was devised for optimal visualization of normal or cancerous cells exfoliated from epithelial surfaces of the body, especially the vagina. This stain can also be used for sperm. This stain is not specific for any substance; rather, it is a polychrome staining reaction.

PROCEDURE. The following are the four main steps for the Papanicolaou staining procedure: fixation, nuclear staining, cytoplasmic staining, and clearing. These steps are interspersed with solutions that hydrate, dehydrate, and rinse the cells.

1. Fixation: Hair spray, 95% (v/v) alcohol, or other acceptable fixatives may be used. Subsequent steps in the Papanicolaou staining method will be effective only if specimens are immediately fixed.
2. Nuclear staining: Hematoxylin, which has an affinity for nucleoproteins, is used. This is one of the few natural stains in laboratory use.
3. Cytoplasmic staining: The purpose of the many colors in the counterstains is to display the many variations of cellular morphology showing degrees of differentiation and metabolic activity. By using solutions of high alcoholic content, the counterstains

provide clear visualization. The following are two cytoplasmic stains:

Orange G (OG-6): This monochromatic cytoplasmic stain is used for staining keratin a brilliant orange and usually does not stain sperm well.

EA (EA-50, 65): This polychromatic cytoplasmic stain is a mixture of eosin, light green, and bismarck brown. Eosin stains mature sperm heads (and nuclei and cilia). Light green stains the cytoplasm of metabolically active cells and sperm.

4. Clearing: This is the final step in the staining procedure, which results in cellular transparency. The solution used will transmit light rays from the microscope illuminations in the same manner as the cell itself, thereby making the cells transparent. Xylene (xylol) is the most commonly used clearing solution.

Successive steps for the immersion of a microscopic slide of fixed seminal fluid are as follows:

1. Water (distilled), 10 minutes
2. Hematoxylin, 2 minutes determined by test slide
3. Wash in distilled water until clean, about 4 to 5 washes
4. 50% (v/v) ethanol, with 3 ml of acetic acid/200 ml ethanol
5. 70% (v/v) ethanol with 3 ml of NH_4OH
6. 80% (v/v) ethanol
7. 95% (v/v) ethanol
8. OG-6, 2 minutes
9. 95% (v/v) ethanol
10. 95% (v/v) ethanol
11. Eosin, 2 minutes (as determined by using test slide for staining)
12. 95% (v/v) ethanol
13. Wash in absolute ethanol until clean
14. Clear in cedar oil and leave in xylene
15. Cover slip using permount adhesive

MATERIALS AND REAGENTS. Since the publication of the first part of Papanicolaou's Atlas in 1954, the EA 65-Eosin-Hematoxylin method used in our laboratory for staining smear preparations has remained essentially the same, except for a few modifications related chiefly to the preparation of the stains and the timing of the staining procedures.

PREPARATION OF STAINS

1. Harris hematoxylin contains the following:
   Hematoxylin (5 g)
   Ammonium aluminum sulphate (100 g)
   Ethyl alcohol (50 g)
   Distilled water (1,000 g)
   Mercuric oxide (2.5 g)

2. EA-65
   a. Stock solutions: First prepare 10% (w/v) aqueous stock solutions of Light Green S.F. Yellowish, Bismark Brown, and Eosin Yellowish (water and alcohol soluble). Then prepare three alcoholic stock stolutions as follows:
      1. Light Green S.F. Yellowish (0.5% solution in 95% ethanol)
      2. Bismark Brown (0.5% solution in 95% ethanol)
      3. Eosin Yellowish (0.5% solution in 95% ethanol)
   b. The EA-65 stain is prepared as follows:
      1. Alcoholic stock solution 1 (180 ml)
      2. Alcoholic stock solution 2 (40 ml)
      3. Alcoholic stock solution 3 (180 ml)
      4. Phosphotungstic acid (2.4 g)
   c. Filter and store in brown bottle.
      (All dyes used in these preparations are National Aniline and Chemical Company certified stains.)
3. Eosin Reagent
   a. Dissolve 10.0 g Light Green S.F. Yellowish in 100 ml glycerine or dissolve 10.0 g Fast Green in 100 ml glycerine. Add 10.0 g Eosin Yellowish dissolved in 100 ml glycerine.
   b. Measure 500 ml of 95% (v/v) ethanol.
   c. Into 1,000 ml flask containing 100 ml of 95% (v/v) ethanol, pipette 20 ml stock eosin reagent. Rinse the pipette in solution. Rotate the flask while pipetting.
   d. Add 4 ml Glacial Acetic Acid to solution.
   e. Into 500 ml flask containing 95% (v/v) ethanol, pipette 5 ml Light Green or 2.5 ml Fast Green. Rinse pipette until clean.
   f. Use remainder of 500 ml of 95% (v/v) ethanol to clean pipette and add to eosin solution.
   g. Add 0.50 g phosphotungstic acid, crystalline to stain.

REFERENCES

1. Keebler, C., Reagan, J., and Wied, G.: Compendium on Cytopreparatory Techniques. 4th Ed. Chicago, International Academy of Cytology, 1976, pp. 10–11.
2. Papanicolaou, G.: Atlas of Exfoliative Cytology. Cambridge, Harvard University Press, 1954, p. 1.
3. Prince, L.: Personal communication, 1979.

SPERMATOZOA STAIN (FOR RAPE CASES)

METHOD. Kernechtrot picroindigocarmine technique.

PRINCIPLE. Identification of presence of human spermatozoa for forensic medicolegal purposes is facilitated by staining the sperm heads red, and the tails red and green.

SPECIMEN. For suspected seminal stains on clothing or bedding, scrape or elute 1-cm square of clothing with about 4 to 5 ml of distilled water into a test tube.

1. Eluate: Centrifuge the eluate, and carefully decant most of the supernatant liquid (the supernatant fluid can be used for acid phosphatase determination!). Smear sediment into microscopic slide.
2. Scrapings: Place scrapings on glass microscope slide and add drop of distilled water.

PROCEDURE

1. To solution containing suspected sperm from sediment, add one drop of Kernechtrot solution (KS) and allow to stand under an inverted 600-ml beaker for about 15 minutes.
2. Using a clean, disposable pipette, place one to two drops distilled water on one side of the KS sample, carefully tilt the glass slide, and remove the effluent with blotter paper. (Do not touch the original area of the sample drop with the blotter paper.) Do this several times carefully until the wash solution is colorless.
3. Place one drop of picroindigocarmine solution (PICS) on the original sample drop area. Be prepared to remove this after no more than 15 seconds.
4. Use the same technique for washing the PICS as given in step 2, but use absolute ethanol.
5. Slide is ready for microscopic examination.

INTERPRETATION. Spermatozoa will be stained as follows: sperm heads, red; and sperm tails, red and green.

DISCUSSION AND CLINICAL SIGNIFICANCE. The color is so marked that it is possible to distinguish sperm from the remaining cellular matter. Mucous membrane (human tissue?) appears to have bright-blue cytoplasm and red nuclei. The nuclei of mucous-membrane epithelial cells are distinctive, even in dried or desiccated material.

In samples that are poorly preserved as a result of putrefaction or moisture, the stain sometimes appears washed out or greenish or violet in color (this also occurs in overcoloration with picroindigocarmine). Nevertheless, the sperm can be recognized. In cases in which the sample is received in such poor condition that the sperm heads are swollen, the tails may be observed.

Fibrous portions of cotton or wool would be stained red or green. Plastics like Dralon and Perlon would not be colored, and the existing sperm are immediately differentiated from extraneous material by morphology.

Exposure to water or bacterial action does not destroy the ability of the sperm to be colored differently in the head and tail portions.

Sperm from chimpanzees, dogs, and horses have morphology distinctively different to be recognized.

MATERIALS AND REAGENTS

1. Microscope with transmitted bright field
2. Microscope slides, 1″ × 3″

3. Disposable glass pipettes
4. Indigo Carmine dye (Matheson, Coleman and Bell, Manufacturers and Chemists, 2909 Highland Ave., Norwood, Oh 45212)
5. Nuclear Fast Red biologic stain (Matheson, Coleman and Bell).
6. Picric acid, reagent grade
7. Absolute ethanol, reagent grade
8. Aluminum sulfate, reagent grade (Sargent-Welch Co., P.O. Box 1026, Chicago, Ill. 60690)
9. Kernechtrot solution (KS): Dissolve 5 g of aluminum sulfate in 200 ml of hot distilled water. Immediately add 0.1 g of Nuclear Fast Red and stir with a glass rod. Allow to cool and filter through filter paper (this solution is stable for about 3 to 6 months).
10. Picroindigocarmine solution (PICS): Place 4 g of picric acid in 300 ml of water in a 600-ml beaker. Cover and allow to stand overnight to produce a saturated solution of picric acid. Dissolve 1 g of Indigo Carmine dye in the solution, filter, and store.
    (Crystals of picric acid may remain).
11. Test tubes, 10 × 100 mm.

REFERENCES

1. Oppitz, E.: A new color method for proof of sperm in moral crimes. Arkiv fur Krimin., *144*:145–148, 1969.
2. Stone, I.: Personal communication, 1976.

ACID PHOSPHATASE (FOR RAPE CASES)

METHOD. Roy thymolphthalein monophosphatase hydrolysis (TMP) procedure modified by ACA.

PRINCIPLE. TMP is hydrolyzed by phosphatase in an acidic medium with calcium salts, producing a thymolphthalein chromogen that is measured in a spectrophotometer at 600 nm after quenching the reaction and converting the anion to an absorbant state with sodium hydroxide. The absorbance of thymolphthalein is proportional to the acid phosphatase in the specimen.

SPECIMEN. Vaginal secretion: 1 ml undiluted liquified secretions. Dried stains: Elute stain with 3 ml saline (on cloth, wood, etc.).

PROCEDURE

1. Place sample cup on input tray of ACA instrument (precise filling of the sample cup is important).
2. Place ACP-1 pack and ACP-2 pack on input tray behind the sample cup, with ACP-1 pack first, and ACP-2 following.
3. The ACA automatically aspirates a 0.3-ml specimen from the sample cup and injects it into the pack, with an injection of 4.7 ml purified water and ACA diluent.
4. The sample reaction is complete within 6 minutes.

5. The thymolphthalein anion chromogen is automatically read at 600 nm.
6. The result is either printed or photographically recorded.

INTERPRETATION. The normal range of acid phosphatase in serum is 0 to 0.8 IU/L. The range of acid phosphatase in seminal fluid is about 100,000 to 600,000 IU/L. Detection of acid phosphatase is evidence of the presence of seminal fluid. Postcoital specimens (<18 hours) contain >2,000 IU/L.

DISCUSSION AND CLINICAL SIGNIFICANCE. In a study done by G. Berry Schumann and Associates, the highest levels of acid phosphatase (>2,000 IU/L) were found in vaginal-fluid specimens taken within 18 hours of intromission of seminal fluid into the vagina. Vaginal acid phosphatase levels were reported to return to normal after 48 hours. In this study, acid phosphatase levels of >300 IU/L were considered "positive for detection of semen" or "recent coitus." In one study, the enzyme has been reported to be within detectable limits up to 7 days postcoital.

The precision of the ACA technique has been reported by the manufacturer to be:

	Day-to-Day CV	*Same-Day CV*
Normal range	about 22%	about 12%
High levels	about 3.7%	about 26%

ACA readouts over 25 IU are nonlinear. The test should be repeated on a diluted specimen and controls should be used.

MATERIALS AND METHODS

1. Dupont ACA (I, II, or III)
2. ACP-1 and ACP-2 packs (store 2 to 8°C; do not expose to sunlight or over 35°C)
3. Sodium chloride, 0.85% (w/v)

REFERENCES

1. ACA brochure (DuPont de Nemours, E.I., & Co., Inc., Wilmington, Del. 19898).
2. Roy, A., Brower, M., and Hayden, J.: Sodium thymolphthalein monophosphate: A new acid phosphatase substrate with greater specificity for the prostatic enzyme in serum. Clin. Chem., *17*:1093, 1971.
3. Schumann, G., Badawy, S., Peglow, A., and Henry, J.: Prostatic acid phosphatase: Current assessment in vaginal fluid of rape victims. Am. J. Clin. Pathol., *66*:944, 1976.

Chapter 8 Cerebrospinal-Fluid Analysis

ALFREDO SUAREZ
JAMES A. FREEMAN

The Egyptian Book of the Dead (ca. 1250 B.C.) regulated funerary and embalming practices, dictating that cranial contents and fluid were to be removed through the nostrils for preservation, not for scientific study. The importance of the brain and the surrounding cerebrospinal fluid was only minimally appreciated in antiquity, but it was acknowledged in the description of an exposed, injured brain in the Papyrus Smith. The Papyrus contained mention of motor deficits that occurred as a result of brain injury and discussions of surgical matters that were similar to descriptions in the Papyrus Ebers. The Papyri may have been teaching manuals. (Apparently, some of the text of the Papyrus Ebers is repeated in the Papyrus Smith and the Papyrus Berlin. Could this have been early plagiarism or even second and third editions?)

George Ebers believed that his Papyrus was the fourth of 66 medical books of the Hermetic collection, a series of writings mentioned in the Christian writings of Alexandria (2nd century A.D.). The writings were considered to be sacred, having been given to mankind by the Egyptian god Toth and containing "all the knowledge of man." The writings became associated with the Greek god Hermes Trismegistos ("thrice great"), and they eventually became known as the Hermetic collection. (Toth was also considered the healing god, until he was replaced by Imhotet about the 6th century A.D.).[1]

The earliest known regulations of the practice of medicine were found in the code developed by Hammurabi (ca. 1700 B.C.), the most famous ruler of the old Babylonian dynasty (ca. 1728–1686 B.C.). The code devotes 10 provisions (out of a total of 282) to the fees of medical practitioners and their punishments for failure (the eye-for-eye, tooth-for-tooth doctrine) for their treatment of people and animals! Although they were relatively highly paid, one wonders how a practitioner mustered enough courage to administer to the ill—unless punishments (such as cutting off one's hands) were more bureaucratic rhetoric than actual practice. Much of the text was devoted to the surgical treatment of tumors and to diseases of the eye, with only slight mention of the fluid surrounding the eye.

Trephination was known to the Babylonians and later to the Egyptians as a technique to relieve the afflicted of evil spirits (permitting the decompression of brain and removal of cerebrospinal fluid) and was practiced more for religious than for medicinal reasons (Fig. 8–1). This spiritual purity was a significant precept of the Judeo-Christian era (the precept "cleanliness is next to Godliness" probably stems from reference to personal hygiene in the Jerusalem Talmud [Avoda Zara]).

Rhazes (Abu-Baker Mohammed ibun-Zakirya al-Razi, ca. 850–923 A.D.) inspired the following Hebrew aphorisms of Isaaic Judaeus, when describing illness, brain disease in particular:

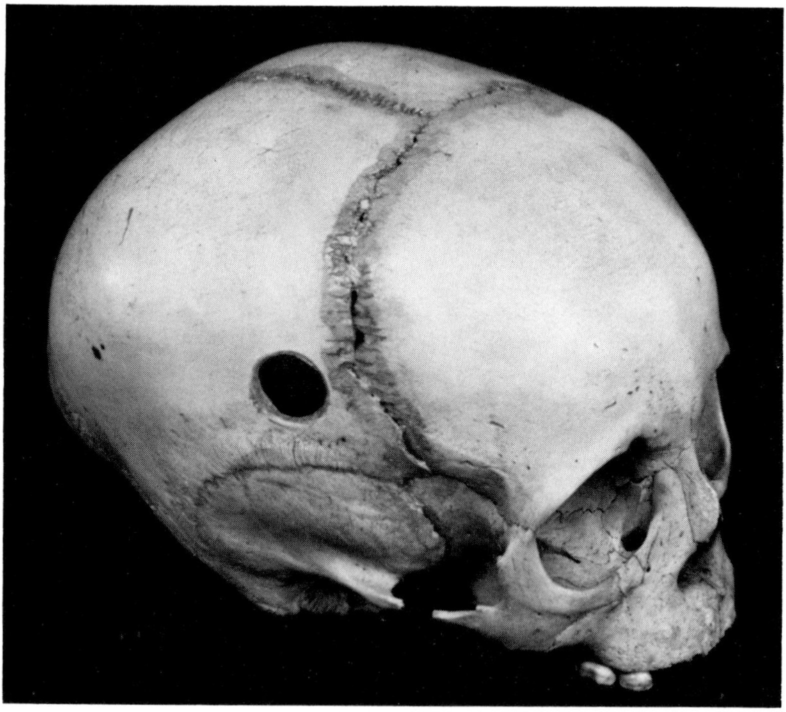

Fig. 8–1. Skull found in Peru that showed evidence of trephination, probably in the pre-Columbian era. (Courtesy of Dr. Robert Hudson, Department of History and Philosophy of Medicine, University of Kansas Medical Center, Kansas City, Kan. 66103.)

Most illnesses are cured without physician help through the aid of nature;
If you cure the patient by dietary means, do not turn to drugs;
Do not rely on cure-alls for they mostly rest on ignorance and superstition;
Always make the patient believe he will be cured when you are not convinced of it, for it aids the healing extent of nature.[1]

J. Leonard Corning was credited with the first therapeutic injection of chemicals in the subarachnoid space in 1885, but it was not until 1891 that Heinrich Quincke first obtained cerebrospinal fluid by lumbar puncture for diagnostic purposes. From that time, the development of cerebrospinal-fluid analysis slowly evolved into a useful diagnostic procedure when it was realized that pathologic changes on the surface of the brain may be detectable by study of the cerebrospinal fluid "bathing" the brain.

PHYSIOLOGY AND FORMATION OF CEREBROSPINAL FLUID

Approximately two-thirds of the cerebrospinal fluid are formed in the capillary tufts of the choroid plexus, mostly in the larger plexus of the floor of the lateral ventricles and in the smaller plexes in the roof of the third and fourth ventricles. The remainder of the cerebrospinal fluid is produced by the ependymal cells of both the ventricles and of the subarachnoid space (Fig. 8–2). Secretion is an energy-consuming process, catalyzed by carbonic anhydrase and requiring ATP. The cerebrospinal-fluid chemical components differ from those of an ultrafiltrate of blood.[2]

The production of cerebrospinal fluid is altered in certain pathologic states. Cerebrospinal-fluid production is increased in the following instances:

1. Choroid plexus papillomas
2. Congenital/obstructive hydrocephalus
3. Ouabaine administration
4. Spironolactone diuretic administration

The following can cause decreased production of cerebrospinal fluid:

1. Hypothermia
2. Alkalosis, both respiratory and metabolic
3. Medication administration (acetazolamide, furosemide, amphotericin, vasopressin, etc.)
4. Experimental intracerebral kaolin administration

The total volume of cerebrospinal fluid in adults has been estimated to be approximately 140 to 170 ml. The fluid constantly moves through the ventricles into the subarachnoid space and is ultimately absorbed into the bloodstream through the arachnoid villi into the cerebral veins. The fluid leaves the lateral ventricles through the interventricular foramen (foramina of Munro) into the third ventricle, then via the narrow passage of the cerebral aqueduct (aqueduct of Sylvius) into the fourth

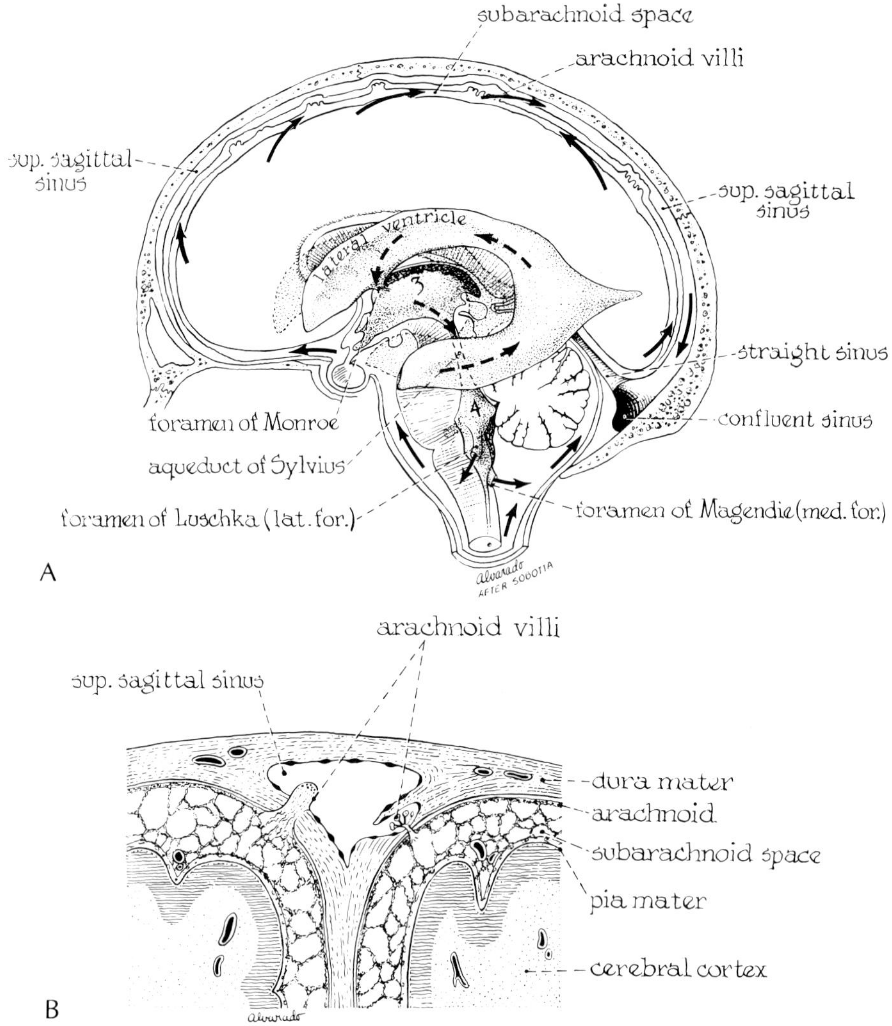

Fig. 8–2. A, Circulation of cerebrospinal fluid. **B,** Anatomic relationship of cerebrospinal space to brain.

ventricle. From the fourth ventricle, the fluid exits through the foramina of Magendi and Lushka into the cisterna magna at the inferior surface of the cerebellum and medulla. This cistern is contiguous with the subarachnoid space that surrounds the cord. Cerebrospinal fluid diffuses unidirectionally from the cisterna magna upward around the hemispheres into the arachnoid villi (in the walls of the superior barrier). Seventy percent of the fluid can be found in the lateral ventricles, 20% in the subarachnoid space, and 10% surrounding the spinal cord. Passive movement of fluid occurs with locomotion and position of the body; a constant flow is not ensured because of the lack of an active pumping mechanism.[3] Other routes of absorption are minor (such as the veins and capillaries of pia mater or the spaces of Virchow-Robin surrounding the vascular walls of arterioles).

Because the brain and cerebrospinal fluid are encased within a rigid, bony structure (the cranium), the volumes of brain substance, the cerebrospinal fluid, and the intercranial blood vascular system must be maintained at a constant level. Any increase in the volume of one component will be at the expense of the other. Consequently, with increases in pressure of the cerebrospinal fluid, the function or anatomic integrity of the brain or the vasculature structures suffer. Excessive volume of cerebrospinal fluid occurs mainly because of obstruction to outflow and absorption and not necessarily as a result of increased fluid production. Such an increase in fluid volume is termed hydrocephalus. In congenital hydrocephalus, the Sylvian aqueduct frequently fails to develop normally, and although the head is normal size at birth, a disproportionate enlargement occurs with pressure on the brain substance from the rapidly enlarging ventricles. In the first year of life, while the bony sutures are opened, there is little resistance to growth by the thin-walled skull. Obstruction to the outflow of cerebrospinal fluid after infancy causes a pressure increase and dilatation of ventricles with compression of both brain substance and dura mater around the optic nerve, thus producing dilatation of the retinal veins and compression of the optic nerve ("choked disc" or papilledema). Persistent papilledema will damage the optic nerve. Such a clinical manifestation can be viewed by the physician utilizing funduscopic examination of the retinae. The most common cause of papilledema is compression of the ventricular system (usually by hemorrhage, tumor, or penetrating injury). Also, acute arterial-blood-pressure elevation can produce increased intracranial pressure (hypertensive encephalopathy).

The following are pathologic changes that can alter the volume of cerebrospinal fluid:

1. Inflammation (meningitis, encephalitis, arachnoiditis)
2. Intracranial hemorrhage (brain, subarachnoid)
3. Intracranial mass (arterial aneurysm, brain and metastatic tumors and abscesses)
4. Spinal canal blocks (spinal-cord tumors, foreign bodies)
5. Cerebral edema (congestive heart failure, crush injuries, head and neck venous and acute arterial outflow obstructions, thrombosis)
6. Subarachnoid space obstructions (congenital and other types of hydrocephalus)
7. Hypo-osmolality (dehydration, hemolysis, hemodialysis, diabetes insipidus)
8. Toxic shock syndrome

The volume of cerebrospinal fluid can be decreased by the following pathologic changes:

1. Acute dehydration
2. Circulatory collapse (hemorrhage, shock)
3. Fractured cranium and dural tears (with leak fluid outside subarachnoid space)
4. Hyperosmolar crisis (diabetes mellitus, monoclonal or polyclonal gammopathy)

The normal cerebrospinal-fluid pressure measured at the lumbar area is approximately 100 to 150 mm of water with the body in a recumbent position; with the body in a sitting position, the pressure will rise to 200 to 300 mm of water. The buoyancy of this cerebrospinal fluid is indicated by the fact that a brain weighing 1,500 g in air will only weigh about 50 g when immersed in cerebrospinal fluid.[2]

The rate of formation of cerebrospinal fluid is independent of the fluid pressure, but resorption into the venous system depends on the pressure gradient between the cerebrospinal fluid and the venous blood in the dural sinuses (superior sagittal sinus). The rate of formation of the cerebrospinal fluid has been estimated to be approximately 600 to 700 ml/day in man.[3] In pathologic cases in which basilar skull fractures permit fluid "leaks" through the sphenoid wing of the temporal bone into the ear or into the retro-orbital space, several liters of spinal fluid may be lost in a day. The rate of production of cerebrospinal fluid permits a daily replacement of the entire volume about every 4 hours (if all fluid were removed instead of being reabsorbed). Samuel Heisey, in 1962, established that the rate of absorption of cerebrospinal fluid normally varies directly with the pressure gradient (usually up to 5 mm of mercury); hence, the greater the pressure, the greater the rate of absorption.[4]

The cerebrospinal fluid probably has nutritive functions in addition to serving as a vehicle for the removal of the waste products of neuronal metabolism. Offering mechanical cushioning to the brain is probably the most important reason for the fluid location and distribution.

INDICATIONS FOR CEREBROSPINAL TAP (LUMBAR PUNCTURE)

Lumbar punctures should be performed if they are likely to contribute to accurate diagnosis, improved management, or prognosis of a patient. The procedure, however, is not ordinarily considered routine. In modern medicine, lumbar puncture is not a sole diagnostic aid, but the technique can provide useful information. Because of the technical ease of lumbar puncture and the fact that it can be performed by the physician, it is frequently one of the earliest investigations to be done in a patient with cerebrovascular disease.[5] The complications in such a blind procedure are minor, but they should always be considered.

The indications for lumbar puncture include:

1. Diagnostic analysis of cerebrospinal-fluid components
2. Evaluation for cerebrovascular hemorrhage (ruptured aneurysms)
3. Detection of infectious disease (meningitis, encephalitis)
4. Administration of therapeutic compound (chemotherapy)
5. Reducing intracranial pressure
6. Diagnosis of immune disorders (multiple sclerosis)
7. Determination of the effectiveness of therapy (neurosyphilis, tumors, leukemias, etc.)
8. Detection of spinal cord compression or of subarachnoid blocks
9. Administration of diagnostic media compounds (myelography)
10. Differential diagnosis of cerebral infarction vs. cerebral hemorrhage
11. Administration of air for diagnostic testing (pneumoencephalography, ventriculography)

SPECIMEN COLLECTION AND PRESERVATION[6]

Cerebrospinal fluid is most commonly collected by "blind" needle aspirations into the lumbar cistern of the lower spinal canal. The procedure is technically simple and is taught to medical students in most schools in the United States. Needle punctures into the lumbar cistern are directed between the third and fourth (L3 and L4) or second and third lumbar (L2 and L3) vertebra in adults. The spinal cord terminus is above this level (about L2); therefore, there is little danger of damaging the spinal cord. In infants, however, aspiration should be done lower (between L4 and L5), because the spinal cord may extend more caudally. The nerve roots of cauda equina, which are present at the level of aspiration in the lumbar cistern, have little chance of being damaged. With the patient relaxed in a recumbent, decubitus position after having had the fundamentals of the technique explained to him, his skin is cleansed with the appropriate solution (Betadine, merthiolate, or other agents) to provide a sterile and aseptic area for puncture. A particularly anxious patient may need some sedation or analgesia prior to the procedure. The patient is draped in sterile manner. A no. 25 needle fitted to a 2-ml syringe should have enough volume to inject 1 to 2 ml of 1 to 2% lidocaine or other analgesic beneath the dermal margin to produce local analgesia of the dermocutaneous nerves. It is not necessary to infiltrate analgesic beneath the cutaneous nerves of the reticular dermis because pain nerve endings are not present below this area. The needle used for injection for the local anesthetic is withdrawn, and a $2^5/_8$-inch spinal needle is inserted into the same location being careful to enter between bony parts of the vertebra (Fig. 8–3). Two barriers to puncture

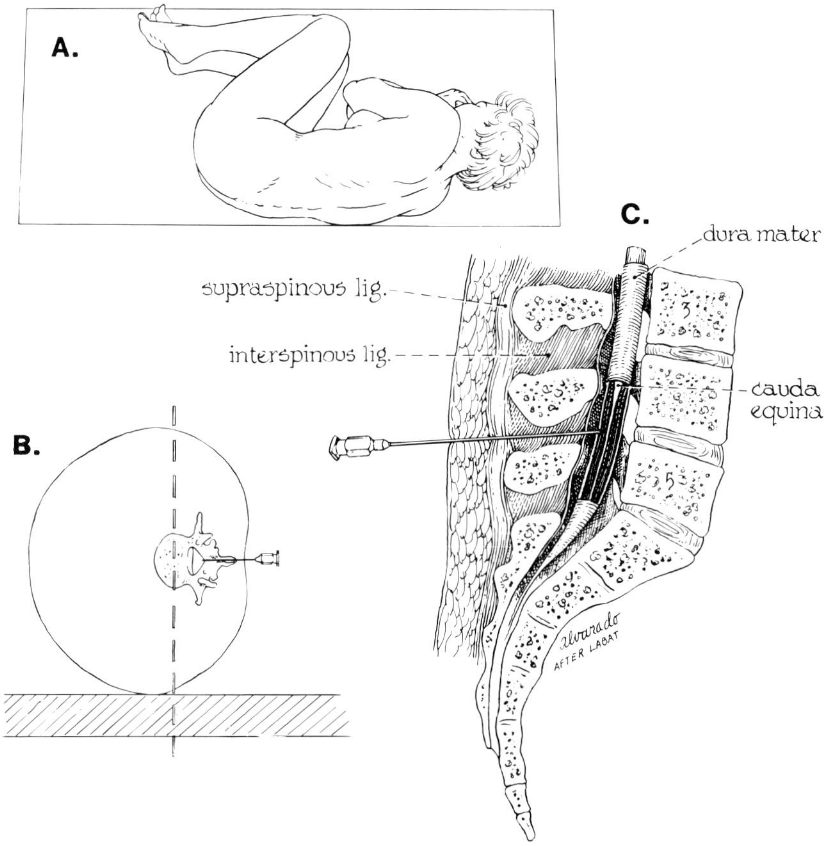

Fig. 8–3. Performance of lumbar spinal tap. **A,** The patient is positioned on side with knees drawn upward as far as possible and head and back flexed. **B,** The needle should be perpendicular to the spinal column to reach the subarachnoid space of the spinal canal. **C,** The spinal needle is inserted through skin, supraspinous ligament, interspinous ligaments, dura mater into subarachnoid space.

can be felt with the experienced, sensitive fingers: perimuscular fibrous tissue bundles and the dura mater.

Once the dura mater is penetrated, one can feel the pressure "pip" of the advancing needle; one should stop at this point, remove the stylet, and determine if cerbrospinal fluid is exuding. A 3-way stopcock should be fitted to the needle. A pressure manometer is then fitted to the stopcock, using sterile precautions, to measure and record the initial "opening" pressure of the cerebrospinal fluid. In cases in which there is increased pressure one should not perform venous obstructive maneuvers (Queckenstedt maneuvers), because herniation of the cerebellum and medulla may occur through the foramen magnum, producing compression of the cardiorespiratory center and immediate death. Once pressure is measured with the manometer, the stopcock is closed, and the fluid permitted to flow into a test tube. Fluid is permitted to flow freely into the test tubes, although one must be careful not to withdraw a large amount of fluid (usually over 10 ml). Withdrawal of large amounts of fluid will produce contracted volume, which will cause the patient to experience a severe basilar-occipital headache. One to two ml of fluid can be obtained in each of three sterile test tubes (labeled tubes no. 1, no. 2, and no. 3).

When the needle is placed correctly, pulsation of the column of cerebrospinal fluid can be visualized concurrent with heartbeat; minor variations occur with respirations. Determining the technique of exact needle placement and rapid measurement of cerebrospinal-fluid pressure come with experience. If initial pressure is above 200 mm, only 1 to 2 ml of fluid should be removed. The pressure should be measured at the end of the procedure (closing pressure) and recorded.

If there is a 50% fall in pressure after removing the 1 to 2 ml of fluid, one should suspect the following problems, and the procedure should be abandoned immediately:

1. Compression at the puncture site
2. Blockage of fluid dynamics
3. Cerebellar herniation
4. Spinal-cord compression

Ordinarily, the cerebrospinal-fluid pressure will not fall more than 10 to 20 mm between the time of opening and closing with removal of less than 10 ml of cerebrospinal fluid.

The tubes should be labeled no. 1, no. 2, and no. 3. Each tube should be utilized for testing as follows:

Tube no. 1: Chemistry, serology, and special studies
Tube no. 2: Bacteriologic study (Gram stain should be performed STAT on centrifuged specimen)
Tube no. 3: Cell count (should be performed immediately on uncentrifuged specimen)

Do not discard unused fluid, because it may not be obtainable again. Store by refrigeration for any future testing needs.

The Queckenstedt procedure is not a routine procedure. Queckenstedt is performed by compression of the jugular vein for 10 seconds to determine if there is a rapid rise in pressure in the manometer and a return to normal within 15 seconds (negative test), or if little change occurs (positive test).[5] In patients suspected of having increased intracranial pressure, a small bore needle should be used to slow removal of fluid and prevent brain herniation. Compression of both jugular veins will cause a rapid increase of cerebrospinal-fluid pressure over 300 mm, but will return to normal when compression ceases. The test depends on creating an increase in pressure within the veins, with retrograde increases in pressure from the jugular veins to the dural sinuses, to the arachnoid villi, and then into the cerebrospinal fluid.

In some cases, the delayed positive test occurs when there is obstruction in the spinal canal at the foramen magnum. The Müeller maneuver will produce increased cerebrospinal-fluid pressure in such a case (held inspiration producing increased intra-abdominal pressure). Most patients with compression of the spinal cord will have a positive Queckenstedt.

After removal of the fluid, the stopcock is closed and the stylet is replaced into the needle; then the needle is gently removed from the spinal canal and back.

If a test is properly performed, the patient will have relatively little discomfort. On occasion, if a portion of the cauda equina is touched or struck by the needle within the lumbar cistern, the patient may experience a sharp "electric-shock" pain radiating down a leg. If this occurs, withdrawal of the needle a fraction of a millimeter will relieve the pressure on the nerve root.

Preservatives or additives to the fluid are not used, because spinal-fluid testing procedures should be considered STAT tests and the specimen sent to the clinical laboratory immediately. However, fluid not used for testing should be refrigerated for any future chemical testing. Refrigeration will destroy Neisseria meningitidis; therefore, bacteriologic culture should be done on fresh, unrefrigerated specimens. Also, factitious meningitis has been detected by Gram-stained smears of nonviable bacteria within sterile, plastic specimen tubes supplied in a commercial lumbar-puncture tray, so the laboratory beware![7] Injection through or into an area of infection should not be done.

Small oscillation of the fluid level in the manometer arises from transmission of the cerebral arterial pulsation, which indicates free communication is present and usually mitigates against a blockage in cerebrospinal-fluid dynamics.[5]

Only experienced physicians should attempt aspiration of spinal fluid at the base of the skull from the cisterna magna via the atlanto-occipital axis; or in infants, from the subarachnoid space.

Most hospital staff regulations require a signed statement indicating informed consent prior to any spinal tap, because the technique is considered an invasive surgical procedure.

Complications[5–6]

The hazard of lumbar puncture is small when the procedure is performed using proper sterile techniques by an experienced physician; nevertheless, the procedure should not be considered routine, because complications can occur.

Cerebellar tonsillar and medullary herniation through the foramen magnum can occur in patients with increased intracranial pressure when a large bore needle is used or when fluid is removed rapidly. The risk can be reduced simply by using a small bore needle and removing fluid slowly. The admonition that spinal tap should not be done in patients with increased intracranial pressure is not a dictum!

The risk of infection is almost nonexistent today because of the use of sterile, commercial lumbar-puncture kits. Nevertheless, arachnoiditis can occur with multiple needle punctures through the dura and pia as a result of multiple procedures, or with poor technical performance during a single procedure.

Damage to the intervertebral disc has been reported, but this should not occur if the needle is not passed too deeply through the spinal canal. Any resistance should not be forcibly overcome. A sense of pride in one's performance of the techniques should never lead to persistent efforts to obtain the specimen when problems occur; it is better to abandon the procedure and try again on another occasion.

Dermoid tumor, which is actually an epidermal inclusion cyst, can occur when a needle is used without a stylet. In such an instance, a "punched" portion of skin may be carried deep into the needle tract and graft into the depth of the tissue. The use of stylet obviates this.

Spinal headache can occur as a result of the removal of too much fluid (generally over 10 ml) or the too rapid removal of fluid. These problems can be overcome by removing small volumes and using a small bore needle. The headache is a function of contracted cerebrospinal-fluid volume; it usually can be alleviated by rapid intravenous fluid replacement or sometimes by oral fluid replacement (we prefer Gatorade, which is inexpensive and palatable to a person in severe pain).

The pain may be extremely severe and produce vertigo, vomiting, and prostration. In such cases, treatment with 40 units of ACTH gel, elevation of the foot of the bed, and the administration of intravenous fluids and narcotics may be needed. The spinal headache is characterized by a constant, sharp, tearing, occipito-basilar pain that can be aggravated by the simplest motions, even raising the head from the pillow. It can be emotionally devastating to the patient, because few laymen understand the problem even after adequate explanation by the physician.

Paralysis secondary to spinal-cord injury will not occur as a result of the usual procedure if the lumbar-puncture site is below the terminus of the spinal cord. The same cannot be said of the injection of substances into the spinal cord (such as myelography techniques or chemotherapy instillation), for there have been recorded instances of either immediate paralysis or an ascending-type paralysis (Guillain-Barré type syndrome, for example).

Infant deaths have occurred from asphyxiation due to excessive restraint or by tracheal obstruction caused by pushing the head forward. This is not understandable.

Lumbar puncture is no longer the sole diagnostic aid for the physician because of the advent of computerized tomography and other noninvasive diagnostic techniques; nevertheless, it remains a useful procedure that needs to be performed with care in order to prevent these complications.

ROUTINE CEREBROSPINAL-FLUID TESTING

Ten years ago, cerebrospinal-fluid testing consisted of a battery of tests that was hallowed by custom, if not sanctioned by wisdom. With the rapid development of new testing parameters in the laboratory, this battery has been altered.

Cerebrospinal fluid is a valuable specimen, not obtained with impunity; therefore, the testing procedure should be selected to fulfill the greatest need of patient care by the clinical staff of the hospital. With the ever increasing demand for financial frugality being made on most laboratories, the cost effectiveness of routine tests needs to be kept under review.

The usual cerebrospinal-fluid routine tests performed in our laboratories include:

1. Visual inspection (color, clarity, turbidity, coagulation)
2. Protein
3. Glucose (only sometimes ordered)
4. Lactic acid (only ordered in cases suspected of having bacterial meningitis)
5. Enzyme studies (LDH, CPK, and/or AST)
6. Differential cell count and morphologic evaluation (leukocytes, erythrocytes, malignant cells, other cells)
7. Bacteriologic, mycobacteriologic, fungal studies

pH can be measured for academic interest, but knowledge of the pH value has no clinical relevance. Determination of cerebrospinal-fluid chloride does not have significant clinical value in modern medicine.

Speciality tests performed under selected circumstances include the following:

1. Protein electrophoretic fractionation (multiple sclerosis and monoclonal gammopathies)
2. Oligoclonal IgG (multiple sclerosis)
3. Syphilis testing (neurosyphilis)
4. Protein fragment determinations, such as myelin basic protein, encephalitogenic protein, and lymphocyte adherence (multiple sclerosis)
5. Glutamine and ammonia (hepatic failure or encephalopathy)

6. Biogenic Amines, such as homovanilic acid, 5-hydroxytryptamine, and dopamine (Parkinsonism and depressive illnesses)
7. Biochemical markers of malignancy:
   carcinoembryonic antigen (metastatic entodermal carcinoma and tumor chemotherapy)
   beta glucuronidase (metastatic carcinoma and chronic "infectious" meningitis)
   adenylate kinase (metastatic tumors)
   polyaminase, which includes putrescine and its metabolites (degenerating neural tissue and tumor chemotherapy)
8. Limulus assay (bacteriologic Gram-negative endotoxin)
9. Pap-stained cells (primary and metastatic tumor)

VISUAL INSPECTION OF CEREBROSPINAL FLUID

Cerebrospinal fluid is clear and colorless. The fluid should be visually inspected immediately after extraction and preferably against a dark background. One should inspect the fluid for:

1. Color
2. Clarity/turbidity
3. Viscosity/observation for coagulation

Color

Cerebrospinal fluid is crystal clear, not unlike a perfect, "flawless D" diamond. In some pathologic conditions (diabetes, epilepsy, lead poisoning, Guillain-Barré syndrome, multiple sclerosis, poliomyelitis, rabies, neurosyphilis, brain tumors, etc.), the fluid may retain the same color (and clarity). Cloudiness may be perceived at concentrations of 3,000 red blood cells/cumm.[8] Red-blood-cell concentrations of 6,000 cells/cumm in the cerebrospinal fluid produce a visual color change.

When small dermocutaneous veins or the anterior cervical venous plexus is pierced during spinal-tap procedure, gross blood may be visible or a smokey red color may be imparted to the fluid. In specimens that are grossly bloody, one should centrifuge the specimen and observe the supernatant to determine if there are abnormal colors present.[9] In cases of subarachnoid hemorrhage, the red cells are usually lysed in vivo and will produce a yellow to yellow-red color (xanthochromia).[10]

If blood is obtained as a result of the lumbar-puncture procedure (a "traumatic tap"), the supernatant should be crystal clear after centrifugation. With this procedure, it is not possible to distinguish between an immediate subarachnoid hemorrhage and a traumatic spinal tap. Red blood cells from such specimens can be crenated in both instances; the detection of crenated red blood cells is not reliable for distinguishing a traumatic tap from a true subarachnoid hemorrhage. In the event of a traumatic tap, different amounts of blood may be collected in each tube, with a great amount being collected in test tube no. 1 and less in test tube no. 3.

Assessment of the degree of xanthochromia obtained from lumbar puncture is usually accomplished by visual observation of the supernatant after centrifugation of the specimen (within an hour of collection). Quantitative spectrophotometric analytic study can be done at 415 to 460 mm to detect bilirubin (similar to Δ OD 450 analysis for bilirubin pigment in amniotic fluid). The analytic information gained by spectrophotometric analysis has no additional clinical value—that is, it is just as clinically relevant to know that xanthochromia is present as it is to affix a chemical value or arbitrarily estimate the depth of intensity.

Xanthochromia may be due to the presence of pigments of:[10]

1. Oxyhemoglobin
2. Bilirubin
3. Methemoglobin
4. Carotenoids
5. Melanin
6. Proteins
7. Diverse substances (including contamination by merthiolate or betadine in specimen collection)

In cases of cerebral laceration or hemorrhagic cerebral infarctions, the amount of oxyhemoglobin generally is high initially and decreases when the hemoglobin is converted to bilirubin. When oxyhemoglobin appears in the cerebrospinal fluid, it reaches a peak in 24 to 26 hours (producing a mildly pink color) and gradually decreases to approximately 1 week. When there is subarachnoid hemorrhage, the yellow xanthochromia that is due to bilirubin reaches a peak generally 2 to 4 days after the initial bleeding episode and gradually disappears in 4 weeks.[8,11] Some oxyhemoglobin may persist up to a month after the initial cerebral bleeding episode, because of sequestration of the pigment in the central nervous system.

Carotenoids in cerebrospinal fluid occur with generalized carotenemia, which usually occurs in newborn infants who are being fed carotene-containing compounds (carrots, squash, etc.), and have no pathologic significance.[10] Premature infants and newborns also may have transient xanthochromia when nonpathologic, "physiologic jaundice" occurs. Melanin or colorless melanogens in cerebrospinal fluid is secondary to melanin-producing tumors (metastatic melanomas). Melanin can be detected using the same procedures that are used in testing urine for melanin: the Thörmahlen test, Ehrlich test, ferric chloride test, or chromatographic procedure. Methemoglobin is formed when the iron in reduced (deoxygenated) hemoglobin is oxidized to the ferric form. In this form, the hemoglobin cannot be reoxygenated. The detection of methemoglobin requires a spectrometer or a spectrophotometric technique.

Clarity/Turbidity

Abnormal spinal fluid may be characterized as cloudy, smokey, hazy, or turbid. Turbidity can be caused by an increased number of erythrocytes, bacteria, fungi, parasites, leukocytes, and even radiographic contrast media. Cloudiness may be perceived visually at concentrations of 3,000 red blood cells/cumm.[6,8] Marked elevations of cerebrospinal-fluid protein may produce not only turbidity but also gel formation of fluid after standing. The latter, combined with xanthochromia, can occur in Froin's syndrome.

Grading of clarity or turbidity can be arbitrarily fixed as follows:

- 0 = Crystal-clear fluid
- 1+ = Faintly cloudy fluid
- 2+ = Turbidity evident, but newsprint can be read through the test tube containing fluid
- 3+ = Turbidity great enough to barely read newsprint through test tube
- 4+ = Marked turbidity, which does not allow newsprint to be read through the test tubes

Such a semiquantitative evaluation may have academic interest, but it has no clinical relevance to the physician handling the patient; therefore, it is more an exercise in mental gymnastics than in relevant laboratory medicine. Thus, grading turbidity is not suggested by the authors, assuming that analytic procedures such as protein determination and morphologic evaluation are to be performed. If leukocytes, red blood cells, and protein are present, they may contribute to the development of turbidity. To estimate the importance of each element is sheer folly. A practicing physician who visualizes a turbid specimen while performing the spinal-tap procedure is likely to deliver the specimen to the laboratory immediately for STAT testing procedures. Thus, the turbidity has forewarned him that there are abnormal elements present; this is as much clinical information as the clinician needs to know about turbidity.

Coagulation

Unusually rapid clot formation is generally indicative of increased fibrinogen, which may occur in traumatic tap, subarachnoid block, bacterial meningitis, tuberculous meningitis, and many other conditions. With abnormal components present, the specimen is more likely to clot; this is an even greater reason for performing STAT procedures.[3]

In marked protein elevation, gel formation or clotting occurs when the specimen stands at room temperature. The time lapse with formation of clotting depends on the disease process (purulent meningitis and viral meningitis, for example) as well as the type of proteins present (immunoglobulins, albumin). In purulent bacterial meningitis, the clot generally forms in a short period of time, whereas in tuberculous meningitis, it may take 24 hours for a clot to become visible. Fine clots or pellicles (strands) may be seen on the surface of spinal fluid after refrigeration for 12 to 24 hours in cases of tuberculosis and neurosyphilis.

pH

Hydrogen-ion concentration of the spinal fluid is maintained within pH limits of 7.40 to 7.24. The cerebrospinal fluid contains only negligible concentrations of buffer system other than bicarbonate.[12] Thus, it can be understood why carbon-dioxide retention in patients with pulmonary ventilatory insufficiency may produce a low cerebrospinal fluid pH and aggravate acidosis. While mild metabolic alkalosis is rarely accompanied by a change in pH in spinal fluid, severe metabolic alkalosis will cause an increase in cerebrospinal fluid pH and consequently, will lower bicarbonate.

Lumbar and cisternal pHs differ. The lumbar cerebrospinal fluid has a slightly higher pCO_2 and consequently, a lower pH, than does the cisternal cerebrospinal fluid. Cisternal cerebrospinal fluid pH ranges from 7.51 to 7.27.

CHLORIDE

The determination of cerebrospinal-fluid chloride does not have significant clinical value. In the past, chloride values were noted to be reduced in patients with tuberculous meningitis. In such a pathologic condition, the reduction in chloride content is secondary to cerebrospinal-fluid protein elevation, systemic hyponatremia, and hypochloremia. Relying solely on a low chloride value to make or suspect a diagnosis of tuberculous meningitis would be poor clinical judgement. Normal cerebrospinal fluid also contains other inorganic substances, such as phosphorous, sodium, potassium, magnesium, and calcium, but with few exceptions, measurement of such compounds has little clinical diagnostic value.

PROTEIN

Protein diffuses from the blood to the cerebrospinal fluid across the CSF/blood barrier; thus, most serum proteins found in blood are found in the cerebrospinal fluid.[13] The ratio of blood to cerebrospinal-fluid protein is about 230:1 to 800:1. Selective osmotic transport and molecular filtration, however, favor the proteins of small molecular size and dimension (transferrin, prealbumin, albumin, for example). The total protein content of cerebrospinal fluid is the lowest of any organic fluid in the body, except the aqueous humor in the eye. The upper limit of normal cerebrospinal-fluid protein in the neonatal period has been reported to be from 140 to 170 mg/dl. By age 6 months, the values fall below normal adult levels to 10 to 30 mg/dl. Adults levels of cerebrospinal-fluid proteins are achieved after age 10, ranging from 25 to 45 mg/dl. There is, however, a gradient between the ventricular fluid (where the mean protein level is 15 mg/dl), the fluid in the cisterna magna (about 30 mg/dl), and the fluid in the lumbar cistern (where the values may be 45 mg/dl).

Increased concentration of protein in cerebrospinal fluid may be seen in patients with

1. Traumatic tap
2. Obstruction to the circulation of cerebrospinal fluid
3. Tissue degeneration and necrosis of neural substance
4. Increased synthesis of protein within the cerebrospinal fluid
5. Increased permeability of the CSF/blood barrier

The increase in cerebrospinal-fluid protein is easily explained with a traumatic tap, the protein being derived from the plasma (which has more than a hundred fold greater amount of protein). Increased permeability of the blood/cerebrospinal fluid barrier is a common cause of increase in cerebrospinal-fluid total protein. In patients with meningitis, the elevated protein content is the result of multiple factors: the leakage of serum proteins, the release from the meninges of products of inflammation, and the breakdown of leukocytes introduced during the infectious process. High levels of protein in the fluid are found with intraspinal block usually complicating more chronic forms of meningitis (tuberculosis, cryptococcus). Excessive concentrations in ventricular fluid are suggestive of a block in the internal circulation of spinal fluid most commonly due to obstruction of the Sylvian aqueduct. Froin's syndrome refers to xanthochromic cerebrospinal fluid with high protein content, which may clot spontaneously. This syndrome is due to obstruction of the spinal subarachnoid space. It was initially thought to be pathognomonic of spinal tumors, but a more modern concept is that the syndrome can be seen in any lesion (inflammatory or neoplastic) that compresses the spinal subarachnoid space and produces stagnation of spinal fluid as well as passive congestion of the meninges.

Decreased concentration of protein may be found with leakage of fluid from a dural tear as a consequence of trauma with removal of large volumes of cerebrospinal fluid.

The different turbidimetric methods of protein determination (trichloroacetic acid, biuret, etc.) show variations in reactivity with albumin and globulin.[14–15] These methods are widely used because they are simple and have no interference from drugs. Interference, however, may occur with xanthochromia and from some chemotherapeutic agents, such as methotrexate. The upper limit of normal protein with turbidimetric methods is about 40 mg/dl.

At 210 nm, the transmittance wavelength of peptide bonds, protein solutions can be measured spectrophotometrically. Interfering low molecular weight substances can be eliminated by either chromatography or ultrafiltration. Ultrafiltration is used, also, to produce a concentrated fluid protein for electrophoresis.[16] These methods require between 100 to 200 μL of cerebrospinal fluid. Such methods are better than the turbidimetric methods but are more time consuming and cumbersome. Upper limit of normal can be as high as 60/dl, depending upon the procedure.[17–19]

Reduction of phosphotungstic acid and phosphomolybdic by a copper protein complex, or the biuret technique, is simple and widely used in clinical laboratories. This method requires between 100 to 200 μL of cerebrospinal fluid. However, drug interference (salicylates, chlorpromazine, tetracyclines, sulfa drugs) is common. The upper limit of normal with this method is about 35 mg/dl.

Immunologic binding and dye binding are less widely used because they are either time consuming or more difficult to perform.

PROTEIN ELECTROPHORETIC FRACTIONATION[19–20]

Cerebrospinal fluid protein can be fractionated using electrophoretic techniques or immunoglobulin measurement, in much the same fashion as with blood protein. Of course, concentration of the minute amount of protein is necessary prior to electrophoretic migration. The electrophoretic analysis of cerebrospinal fluid proteins is a routine diagnostic procedure.[3,21–22] The support media varies, but may include cellulose acetate, agar gel, and polyacrylamide gel. Cellulose acetate is still the most widely used, but it is being replaced by the agarose gel. Electrophoretic analysis on cellulose acetate membranes yield the following mean values on normal spinal fluids:[21–22]

1. Prealbumin (4.1%)
2. Albumin (62.4%)
3. Alpha globulin (5.3%)
4. Alpha II globulin (82.0%)
5. Beta I and beta II globulin (12.8%)
6. Gamma globulin (7.2%)

On agarose-gel electrophoresis, the cerebrospinal-fluid protein pattern may differ from that obtained on cellulose acetate (Fig. 8–4). An additional band sometimes appears between albumin and alpha I globulin. The tau fraction separates from the beta I globulin and migrates slower than the beta II band of serum, which is usually absent in cerebrospinal fluid.[18] While gamma globulin is easily identified on both cellulose acetate and agarose gel, pathologic gamma globulin bands can

EARL K. LONG MEMORIAL HOSPITAL
5825 AIRLINE HIGHWAY
BATON ROUGE, LOUISIANA 70805

DEPARTMENT OF PATHOLOGY

		CSF Patient's Results	SERUM Normal Ranges	
Fraction	Grams/100ml		Grams/100ml	%
PRE-ALBUMIN		10%		
Albumin		59 %	3.5—5.0	52 — 63
Globulins Alpha$_1$		3%	0.2—0.4	3.3—5.7
Globulins Alpha$_2$		8 %	0.6—1.0	10.0—12.5
Globulins Beta		16 %	0.6—1.0	10.0—12.5
Globulins Gamma		7 %	0.7—1.3	10.7—16.3
Total Protein			6.0—8.0	

CSF PROTEIN ELECTROPHORESIS

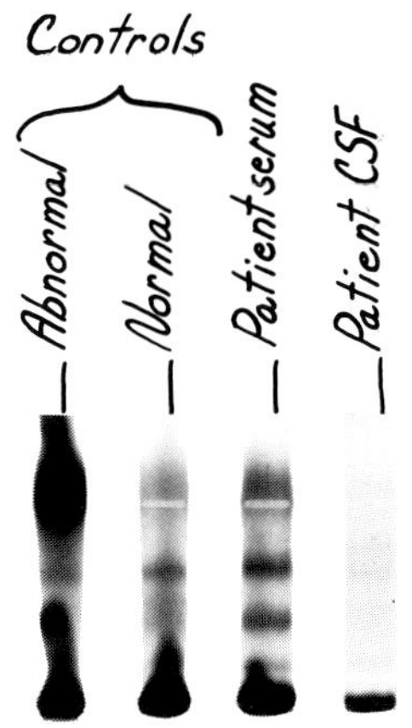

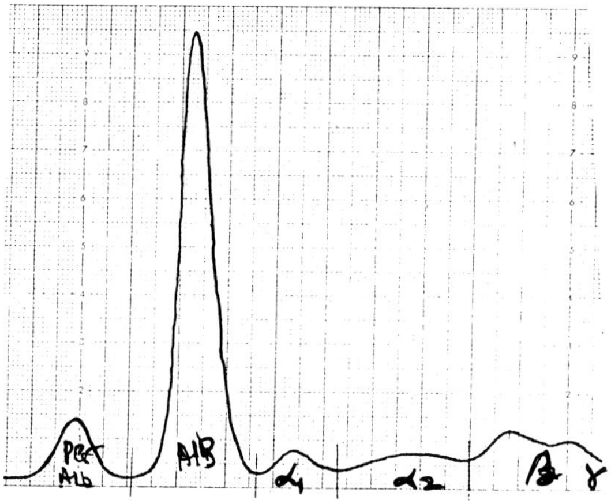

DATE RECEIVED 1-12-81 DATE REPORTED 1-15-81

Comments: ESSENTIALLY NORMAL SPINAL FLUID PROTEIN PATTERN (NO EVIDENCE OF OLIGOCLONAL IgG)

1/15/81
PATHOLOGIST: [signature]

PATIENT

NO. 210-2

Fig. 8–4. Normal cerebrospinal fluid protein electrophoretic pattern on agarose gel.

be demonstrated better on agarose gel. Agar-gel electrophoresis reveals two or more bands in the gamma globulin region in approximately 90% of patients with multiple sclerosis (oligoclonal IgG).[23] These bands are not simultaneously seen on electrophoresis of the patient's serum.[24]

Polyacrylamide gel electrophoresis provides the greatest resolution. It has the advantage of not requiring previous concentration of the cerebrospinal fluid. Normal fluids usually reveal 16 to 18 discrete bands, the complete diagnostic significance of which is not clear. In cases of purulent meningitis, one sees a distinct shift of protein fractions toward gamma globulin. In certain cases, this technique may permit the identification of hemoglobin and haptoglobin bands: hemoglobin precedes beta globulins, and haptoglobin bands migrate in area before gamma globulins. This technique may be of diagnostic importance in cases of blood/brain barrier disturbances.

In 1942, Elvin Kabat and coworkers first noted that the cerebrospinal-fluid gamma globulin content was elevated in some patients with multiple sclerosis and neurosyphilis.[13] Since then, various methods have been described in the search for a rapid, simple, reliable, sensitive test that would quantitate the cerebrospinal fluid immunoglobulins.[25] An electroimmunodiffusion method described in 1966 by Thomas Hartley used minute volumes of unconcentrated cerebrospinal fluid. Using this method, Stuart Schneck and Henry Claman reported 56% of multiple sclerosis patients had a level of gamma globulin greater than 14% of the total cerebrospinal-fluid protein.[26] In those patients with multiple sclerosis and a normal total cerebrospinal-fluid protein, 71% had an abnormally high gamma G (oligoclonal IgG), and only 12.7% had other neurologic illnesses (other than neurosyphilis, the Guillain-Barré syndrome, and optic or retrobulbar neuritis).

There is no perfect test for multiple sclerosis.[24] The most accepted laboratory finding in multiple sclerosis is that of localized synthesis of oligoclonal immunoglobin IgG within the central nervous system.

The highest incidence of positive findings (over 95%) is demonstrated by the oligoclonal pattern of the gamma globulin subfractions in cerebrospinal fluid. This abnormality, first seen on agar-gel electrophoresis by Lowenthal, in 1964, may be detected even when the percentage of IgG is normal. In 1979, Margo Gerson and Benjamin Orr evaluated the presence of oligoclonal bands and the quantitation of IgG in cerebrospinal fluid as indicators of multiple sclerosis.[23] They found oligoclonal bands present in 77% of the multiple-sclerosis positive group while elevation of IgG was present in only 20%. They concluded the presence or absence of oligoclonal bands in agarose electrophoretic patterns is sensitive (77%) and very specific (99%) with respect to multiple sclerosis.

More recently, elevation in IgA has been found in cerebrospinal fluid during exacerbation of the disease. An increased ratio of the kappa: lambda immunoglobulin light chains (indicating an exaggerated synthesis of IgG molecules with light chains) within the central nervous system is found in about 50% of patients with multiple sclerosis. Jan Olsson and Hans Link in 1973 reported significantly higher kappa:lambda light-chain ratios in the cerebrospinal fluid when compared with the serum during exacerbation as well as remissions.[27–28] The determination of the kappa:lambda light-chain ratio is a rather crude measure, and the finding of a normal cerebrospinal fluid kappa:lambda ratio does not exclude the presence of an oligoclonal immunoglobulin.

The immunologic methods of determination of albumin and IgG have become very popular for evaluating the integrity of the blood/CSF barrier and synthesis of IgG within the central nervous system.[29] This CSF/plasma albumin ratio is considered to reflect functional integrity of CSF/blood barrier. Variation in plasma albumin may affect the cerebrospinal-fluid albumin concentration, but it does not significantly affect the CSF/plasma albumin ratio. This ratio is high immediately after birth, which reflects the immaturity of the CSF/blood barrier.

Oligoclonal/immunoglobulin abnormality can be found in inflammatory diseases of the central nervous system such as:[27–28]

1. Neurosyphilis
2. Subacute sclerosing panencephalitis
3. Meningitis
4. Encephalitis
5. Guillain-Barré syndrome
6. Toxoplasmosis

Generally, these bands will not show on cellulose acetate electrophoresis. It has been argued that the oligoclonal pattern on electrophoresis is not as subjective as the IgG determination.[31] Hence, the amount of IgG in cerebrospinal fluid has been related to the amount of albumin and corrected for the respective serum values to generate a quotient (Fig. 8–5).

Another ratio of importance is the CSF/plasma IgG ratio, which reflects the synthesis of IgG within the central nervous system. In order to correct the cerebrospinal fluid-IgG measurement for significant variations in plasma IgG and for permeability of the CSF/blood barrier, IgG may be expressed as a percentage of cerebrospinal-fluid total protein or cerebrospinal fluid albumin. Normal value are approximately 8% for the former and 12% for the latter.

The cerebrospinal-fluid-IgG index is more reliable than electrophoretic fractionation or isoelectric focusing for diagnosing multiple sclerosis, according to Linda Hershey and John Trotter (Fig. 8–6).[24] The index is a secondary ratio:

$$\frac{\text{CSF IgG/CSF albumin}}{\text{serum IgG/serum albumin}}$$

All these determinations should be performed simultaneously, because there is neither a definite nor a perfect test for multiple sclerosis.[32] However, the determination of cerebrospinal fluid-IgG index requires less cerebrospinal fluid and serum, less technologist time, and less

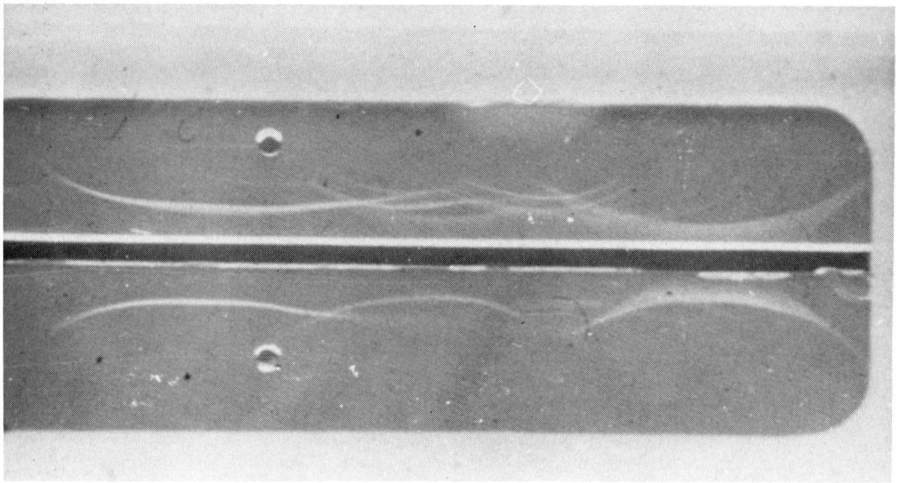

Fig. 8–5. Immunoelectrophoretic pattern of oligoclonal IgG in cerebrospinal fluid (top trough) and serum (bottom trough) of a patient with multiple sclerosis (Courtesy of Dr. Carl E. Speicher, Department of Pathology, Ohio State University Hospital, Columbus, Oh. 43201.)

technical experience and skill, than ultrafiltration and electrophoretic procedures, with equivalent diagnostic information.

GLUCOSE

The transfer of glucose from blood to spinal fluid is mediated by two processes: passive diffusion and carrier facilitated diffusion. Within normal ranges of blood sugar, the cerebrospinal-fluid glucose is about two-thirds of the blood value. When blood sugar rises above 200 mg/dl, the ratio falls progressively to 50% or less, because the pinocytotic transport mechanism for glucose is overwhelmed. Passive diffusion of glucose from plasma to cerebrospinal fluid is influenced by the level and duration of elevated plasma glucose. Following a change in plasma glucose, the cerebrospinal fluid glucose rises or falls slowly over a 2-hour time interval.[3,11] In the neonatal period, the CSF/plasma glucose ratio approaches 1.

When feasible, a blood sugar should be drawn 2 hours prior to a lumbar puncture, as it has been estimated that this is the time period necessary for equilibration of blood and cerebrospinal-fluid glucose. A fasting blood sugar determination at the time of the lumbar puncture may suffice.[33] As with protein, there is a difference between ventricular and lumbar values, levels of glucose being higher in the ventricles than in the lumbar cistern.

Reduction of the concentration of glucose in the spinal fluid is usually but not always observed in the active, untreated phase of bacterial

CLINICAL IMMUNOLOGY LABORATORIES, INC.
2122 Granville Ave.
Los Angeles, California 90025
Telephone (213) 478-1295
Toll Free outside California 1-800-421-7110

CLIA	04-1171
MEDICARE	05-9103
CA	ID 02586
CAP	90404-003-011

REPORT SENT TO SUBMITTING LABORATORY/PHYSICIAN:

PATIENT'S NAME

Address or Rm. Number

Med Record/Unit/Lab No's

Physician

DATE Drawn			
DATE Received			
DATE Reported			
CIL LOG #			
ACETYLCHOLINE RECEPTOR ANTIBODY	N = < 1 Unit		
ANTISTRIATIONAL ANTIBODY	N = < 1/10		
BETA$_2$-MICROGLOBULIN CSF SERUM	N = < 2.4 mg/l N = < 2.4 mg/l		
CSF BETA-GLUCURONIDASE	N = < 40 mU/ml		
CSF CEA	N = < 0.9 ng/ml		
CNS IgG SYNTHESIS RATE	N = −9.9 to +3.3 mg/24 hrs.		
CSF IgG	N = 0.5-6.1 mg/dl		
CSF ALBUMIN	N = 13-24 mg/dl		
IgG INDEX	N = < 0.7		
MYELIN BASIC PROTEIN (CSF)	N = < 4 ng/ml		
OLIGOCLONAL IMMUNOGLOBULINS (CSF)	N = No abnormal bands detected		

COMMENTS
For Multiple Sclerosis Panel (includes CNS IgG Synthesis rate, Oligoclonal Immunoglobulins and Myelin Basic Protein) CIL micromethods now require only 3.5cc CSF and 0.5cc Serum.

0661BR SEE REVERSE SIDE FOR DISCUSSION

Fig. 8–6. Laboratory report form for test "panel" in workup of a patient suspected of having multiple sclerosis. (Courtesy of Clinical Immunology Laboratories, Inc.)

meningitis. Levels may be normal in the very early stages of disease, but they decrease as the infection progresses.[34] The metabolic demands of the bacteria or of the leukocytes alone do not account for the lower levels of glucose. Interference with the transport of glucose from blood to cerebrospinal fluid appears to be the major factor contributing to lowering of the concentration of glucose in the spinal fluid.

Reduction of cerebrospinal-fluid glucose has also been reported following subarachnoid hemorrhage in patients with fungal diseases, and in cases of carcinomatous meningitis. In all of these conditions, the cerebrospinal-fluid glucose may remain depressed for days following resolution of CSF/cellular pleocytosis and protein elevations. A cerebrospinal-fluid glucose level below 40 mg/dl should always be considered abnormal regardless of the blood sugar.[33] In infants, a low level of glucose does not necessarily indicate infection; instead, it may reflect hypoglycemia due to vomiting or poor food intake.

An elevated cerebrospinal-fluid glucose level indicates hyperglycemia 2 to 4 hours prior to lumbar puncture. It is present in diabetes mellitus as well as in other diseases that produce marked hyperglycemia. Various levels of increased cerebrospinal-fluid glucose can be seen in cases of encephalitis and poliomyelitis.[34] Increased levels have been recorded in diseases that increase the cerebrospinal-fluid pressure, such as cerebral abscesses, cerebral tumors, and convulsive states; the increase may be slight and of little laboratory diagnostic value.

Glucose values have the same clinical significance and almost the same range of normal values whether measurement is performed by oxygen tension electrode, orthotolidine, or glucose hexose monophosphate shunt techniques. Minor variations are not clinically significant.

LACTIC ACID

The lactate content of cerebrospinal fluid has been known, since 1924, to be elevated in patients with bacterial meningitis. The assay of lactic acid, therefore, may be useful in differentiating bacterial meningitis from aseptic (viral) meningitis.[35–36] In addition, serial lactic-acid levels at different stages of treatment offer a significant indicator for the determination of efficacy of antibiotic therapy. However, lactic-acid levels may not have relevance in medical decision-making, according to physicians of Joe Rutledge's group at the University of Washington at Seattle. The predictive value of the test from their study was only 27%.[37] Normal lactic-acid levels vary between 10 to 25 mg/dl (0.11 to 0.28 mmol/L). Over 90% of the patients with bacterial meningitis will have an elevated cerebrospinal-fluid lactic acid above 25 mg/dl. Less than 15% of the patients with severe aseptic meningitis will have lactate levels above this value.

Moderate elevations (over 25 mg/dl) of lactic acid have been found in patients with:[39]

1. Hydrocephalus
2. Brain abscess
3. Cerebral ischemia
4. Severe metabolic acidosis
5. Increased intracranial pressure
6. Reduced cerebral blood flow

Elevation of lactic acid correlates best with granulocyte pleocytosis, not with protein elevation. An increase in intracranial pressure or a significantly reduced cerebral blood flow may elevate lactic-acid levels.[35] In such cases, the brain's metabolic processes may shift from aerobic to anaerobic metabolism with the subsequent rise in the lactic-acid levels of the cerebrospinal fluid.

Modern methods for the determination of lactate levels are enzymatic techniques employing oxidation of lactate to pyruvate and not requiring deproteinization. A popular and reliable method is used in the Dupont Automatic Clinical Analyzer chemistry system. Because of the rapidity of the technique (6 minutes), the Dupont ACA is unsurpassed in providing STAT results for lactic-acid levels. Gas-liquid chromatographic methodology has been used in the past, but these methods are not available for STAT testing.

LACTIC DEHYDROGENASE

The lactic dehydrogenase (LDH) enzyme is widely found in the cytoplasm of cells throughout the body, especially in the brain, kidney, liver, heart, and muscle. The enzyme catalyzes the reversable oxidation of lactate to pyruvate in the terminal phases of the Embden-Meyerhoff (glycolytic) pathway of intermediary metabolism. The elevated activity of enzyme in the cerebrospinal fluid (the same as in plasma) in disease states is due to leakage from damaged cells and bacteria.[73] The lactic dehydrogenase level in the cerebrospinal fluid is about one tenth that found in blood: cerebrospinal-fluid lactic dehydrogenase is less than 20 IU/L and serum is 200 IU/L.[36,38]

Increased cerebrospinal-fluid LDH has been reported in the following instances:

1. Patients with bacterial meningitis
2. 10% of the patients with aseptic (viral) meningitis
3. Subarachnoid hemorrhage
4. Lymphomas
5. Leukemias
6. Metastatic tumors involving the central nervous system

An elevated LDH is a more sensitive index of neurologic disorder than is an elevated cerebrospinal-fluid protein alone. Nevertheless, LDH assay has no specific diagnostic importance other than it raises a suspicion of increased tissue destruction. Total LDH correlates best with presence of meningitis or tumor—that is, those conditions that will cause cellular necrosis with the release of intracytoplasmic enzymes (a sensitivity of about 50% but a specificity of about 94%). Such information—along with protein and lactic-acid determinations—may be valuable in assessing the total picture, before bacteriologic culture results are available.[39] Children who have had febrile convulsions do not necessarily have increased LDH in the cerebrospinal fluid.

The isozymes of LDH can be determined in cerebrospinal fluid by concentration and subsequent electrophoresis, as they are in blood.[39] LDH isozymes, however, offer no additional diagnostic information. It is known that different isozymes predominate in various tissue. For example, LDH I and II predominate in neural brain tissue, LDH III and IV in blood lymphocytes, and LDH IV and V in blood granulocytes. Therefore, in cases of leukemias and lymphomas of the central nervous system, there is an increase in isozymes III and IV. Elevated LDH I and II without the presence of cellular components indicates neural tissue damage.

Most currently available two-point assays or rate-kinetic assays of LDH methodologies that utilize serum can utilize urine and cerebrospinal fluid as the specimen substrate. Because cerebrospinal-fluid testing is done on a STAT basis, the Dupont ACA technique, which requires only 6 minutes of "bench" working time, is particularly useful.

CREATINE KINASE

The creatine-kinase molecule consists of only two subunits: B and M fractions. Each subunit may have two forms, each of which predominates in different tissues. The MM form, for example, predominates in skeletal muscle tissue, the MB form in heart muscle tissue, and the BB form in brain tissue.

The hybrid MB form, which is a minor fraction, is a diagnostically important component of the heart-muscle enzyme. The synthesis of the subunits is controlled by separate genes, thereby qualifying these fractions as isoenzymes (isozymes) as defined by the International Union of Biochemistry. Isoenzyme composition of enzymes produced by tumors is more fetal than adult in molecular composition or configuration; hence, it is not surprising to find tumors elaborating the BB isozyme of creatine kinase.

It has been assumed that the presence of elevated creatine kinase (CK) in cerebrospinal fluid is indicative of neural damage.[40–41] CK isozyme studies on cerebrospinal fluid may fail to reveal increased BB fraction, CK, while MM is seen in nearly all patients with strokes. This has led some observers to suggest that CK originates from skeletal muscle. However, alterations in electrophoretic migration pattern of creatine-kinase isozymes have been observed, under experimental conditions, to produce changes of migration pattern from BB to MM (Cave, S.: Unpublished Master's thesis. Louisiana State University, 1978.).

Creatine kinase has been reported to be elevated in cerebrospinal fluid in the following instances:[41]

1. All types of stroke (subarachnoid hemorrhage, cerebral thrombosis, intracerebral hemorrhage)
2. Multiple sclerosis
3. Degenerative disorders
4. Primary brain tumors

5. Viral and bacterial meningitis
6. Patients with epileptic seizure

The terms "creatine kinase" and "creatine phosphokinase" (the latter an older term) are synonymous.

ASPARTATE AMINOTRANSFERASE

In addition to increased levels of creatine kinase, increased levels of aspartate aminotransferase (AST) (or, in the older terminology, glutamic oxaloacetic transaminase (GOT)) have been reported in:

1. Intracerebral hemorrhage
2. Subarachnoid hemorrhage
3. Patients with bacterial meningitis

Whether differentiation of the mitochondrial and cytosolic forms of aspartate aminotransferase has any chemical significance remains to be determined.

The techniques for enzyme measurements are identical to those used in routine analytical chemistry in clinical laboratories. The Dupont ACA procedure is analytically accurate and rapid enough to warrant use as a STAT procedure.

SYPHILIS TESTING

Spinal manifestations of syphilis are uncommon today, but cases of late or latent syphilis continue to occur. Whether lumbar puncture should be performed solely for serologic testing of cerebrospinal fluid for syphilis is controversial. The diagnostic significance of a "positive" serologic test for neurosyphilis may not be enough information to warrant a diagnosis of syphilis, with its attendant social stigma.

Antibodies in patients with syphilis are generally considered to be in two classes: nonspecific reagins arising in response to treponemal lipid antigens or the products of interaction of treponemes in tissue and specific antibodies arising in response to Treponema pallidum and other treponemes.

Antibodies reacting with cardiolipin-lecithin antigen are a combination of immunoglobulins 19^S (IgM), which reacts in the flocculation tests, and 7^S (IgG) component, which is necessary for complement fixation reactions.[42,43] No serologic test identifies the presence of syphilis; rather, it reflects the patient's immunologic status. Consequently, the recommended serologic tests for syphilis fall into two categories: the nontreponemal and the treponemal procedures. The recommended nontreponemal procedures are the Venereal Disease Research Laboratories (VDRL) test (developed at the Communicable Disease Center, DHEW, Atlanta, Ga. 30300), the automated reagin test (ART), or the rapid plasma reagin (RPR) test.[44] Because the VDRL may be negative in approximately half the patients with neurosyphilis, treponemal tests have been developed. The antigen stimulant for the reagin antibody is thought to be present in destroyed cell membranes.

The physician must evaluate the sensitivity and specificity of tests for the detection of syphilis. Sensitivity is the ability of a test to react in the presence of syphilitic antibodies, while specificity is the ability of the test not to react in the absence of syphilitic antibodies. The VDRL has a high degree of sensitivity, but a low degree of specificity, because the reaction will occur in diseases other than syphilis (Figs. 8–6 and 8–7) such as:

1. Yaws
2. Pinta
3. Pregnancy
4. Autoimmune states
5. Infectious hepatitis
6. Lepromatous leprosy
7. Malaria
8. Miliary tuberculosis
9. Atypical pneumonias
10. Immunodeficiency diseases
11. Periarteritis nodosa
12. Smallpox vaccinations

The VDRL test, developed by the Communicable Disease Center in 1955, is a screening test and does not indicate that the patient has active syphilis. In general, the higher the titer of the VDRL the more likely the diagnosis is syphilis. The titers of cardiolipin tests are usually highest in secondary syphilis. Early latent syphilis (that is, 1 to 2 years following the initial infection) is associated with high or beginning diminishing titers. Adequate treatment in the early infectious stage usually leads to a fall in titer, but treatment in the latter stage may be associated with unchanged or slowly decreasing titers. There is no constant relationship for the titers to late latent syphilis with cardiovascular and neurologic components. It takes approximately 2 weeks or more for the VDRL tests to become positive after the initial infection; therefore, the VDRL should not be relied upon to make the diagnosis of syphilis shortly after suspected contact (Fig. 8–7 and Table 8–1).

The VDRL is frequently followed by a treponemal antigen test, especially the Reiter test, which uses a nonpathologic strain of treponemes, treponemal tests, or others that use live pathogenic T. pallidum from rabbit testicular syphilomas. The treponemal tests lack sensitivity but have a high degree of specificity; therefore, the VDRL may be positive and the FTA may not yet be positive in the patient with early active syphilis. If the FTA is positive, however, the patient has had syphilis (Fig. 8–7). The specificity and the sensitivity are superior to the VDRL slide test.[45] False-positive FTA reactions have been reported

TABLE 8–1. General Comparison of Specificity and Sensitivity of Some Current Serologic Tests for Syphilis and an Index of Their Therapeutic Usefulness.

Test	Test Principle	Sensitivity		Specificity	Use as Therapeutic Index Response
		Early Syphilis	Late Syphilis		
Nontreponemal:					
VDRL	Microflocculation slide screening test	High	Low	Low	Yes
RPR	Reagin test	High	Low	Low	No
RCFP	Kolmer complement fixation using extract of Reiter treponeme	High	Low	Low	No
Treponemal:					
FTA-ABS	Fluorescent test with T. Pallidum as antigen	Equal to Nontreponemal	Equal to Nontreponemal	High	No
TPI-IgM	Hemabsorption	Highest	Highest	Highest	Yes

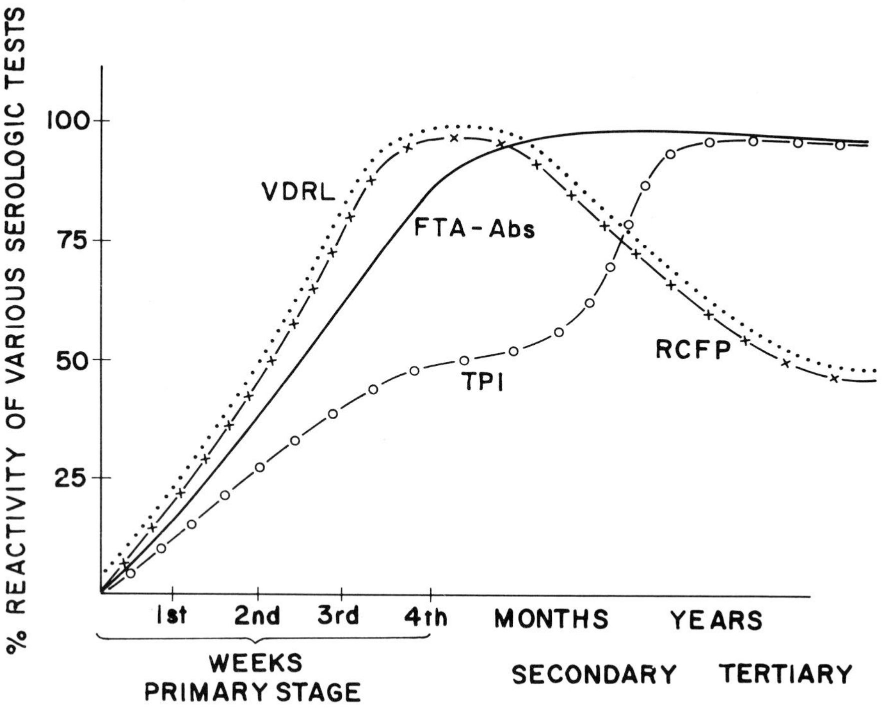

Fig. 8–7. The reactivity of serologic tests for syphilis with the stage of the disease and the length of infection after the appearance of a primary lesion.

in patients with macroglobulinemia, and possibly in patients with lupus erythematosus producing antinuclear antibodies. False-positive cerebrospinal fluid FTA tests can occur in patients with high serum treponemal antibodies when the immunoglobulins may diffuse from serum into the cerebrospinal fluid. Although it has been widely held that these tests are positive in 95% cases of suspected neurosyphilis, recent studies have indicated the specificity ranging only from 66 to 89%. Serial studies of cerebrospinal fluid reactivity in chimpanzees infected with treponema for 4 years previously, suggest that antibody reactivity is not proportional to the intensity of reaction in the serum, but reflects instead a separate response to antibodies within the cerebrospinal fluid. Persistence of T. pallidum antigen after penicillin G therapy in (two) adults with normal neurologic and cerebrospinal fluid examination may be demonstrated by treponemal tests only.[47]

T. pallidum specific IgM antibody develops rapidly after acute infection of syphilis, the antibody titer correlating with the activity of the disease.[46] The effectiveness of therapy also can be judged by this antibody, because it usually disappears with adequate treatment. In contrast, however, the T. pallidum specific IgG may persist throughout life (Table 8–1).

The VDRL procedure is recommended for nontreponemal testing. The solid-phase hemabsorption test for T. pallidum specific 19^S IgM is the most highly specific and most highly sensitive of the serologic tests for syphilis; the test also obviates the problems of fluorescence.

Nevertheless, as Ray Gambino points out, the diagnosis of neurosyphilis and the decision regarding therapy still require consideration of clinical findings in individual patients and are not based solely on laboratory data.[46]

MYELIN BASIC PROTEIN FRAGMENTS

Using electron microscopy, Robert Herndon and Marjorie Johnson reported, in 1970, the presence of myelin fragments in the cerebrospinal fluid of two out of three patients with active multiple sclerosis; patients with other neurologic diseases and with multiple sclerosis in remission did not show such fragments in their cerebrospinal fluid. After their work was published, a radioimmunoassay method of silica-gel absorption for the protein fraction of myelin (myelin basic protein) was designed by Steven Cohen and Robert Herndon.[48–49] Patients with multiple sclerosis in acute exacerbation had high levels of myelin basic protein (17–100 ng/ml); those with slowly progressive multiple sclerosis had lower levels (6–16 ng/ml); and those in remission had less than 4 ng/ml (comparable to the control population). Myelin basic protein is usually not detectable (>10 ng/ml) in normal cerebrospinal fluid.

ENCEPHALITOGENIC PROTEIN FRAGMENTS

In 1977, John Whitaker developed a double antibody radioimmunoassay technique for unconcentrated cerebrospinal fluid to detect encephalitogenic (EP) protein fragments in patients with multiple sclerosis.[50–51] EP appears to be a structural element of the myelin sheath that can induce experimental allergic encephalomyelitis in a variety of laboratory animals. These fragments have been called EP-P1. In acute or active cases of multiple sclerosis, the EP-P1 fragments can rise to levels of 3.4 to 15.4 mg/ml. These fragments were not found in patients with multiple sclerosis in remission or in patients who had the slowly progressive form of the disease. Review of the original control group revealed that 6 of 117 individuals without multiple sclerosis exhibited detectable levels of the EP-P1 protein. Two of these patients had levels in the same range as patients with acute multiple sclerosis; one of these patients had had a recent cerebral infarct; and the other was in a diabetic coma.

LYMPHOCYTE ADHERENCE

The Whitaker test (EP-P1) appears to be more specific than the myelin basic protein test, and both procedures are more specific than the lymphocyte adherence determination (LAD).[50,52] The LAD test uses peripheral lymphocytes from the blood of multiple sclerosis patients; when these lymphocytes are incubated with human epithelial (HEp-2) cells infected with measles virus, they produce adherence to lymphocytes. The LAD is greater in multiple sclerosis patients than in healthy persons or patients with neurologic disorders other than multiple sclerosis.

GLUTAMINE AND AMMONIA

Ammonia originates from ingested nitrogenous protein metabolism and hydrolysis of urea in the gastrointestinal tract. Thirty to 40% of urea produced in the liver is hydrolyzed to ammonia in the intestine and can contribute to the "ammonia load" (composed of free ammonia and amino acids, especially alanine and glutamine). Small rises in glutamine or alanine levels in the blood can produce a "buffering" of large rises in ammonia levels, but this effect does not alter ammonia excretion or inhibit ammonia toxicity.

Deficiency of the urea-cycle enzymes—specifically, a congenital deficiency of ornithine aminotransferase activity— can cause hypoammonemia, which is manifest by gyrate atrophy of the choroid plexus and retina, with hyperornithenemia. Hyperammonemia can occur in a patient with any severe liver disease that interferes with urea metabolism, but it especially occurs in patients with

1. Acute hepatitis
2. Cirrhosis
3. Liver failure of any etiology
4. Reye's syndrome

Hyperammonemia has been reported in severely infected, obstructed urinary tracts in which a urea-splitting organism, Proteus, is the offending organism.

In patients with hepatic failure, the ammonia levels increase in cerebrospinal fluid, as well as in the blood, by crossing the blood/CSF barrier. Although the process is not well understood, elevated ammonia levels cause neurotoxic effects. In the cerebrospinal fluid, ammonia undergoes combination with alpha-ketoglutarate, a vital enzyme in the Kreb's tricarboxylic acid cycle, to form glutamic acid, which then recombines with the ammonium ion to form glutamine. Alternately, the elevated glutamine may be converted in part to alpha-ketoglutamate, which is neurotoxic. The end result of the reaction creates consumption of adenosine triphosphate (ATP) and produces depletion of alpha-ketoglutarate. The reduced levels of alpha-ketoglutarate correlate with the increased levels of glutamine. Coma, it is proposed, develops from this reduced Kreb's cycle activity. Thus, it is presumed that measurement of glutamine reflects the state of consciousness as well as the degree of "hepatic encephalopathy" (liver disease producing brain symptoms).[53] Since the demonstration of elevated glutamine levels in hepatic encephalopathy by Thomas Whitehead and Steven Whitaker, in 1955, glutamine determination has been in vogue in the United States for detecting hepatic encephalopathy with coma. There are conflicting reports, however, regarding elevated glutamine levels in patients with hepatic encephalopathy but without coma.

Most cases of Reye's syndrome have increased cerebrospinal-fluid glutamine although there is no correlation between glutamine levels and the clinical outcomes in these patients.

In normal patients, the glutamine ranges from 5 to 19 mg/dl; in those patients with chronic liver disease but without evidence of encephalopathy, however, glutamine values of 13 to 39 mg/dl are detected. As the degree of encephalopathy increases, so does the mean cerebrospinal-fluid glutamine level. There is a better correlation of glutamine levels in the cerebrospinal fluid than in the blood of patients with hepatic encephalopathy and coma. Benjamin Hourani and associates have found a mean level of 40.3 $\pm$ 14 mg/dl. There is some indication that the glutamine level may rise prior to the clinical recognition of asterixis (tension tremors) in patients with hepatic encephalopathy and coma.

The phenol-hypochloride modification of the Nesslerization procedure is simple enough to be performed in practically any clinical laboratory.

BIOCHEMICAL MARKERS OF MALIGNANCY

Elevation of beta glucuronidase and carcinoembryonic antigen (CEA) levels have been reported to reliably reflect the infiltration of leptomeninges by metastatic carcinoma.[55] They are not elevated in patients with leptomeningeal infiltration by malignant lymphoma. Neither do patients with tumor colonization in the brain parenchyma or spinal epidural space exhibit elevated levels. Beta glucuronidase alone has been found to be slightly elevated in cerebrospinal fluid in cases of chronic "infectious" meningitis. Both these biologic markers approach control levels after effective treatment. Elevated adenylate kinase has been demonstrated in patients with metastases to areas of brain "bathed" by cerebrospinal fluid.[56]

The polyamines putrescine and its metabolites spermine and spermidine are liberated from rapidly growing and dying cells. This measurement of increased polyamines in cerebrospinal fluid has been proposed as a monitor for patients with brain tumors since 1971, when increased excretion of polyamines in urine of human cancer patients was reported. Enzymatic, chemical, thin-layer chromatographic and high-performance liquid chromatographic analyses for measuring the polyamines are within the technical capabilities of most clinical laboratories.

IMMUNOCYTOLOGIC MARKERS

Immunologic and cytochemical marker procedures can be used to differentiate and identify B and T lymphocytes, cells from the monocyte-macrophage series, and precursor cells of polymorphonuclear leukocytes. Using these methods, B lymphocytes predominate in multiple sclerosis and T lymphocytes predominate in tuberculous meningitis. Varying quantities of B and T lymphocytes are found in viral meningitis.[57] In cases of plasmacytoma tumor cells in the cerebrospinal fluid, the lymphocytes are usually identified as type B.

BIOGENIC AMINES

Cerebral amine metabolic studies have shown that different biogenic amines may serve as synaptic transmitters or modulators of neuronal activity in distinct brain systems.[54] Hydroxytryptamine, for example, functions in the limbic system; dopamine in the extrapyramidal system; and noradrenaline in the autonomic and "alerting" system. The main metabolite of 5-hydroxytryptamine is 5-hydroxyindoleacetic acid (5-HIAA), and the main metabolite of dopamine is 3-methoxy, 4-hydroxymandelic acid and homovanillic acid. Reduction of homovanillic acid and of 5-HIAA have been reported in cases of Parkinson's disease and depressive illnesses, suggesting impairment of dopamine and 5-hydroxytryptamine metabolism in those disease processes. The determination of these biogenic amines can be done in most clinical laboratories, but the diagnostic significance of the determinations is more of research interest than of diagnostic, clinical value at this time.

DIFFERENTIAL CELL COUNTS AND MORPHOLOGIC EVALUATION OF CELLS

Cerebrospinal-fluid white cell (leukocyte) counts should be performed on the uncentrifuged specimen (tube no. 3) during the first hour after specimen collection, since all cells begin to lyse rather rapidly. It is almost completely agreed upon that a cell count in excess of 5 mononuclear cells/μL is abnormal in adults.[58] Normal values in neonates may go slightly higher—between 0 and 30 mononuclear cells/μL.

Due to the low cellularity of normal spinal fluid, the coefficient of variation in the counting technique is expected to be high and is in most laboratories.[59] Precision in the technique can be improved by counting larger numbers of cells. Because the cerebrospinal fluid is contaminated with peripheral blood in a traumatic tap, one may assume that there is one white blood cell (WBC) and 1 mg protein in the cerebrospinal fluid for every 750 red blood cells.

In cases of abnormal cell counts in peripheral blood, one may use the following formula:

$$\text{WBC} = \frac{\text{Peripheral blood WBC count} \times \text{CSF RBC count}}{\text{Peripheral blood RBC count}}$$

Since the percentage of cells present in the cerebrospinal fluid is usually considerably lower than that in most other body fluids, it may be necessary to concentrate the specimen for staining techniques and morphologic identification.

Different methods for concentrating cerebrospinal-fluid cells include:

1. Centrifugation
2. Millipore or filter techniques
3. Sedimentation methods
4. Cytocentrifugation

The method used depends on the specific needs of the laboratory. For quantitative and more precise qualitative profiles of cerebrospinal-fluid cells, the sedimentation and filtration methods are superior to the counting chamber, direct smear, and centrifugation procedures.[60] The filtration method is more than adequate for cytologic identification of central-nervous-system neoplasm (primary or metastatic). Better cellular details are obtained with a sedimentation technique, and the procedure is rapid and technically simple.[61] Cytocentrifuge methods are simple, provide excellent cell preservation (but not as good as sedimentation methods), and good recovery of cells. The main disadvantages of the cytocentrifuge method are the need for special equipment and use of a larger volume of fluid that may obviate other tests and some chemical analysis.

The cell types of leukocytes in cerebrospinal fluid can be separated morphologically into the following categories:

Normal

1. Lymphocytes
2. Neutrophils (<5%)
3. PAM cells

Abnormal

1. Neutrophils (>5%)
2. Eosinophils
3. Plasma cells
4. PAM cells
5. LE/reticular cells
6. Leukemic cells
7. Malignant cells
8. Lymphocytes (when increased)

The technique of cell counting and morphologic identification is essentially the same methodology as the peripheral blood white-blood-cell count using the Fuchs-Rosenthal counting chamber with Neubauer ruling (Fig. 8–8). Under phase microscopy with undiluted cerebrospinal fluid, cytologic differentiation can be made accurately after an acidified crystal violet stain.

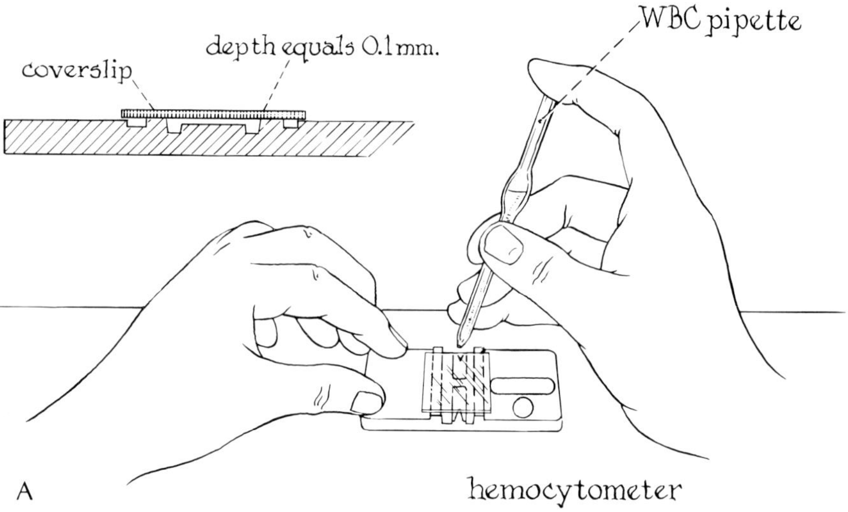

A

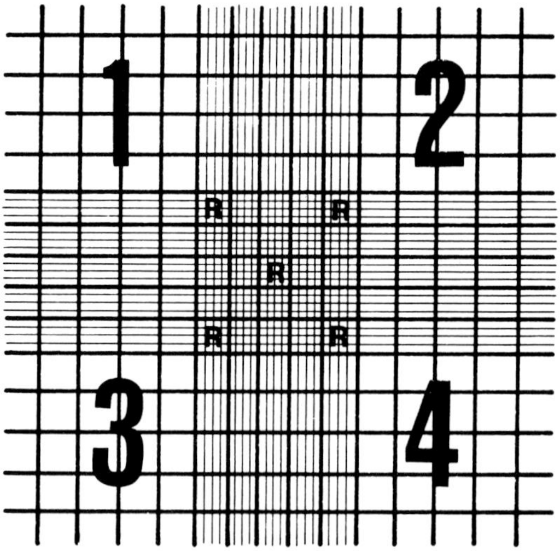

B

Fig. 8–8. A, Hemocytometer counting chamber with Neubauer ruling for cell-counting technique. **B,** The cells in the outer four squares (nos. 1, 2, 3, 4) are counted under the conventional light microscope.

Lymphocytes

Lymphocytes represent the predominant cell in the normal cerebrospinal fluid (62% ± 34). The rest of normal cellular constituents are represented to be pia-arachnoid cells, mesothelial cells, and monocytes (PAM cells) (36% ± 20).[64] Elevated lymphocyte counts are found in association with:

1. Viral meningoencephalitis
2. Fungal meningitis (crytococcosis, coccidioidosis, chromoblastomycosis)
3. Tuberculosis
4. Syphilis
5. Cystospyrosis involving meninges
6. Parasitic disease (toxoplasmosis, cysticercosis)
7. Aseptic meningitis

Neutrophilic Leukocytes

Some authors consider the detection of one neutrophil to be abnormal, while others consider neutrophils up to 5% of the total cell count to be normal in neonates. Increased numbers of neutrophilic leukocytes are found in cases of:

1. Bacterial meningitis
2. Early viral meningitis
3. Tuberculous or mycotic meningitis
4. Amebic encephalomyelitis
5. Aseptic meningitis
6. Early syphilis
7. Hemorrhage
8. Toxic meningitis
9. Reactions to repetitious lumbar puncture
10. Necrotic tumors
11. Some leukemias

Cell counts are usually in excess of 1,000/cumm with 90% neutrophils in cases of bacterial meningitis. In cases of viral meningitis, however, cell counts are usually between 100 to 500 cells/cumm, with lymphocytic predominance. A pleocytosis may not be characteristic of the differential cell count in patients with partially treated bacterial meningitis; there might be a mixed reaction of neutrophils, lymphocytes, and monocytes. In such cases, demonstration of elevated lactic acid would be diagnostically valuable.

Eosinophilic Leukocytes[64]

Eosinophilic pleocytosis in the cerebrospinal fluid was first associated with neurosyphilis. Increased eosinophilic leukocytes also occur as a result of:

1. Helminthic infections (cysticercosis, schistosomiasis, ascariasis, echinococcosis, visceral larval migrans infestation, trichinosis)
2. Fungal infections (coccidioidomycosis)
3. Bacterial infections (tuberculosis)
4. Some malignant lymphomas
5. Drug reactions
6. Food allergies and atopic conditions

Plasma Cells

In vivo development of plasma cells has been demonstrated in the central nervous system in cases of plasmacytomas.[65] Plasma cells in spinal fluid have been described in cases of:

1. Plasmacytomas
2. Multiple sclerosis
3. Viral infections
4. Cysticercosis
5. Granulomatous diseases
6. Neurosyphilis
7. Subacute sclerosing panencephalitis (SSPE)

Pia-arachnoid, Mesothelial, and Monocytic Cells

The pia-arachnoid, mesothelial, and monocytic cells (PAM cells) are grouped together for purposes of laboratory evaluation.[60,63] PAM cells have been described as monocytoid—that is, young monocytes whose nuclei are round and compact with cytoplasm that is more basophilic than mature monocytes. Macrophages in the cerebrospinal fluid are sometimes considered to be in the general group of monocytes and PAM cells.

An elevated number of PAM and monocytes has been seen as mixed reactions with granulocytes and lymphocytes in:

1. Bacterial meningitis
2. Tuberculous meningitis
3. Fungal meningitis
4. Ruptured brain abscess
5. Amebic encephalomyelitis

Increased numbers of ependymal cells have been described in hydrocephalic children, especially in the cerebrospinal-fluid specimens obtained by cisternal or ventricular tap. Monocytes, in the form of phagocytes occurring singly or in the form of giant cells, can be seen in cases of tuberculosis or mycotic meningitides. Erythrophagocytosis and hemosiderin-laden macrophages have also been identified in association with acute and chronic subarachnoid hemorrhage.

Choroid Plexus and Ependymal Cells

Neuroectodermal cells such as choroid plexus and ependymal cells (Fig. 8–9) are infrequently found in cerebrospinal fluid. These cells can be found in a variety of conditions, including ventricular and cisternal punctures, central nervous system trauma, or surgery, following myelography, and with ischemic infarction of the brain. The distinction between choroid plexus and ependymal cells is probably not clinically beneficial, and the presence of these cells is of little diagnostic significance; however, they must be differentiated from metastatic and primary brain tumor cells. Neuroectodermal cells usually appear "bland," lack uniform nuclei or nucleoli, and have low nuclear-cytoplasmic ratios.

Choroid plexus cells are usually found in cell clusters and have relatively abundant cytoplasm that is usually slightly basophilic. The cytoplasmic borders often show vacuolization, and fine cilia may be identified in well-preserved specimens. The nuclei are round with a smooth nucleus membrane. The chromatin is finely granular and evenly distributed throughout the nucleus. Nucleoli are usually not evident.

Ependymal cells also occur in cell clusters and may be difficult or impossible to distinguish from choroid plexus cells. Cytoplasm is relatively abundant, amphophilic to lightly basophilic, and usually lacks peripheral vacuolization. Cilia may occasionally be found at the periphery. The nucleus is round to oval and similar to choroid plexus nuclei.

Lupus Erythematous Cells and Reticular Cells

The presence of lupus erythematous cells (LE cells) have been reported to occur spontaneously in very rare cases.[66] In addition, abnormal histiocytes have been seen in cases of histiocytosis X. Abnormal reticular cells have been seen in the cerebrospinal fluid of patients with lymphomatoid granulomatosis involving the central nervous system.

Leukemic Cells

Fifty percent of children with lymphocytic leukemias without previous treatment have central nervous involvement.[67] Even with adequate treatment, 5% of these patients will have continued involvement during the course of their disease. Once leukemic cells enter the cerebrospinal fluid from the blood they can undergo uninhibited proliferation. Leukemic cells in cerebrospinal fluid may be found in just a few numbers or in more than 1,000/μL. The morphologic appearance of

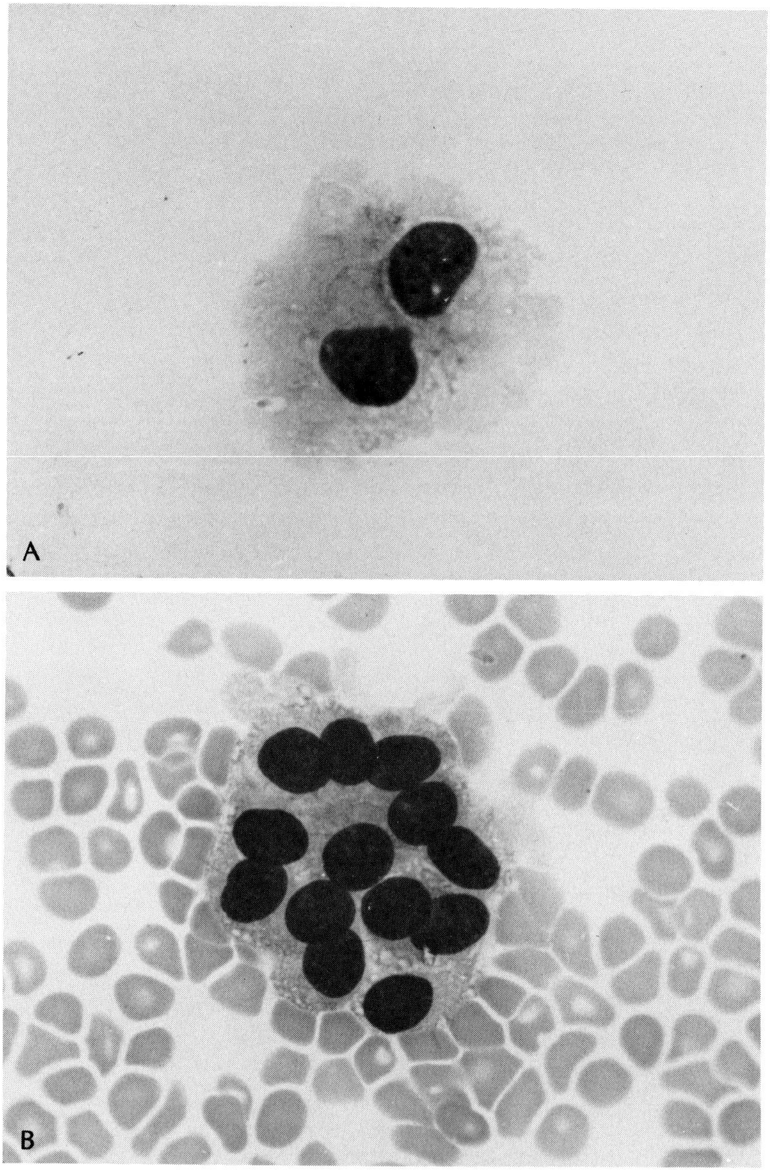

Fig. 8–9. Neuroectodermal cells in spinal fluid prepared with cytocentrifuge technique. **A,** Ependymal cells (× 750). **B,** Choroid plexus cells (× 750). (Courtesy of Dr. John Brandt, Department of Pathology, Ohio State University Medical Center.)

these cells in a well preserved specimen is similar to that of the same cells in bone marrow, peripheral blood, or urine. Adults can have leukemic cells in the cerebrospinal fluid in cases of acute myeloblastic and promyelocytic leukemia, commonly having meningeal involvement. Lymphosarcoma cell leukemias can spread to the meninges.

Malignant Cells

Malignant cells in cerebrospinal fluid have been encountered in 20 to 40% of patients with malignant tumors of the central nervous system.[68–71] The presence of malignant cells implies that the leptomeninges have been seeded widely by viable tumor. Absence of malignant cells in the cerebrospinal fluid does not rule out that diagnosis. Most cases of false-positive cytology in cerebrospinal fluid have been due to immature or reactive lymphocytes being misdiagnosed as lymphoma cells. Repeated cytologic evaluation for tumor cells is useful in assessing the results of therapy (Fig. 8–10).

Among the primary intracranial tumors that can produce cells in the cerebrospinal fluid are:

1. Astrocytomas
2. Ependymomas
3. Choroid plexus carcinomas
4. Tumors of the medulloblastoma-retinoblastoma category
5. Chromophobe adenomas
6. Craniopharyngiomas

Metastatic cells can come from tumors of the lung, gastrointestinal tract, breast, and skin. In meningeal metastasis from colorectal carcinoma, the finding of elevated carcinoembryonic antigen (CEA) in the cerebrospinal fluid can be used in conjunction with the cytologic examination to diagnose and to evaluate response to therapy.

MICROSCOPIC EXAMINATION OF MICROORGANISMS

Gram Stain

The classic method of detection of bacteria involves microscopic examination of the gram-stained dried smear of cerebrospinal fluid on a 1″ × 3″ glass microscopic slide. When this stain is made on cerebrospinal fluid containing 10^5 bacteria/μL, there will be about one bacterium/oil immersion field. Centrifugation and concentration of the cerebrospinal-fluid sediment may increase the organism concentration and improve the efficiency of bacterial detection. The Gram stain remains one of the most useful STAT procedures for the detection of bacteria.[62] Observation for organisms should especially be directed to any leukocytes present. A positive Gram stain should be reported to the physician immediately.

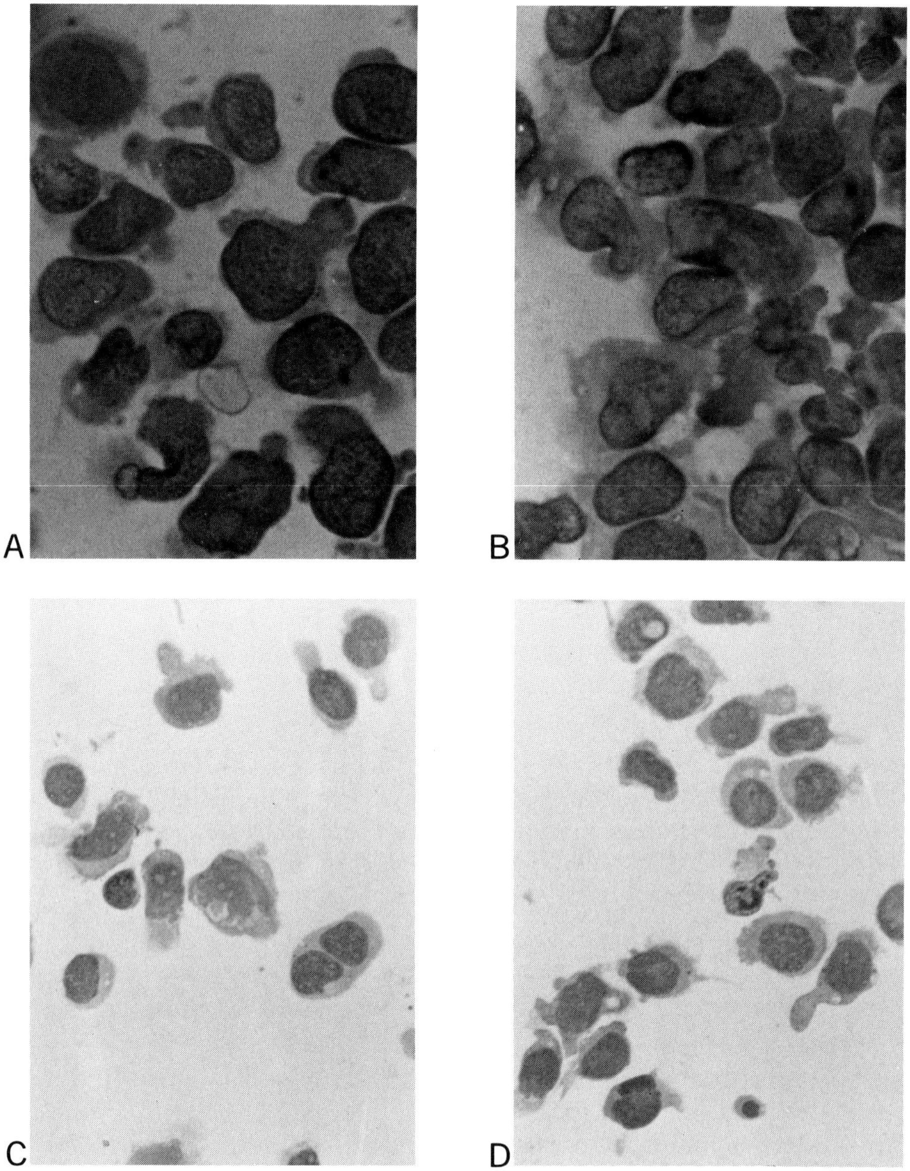

Fig. 8–10. Malignant cells found in cerebrospinal fluid of patient with a lymphoblastic lymphoma, isolated by cytocentrifugation, and stained with PAP technique (**A** and **B,** ×5000) and Wright's stain (**C** and **D,** ×3000).

The most common organisms found in pathologic cerebrospinal fluid are:

1. Streptococcus pneumoniae
2. Neisseria meningitidis
3. Haemophilus influenzae, type B
4. Staphylococcus aureus
5. Cryptococcus neoformans

The presence of these organisms can be strongly suspected by the trained technologist with visual identification of the Gram-stained specimen (with the exception of the cryptococcus species). This can be a true STAT observation (Fig. 8–11). Consequently, delay in culture reporting will not retard the clinician's decision for specific STAT therapeutic measures. The final bacteriologic culture report is truly a confirmatory measure and does not help the physician decide whether or not to initiate therapy.

India-Ink Preparation

Cryptococcus species will produce a gelatinous capsule that can be "negatively" detected by surrounding the gelatinous capsule with carbon particles in suspension, using India ink. The gelatinous capsule will displace the particles, leaving a clear halo. Thus, single budding yeast can be readily detected in Cryptococcus neoformans (Fig. 8–12).

There has been much discussion about the quality of India ink to be

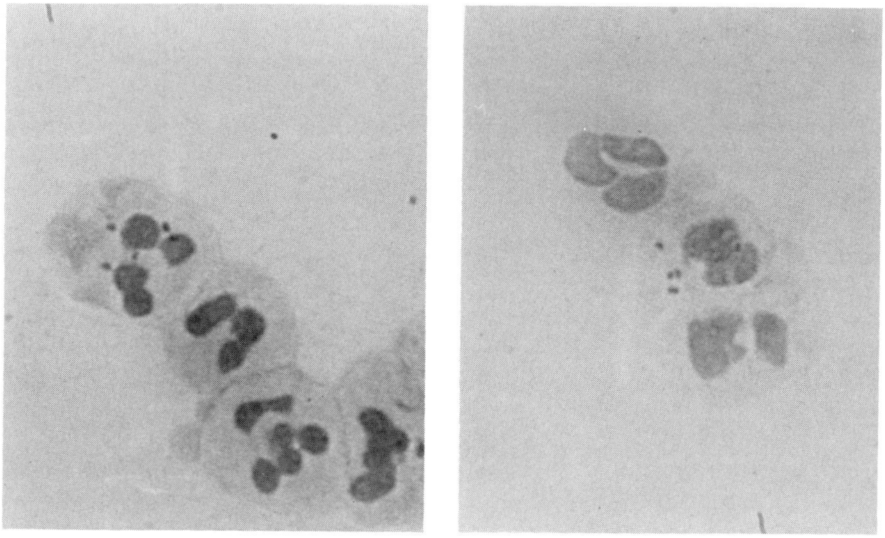

Fig. 8–11. Gram stain of cerebrospinal fluid sediment revealing intracellular gram-negative cocci within polymorphonuclear leukocytes. ×1000.

A 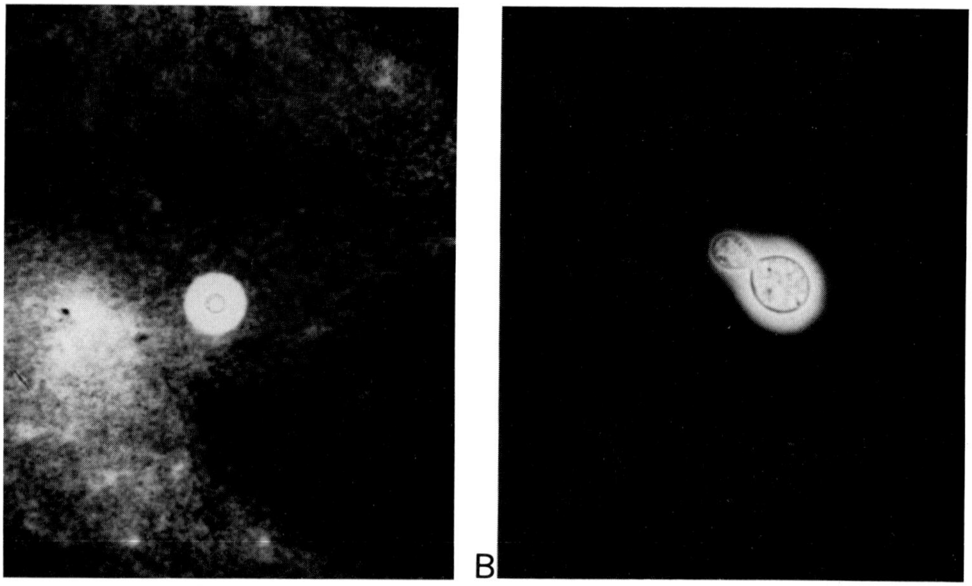 B

Fig. 8–12. India-ink preparation of Cryptococcus neoformans from cerebrospinal fluid in 48-year-old Caucasian female with headache. Lumbar spinal tap revealed a normal CSF protein, lymphocytic pleocytosis, and negative bacteriologic cultures. **A,** Thick gelatinous capsule. **B,** Single budding yeast (about ×4000).

used for this procedure, primarily because the inks contain other yeast, which may produce a capsule that mimicks cryptococcus. In the past, the recommended ink was manufactured by Günther Wagner of Hanover, Germany. Perlikan India ink, with a small-sized carbon particle, contains enough phenol to inhibit growth of yeast to provide good enough preparation for microscopic evaluation of the capsule of the yeast form of cryptococcus. The Latex test for cryptococcus antigen is positive in titers of 1:10 or greater in the cerebrospinal fluid of some 99% of patients with cryptococcal meningitis. The test is also positive in the serum of about 60% of patients with active pulmonary cryptococcosis.

Other Stains and Preparations

Ziehl-Neilsen's and Fite's stains for acid-fast organisms are widely used to detect tuberculous meningitis. These acid-fast stains depend on phenol (in carbolfuscin) penetrating the lipophilic cell wall, with subsequent dye binding of the cell wall of the bacterium. The Fite stain was devised to permit a "light" acid-alcohol decolorization that can be used for Mycobacterium leprae, as well as for all other mycobacterium. It is the standard acid-fast stain used in our laboratories. George Fite developed the stain for detecting Hansen's bacillus in any tissue. However, there has never been a case of central-nervous-system Hansen's disease found at the U.S. Public Health Service Hospital, National Leprosy Center, Carville, La. 70721, since Fite's stain has been in use since 1955.

Additional stains for fungi include Gomori's methenamine silver (GMS), Periodic Acid Schiff (PAS), and mucicarmine stains. These stains are commonly employed in most histology sections of clinical laboratories and their "cookbook" performance has been well presented in the Manual of Histologic Staining Methods of the Armed Forces Institute of Pathology (Luna, L. (ed): American Registry of Pathology. New York, McGraw-Hill Book Company, 1980).

BACTERIOLOGIC CULTURES FOR DETECTION OF MENINGITIS

The confirmation, if not the recognition, of meningitis in patients requires the examination of the cerebrospinal fluid obtained by lumbar puncture. This is especially true in recognizing the occurrence of meningitis, which may be classed as follows:

1. Bacterial meningitis
2. Viral meningitis
3. Granulomatous meningitis

The expected cerebrospinal-fluid abnormalities associated with each of the main types of meningitis are shown in Tables 8–2 and 8–3.[62] The cerebrospinal-fluid changes associated with tuberculous, fungal, and viral meningitis overlap and make it difficult to separate these entities. Detection of bacterial meningitis is generally made more readily. In most instances, other clinical findings and judgment, coupled with x-ray and laboratory data, provide the physician with enough information to establish a classification of meningitis. The major concern in the laboratory evaluation for acute bacterial meningitis is STAT diagnosis to permit rapid institution of appropriate therapy. The sequelae of meningitis may be disastrous—acute gross neurologic defects, long-term, subtle personality problems, behavioral aberrations—and may be prevented by rapid diagnosis and treatment. In fact, therapy should be administered within a short time (less than 1 hour) after diagnosis of acute bacterial meningitis. There is no reason for withholding therapy, even in patients from whom cerebrospinal fluid cannot be obtained. Admittedly, such therapy will be "shotgun" in character, but might make the difference in a patient's long-term physical and mental well being. Cerebrospinal-fluid changes in patients with bacterial meningitis are modified relatively little by a few hours therapy.[62] Even failure to find bacteria on a Gram stain of cerebrospinal-fluid sediment in which there are polymorphonuclear leukocytes should not inhibit the clinician from therapy. It is not uncommon to find large numbers of polys with a negative Gram stain in patients with cerebrospinal fluid infected with N. meningitidis.[62]

TABLE 8–2. Classification, Pathogenesis, and Etiology of Infections of the Central Nervous System.*

Type of Infection and Specific Examples		Pathogenesis	Most Frequent Causative Microorganisms
Acute bacterial infections	Abscesses: Brain, Epidural, Subdural	Blood borne (lung, intestinal tract, skin, paranasal sinuses) or direct invasion (trauma or ENT, neuro-orthopedic surgery)	Peptostreptococci; Bacteroides; Staphylococci; and Streptococci, group A or D
	Meningitis: Infants (2 months)	Blood borne (intestinal tract) or direct invasion (birth canal)	Escherichia coli and Streptococci, group B
	Children (2 months to 5 years)	Blood borne (orpharynx); rarely by direct invasion	Haemophilus influenzae, type B; Streptococcus pneumoniae; and Neisseria meningitidis
	Adults	Blood borne (oropharynx); rarely by direct invasion	Streptococcus pneumoniae; Neisseria meningitidis; and Haemophilus influenzae, occasionally in adults
	All ages	Direct invasion secondary to head trauma (old or recent), congenital neuromalformations, neurodiagnostic procedures, and neuro-orthopedic surgery	Staphylococci; Streptococci, group A; Streptococcus pneumoniae; and Pseudomonas aeruginosa
Granulomatous meningitis	Tuberculous meningitis	Blood borne (lung)	Mycobacterium tuberculosis
	Cryptococcal meningitis	Blood borne (lung)	Cryptococcus neoformans
Acute viral infections	"Aseptic" meningitis	Blood borne (intestinal tract or oropharynx)	Enteroviruses and mumps virus
	Viral encephalitis	Blood borne (intestinal tract) or arthropod vector feeding	Mumps virus, herpesvirus, enteroviruses, and arboviruses

*Reproduced with permission from Youmans, G., Patterson, P., and Sommers, H.: The Biologic and Clinical Basis of Infectious Diseases. Philadelphia, W.B. Saunders, 1975, p. 532.

Table 8–3. Cerebrospinal Fluid Abnormalities Associated with Meningitis.

Type of Meningitis	Predominant Cell Type	Glucose (mg/dl)	Protein	Stained Smear	Result of Culture
Bacterial	Segmented neutrophils	Low (<5–20)	Elevated	Usually positive*	Usually positive*
Tuberculous	Mononuclear cells (neutrophils early)	Low (20–40)	Elevated	Usually negative	Usually negative
Fungal	Mononuclear cells	Low (20–40)	Elevated	Often positive	Usually positive
Viral (aseptic)	Mononuclear cells	Normal (60–90)	Slightly elevated early	Negative	Negative

*A major exception is bacterial meningitis caused by *Neisseria meningitidis,* in which the Gram stain of cerebrospinal fluid sediment often fails to reveal microorganisms and cultures may be negative for growth. (Reproduced with permission from Youmans, G., Paterson, P., and Sommers, H.: The Biologic and Clinical Basis of Infectious Disease. Philadelphia, W.B. Saunders, 1975, p. 537.)

Acute bacterial infections of the central nervous system can be divided into focal abscesses or diffuse inflammatory processes. Abscess of meningeal inflammation may result from direct invasion of the nervous system of the subarachnoid space by bacteria or seeding of central nervous system by microorganisms through the blood/brain barrier.

Examination of cerebrospinal fluid in patients with suspected brain abscesses usually yield little assistance. Remember, removal of even minute amounts of cerebrospinal fluid with increased intracranial pressure may promote herniation of the brain stem into the foramen magnum, producing cardiorespiratory failure with pressure on the medulla, or transtentorial herniation of the cerebral hemispheres into the posterior fossa, producing death. Brain abscesses frequently develop in conjunction with traumatic head injury or contiguous infection from the mastoid sinuses, vertebral body, or spinal column. Fractures through the petrous portion of the temporal bone rarely heal, thus providing ready access to the cerebrospinal fluid from the middle ear or mastoid sinus infections. Fractures of the cribriform plate of the orbit represent another source of bacterial invasion from the paranasal sinuses. Constant leakage of small amounts of cerebrospinal fluid through the nasal sinuses produces a watery nasal discharge; leakage through the external otic canal produces a similar discharge. For rapid evaluation of discharge from these areas to determine if, in fact, cerebrospinal fluid is leaking, utilize a Dextrostix to determine the glucose content of the fluid, which of course, is higher than that of serous discharge from infectious processes. This is a favorite evaluation performed by the astute emergency room physician.

Bacterial Meningitis

The types of bacteria commonly encountered with acute bacterial meningitis depend on the type of infection, the site of infection, the pathogenesis, and the age of the patient (Table 8–2). The immune response of the individual is all important in the defense mechanisms of bacterial infection. Bacteria that most often cause brain, epidural, and spinal abscesses are the peptostreptococci, bacteroides species, staphylococci, and streptococci. In premature and newborn infants, meningitis is most often associated with intestinal bacteria, especially Escherichia coli. Since the opsonizing antibody for K1 antigen (an IgG_2 immunoglobulin) passes transplacentally only during the last stages of full-term gestation, it may not be present in premature infants, making it less likely that there is a protective level of antibody against E. coli. The serum levels of opsonizing bactericidal antibody are critical for the immune process at this age.

Invasion of the central nervous system by bacteria in patients with septicemia or bacteremia from a distant primary infection is probably the most common cause of acute bacterial meningitis. In infants this is most certainly true, bacteria usually disseminating from the oropharynx.[74] The following are the bacteria that most commonly cause meningitis in this age group:

1. Haemophilic influenzae, type B
2. Streptococcus pneumoniae
3. Neisseria meningitidis
4. Streptococcus, group B

In adults, meningitis is also most commonly a result of direct dissemination of bacteria from the oropharynx. The most common organisms infecting this age group are:

1. Streptococcus pneumoniae
2. Neisseria meningitidis
3. Haemophilic influenzae (in the elderly)

In patients with fractures of basilar bones of the skull or paranasal sinuses, with congenital malformations of the central nervous system, and after diagnostic invasive procedures of the central nervous system or brain, the most common bacteria causing meningitis (by direct invasion) are the following:

1. Staphylococcus aureus
2. Streptococcis, group A
3. Streptococcus pneumoniae
4. Pseudomonas aeruginosa
5. Strains of enterobacteriaceae
6. Staphylococcus epidermidis, which may be pathogenic

Granulomatous Meningitis

Granulomatous meningitis is characterized by a histologic response to injury by the organism—that is, accumulation of lymphocytes and mononuclear histiocytes with development of epithelioid (multinucleated giant) cells. The most common causes of granulomatous meningitis in adults are Mycobacterium tuberculosis (var. humanis) and Cryptococcus neoformans.

The infection is usually from the lungs; it is either hematogenous or a result of aerosol inhalation of the organisms. Frequently, the first manifestation of cryptococcal disease is from the central nervous system and not the respiratory system. Furthermore, undetected granuloma in tuberculosis sometimes is discovered only after the patient presents with tuberculous meningitis.

Viral Meningitis

Acute central-nervous-system infections of viral origin are usually either aseptic meningitis or encephalitis. Viremia produces seeding of the subarachnoid space and the cerebrospinal fluid, the source usually being the intestinal tract, the oropharynx, or dermal vessels injected by feeding arthropods. Viruses producing meningitis are listed in Table 8–2.

CONDITIONS SIMULATING MENINGITIS

Focal brain abscesses often masquerade as tumorous processes, because they produce increased intracranial pressure. With the advent of computerized axial tomography, differentiating cystic abscesses from solid tumors is easier. Focal necrosis of tumors may elude diagnostic differentiation—that is, neoplastic metastasis involving the meninges may produce a clinical picture simulating granulomatous or bacterial meningitides. In such cases, the abnormalities of cerebrospinal fluid may be identical to those characterizing meningitis and may be distinguished only by detection of malignant cells in the spinal fluid.

BACTERIOLOGIC PLATING

It is urgent that the physician initiate specific and rapid therapy and that the laboratory personnel share this urgency when plating cerebrospinal fluid for bacteriologic culturing. Bacteriologic plating techniques are routine in most laboratories, however, and include the following media:

1. Blood agar plate, to detect Neisseriae meningitidis, Streptococcus pneumoniae, Escherichia coli, Streptococcus, group B, and Cryptococcus neoformans
2. Chocolate agar plate, to detect Haemophilis influenzae and hemophilis species and Neisseria meningitidis
3. Brain-heart infusion (with para-aminobenzoic acid and 0.1% (w/v) agar), to detect anaerobic organisms

Cerebrospinal fluid for fungal cultures are plated on Sabouraud's dextrose agar and microbiotic agar.

LIMULUS TEST

Gram-negative septicemia with central-nervous-system involvement remains a major infectious disease problem for any hospitalized patient, especially the elderly. The Gram stain of cerebrospinal-fluid sediment, when positive, is probably the quickest way to provide the physician with enough information to make a tentative diagnosis. Detection of endotoxin produced by bacterial organisms is now technically feasible and has gained medical popularity since the early 1970s. Because patients suspected of having septic meningitis require immediate therapy, STAT or rapid laboratory procedures become diagnostically invaluable.

The limulus test promises rapid (about 1 hour) detection of a Gram-negative bacterial infection.[75,76] The test is considered to be most reliable in detecting endotoxin in the cerebrospinal fluid but can be used effectively with blood and any other body fluids. The test is made on the protein containing fluid derived from lysates of blood cells (amebocytes) of Limulus polyphenrus (the horseshoe crab). This method can detect as little as 0.0005 mg of endotoxin/ml of cerebrospinal fluid, blood, or other body fluids. Cerebrospinal fluid that yields a positive limulus test may not yield a positive bacteriologic culture for Gram-negative organisms. However, a cerebrospinal fluid cultured positive for Gram-negative organisms will more often have a positive limulus test; thus, a positive limulus test with cerebrospinal fluid is indicative of a bacterial infection that is probably caused by Gram-negative organisms. This information can be the basis of rapid aggressive therapy in view of the high mortality associated with this type of septic meningitis.

The test is not meant to be the only parameter considered in therapeutic decision-making; other relevant judgemental, laboratory, and clinical parameters must be taken into consideration.

REFERENCES

1. Lyons, A., and Petrucelli, R.: Medicine: An Illustrated History. New York, Harry N. Abrams, 1978.
2. Clark, R.: Manter and Gatz's Essentials of Clinical Neuroanatomy and Neurophysiology. 5th Ed. Philadelphia, F.A. Davis, 1975, p. 167.
3. Plum, F., and Siegjo, B.: Recurrent advances in CSF physiology. Anesthesiology, *42*:708, 1975.
4. Heisey, S., Held, D., and Pappenheimer, J.: Bulk flows and diffusion in the CSF system of the goat. Am. J. Physiol., *203*:775, 1962.
5. Davis, J., and Mason, C.: Neurologic Critical Care. New York, Van Nostrand Reinhold, 1979.
6. Marshall, J.: Lumbar puncture. Br. J. Hosp. Med., *3*:216, 1970.
7. Weinstein, R., et al.: Factitious meningitis: Diagnostic error due to nonviable bacteria in commercial lumbar puncture trays. J.A.M.A., *233*:878, 1975.
8. Patten, B.: How much blood makes the cerebrospinal fluid bloody? J.A.M.A., *206*:378, 1968.
9. Walton, J.: Subarachnoid Hemorrhage. Edinburgh, Livingstone Press, 1956.
10. Van der Meuler, J.: Cerebrospinal fluid xanthochromia: An objective index. Neurology, *16*:170, 1966.
11. Cole, M.: Pitfalls in cerebrospinal-fluid examination. Hosp. Pract., *4*:47, 1969.
12. Diem, K., and Lentner, C. (eds.): Documenta Geigy Scientific Tables. 7th Ed. Basle, Ciba-Geigy, 1970, p. 635.
13. Kabat, E., Moore, D., and Landow, H.: An electrophoresis study of the protein components in cerebrospinal fluid and their relationship to the serum proteins. J. Clin. Invest., *21*:571, 1942.
14. Kluge, H., Winkler, G., and Weiczorek, V.: Results of the comparison of different methods of total protein in CSF. Dtsch. Gesundh., *23*:2039, 1968.
15. Gilland, O.: Cerebrospinal fluid paper electrophoresis in healthy volunteers. Acta Neurol. Scand., *43*:403, 1967.
16. Werner, M.: A combined procedure for protein estimation and electrophoresis of cerebrospinal fluid. J. Lab. Clin. Med., *74*:166, 1969.
17. Salo, E., and Honkavaara, E.: A linear single reagent method for determination of protein in cerebrospinal fluid. Scand. J. Clin. Lab. Invest., *34*:283, 1974.
18. Kawa, T.: Clinical Aspects of the Plasma Proteins. Tokyo, Igaki Skoin, 1973, p. 125.

19. Igou, P.: An evaluation of gel-filtration spectrophotometric method for spinal fluid proteins. Am. J. Med. Technol., *33*:354, 1967.
20. Wald, D.: Disc electrophoresis of cerebrospinal fluid proteins on polyacrylamide gel. Polish Med. J., *8*:2, 1969.
21. Sherwin, M., and Moore, G.: Microzone electrophoresis of unconcentrated cerebrospinal fluid using cellulose acetate strips and nigrosin dye. Am. J. Clin. Pathol., *55*:705, 1971.
22. Hordynsky, W.: Importance of prealbumin, alpha, alpha 2, and tau fraction in cerebrospinal fluid. Am. J. Clin. Pathol., *57*:251, 1972.
23. Gerson, M., and Orr, B.: Oligoclonal bands and quantitation of IgG in cerebrospinal fluid as indicators of multiple sclerosis. Am. J. Clin. Pathol., *73*:87, 1980.
24. Hershey, L., and Trotter, J.: The use and abuse of the cerebrospinal fluid: IgG profile in the adult. Ann. Neurol., *8*:426, 1980.
25. Johnson, K., Arrigo, S., Nelson, B., and Ginsberg, A.: Agarose electrophoresis of cerebrospinal fluid in multiple sclerosis. Neurology, *27*:273, 1977.
26. Schneck, S., and Claman, H.: CSF immunoglobulins in multiple sclerosis and other neurologic disorders. Arch. Neurol., *20*:132, 1969.
27. Gordon, R.: Diagnostic criteria for Guillain-Barré meningitis caused by hemophilis influenzae. J.A.M.A., *240*:1709, 1978.
28. Link, H., and Muller, R.: Immunoglobulins in multiple sclerosis and infection of the nervous system. Arch. Neurol., *25*:326, 1971.
29. Olsson, J., and Link, H.: Immunoglobulin abnormalities in multiple sclerosis. Arch. Neurol., *28*:372, 1973.
30. Ganrot, K., and Laurell, C.: Measurement of IgG and albumin content of cerebrospinal fluid, and its interpretation. Clin. Chem., *20*:571, 1974.
31. MacPherson, C., and Cosgrove, J.: An unusual IgG globulin. Arch. Neurol., *19*:503, 1968.
32. Gambino, R.: CSF immunoglobulins: Use and abuse of CSF protein studies in the diagnosis of multiple sclerosis. Lab Reports for Physicians, *3*:42, 1980.
33. Kaplinsky, N., and Frankl, O.: The significance of cerebrospinal fluid examination in the management of chlorpropamide–induced hypoglycemia. Diabetes Care, *3*:248, 1980.
34. Smith, D. (ed.): Bacterial meningitis: A symposium. Pediatrics, *52*:586, 1973.
35. Controni, G., et al.: Cerebrospinal fluid lactic acid levels in meningitis. Pediatrics, *91*:379, 1977.
36. Feldman, W.: Cerebrospinal fluid lactic acid dehydrogenase activity. Am. J. Dis. Child, *129*:77, 1975.
37. Rutledge, J., Benjamin, D., Hood, L., and Smith, A.: Is the CSF lactate measurement useful in the management of children with suspected bacterial meningitis? J. Pediatr., *98*:20, 1981.
38. Nishimura, K.: The lactic acid content of blood and seminal fluid. Proc. Soc. Exp. Biol. Med., *22*:322, 1924.
39. Nelson, P., Carey, W., and Pollard, A.: Diagnostic significance and source of lactate dehydrogenase and its isoenzymes in cerebrospinal fluid of children with a variety of neurological disorders. J. Clin. Pathol., *28*:828, 1975.
40. Greenblatt, S.: Cerebrospinal fluid creatine phosphokinase in acute subarachnoid hemorrhage. J. Neurosurg., *11*:50, 1976.
41. Morrison, J., et al.: Enzyme levels in the serum and cerebrospinal fluids in eclampsia. Am. J. Obstet. Gynecol., *110*:619, 1971.
42. Gambino, R.: Tips on Technology: Value of LDH in spinal fluid. Med. Lab. Observer., *7*:13, 1975.
43. Manual of Tests of Syphilis 1969. U.S. Public Health Service Publication no. 411. Washington, D.C., G.P.O., 1969.
44. Feldman, Y., and Nikitas, J.: Syphilis serology today. Arch. Dermatol., *116*:84, 1980.
45. John J., and Cuetter, A.: Spinal syphilis: The problem of the fluorescent treponemal antibody in the cerebrospinal fluid. South Med. J., *70*:309, 1977.
46. Gambino, R. (ed.): Syphilis serology—look for IgM. Lab Reports, *3*:12, 1981.
47. Tramont, E.: Persistence of Treponema pallidum following penicillin G therapy. J.A.M.A., *236*:2207, 1976.

48. Cohen, S., Herndon, R., and McKhann, G.: Radioimmunoassay of myelin basic protein in spinal fluid. N. Engl. J. Med., *295*:1455, 1976.
49. Thompson, E.: Laboratory diagnosis of multiple sclerosis. Immunological and biochemical aspects. Br. Med. Bull., *33*:28, 1977.
50. Pribor, H., and Publiese, P.: New laboratory procedures for multiple sclerosis. Laboratory Management: 27, 1980.
51. Whitaker, J.: Myelin encephalitogenic protein fragments in cerebrospinal fluid of persons with multiple sclerosis. Neurology, *27*:911, 1977.
52. Levy, N., Auerbach, P., and Hayes, E.: A blood test for multiple sclerosis based on the adherence of lymphocytes to measles infected cells. N. Engl. J. Med., *294*:1423, 1976.
53. Hourani, B., Hamlin, E., and Reynolds, T.: Cerebrospinal fluid glutamine as a measure of hepatic encephalopathy. Arch. Intern. Med., *127*:1033, 1971.
54. Moir, A., et al.: Cerebral metabolites in cerebrospinal fluid as a biochemical approach to the brain. Brain, *93*:357, 1970.
55. Schold, S., et al.: Cerebrospinal fluid biochemical markers of central nervous system metastasis. Ann. Neurol., *8*:597, 1980.
56. Ronquist, G., Frithz, G., Ericsson, P., and Hugosson, R.: Malignant brain tumors associated with adenylate kinase in cerebrospinal fluid. Lancet, *1*:1284, 1977.
57. Oehmichen, M., and Hüber, H.: Supplemental cytodiagnostic analyses of mononuclear cells of the CSF using cytological markers. J. Neurol., *218*:187, 1978.
58. Sornas, R.: The cytology of the normal cerebrospinal fluid. Acta Neurol. Scand., *48*:313, 1972.
59. Sheth, K.: Cerebrospinal and body fluids cell morphology. Workshop Manual. Chicago, American Society of Clinical Pathologists, 1977.
60. Krentz, M., and Dyken, P.: Cerebrospinal fluid cytomorphology. Arch. Neurol., *26*:253, 1972.
61. Chu, J., Freiling, P., and Wassilak, S.: Simple method for cytological evaluation of cerebrospinal fluid. J. Clin. Path., *30*:486, 1977.
62. Youmans, G., Patterson, P., and Sommers, H.: The Biologic and Clinical Basis of Infectious Diseases. Philadelphia, W.B. Saunders, 1975.
63. McIntosh, K.: Recent advances in viral diagnosis. Arch. Pathol. Lab. Med., *104*:3, 1980.
64. Kuberski, T.: Eosinophils in the cerebrospinal fluid. Ann. Intern. Med., *91*:70, 1979.
65. Glasser, L., Payne, C., and Corrigan, J.: The in vivo development of plasma cells: A morphologic study of human cerebrospinal fluid. Neurology, *27*:448, 1977.
66. Nosanchuk, J.: Lupus erythematosus cells in CSF. J.A.M.A., *236*:2883, 1976.
67. Simone, J.: Childhood leukemia: The changing prognosis. Hosp. Pract., *9*:59, 1974.
68. Shankar, S., Dawar, R., Roy, S., and Verma, D.: Exfoliative cytology of cerebrospinal fluid in diagnosis of neoplasm of the CNS. Indian J. Med. Res., *68*:829, 1978.
69. Glass, J., Melamed, M., Chernik, N., and Posner, J.: Malignant cells in cerebrospinal fluid (CSF): The meaning of a positive CSF cytology. Neurology, *29*:1369, 1979.
70. Balhuizen, J., Bots, G., Schaberg, A., and Bosman, F.: Value of cerebrospinal fluid cytology for the diagnosis of malignancies in the central nervous system. J. Neurosurg., *48*:747, 1978,
71. Baten, M., and Vennucci, C.: Intraspinal metastatic disease in childhood cancer. J. Pediatr., *90*:207, 1977.
72. Bartlett, R., et al.: Quality assurance of gram-stained direct smears. Am. J. Clin. Pathol., *72*:984, 1979.
73. Feldman, W.: Concentrations of bacteria in cerebrospinal fluid of patients with bacterial meningitis. J. Pediatr., *88*:549, 1976.
74. Feldman, H.: ASCP Check Sample Microbiology No. MB-89. *Neisseria Meningitidis*. Chicago, American Society of Clinical Pathologists, 1977.
75. Tuazon, C., Perez, A., Elin, R., and Sheagren, J.: Detection of endotoxin in cerebrospinal and joint fluid by limulus assay. Arch. Intern. Med., *137*:55, 1977.
76. Nachum, R., Lipsey, A., and Siegel, S.: Rapid detection of gram-negative bacterial meningitis by the limulus lysate test. N. Engl. J. Med., *289*:981, 1973.

TOTAL PROTEIN

METHOD. Modification of Mestrezat method.

PRINCIPLE. Trichloroacetic acid precipitates the protein in the spinal fluid, resulting in decreased light transmission and increased light scattering. The amount of light scattering is proportional to the original concentration in the sample, and it is measured using the 2-filter technique at 340 and 540 nm.

PROCEDURE

1. Place the sample cup on the input tray of the ACA instrument (precise filling of cup is important).
2. Place CFP pack behind the sample cup, then place the reagent pack on input tray following method.
3. Press operate mode.
4. The ACA automatically aspirates 0.3 ml of sample and injects it into the pack along with 4.7 ml of water.

INTERPRETATION. Normal cerebrospinal-fluid total protein should be 25 to 45 mg/dl. Each laboratory should establish its normal range if possible.

DISCUSSION AND CLINICAL SIGNIFICANCE. Increased protein in the cerebrospinal fluid is seen with tissue degeneration and necrosis of neural tissue and other substances. In infectious processes, such as meningitis, the elevated protein is usually a result of many factors, including leakage of serum protein, release of proteins from breakdown of leukocytes, and release of proteins from cells as byproduct of inflammation. Elevated protein, therefore, is a nonspecific finding. Nevertheless, a markedly elevated protein alerts the clinician to the need for other diagnostic procedures, such as protein electrophoretic fractionation.

The procedure is linear to 200 mg/dl. Above this value, the specimen should be diluted and the test performed again. Specimen should be diluted with purified water or 0.85% (w/v) saline.

The trichloroacetic acid (TCA) method is less sensitive to turbidity differences between albumin and globulin than is a sulfosalicylic acid method. Temperature variation can also cause differences in the results of these two techniques. The ACA technique and anion exchange column spectrophotometric procedures give a correlation coefficient of 0.964.

The technique is rapid (about 6 minutes); therefore, it can be defined as a STAT procedure. The precision of the ACA technique has been reported by the manufacturer to be:

	Day to Day CV	*Same Day CV*
Normal range	about 4.2%	about 2.8%
High range	about 2.0%	about 1.0%

MATERIALS AND METHODS

1. Dupont ACA (I, II, III)
2. CFP pack (store to 2–8° C and do not freeze or expose to temperatures above 35° C)
3. Sodium chloride, 0.85% (w/v)

REFERENCES

1. ACA brochure (Dupont de Nemours, E.I., & Co., Inc. Wilmington, Del. 19898)
2. Mestrezat, W.: Echelle diaphanometritue de nature albuminoide pour le dosage rapide et precis de l'albumine dansile liquide cethalorachieien. Compt. Rend. Soc. Biol., *84*:382, 1921.
3. Tietz, N.: Fundamentals of Clinical Chemistry. Philadelphia, W.B. Saunders, 1970, p. 206.

PROTEIN CONCENTRATION

METHOD. Minicon ultramicrofilter.

PRINCIPLE. A disposable dialysis chamber with a semipermeable membrane and a solvent in a well is used to dialyze and concentrate body-cavity fluids, including cerebrospinal fluid. Different semipermeable membranes are used depending upon the molecular weight of proteins to be dialyzed. The capacity of the absorbent is about 3 times the total sample volume, and the chamber is graduated at various levels 5× through 100×, indicating concentration ratio. It takes approximately 3 hours to concentrate a sample 100 times.

SAMPLE. Concentration requires a Minicon B-15 filter, which has a molecular weight cut-off of about 15,000.

PROCEDURE. A small aliquot sample can be tested with a couple drops of salicylic acid to determine whether protein is present. Sulfosalicylic acid will precipitate all proteins, including immunoglobulins, Bence-Jones, hemoglobin, and myoglobin. It is fruitless to try a concentration in the event that no protein is present.

1. Determine the required concentration level with protein dipstick tests (Multistix, Labstix, Chemstrips). The percentage of recoverable macrosolute decreases with the degree of concentration.
   Examples: A dipstick determination of 100 mg/dl is found as the protein content of a concentrated protein. Analysis by electrophoresis or immunoelectrophoresis requires that the macrosolute content be at least 2.5 g/L. Concentration by dialysis to 50% (v/v) assures the required degree of enrichment for analysis.
   To achieve concentrations above 100×, fill chambers 1 through 5 with 5 ml of sample and allow concentration of 25× in each chamber. This reduces the volume in each chamber to 0.2 ml. Pool the concentrated samples (1 ml) and transfer to chamber 6. Allow to concentrate an additional 10% (v/v) and withdraw. The final concentrate is 250×.
2. Insert sample to level no higher than FILL line using a Pasteur

pipette or syringe. Care should be taken to avoid scratching the membrane surface. Mark chamber numbers on sample identity record.

3. Sample volume will decrease to approximately 100×. Volume at each graduation line is shown below. For samples smaller than 5 ml, graduations are determined proportionally.
4. To recover sample, insert pipette or syringe to base of chamber and withdraw. Mixing the sample by drawing in and out of the pipette or syringe several times improves recovery.

INTERPRETATION. Protein concentrated in the chamber is spotted for electrophoretic or chromatographic techniques.

DISCUSSION AND CLINICAL SIGNIFICANCE. Retention of protein in the Minicon-B Concentrator is closely related to molecular size, shape, and especially molecular weight, which is a more convenient parameter. Proteins whose molecular weights are close to the membrane cut-off are partially retained. A typical concentration of urine with the Minicon B-15 filter is discussed in the section on protein concentration in Chapter 1. There is some nonspecific binding of solute (protein) on the membrane, and there is nonrecoverable loss through the wetting of the chamber; hence, the Minicon B-15 filter is not recommended when analytically exacting results are required. The technique is, however, suitable for qualitative or semiquantitative evaluations and for electrophoretic or chromatographic migrations.

MATERIALS AND REAGENTS

1. Minicon filter systems (Amicon Corporation, 21 Hartwell Ave., Lexington, Mass. 02173)
2. Pasteur pipettes and bulbs
3. Sulfosalicylic acid, 20% (v/v)
4. Albustix, Combistix, or Labstix (Ames Company, Div. Miles Lab., Inc., P.O. Box 70, Elkhart, Ind. 46514); Chemstrips (Bio-Dynamics, 9115 Hague Road, Indianapolis, Ind. 46250).

REFERENCE

1. Minicon brochure (Amicon Corporation, 21 Hartwell Ave., Lexington, Mass. 02173)

PROTEIN ELECTROPHORESIS

METHOD. Agarose gel electrophoresis.

PRINCIPLE. A concentrated ultrafiltrate of cerebrospinal fluid is electrophoresed for 35 minutes at 90 volts. The strip is stained and checked for a distinct band in the Gamma region of the cerebrospinal fluid that is not present in concomitant serum electrophoresis.

SAMPLE. Uncentrifuged cerebrospinal fluid.

PROCEDURE

1. CSF is concentrated 80 times (Minicon CS-15) by placing 2 ml of CSF in a concentrator until the desired concentration is reached.

2. Special barbital buffer is prepared.
3. Add 95 ml of special buffer to each side of the electrophoresis cell. Tip to obtain equal levels.
4. Apply 2 μL of concentrated CSF, 1 μL at a time, to universal electrophoresis film.
5. 1 μL of patient serum is applied adjacent to the CSF. Two controls are also placed on wells 7 and 8 of plate.
6. Process the film in the power supply for 35 minutes.
7. The film is immediately stained for 10 minutes with Amido Black 10-B stain.
8. The film is destained by immersing in acetic acid solution, 5% (v/v) for 2 minutes. The step is repeated twice or until no more patches of stain remain.
9. The gel is dried in the incubator oven for 20 to 25 minutes or until the film is no longer sticky.
10. The film is destained again in acetic acid solution, 5% (v/v) for 2 minutes. This step is repeated until the background is clear.
11. The film is then dried in the incubator oven for 5 minutes.
12. The film is scanned using the 610 nanometer filter.

INTERPRETATION. A simultaneous serum protein electrophoresis on agarose gel must be performed. This is compared to the CSF agarose electrophoretic plate and an interpretation is rendered by the pathologist. Typical interpretation would include:

Pattern	*Interpretation*
Normal CSF total protein; normal electrophoretic	Normal protein fractionation
Increased CSF total protein; normal fractionation (nontraumatic tap)	Increased blood-brain permeability or impaired CSF resorption
CSF polyclonal gammopathy; normal serum fractionation	Active inflammatory or neoplastic disease
Oligoclonal bands in CSF; normal serum study	Suggestive of multiple sclerosis

DISCUSSION AND CLINICAL SIGNIFICANCE. Fractionation of CSF protein by agarose-gel electrophoresis can provide valuable information, particularly in the diagnosis of multiple sclerosis and the differential diagnosis of increased cerebrospinal-fluid protein. Oligoclonal bands are seen as multiple, discrete lines in the gamma zone. These are thought to result from the localized synthesis of immunoglobulins of limited specificity by lymphocytes in the central nervous system. Oligoclonal bands are found in fluid of 77 to 95% of patients with multiple sclerosis. The specificity of this finding, however, has been questioned by some authors who have found a high frequency of oligoclonal bands in other neurologic diseases, particularly subacute sclerosing panencephalitis (SSPE). Nevertheless, in a large series including multiple neurologic diagnosis, Benjamin Gerson and Margo Orr demonstrated the presence of oligoclonal bands to have a sensitivity of 77% and specificity of 99% in the diagnosis of multiple sclerosis. Agarose-gel electrophoresis appears to have more sensitivity than cellulose acetate in detecting oligoclonal bands (77% compared to 51%). Comparison to the serum is imperative to rule out oligoclonal or monoclonal components crossing the blood-brain barrier.

MATERIALS AND REAGENTS

1. Corning cassette electrophoresis cell, no. 470130
2. Corning power supply, no. 470134
3. Corning incubator oven, no. 470144
4. Corning special barbital buffer
5. Corning agarose universal purpose electrophoresis film
6. Corning sta-moist filter paper, no. 470158
7. Amido Black 10-B protein stain
8. Acetic acid, 5% solution
9. Hamilton syringe with chaney adapter
10. Minicon CS-15 (Amicon Corporation, 21 Hartwell Ave., Lexington, Mass 02173)

REFERENCES

1. Corning Electrophoresis Products, 490 San Antonio Rd., Palo Alto, Ca. 94306)
2. Gerson, B., and Orr, M.: Oligoclonal bands and quantitation of IgG in CSF as indicators of multiple sclerosis. Am. J. Clin. Pathol., *73*:87, 1980.
3. Johnson, K., Arrigo, S., and Nelson, B.: Agarose electrophoresis of CSF in multiple sclerosis. Neurology, *27*:273, 1977.

IMMUNOGLOBULIN M (IgM) AND G (IgG) AND A (IgA)

METHOD. Single radial immunodiffusion (Mancini) quantitative determination, using low-concentration plates.

PRINCIPLE. Cerebrospinal fluid containing antigen, applied to a cylindric well, diffuses radially into a gel matrix containing a known concentration of IgM, IgG, or IgA antibody. The antigen-antibody reaction produces a precipitin ring whose diameter correlates directly with the amount of antigen present in the cerebrospinal fluid.

SPECIMEN. Undiluted cerebrospinal fluid.

PROCEDURE

SETTING UP THE DIFFUSION PLATES

1. Bring plates, control plasma, and patient samples to room temperature.
2. Mix elements in step 1 by inverting several times.
3. Remove plate from aluminum foil envelope and open by pressing thumbs firmly on the center of the lid while holding the lid at the periphery. Allow the plate to stand open at room temperature for

5 minutes, to allow for the evaporation of any moisture that may have condensed in the wells.

4. For the construction of the reference curve, dilute the standard human serum with normal saline to produce three solutions, according to the instructions provided in the standard human serum package insert enclosed in the kit.
5. Using a Drummond microliter syringe, deliver 20 μL of standard human serum to the first well (dilution 1).
6. Wipe excess from the outside of the Drummond syringe with a tissue to ensure accuracy. Repeat this step after filling each well.
7. To the second well, deliver 20 μL of standard human serum (dilution 2).
8. To the third well, deliver 20 μL of standard human serum (dilution 3).
9. Repeat step 6.
10. Fill the fourth well with control, diluting control to fall within any range of plates.
11. Fill wells 4 to 12 with 20 μL of patient samples.
12. Tightly close the plate by placing a lid over the plate and pressing firmly in the center.
13. State the date and time the wells are filled on the worksheet.
14. Incubate at room temperature in a moist chamber.
15. Determination may be made after a minimum diffusion time of 60 to 72 hours.

READING DIFFUSION PLATES

1. Anytime after the minimum diffusion time (60–72 hours), measure the diameter (d) of the precipitin rings to an accuracy of 0.1 mm, using the calibrated measuring ruler or a calibrated magnifier. Square the diameter readings (d^2). Construct a standard reference curve and read the immunoglobulin concentrations from this curve.
2. Construction of reference curve:
   a. Measure the diameter (d) of the precipitin rings to 0.1-mm accuracy.
   b. Calculate d^2 (mm^2).
   c. Plot the squared diameter (d^2) of the precipitin rings obtained from the standard human serum dilutions (ordinate) against their respective concentrations (abscissa) on linear graph paper. A straight line is drawn that should intercept the ordinate at 22 ± 3.5 mm. The values for the patient's samples are determined by interpolation from the reference curve.
3. If the precipitate is too faint to measure accurately, it is recommended that the gel plate be treated with tannic acid (tannin). Rinse the plate with phosphate-buffered saline for at least 1 to 3 days if the concentration of accompanying proteins is higher. The

removal of nonprecipitated proteins from the agar-gel can be speeded by repeatedly changing the rinsing liquid and constantly stirring with a magnetic stirrer. Once the rinsing procedure is finished, cover the gel surface with an aqueous solution of tannic acid for 30 minutes and then put the plate into a water-filled container for 1 hour. After this treatment, the precipitin rings can be easily measured.

4. Sample Calculation:
   d for the patient's sample = 7.9 mm
   d^2 for the patient's sample = 62.4 mm
   d^2 is plotted on the ordinate, and the unknown concentration (C) in the test sample is read from the abscissa using the reference curve.
5. The assay range of the IgG plates is indicated by the manufacturer or printed on the label. In cases in which the IgG concentrations exceed the upper limit of the assay range, the test should be repeated with appropriate dilutions of the specimen. When the IgG concentrations are below the assay range, the sample should be concentrated before assay.
6. Complete the worksheet as to the date and time the rings are measured. When reading the concentration value, be sure to multiply by the dilution factor or divide by the concentration factor if indicated.
7. Partly used IgM, IgG, or IgA plates can be used again (prior to the expiration date listed on the label if the plate has been properly closed after initial use, stored in a refrigerator at 4°C, and sealed in a polyurethane bag).
8. The standard curve is good for 2 weeks (if more than 2 weeks have elapsed since the first use, a new reference curve should be constructed).

QUALITY-CONTROL REAGENTS

1. Record results of controls each day in quality-control book.
2. If the reference curve is not linear or does not intersect the ordinate at 22 ± 3.5 mm, repeat the procedure. Errors in technique or product instability due to improper handling should be considered.
3. If control fails to react as indicated, be sure wells were not over filled or damaged while filling them.
4. If control still fails to react properly, use a new control and/or plates of a new lot number.
5. Record all testing results.

INTERPRETATION AND CLINICAL SIGNIFICANCE. Normal CSF IgA concentration is less than 1.6 mg/dl; IgG concentration is less than 5.5 mg/dl; and IgM is normally not detected.

DISCUSSION AND CLINICAL SIGNIFICANCE. IgG levels may be

elevated in multiple sclerosis. IgM levels are sometimes found in parasitic diseases. Decreased levels may be found in protein-losing enteropathics and in congenital and acquired immunoglobulin deficiencies.

Increased IgG levels may be present in collagen diseases, cerebrospinal infections, multiple myeloma, monocytic leukemia, and Hodgkin's disease. Decreased levels may be found in nephrotic syndrome and in congenital and acquired immunoglobulin deficiencies. Elevated levels of IgA are sometimes found in bacterial meningitis and some encephalopathies.

MATERIALS AND REAGENTS

1. Partigen-low concentration IgM, IgG, and IgA radial immunodiffusion plates (Calbiochem-Behring Corp., La Jolla, Ca. 92039)
2. Standard human serum
3. Control plasma (diluted within assay range)
4. Normal saline
5. Drummond μL syringe
6. Capillary tubes
7. Chamber (for incubation)
8. Worksheets
9. Measuring ruler (calibrated)
10. Light source
11. Tissue wipes
12. Sealer
13. Polyurethane bags
14. Tannic acid, 4% w/v aqueous solution
15. Phosphate buffered saline, pH 7.2
    $NaCl$, 0.85% (w/v)
    $NaHPO_4$, $2H_2O$, 0.86% (w/v)
    NaH_2PO_4, 0.25% (w/v)
16. Distilled water

REFERENCES

1. Calbiochem-Behring Corp. test brochure
2. Henry, J. (ed.): Clinical Diagnosis by Laboratory Methods. 16th Ed. Philadelphia, W.B. Saunders, 1979, p. 1214.
3. Miale, J.: Hematology. 7th Ed. St. Louis, C.V. Mosby, 1979.

GLUCOSE

METHOD. Stein method.

PRINCIPLE. Hexokinase catalyzes the phosphorylation of glucose by adenosine-5-triphosphate (ATP) to glucose-6 phosphate, which is oxidized to 6 phosphoagluconolactone by glucose-6-phosphate dehydrogenase (G-6-PD) with simultaneous reduction of nicotinamide-adenine dinucleotide. One mole of NAD is reduced for each mole of glucose present. The Absorbance of the reduced NAD can be determined using a two-filter technique at 340 to 383 nm.

PROCEDURE

1. Fill sample cup and place on ACA input tray.
2. Place glucose pack behind sample cup.
3. Activate operate mode.
4. The ACA automatically aspirates 40 μL of sample from the cup and injects it into the pack along with 4.96 μL of purified water (the sample cup must contain sufficient amount of specimen but precise filling by the technologist is not required).
5. Reagents should not be frozen but should be stored under refrigeration (2–8° C) and not exposed to temperatures above 35° C.
6. The machine automatically determines the results and records value either photographically or by impact printing.

INTERPRETATION. Normal range of cerebrospinal-fluid glucose is 60 to 90 ml/dl.

DISCUSSION AND CLINICAL SIGNIFICANCE. It has been known, almost since lumbar puncture for obtaining cerebrospinal fluid was devised by Heinrich Quincke in 1895, that glucose levels are depressed in cerebrospinal fluid if bacterial meningitis is present. The finding is nonspecific and should be considered only with other, probably more important, laboratory and clinical features of meningitis.

The hexokinase method is one of the most specific methods for measuring glucose, and the values may be 5 to 10% lower than the values obtained by chemical reducing methods. The procedure is linear to a 500 mg/dl glucose.

The precision of the technique is reported by the manufacturer to be:

	Day-to-Day CV	*Within-Day CV*
Normal range	about 1.9%	about 1.6%
High range	about 0.8%	about 0.5%

MATERIALS AND REAGENTS

1. Dupont Automatic Clinical Analyzer I, II, or III (DuPont de Nemours, E.I., & Co., Inc., Wilmington, Del 19898)

REFERENCES

1. Speicher, C., et al.: An automatic clinical analyzer: A critical evaluation. Am. J. Clin. Pathol., 57:643, 1972.
2. Stein, M., and Bergmeyer, J.: Methods of Enzymatic Analysis. New York, Academic Press, 1963, p. 117.

LACTIC ACID

METHOD. Marbach and Weil method, modified.

PRINCIPLE. Lactic acid dehydrogenase (LDH), which is made from rabbit skeletal muscle, catalyzes the oxidation of L-lactate to pyruvate with simultaneous reduction of nicotinamide-adenine dinucleotide (NAD). One mole of NAD is reduced for each molar equivalent of lactate present. The absorbance gain of the reduced NAD, which is directly proportional to the lactate concentration, is measured by a two-filter technique at 340 and 383 nm.

SPECIMEN. Uncentrifuged cerebrospinal fluid.

PROCEDURE

1. Place filled sample cup on input tray of ACA track.
2. Place LA pack behind sample cup on tray.
3. Activate operate mode.
4. The ACA automatically aspirates 40 μL of cerebrospinal fluid into the sample cup and injects it into the pack, along with 4.96 ml of tris buffer. (The sample cup must contain a sufficient quantity of specimen to accommodate a 40 μL sample size plus the 120 μL reservoir volume of cup. Precise filling of the cup by the operator is not required. (Microsample cups insert, with total 500 μL of sample with a dead volume of 10 μL, may be used.)
5. The machine automatically records the result by either photographic means or an impact printer.

INTERPRETATION. Normal lactic acid is 0.11 to 0.28 mmol/L (10 to 25 mg/dl).

DISCUSSION AND CLINICAL SIGNIFICANCE. Lactic acid has been found to be elevated in patients with bacterial meningitis, especially those who have leukocytes in their cerebrospinal fluid.

Accumulation of lactic acid causes a pH shift—because lactic acid is a strong acid (pK 3.08)—with a subsequent reduction in bicarbonate iron, leading to a metabolic acidosis (lactic acidosis). Acidosis from whatever cause can produce altered consciousness and potentially death. Although the clinical relevance of the knowledge of lactic-acid level has come under criticism lately, it can be used effectively in conjunction with other laboratory parameters and with appropriate clinical judgement to help rule in or rule out the probability of bacterial meningitis. The analytic correlation between this technique and manual enzymatic methods is good. Because measurement of lactic acid in cerebrospinal fluid should be a STAT procedure, there is no reason to hold the specimen in refrigeration. The precision of the technique according to the manufacturer is:

	Day-to-Day CV	*Within-Day CV*
Normal range	about 8.7%	about 3.6%
High range	about 3.1%	about 0.8%

MATERIALS AND REAGENTS

1. Dupont Automatic Clinical Analyzer I, II, or III (DuPont de Nemours, E.I., & Co., Inc., Wilmington, Del 19898)

REFERENCES

1. Marbach, E., and Weil, M.: Rapid enzymatic measurement of blood lactate and pyruvate. Clin. Chem., *13*:314, 1967.
2. Westgard, J., Lahmeyer, B., and Birnbaum, L.: Use of the DuPont Automatic Clinical Analyzer in direct determination of lactic acid in plasma stabilized with sodium fluoride. Clin. Chem., *18*:1334, 1972.

LACTIC DEHYDROGENASE

METHOD. Modified Wacker method.

PRINCIPLE. Lactic dehydrogenase (LDH) in the specimen catalyzes oxidation of L-lactate to pyruvate with the reduction of nicotinamide-adenine dinucleotide (NAD), the latter of which is measured at 340 nm in a spectrophotometer. The amount of NADH (reduced NAD) is proportional to the amount of LDH in the specimen.

PROCEDURE

1. Place sample cups on input tray of ACA instrument (precise filling of the cup is necessary).
2. Place LDH pack behind sample cup on tray.
3. Press operate mode on instrument.
4. The ACA automatically aspirates 0.2 ml of specimen from the sample cup and injects it into a pack with 4.8 ml tris buffer.
5. The NADH appearance is measured at 340 nm. The results are either printed or recorded photographically.
6. If the result is over the linear limit (in our laboratory 500 IU/L) the specimen should be diluted with 6% (w/v) albumin and reprocessed.

INTERPRETATION. Normal cerebrospinal fluid LDH should be less than 20 IU/L (or about 1/10 that of serum value).

DISCUSSION AND CLINICAL SIGNIFICANCE. Any pathologic process that causes destruction of cells, and especially neural tissue necrosis, will permit "leakage" of the enzymes of the cellular cytoplasm into the cerebrospinal fluid. LDH is involved in the Embden-Meyerhoff glycolytic cycle metabolism.

The finding of the elevated LDH is a sensitive index of a neurologic disorder and is probably more important than the finding of an isolated protein elevation. Nevertheless, the assay has no other specific diagnostic importance than raising a suspicion of increased tissue destruction.

Because red blood cells contain large amounts of LDH, a traumatic tap or a bloody spinal fluid renders interpretation valueless.

The precision of the ACA technique reported by the manufacturers is:

	Day-to-Day CV	*Within-Day CV*
Normal range	about 5.6%	about 4.4%
High range	about 1.3%	about 0.7%

MATERIALS AND REAGENTS

1. Dupont Automatic Clinical Analyzer I, II, and III (DuPont de Nemours, E.I., & Co., Inc., Wilmington, Del. 19898)
2. LDH packs (store at 2 to 8° C; do not expose to sunlight or temperatures above 35° C)
3. Albumin, 6% (w/v)

REFERENCES

1. Wacker, W., Ulmer, D., and Valee, B.: Metalloenzymes and myocardial infarction. New Engl. J. Med., *255*:449, 1956.
2. Westgard, J., Hunt, M., and Lahmeyer, B.: Estimates of normal range for 15 determinations on the DuPont Automatic Clinical Analyzer. Wilmington, DuPont de Nemours, E.I., & Co., Inc., 1973.

CREATINE KINASE

METHOD. Modified Oliver and Rosalki method.

PRINCIPLE. Creatine kinase (CK) catalyzes the transphosphorylation of phosphate from creatine phosphate to adenosine-diphosphate (ADP), thus producing adenosine-triphosphate (ATP). The ATP produces phosphorylation of glucose in a hexokinase shunt resulting in glucose-6-phosphate, which is then oxidized to its dehydrogenase (G-6-PDH) form, with the simultaneous reduction of nicotamide dinucleotide (NAD) to reduced nicotamide dinucleotide (NADH). NADH is measured by appearance at 340 nm in the spectrophotometer. The amount of NADH produced is proportional to the amount of CK in the specimen.

PROCEDURE

1. Place sample cup on input tray of ACA instrument (precise filling of cup is important).
2. Place CK packs behind sample tray cup on tray.
3. Press operate mode.
4. The ACA automatically aspirates 0.2 ml of sample from the specimen cup and injects it into the pack, along with 4.8 ml of water.
5. The NADH appearance is measured at 340 nm and photographically recorded or printed.

INTERPRETATION. The appearance of creatine kinase in the spinal fluid is indicative of neural damage.

DISCUSSION AND CLINICAL SIGNIFICANCE. Creatine kinase will be elevated in the cerebrospinal fluid in any condition involving cellular destruction of neural tissue. This is a nonspecific finding. Because the cerebellum contains more creatine kinase than other tissue, small infarcts of cerebellum can create large elevations in levels of creatine kinase. Furthermore, CK can be electrophoretically separated into its isozymes, the CPK I-BB fraction being found in brain. In nearly all patients with strokes, however, it is the CPK III isozyme fraction that is found to be elevated.

The linear limit of this technique is 800 IU/L. Specimens with higher results should be diluted and reprocessed. The precision of the ACA technique has been reported by the manufacturer to be:

	Day-to-Day CV	*Within-Day CV*
Normal range	about 3.2%	about 2.4%
High range	about 4.4%	about 1.8%

MATERIALS AND REAGENTS

1. Dupont Automatic Chemical Analyzer (I, II, and III)
2. CK packs (store at 2 to 8° C; do not expose to sunlight or temperatures above 35° C)

REFERENCES

1. ACA brochure (DuPont de Nemours, E.I., & Co., Inc., Wilmington, Del. 19898)
2. Oliver, I.: A spectrophotometric method for the determination of creatine phosphokinase and myokinase. Biochem. J., *61*:116, 1955.
3. Rosalki, S.: An improved procedure for creatine phosphokinase determination. J. Lab. Clin. Med., *69*:696, 1967.

SEROLOGIC TEST FOR SYPHILIS

METHOD. VDRL slide flocculation test and titers.

PRINCIPLE. Nontreponemal tests for syphilis, such as the VDRL, utilize cardiolipin-lecithin antigen to detect an antibody (reagin) in the cerebrospinal fluid. The antigen-antibody reaction produces a visible flocculation.

SPECIMEN. Clear cerebrospinal fluid is necessary. If fluid is visibly contaminated by blood, it is unsatisfactory for testing. Refrigerate specimen at 4° C ± 2° if there is over a 24-hour delay in testing. The specimen should be brought to room temperature (23°–29°C) before testing.

PROCEDURE

QUALITATIVE

1. Pipette 0.05 ml spinal fluid into one well of an agglutination slide. Place numbered patient samples in corresponding wells of slide.
2. Include prepared reactive, weakly reactive, and nonreactive controls with each batch of tests (all at room temperature).
3. Add one drop (ca. 0.01 ml) of prepared antigen suspension into each well of spinal fluid and control using a 21- or a 22-gauge needle, while holding the syringe perpendicular to the slide.
4. Rotate 8 minutes on mechanical rotator at 180 rpm.
5. After rotating is completed, immediately read for agglutination microscopically, using a 10× objective.
6. Read controls first.

7. If expected results are not obtained, see "Quality Control for Reagents," which is discussed later in this section.

INTERPRETATION

Reading	*Results*
No clumping or slight degree of "roughness"	Nonreactive (N)
Small clumps	Weakly reactive (WR)
Medium and large clumps	Reactive (R)

QUANTITATIVE

1. Retest quantitatively to an endpoint titer all spinal fluids that produce reactive and weakly reactive results in the qualitative procedure.
2. The dilutions of spinal fluids to be tested are: Undiluted 1:1, 1:2, 1:4, 1:8, 1:16, etc.
3. Dilute spinal fluid using normal saline.
4. Pipette 0.5 ml normal saline into four test tubes.
5. Pipette 0.5 ml patient's spinal fluid to tube no. 1. Mix and transfer 0.5 ml to tube no. 2. Continue to tube no. 4 but do not discard.
6. Pipette 0.05 ml of each patient's spinal-fluid dilution to the appropriate well on the slide.
7. Include a weakly-reactive control with each patient to be quantitated. This control is used as a comparison for reporting results.
8. Add one drop (0.01 ml) of antigen suspension to each spinal-fluid dilution and control, using a 21- or a 22-gauge needle and holding the syringe perpendicular to the slide.
9. Rotate slide 8 minutes on mechanical rotator at 180 rpm.
10. Immediately read for agglutination microscopically, using a 10× objective.
11. The endpoint titer is the greatest dilution giving reactive results (not weakly reactive)—that is, reactive 1:2; weakly reactive 1:4; and reported titer 2 dils
12. If still reactive at 1:16, continue diluting until endpoint is reached.
13. If less than 0.5 ml of spinal fluid is received, dilute using smaller amounts of normal saline and spinal fluid.

DISCUSSION AND CLINICAL SIGNIFICANCE. The VDRL procedure performed on cerebrospinal fluid is used to make the diagnosis of neurosyphilis. Degeneration of the spinal cord and nerve trunks and vascular occlusion and infarction lead to paralysis and other nervous-system damage. However, in about a quarter of untreated cases, the tertiary stage is asymptomatic and recognizable only by serologic tests. In almost all cases of neurosyphilis, the serum FTA-Abs-IgG will be reactive, while FTA-Abs-IgM will revert to normal after therapy.

MATERIALS AND REAGENTS

1. Rotating machine—adjustable to 180 rpm, circumscribing a circle $^{3}/_{4}$-inch in diameter, centrifuge and microscope

2. Concave agglutination slides
3. Syringe, 2 ml luer-lock type
4. 21- or 22-gauge hyperdermic needle, without a bevel
5. 0.1 ml, 0.2 ml serologic pipettes or an automatic pipette system
6. VDRL antigen (Sylvana, distributed by Scientific Products, 155 Brookhollow Esplanade, New Orleans, La. 70183)
7. VDRL buffered saline
8. Normal saline
9. Sodium chloride, 10% (w/v)
10. Controls—reactive, weakly reactive, nonreactive

PREPARATION OF CONTROLS

1. Prepare reactive, weakly reactive, and nonreactive controls using a serum of positive reactivity ($\leq$ 1:80).
2. Dilute this serum in normal saline, yielding reactive, weakly reactive and nonreactive results.
3. Freeze controls in small aliquots.

PREPARATION OF 10% (W/V) SALINE

1. Weigh out 10 g NaCl (found in the chemistry lab) and dissolve in 100 ml of distilled water.

PREPARATION OF ANTIGEN

1. Pipette 0.4 ml buffered saline into bottom of a round bottle.
2. Add 0.5 m VDRL antigen (from lower half of a 1.0 ml serologic pipette graduated to the tip) onto saline in a dropwise fashion while gently rotating the bottle on a flat surface.
3. Blow last drop of antigen from pipette.
4. Continue rotating bottle for 10 seconds.
5. Add 4.1 ml buffered saline from a 5 ml pipette.
6. Cover bottle with parafilm and shake vigorously for 10 seconds.
7. Add one part 10% (w/v) saline to one part VDRL slide test antigen suspension (1 ml of each is recommended).
8. Mix gently.
9. Allow to stand 5 minutes.
10. Antigen is good for 2 hours.

QUALITY CONTROL FOR EQUIPMENT

TESTING ACCURACY OF DELIVERY NEEDLES

1. Aspirate 1.0 ml antigen suspension into syringe.
2. Holding syringe perpendicular to bottle, dispense antigen through 21- or 22-gauge needle (without bevel).
3. 100 drops $\pm$ 2 should be obtained from 1.0 ml.
4. If needle fails to deliver proper number of drops, repeat procedure.
5. If still inadequate, discard needle and obtain new one.
6. Repeat procedure using new needle.
7. Record all results in quality control book.

TESTING ROTATIONS OF MECHANICAL ROTATOR

1. Hold a pen vertically and close enough for rotator to strike pen during each rotation.

2. Count rotations (each strike against pen) during 1.0 minute using a stopwatch.
3. 180 rpm (± 2 rpm) should be obtained.
4. If rpms are incorrect, repeat the procedure.
5. If still incorrect, adjust rotator and repeat testing.
6. Record all results in quality control book.

QUALITY CONTROL FOR REAGENTS

1. Record results of controls each day in quality control book.
2. If controls fail to react properly, repeat the procedure using fresh antigen suspension.
3. If controls still fail to react properly, repeat procedure using a new set of controls.
4. Record all testing results.

REFERENCES

1. Bryant, N.: Laboratory Immunology and Serology. Philadelphia, W.B. Saunders, 1978.
2. Henry, J. (ed.): Clinical Diagnosis by Laboratory Methods. 16th Ed. Philadelphia, W.B. Saunders, 1979, p. 654.
3. Manual of Tests of Syphilis 1969. U.S. Public Health Service Publication No. 411. Washington, D.C., G.P.O., 1969.

GLUTAMINE

METHOD. Glasgow and Dhiensiri modification of Whitehead and Whittaker procedure.

PRINCIPLE. Glutaminase is used to deaminate glutamine by hydrolyzation, and the liberated ammonia is then reacted with phenol-hypochlorite and measured at 640 nm.

SPECIMEN. Uncentrifuged cerebrospinal fluid.

PROCEDURE

1. Pipette 0.2 ml glutaminase to test tube.
2. Add 200 μL cerebrospinal fluid.
3. Incubate for 30 minutes at 37° C.
4. Add 1.0 ml phenol reagent to tube and mix thoroughly.
5. Immediately add 1.0 ml alkaline hypochlorite and mix thoroughly.
6. Incubate 30 minutes at 37° C.
7. Read absorbance at 640 nm.
8. Set up standard, and set up reagent blank (using 20 μL water instead of specimen).

INTERPRETATION. Normal cerebrospinal fluid glutamine is 5.8 to 14.1 mg/dl (averaging 8.2 mg/dl).

DISCUSSION AND CLINICAL SIGNIFICANCE. The concentration of glutamine is increased in the spinal fluid of patients with comas of hepatic origin. Most cases of Reye's syndrome have increased cerebrospinal-fluid glutamine (20 of 27 in Glasgow's experience), although there is no correlation between the glutamine levels and the ultimate clinical outcomes of these patients. There is, however, a better correlation of cerebrospinal-fluid glutamine than of blood ammonia with the progress of the disease in patients with hepatic coma. Although the reaction is linear, multiple standards provide greater analytic performance. Recovery experiments averaged 99.8%.

Asparagine is deaminated by glutaminase much more slowly than glutamine, thus the resultant value may be raised by an average of 0.6 mg/dl.

A quantitative procedure measuring the amount of ammonia is also in vogue. A fluorometric analysis based on Whitehead and Whittaker's procedure is also available.

MATERIALS AND METHODS

1. Spectrophotometer, 640 nm
2. Test tubes, 10 × 100 ml
3. Cuvettes
4. Micropipettes, 20 μL
5. Pipettes, 1 ml
6. Incubator, 37° C
7. L-glutamine standards (N.R.C., A grade; Calbiochem-Behring Corp., 10933 North Terry Pines Road, La Jolla, Ca. 92037)
   Dilute to concentrations of 10 mg/dl, 50 mg/dl, 100 mg/dl with water.
8. Phenol reagent

Phenol	50 g
Sodium nitroprusside	0.25 g
H_2O q.s.	to 1000 ml

9. Alkaline hypochlorite reagent (Sigma Chem. Co., P.O. Box 14508, St. Louis, Mo. 63178)

NaOH	25 g
Sodium hypochlorite	2.1 g
H_2O q.s.	to 1000 ml

REFERENCES

1. Glasgow, A.: Clinical application of blood ammonia determinations. Lab. Med., *12*:151, 1981.
2. Glasgow, A., and Dhiensiri, K.: Improved assay for spinal fluid glutamine, and values for children with Reye's syndrome. Clin. Chem., *20*:642, 1974.
3. Stahl, A., Frich, A., Imler, M., and Schlienger, J.: Enzymatic micro-assay for blood glutamine. Clin. Chem., *24*:1739, 1978.

LEUKOCYTE COUNT

METHOD. Hemocytometer method.

SPECIMEN. Undiluted uncentrifuged cerebrospinal fluid (tube no. 2).

PRINCIPLE. The cerebrospinal fluid is pipetted undiluted in a white-blood-cell diluting pipette, and then the fluid is placed on a hemocytometer and the cells are counted. In the event that the fluid is cloudy (with red blood cells creating the cloudiness) a dilution can be made with isoton to count the red blood cells also. If the red blood cells have to be lysed, a 1 to 20 dilution can be made in the white-blood-cell pipette using an acid solution that will destroy the red cells.

PROCEDURE

1. Draw cerebrospinal fluid into the white-blood-cell pipette, using flexible rubber tubing (be careful not to aspirate fluid into the mouth).
2. Discard 1 to 2 drops from pipette.
3. Fill counting chamber and allow cells to settle for several minutes.
4. Place under the microscope and, using the low-power (10×) objective, count the nucleated cells in each of the four large outer corners (4 mm^2).
5. Record the total number of cells counted in the 4 mm^2 area.
6. If over 5 cells are counted, a morphologic differential should be done.

INTERPRETATION. Up to five mononuclear cells (lymphocytes) are considered normal.

DISCUSSION AND CLINICAL SIGNIFICANCE. Almost any increase in cells in the cerebrospinal fluid is considered abnormal. Morphologic identification, therefore, becomes an important parameter for alerting the clinician about the type of cellular response. Comment should also be made about any red blood cells that are present—that is, crenation, intactness, etc. In addition, it is important to know whether the white blood cells are intact or ruptured.

MATERIALS AND REAGENTS

1. White-blood-cell diluting pipette
2. Flexible rubber tubing for white-blood-cell pipette
3. Hemocytometer with improved Neubauer ruling and coverslip
4. Microscope
5. Acetic acid, 2% (w/v)
6. Isoton

REFERENCES

1. Page, L., and Culver, P.: Ham's Syllabus of Laboratory Examinations in Clinical Practice. Cambridge, Harvard University Press, 1961, p. 27.
2. Smith, B.B.: Clinical communication, 1981.

ACID-FAST STAIN

METHOD. Kinyoun method (cold).

PRINCIPLE. The acid-fast stain depends upon the chemical composition of the bacterial cell wall. The mycobacteria are lipophilic and difficult to stain, but once stained, they are resistant to destaining. They are stained with the basic dye, carbolfuchsin (containing phenol, which aids the penetration of the dye through the mycobacterial lipid), decolorized with acid alcohol, and counterstained with methylene blue.

PROCEDURE

1. Make a thin smear from sputum, dry, and fix in flame. Do not overheat.
2. Apply as much carbon-fuchsin as will stay on the slide and stain for 3 to 5 minutes.
3. Wash with water and decolorize with acid alcohol until all the pink color has disappeared from the thinner portions of the smear (at least 5 minutes).
4. Wash and counterstain with methylene blue solution for 3 minutes.
5. Examine microscopically.

INTERPRETATION. Acid-fast organisms retain the red dye. The other organisms and background are blue.

DISCUSSION AND CLINICAL SIGNIFICANCE. The most important mycobacteria are the following:

1. Mycobacteria tuberculosis (human pulmonary tuberculosis organisms), which has a beaded appearance
2. Mycobacterium bovis (bovine visceral and bone tuberculosis)
3. Mycobacterium avis (avian lymph node tuberculosis)
4. Mycobacterium fortuitum (human glandular tuberculosis)
5. Mycobacterium leprae (Hansen's bacillus), which is acid fast, but only slightly so; therefore, little acid-alcohol decolorization should be used when this organism is suspected.

Whenever acid-fast organisms are seen on a smear, suspect tuberculosis and obtain a proper culture. Final diagnosis is based on cultural evidence, except when dealing with leprosy, which is based on a clinical picture and demonstration of organisms by staining smear or histologic section (a smear should be examined thoroughly before calling it negative). However, no case of central-nervous-system leprosy has ever been demonstrated at the National Leprosorium U.S. Public Health Service Hospital, Carville, La. 70721.

MATERIALS AND REAGENTS

1. Kinyoun Carbol-Fuchsin stain

Basic Fuschin stain	4 mg
Phenol	8 mg
95% (v/v) ethyl alcohol	20 ml
Distilled water	100 ml

2. Acid alcohol

Concentrated HCl	3 ml
95% (v/v) ethyl alcohol	q.s. to 100 ml

3. Loeffler's methylene blue

Methylene blue	3 g

95% (v/v) ethyl alcohol, then add	30 ml
0.1% (w/v) aqueous KOH	100 ml

4. Microscope slides, 1″ × 3 ″
5. Coverslips
6. Microscope
7. Inoculating loop

REFERENCE

1. Jolik, W., and Willet, H.: Zinnser Microbiology. 16th Ed. New York, Appleton-Century-Crofts, 1976, p. 25.

INDIA-INK STAIN

METHOD. India-ink method.

PRINCIPLE. India ink is composed of carbon particles in suspension. The organism Cryptococcus will produce a capsule that will displace the particles and leave a clear halo around the single budding yeast.

PROCEDURE

1. Place a drop of India ink on the slide.
2. Flame loop, get a loopful of cerebrospinal fluid, and place in the India ink.
3. Coverslip, let it stand for a while to settle down, then read.

INTERPRETATION. Small, single budding yeast in a large capsule that resembles a halo effect. The halo will be clear, and the background will be black (see Fig. 8–11B).

MATERIALS AND REAGENTS

1. Microscope slides, 1″ × 3″
2. Pelikan India Ink, no. 17 in dropper bottle (Marion Scientific Co., 9233 Ward Parkway, Kansas City, Mo. 64114)
3. Microscope coverslips
4. Inoculating loop
5. Bacti-incinerator

REFERENCE

1. Larone, D.: Medically Important Fungi: A Guide to Identification. Hagerstown, Harper & Row, 1976, p. 117.

GRAM STAIN

METHOD. Burke's modification of Gram's method.

PRINCIPLE. A heat-fixed smear is treated with the basic crystal violet dye, which the organisms absorb. Gram-positive bacteria apparently contain an acidic substance, magnesium ribonucleate, which forms, with the crystal violet and iodine, an insoluble complex that cannot be removed with alcohol-acetine. Gram-negative bacteria apparently lack this substance and the iodine–dye complex; therefore, the bacteria used must be counterstained with safranin to be visualized.

SPECIMEN. Undiluted cerebrospinal fluid.

PROCEDURE

1. Smear a small sample of cerebrospinal fluid on a glass slide and air dry.
2. Cover with crystal violet for 1 minute.
3. Wash with free-flowing water.
4. Cover with Gram's iodine solution for 1 minute.
5. Wash slide with 95% (v/v) alcohol, rocking back and forth and continuing while you can see crystal violet being extracted into the alcohol from the material on the slide. This should take about 30 seconds.
6. Wash with free-flowing water.
7. Counterstain with safranin for 15 to 20 seconds.
8. Dry slide and examine it under microscope for bacteria and cells.

INTERPRETATION. Gram-positive organisms stain blue and gram-negative organisms red. Definitive identification of type requires culture and/or chemical study.

DISCUSSION AND CLINICAL SIGNIFICANCE. The following are important organisms:

1. Gram-positive cocci:
   a. Streptococcus pneumoniae, lancet shaped, encapsulated diplococcus
   b. Streptococcus pyogenes (beta strep), spherical, in chains/pairs
   c. Streptococcus fecalis (enterococcus), round, in chains/pairs
   d. Staphylococcus aureus (pyogenes), round, grapelike clusters.
2. Gram-negative cocci:
   a. Neisseria meningitidis (meningococcus), bean-shaped with adjacent sides flattened, intracellular in polys.
3. Gram-positive bacilli:
   a. Corynebacterium diphtheriae, slightly curved rods, beaded, lying side by side to form "Chinese letter" patterns
   b. Corynebacterium pseudodiphtheriticum and others (diphtheroids), irregular staining, club-shaped, resemble C. diphtheriae.
   c. Listeria monocytogenes, short rods, tend to form "picket-fence pattern"
   d. Clostridium species (tetani, welchi, botulinum, etc.), variable short rods, frequently somewhat curved, with terminal spores (tetani) and subterminal spores (other species)
4. Gram-negative bacilli:
   a. Escherichia coli
   b. Aerobacter aerogenes
   c. Klebsiella pneumoniae (Friedlander's bacillus)
   d. Salmonella typhi
   e. Pseudonomonas aeruginosa

f. Salmonella species
g. Shigella species (dysenteriae, sonnei, flexneri, and others)
h. Haemophilus influenzae and hemophilus species

The mechanism of the Gram stain is related not only to the chemistry but also to the thickness of the cell wall, pore size, and permeability properties of the intact cell envelope. Gram-positive bacteria stain gram-negative if they lose osmotic integrity by rupture of the plasma membrane. Autolyzed, old, or dead Gram-positive cells and isolated cell envelopes stain Gram-negative. A unique bacterial cell-wall chemical composition does not appear to explain the stain, since thick-walled yeast cells, which also stain Gram-positive, have a chemical composition and structure different from Gram-positive bacteria.

MATERIALS AND REAGENTS

1. Solution A contains 4 g of crystal violet and 20 ml of 95% (v/v) ethyl alcohol
   Solution B contains 0.8 g of ammonium oxalate $(NH_4)_2C_2O_4{\bullet}H_2O)$ and 80 ml of distilled water
   Mix equal parts solution A and solution B for use.
2. Gram's iodine is composed of 2 g of KI, 1 g of iodine, and distilled water, q.s. to 100 ml
3. Microscope slides, 1″ × 3″
4. Coverslips
5. Microscope
6. Inoculating loop

REFERENCE

1. Jolik, W., and Willte, H.: Zinnser Microbiology. 16th Ed. New York, Appleton-Century Crofts, 1976, p. 25.

CYTOLOGIC STAIN FOR MALIGNANT CELLS

METHOD. Papanicolaou stain, sedimentation and cytocentrifuge methods.

PRINCIPLE. Cells in cerebrospinal fluid are isolated by centrifugation, dried on a microscope slide, mixed with carbowax, stained with PAP stain, and identified microscopically.

SAMPLE

SEDIMENTATION PREPARATION

1. Make a circle on the opposite end of a frosted microscope slide using a heavy waxed pencil.
2. With a disposable pipette, fill the center of the circle with cerebrospinal fluid (ca. 1 to 2 drops).
3. Place slide in a covered petri dish for 1 hour, permitting cells to sediment.
4. After 1 hour, siphon the excess fluid by touching filter paper to the edge of the specimen near the wax circle.

5. Drop 1 to 2 drops of carbowax into the specimen and permit to dry.

CYTOCENTRIFUGE PREPARATION

1. Centrifuge specimen at 1,500 rpms for 10 minutes.
2. Using a disposable pipette, lift out the sediment before discarding the supernatant.
3. Drop $^1/_4$ to $^1/_2$ ml spinal fluid into the well of the cytocentrifuge and spin for 3 minutes at 2,000 rpms.
4. Immediately remove the slide and fix it with hairspray or carbowax spray.
5. The slide is now ready to be stained by the PAP method (this method is most useful for cerebrospinal fluid with scant numbers of cells).

PROCEDURE. Immerse slides in successive fluids (in Coplin jars or staining racks) as follows:

1. Fixative:

a. Distilled water	10 minutes
b. Hematoxylin	2 minutes
c. Distilled water, wash until clean	4–5 washings
d. 50% (v/v) alcohol	10 dips
e. 70% (v/v) alcohol	10 dips
f. 80% (v/v) alcohol	10 dips
g. 95% (v/v) alcohol	10 dips

2. Staining:

a. Distilled water	6 minutes
b. Filtered hematoxylin	1 $^1/_2$ minutes
c. Distilled water (when finished staining, discard water)	washing
d. Acid alcohol	5–6 dips
e. 50% (w/v) alcohol	5–6 dips
f. 70% (w/v) Ammonium Hydroxide	5–6 dips
g. 80% (v/v) and 95% (v/v) alcohol	5–6 dips
h. OG-6	1 minute
i. 95% (v/v) alcohol	5–6 dips
j. EA-50	2 minutes
k. 95% (v/v) alcohol	5–6 dips
l. Wash 3 times in absolute ethyl alcohol	5–6 dips

3. Clearing:

   a. Wash in absolute alcohol until clean.

b. Clear in 1/2 absolute alcohol and 1/2 xylene for 10 dips.
c. Place in xylene for 30 minutes and repeat for three changes.

4. Mounting:
   a. Coverslip with permount.
   b. Observe under microscope.

INTERPRETATION. Cells will be stained as they are stained with vaginal cytology:

Stain	*Cell Substance*
Orange G (OG-6)	Keratin stains orange Cytoplasm stains blue to yellow
Eosin (EA-50, 65)	Cytoplasm and nucleoli stains red Metabolically active substance stains green

DISCUSSION AND CLINICAL SIGNIFICANCE. Identification of cell types and pathologic changes should be made by trained cytologists and pathologists. A positive finding (malignant cells) is extremely important in diagnosis and decision-making. A more complete discussion of the methodology can be found in Chapter 7, "Seminal-Fluid Analysis."

MATERIALS AND METHODS

1. Pap stain EA-50 (Harleco Co., Gibbstown, N.J. 08027)
2. Harris or Meyers hematoxylin (Harleco Co., Gibbstown, N.J. 08027)
3. OG-6
4. Carbowax 1540 (Applied Scientific Laboratories, Inc., P.O. Box 440, State College, Pa. 16801). Melt to liquidity then make 2% (w/v) in 50% (v/v) ethyl alcohol.
5. Absolute ethyl alcohol
6. Xylene
7. Microscope slides, 1″ × 3 ″
8. Coverslips
9. Permount
10. Microscope
11. Disposable pipettes, 9 in. in length
12. Cytospin 2 (Shandon Southern Instruments, Inc., 575 Broad St., Sewickley, Pa. 15143)

REFERENCES

1. Prince, C.L.: Personal communication, 1979.
2. Scimetries, Inc., 8321 Dunlap Drive, Houston, Tex. 77074.
3. Wied, G., Koss, L., and Reagar, R. (eds.): Compendium on Diagnostic Cytology. 4th Ed. Chicago, International Academy of Cytology, 1976.

BACTERIOLOGIC CULTURE

METHOD. Culture plating/inoculation.

PRINCIPLE. With a loop, cerebrospinal fluid is inoculated into test tubes and onto culture plates containing appropriate bacteriologic media. These test tubes and culture plates are then incubated at 37° C to be visually observed for bacterial colony growth.

SPECIMEN. Uncentrifuged cerebrospinal fluid in sterile test tubes (tube no. 2) from the lumbar spinal puncture collection procedure. Specimen should be plated immediately and bacteriologic culture should be considered a STAT procedure.

PROCEDURE

1. The cerebrospinal fluid is taken by the physician or his designee to the laboratory in numbered, well identified, sterile, closed tubes. The tubes must be accompanied by requisition slips with proper identification.
2. Centrifuge cerebrospinal fluid in clinical centrifuge at 2500 RPM.
3. Remove the supernatant and send to the other parts of the laboratory for chemical testing. Resuspend the sediment by shaking.
4. Inoculate the following blood plates:
   a. Blood agar plate—inoculate for Pneumococcus, N. meningitidis, group B streptococci, E. coli, and cryptococcus
   b. Chocolate agar plate—inoculate for Haemophilus species and N. meningitidis
   c. Brain heart infusion containing PABA and 0.1% (w/v) agar—inoculate for anaerobic organisms

   These combinations permit identification of most pathogenic and nonpathogenic organisms.
5. Gram stain, India-ink prep, and potassium hydroxide preps are routinely set up on specimens. If the Gram stain is positive, the results should be telephoned to the physician immediately.
6. The inoculated plates are incubated for 24 hours in high CO_2 atmospheric 37° C.
7. Plates are removed from incubation after appropriate time and "read out" for organisms.
8. All negative plates should be held for 48 hours before final decision and report.
9. Cerebrospinal fluid for fungal cultures should be set up on Sabouraud's dextrose agar and microbiotic agar.
10. The plates are held for 30 days at room temperature.
11. Cerebrospinal-fluid plates requiring mycobacterial culture are sent to the Louisiana State Board of Health.

INTERPRETATION. The following organisms are most frequently encountered in pathologic cerebrospinal fluid:

1. Haemophilus influenza, type B
2. Neisseria meningitides
3. Streptococcus pneumoniae
4. Cryptococcus neoformans
5. Listeria monocytogenes
6. Staphylococci, streptococci

DISCUSSION AND CLINICAL SIGNIFICANCE. See text on bacterial meningitis.

MATERIALS AND REAGENTS

1. Blood agar plate
2. Chocolate agar plate
3. Brain-heart-infusion broth containing PABA and 0.1% (w/v) agar
4. CO_2 incubator at 37° C
5. Inoculating loop
6. Clinical centrifuge

REFERENCES

1. Finegold, S., Martin, W., and Scott, E.: Bailey and Scott's Diagnostic Microbiology. 5th Ed. St. Louis, C.V. Mosby, 1978, p. 91.
2. Marionneaux, M.: Personal communication, 1981.

LIMULUS TEST

METHOD. Limulus gelation test of Levin.

PRINCIPLE. Endotoxin produced by Gram-negative bacilli will gel a lysate of blood cells (amebocytes) of the horseshoe crab (Limulus). The increase in turbidity, viscosity, or gelation can be visually observed and is indicative of the presence of the bacterial endotoxin.

SAMPLE. Uncentrifuged cerebrospinal fluid.

PROCEDURE

1. Set up pyrogen-free test tubes labeled "cerebrospinal fluid," "negative control," and "positive control." The positive control should be a known endotoxin; the negative can be pyrogen-free saline.
2. Using sterile technique, pipette 0.05 ml of cerebrospinal fluid into a test tube; the same amount of saline into the second tube; and a like amount of endotoxin into the third test tube.
3. Using the same sterile technique, add 0.05 ml of lysate to each tube. Mix thoroughly.
4. Incubate at 37° C in water bath.
5. Observe after 1 hour and again in 4 hours for gelation, increased viscosity, or turbidity.
6. Remove test tubes from water bath and let stand at room temperature until the next morning or for 24 hours.
7. Observe visually (tilt test tube gently to avoid breaking gel, because it is fragile).

INTERPRETATION. The test is considered positive if a solid gel forms or if there is definite increase in viscosity or turbidity; microflocculation is considered negative. Any turbidity or viscosity greater than the negative control indicates the presence of low levels of endotoxin. A negative Limulus test indicates that either Gram-negative or-

TABLE 8–4. Summary of Typical Findings in Pathologic Cerebrospinal Fluid.

	Appearance	Cells	Glucose	Protein	LDH	CPK	Lactic Acid	Other
Normal	Clear, colorless, no clot	0–5 lymphocytes/μL	60–90 mg/dl	20–45 mg/dl	20 IU/L	0	10–25 mg/dl	
Bacterial meningitis: Meningococcal	Milky opalescent to yellow-green, thick clot	1000–2000 95% polymorphonuclear leukocytes (early)	Decrease	Increase	Increase	Normal	Increase	Gram-negative diplococci on smear
Pneumonococcal	Turbid yellow clots	Early slight increase Late 100–5000 95% polymorphonuclear leukocytes (later)	Decrease	Increase	Increase	Normal	Increase	Gram-positive cocci on smear usually easy to find
Haemophilus	Slightly cloudy/turbid clots	200–3000 60–70% polymorphonuclear leukocytes	Decrease	Increase	Increase	Normal	Increase	H. influenzae hard to find on Gram stain
Other Pyogenic	Turbid, thick clot	100–6000 95% polymorphonuclear leukocytes	Decrease	Increase	Increase	Normal	Increase	Streptococcus, staphylococcus, typhoid, E. coli, etc., on Gram stain
Tuberculous meningitis	Clear, opalescent, or white; fibrin web	Early 10–100 Late 100–100 70–90% lymphocytes (Adults, less)	Decrease	Slight increase	Normal	Normal	Normal	Increased fluid; AFB in web
Viral meningitis: Lymphocytic choriomeningitis	Clear/opaque	Early 10–100 Late 100–500 (lymphocytes)	Normal	Slight increase	Slight increase	Slight increase	Normal	No organisms found with Gram stain
Poliomyelitis	Clear-to-milky; occasional fibrin clot	15–2000 (polymorphonuclear leukocytes) preparalytic; 10–100 (lymphocytes) paralytic	Normal	Slight increase	Normal	Increase	Normal	Less than 10 after third week

Epidermic encephalitis	Normal fibrin clot	10–200 (lymphocytes) 30% less than 10 cells	Normal	Slight increase	Normal	Increase	Normal	Slight increase in fluid
Neurosyphilis: Acute meningitis	Clear-to-turbid	10–500 90% monocytes/ lymphocytes	Normal	Slight increase	Normal	Normal	Normal	CSF STS negative
Chronic meningitis	Clear fibrin clot	10–60 monocytes	Normal	Slight increase	Normal	Normal/increase	Normal	10–15% positive CSF STS
Tabes dorsalis	Normal	10–75 monocytes	Normal	Normal/slight increase	Normal	Normal	Normal	60–70% positive CSF STS
Paresis	Normal small clot	20–400 monocytes	Normal	Normal	Normal	Normal	Normal	100% positive CSF STS
Brain abscess	Normal or slightly turbid	Rupt. 10–100 7–75% polymorphonuclear leukocytes; Unruptured 5–30 90–95% (monocytes)	Normal	Normal/increase	Normal/increase	Normal/increase	Normal/increase	Organisms usually found on Gram stain
Brain tumor	Normal or slight xanthochromia	Normal 10–80	Normal	Increase	Increase	Normal/increase	Normal/increase	20% of cases normal
Subarachnoid hemorrhage	Bloody or xanthochromia	Increase due to blood	Normal	Increase	Increase	Normal/increase	Normal	Changes due to blood
Spinal-cord compression	Clear or slight xanthochromia	Normal increase monocytes	Normal	Normal	Normal/increase	Normal	Normal/increase	Fluid decrease in block
Multiple sclerosis	Normal	Normal/slight increase monocytes	Normal	Normal	Normal	Normal	Normal	Usually normal oligoclonal IgG

ganisms are not present or that these organisms have not produced enough endotoxin to reach detectable levels.

DISCUSSION AND CLINICAL SIGNIFICANCE. The limulus test is a qualitative measure of a biologic activity of endotoxin. It does not accurately measure concentrations of endotoxin in the specimen. Serial dilutions, however, can be used as semiquantitative measures of rising and falling levels of endotoxin. In this instance, a series of decreasing concentrations of endotoxin could be tested and the end points compared with the tests of the cerebrospinal fluid. The detection of endotoxin indicates the presence of a component from Gram-negative bacteria in the sample, but a positive limulus test does not necessarily indicate that viable Gram-negative bacteria are also present in the body fluid tested.

Clinical manifestations of Gram-negative sepsis (especially those produced by E. coli, proteus species, klebsiella species, and pseudomonas species) appear to be predominantly the result of endotoxins produced. Because hypotension and death occur twice as frequently in patients with detectable endotoxemia as in patients without, detection of endotoxin becomes valuable information for aggressive clinic therapy and prognostication of mortality. Jack Levin and associates found endotoxemia in 14% of patients with Gram-negative sepsis; 7% also had endotoxemia and bacteremia. The mortality rates were 70% in patients who had a positive limulus test and a bacteriologic blood culture for Gram-negative organisms, while the rate was 58% in patients with a positive limulus test alone. Septic patients, for whom both tests were negative, had a 15% mortality.

Endotoxins have been reported to exert an effect on the blood-coagulation system (including the Hageman factor), the complement system, the fibrinolysin system, and the kallikrein-kinin system.

The rate and the extent of the reaction with amebocyte lysate are dependent upon the concentration of the endotoxin in the sample. With low endotoxin levels, it may take a longer time for the assay to become positive; consequently, one should retain the sample until the next morning for visual observation.

Although manufacturers of lysates indicate that sensitivity to endotoxin and control curves are helpful, it is important to note that chemically pure endotoxin is not available; therefore, apparent concentrations of endotoxins are arbitrary. The commercially prepared lysate is stable for about 10 months if stored at 4° C in sterile, pyrogen-free glass containers. The method described above can detect as little as 0.0005 μg endotoxin/ml blood. However, inhibitors must be removed from samples of plasma before attempting to detect endotoxin in the blood. The limulus test can be used to detect endotoxin in cerebrospinal fluid, other body fluid, parenteral fluids, and drugs.

Nephelometric or spectrophotometric methods can be used to derive a value to compare with the control values, but at the present time, this level of analytic excellence has no additional clinical relevance.

MATERIALS AND REAGENTS

1. Waterbath at 37° C
2. Pipettes, 0.1 ml, sterile pyrogen-free
3. Test tubes, 2 ml, sterile, and pyrogen-free. If glass test tubes are used, this can be achieved by subjecting them to dry heat at 180° C for at least 2 hours; plastic test tubes, which are suitable for tissue culture, are usually endotoxin-free and sterile.
4. Limulus amebocyte lysate (Associates of Cape Cod, 10 Rose Morrin Drive, Falmouth, Mass. 02540; M.A. Bioproducts, Biggs Ford Road, Building 100, Walkersville, Md. 21793; and Mallinckrodt Chemical Co., P.O. Box 5840, St. Louis, Mo. 63134)
5. Endotoxin standard of E. coli extraction. (Difco Laboratories, P.O. Box 1058A, Detroit, Mich. 48232)

REFERENCES

1. Levin, J.: The Limulus test: A status report. *In* Biomedical Applications of the Horseshoe Crab (Limulidae). Edited by E. Cohen, B. Bang, and J. Levin. New York, Alan R. Liss, 1979, p. 235.
2. Levin, J., et al.: Gram-negative sepsis: Detection of endotoxemia with the limulus test. Ann. Intern. Med., *76*:1, 1972.
3. Levin, J., Tomasulo, P., and Oser, R.: Detection of endotoxin in human blood and demonstration of an inhibitor. J. Lab. Clin. Med., *75*:903, 1970.
4. Levin, J., and Bang, F.: Clottable protein in Limulus: Its localization and kinetics of its coagulation by endotoxin. Thromb. Diath. Haemorrh., *19*:186, 1968.

Chapter

9 The Microscope and Microscopy

JAMES A. FREEMAN

The microscope is, perhaps, the single most important instrument associated with development of a scientific approach to medicine. Simple magnifying lenses, of course, had been known to the Romans in the 1st century A.D., but they were used for reading and starting fires. For many years, the Dutch "spectakelmaker" father-and-son team Hans and Zacharias Janssen were credited with devising the first workable microscope in 1590.[1] However, recent evidence tends to date the invention before the time of the Janssens. The maker of this earliest instrument is still unknown, but a microscope is known to have been found about 1590 in Middelburg, Holland. An unknown Italian engraved the words Anno 1590 on a crude telescope (microscope?) thought to have been exported from Italy to Holland (possibly the microscope just referred to). This fact, coupled with recent recovery of Leonardo da Vinci's drawings of a functional two-lens telescope, leads one to surmise that the unknown Italian may have learned the principles of the instrument from da Vinci's invention.[2] If we take into consideration that in the 16th century the laws of refraction had not yet been formulated and that the theory of lens structure and function was unknown, this would certainly be additional evidence of the phenomenal genius of da Vinci. Even Galileo Galilei, who is given credit for being the first to construct a telescope (in 1609), admitted, correctly, that a

This chapter was revised, adapted, and reproduced with permission from Freeman, J.: The Microscope. *In* Clinical Diagnosis by Laboratory Methods. 14th Ed. Edited by I. Davidsohn and J. Henry. Philadelphia, W.B. Saunders, 1969. Figures 9–1 through 9–13 of this chapter were reproduced from Davidsohn and Henry.

Hollander (or someone prior to him) deserved the title of inventor of the instrument.

The word "microscope" (from the Greek *mikros*, small, and *skopein*, to see) was introduced by Giovanni Farber in a letter dated April 13, 1625, to the Academy of Lincei. Serious use of the early crude instruments was slow to develop. Insects were, at first, the most "incredible" wonder studied by the "flea glass," a designation used by some wags of the day. Acuity of scientific observation with the microscope was given important documentation in 1665, when Robert Hooke published Micrographia in which he introduced the term "cell" (Fig. 9–1A). This book was the first printed observation of microscopic plant and animal life. Peering through the wrong end of the telescope devised by Galileo, an "eccentric" of the day, Marcello Malpighi, achieved the effect of a microscope with some 30-fold magnifying power. In a series of more than 200 rather unusual "letters" laced with crotchety commentary about his neighbors' health and wealth that were sent to the Royal Society of London (1673 to 1723), a dry goods clerk of Delft, Anton van Leeuwenhoek, reported observing of "animalcules"—protozoa and microorganisms—observed with a compound microscope of his own de-

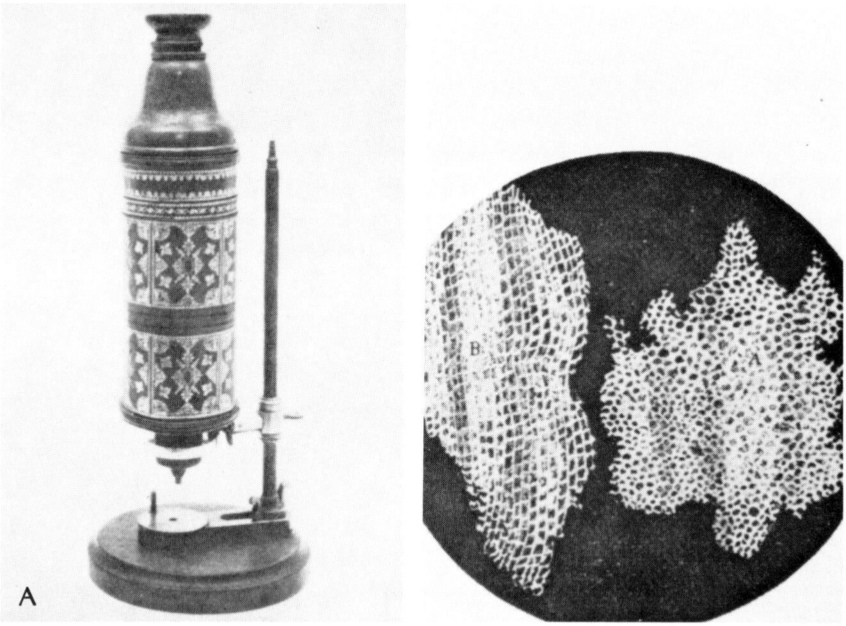

Fig. 9–1A. *Left,* Microscope of the type designed and used by Robert Hooke in preparing his epochal work, Micrographia, in 1665. (Courtesy of The Billings Microscope Collection of the Medical Museum of the Armed Forces Institute of Pathology. Washington, D.C., The American Registry of Pathology, p. 2 [AFIP #49004-66-1836-1], 1967.) *Right,* Drawings from Hooke's work.

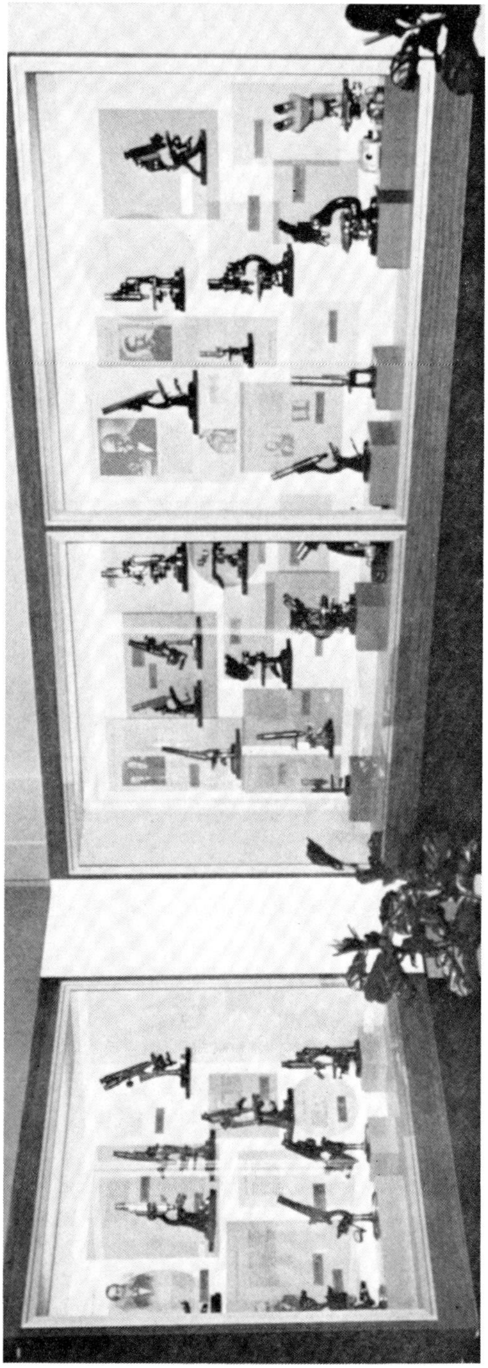

Fig. 9–1B. A portion of the Billings collection of microscopes of the Armed Forces Institute of Pathology, Washington, D.C., which at present contains an excess of 556 microscopes with the recent acquisition of the Koss collection. A facsimile of the microscope designed and used by Robert Hooke (but constructed by Christopher Cock of London) can be viewed in the collection. (Courtesy of Medical Museum Branch, Armed Forces Institute of Pathology, 1972, personal communication.)

sign notable for the short focal length of its lenses. Leeuwenhoek's studies generated a totally new concept of the structure of living matter (although it remained for the Germans Matthias Schleiden and Theodor Schwann, about 1839, to apply Hooke's cell theory to all animals and plants). By the early 19th century, the microscope was in common use among scientists—both in the life sciences and in the physical sciences (Fig. 9–1). Today we realize that the instrument is not only important to pathologic study, but that it actually makes possible the very existence of this field as we know it.

STRUCTURE OF THE MICROSCOPE[3]

Basically the microscope serves its purpose by increasing the visual angle either by means of lenses, to enable the eye to form a sharp image on the retina when the eye is too close to an object to visualize it clearly (usually less than 250 mm); or by means of visible projection to produce an enlarged image independent of the eye. In the first manner, the image is formed in the eye by light waves emanating directly from the instrument (optical microscope); and in the second, by light waves focused on a screen or other surface onto which the image is projected (movie projector) (Fig. 9–2).

A modern microscope consists of an illuminator system, a substage condenser system, an objective system, a projector (eyepiece or ocular) system, an iris diaphragm, Nicol prisms, a tubular barrel (monocular or binocular bodies), and a mechanical stage.

In the compound microscope, a combination of lenses—the objective lens system (lens closer to the object) and the ocular lens system (lens closer to the eye)—are used to form the image on the retina. The objective lens acts much like a small projection lens, but instead of projecting an image onto a screen, it projects an enlarged image, appearing to the observer to be formed below the lens barrel, into the air (aerial image). The final image formed on the retina appearing to be below the plane of the subject is called a virtual image. Light rays do not actually come from this image, they merely appear to be doing so as a result of magnification of the image (Fig. 9–3).

MAGNIFICATION

There is no theoretical actual limit to the magnification that can be produced by a microscope (disregarding limitations imposed by the light energy source), but there is a limit to useful magnification that can be achieved.[4] Useful magnification, in essence, depends upon resolving power, or the ability of the microscope to render fine details of an object visible, which is in turn dependent upon the numeric aperture of the lens systems. If the resolving power is limited, increased magnification renders the image indistinct or fuzzy, so that fine detail

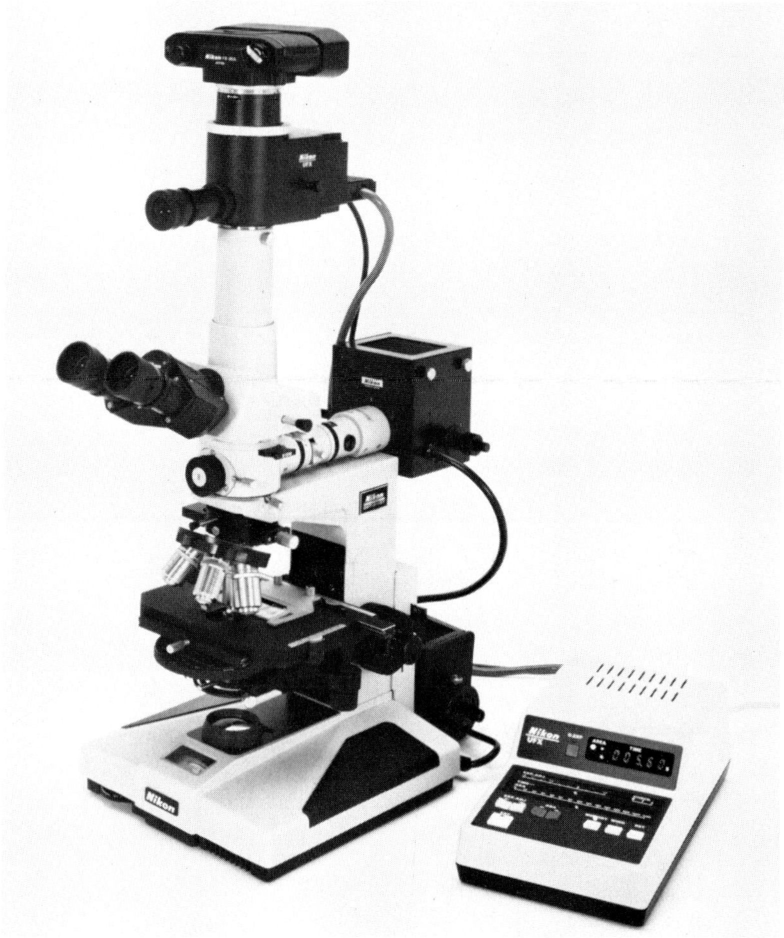

Fig. 9–2. Modern Microscopic (Nikon Optiphot with Normonski phase), reflected fluorescence and photographic attachments, used by one of the authors. (Courtesy of Nikon, Inc., Garden City, N.Y. 11530, through Mr. Steve Edgett, Advanced Scientific Inc., Chalmette, La. 70043.)

cannot be visualized. Such a useless increase in magnification is called empty magnification.[4]

The degree of magnification should be described by diameters not by the expression times (×), the latter being a misleading term. Diameter, as the word implies, refers to an increase in diameter; times refers to an increase in area. The comparatively low magnification of 100 diameters is the same as the apparently enormous magnification of 10,000×.

In this country, objectives are designated by their focal length, which

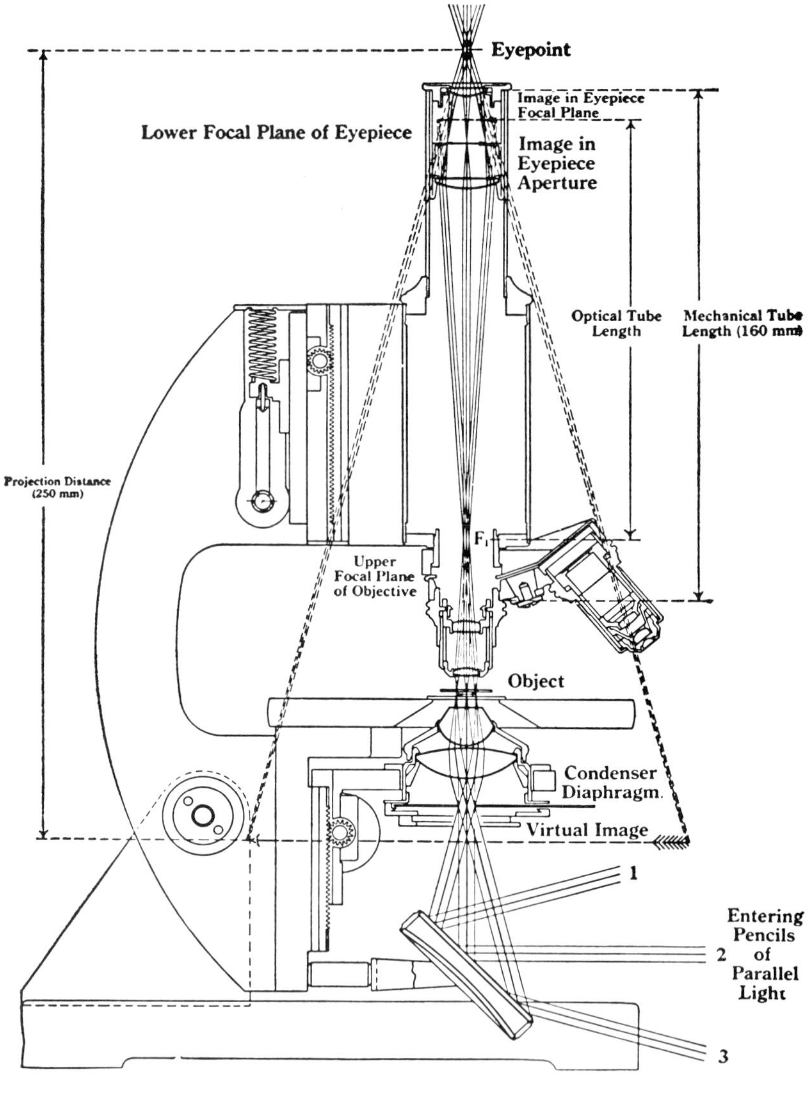

Fig. 9–3. Path of light through the microscope with projection of the virtual image.

is expressed in millimeters, or by their initial magnification. Oculars are designated by their magnifying power, indicated by an "×."

According to the rating system of magnification used in this country, the magnifying power of an objective is determined by dividing the optical tube length by the focal length of the objective lens. The optical tube length is usually somewhere near 165 mm in binocular microscopes, but it varies and the manufacturer's catalog should be consulted. Some manufacturers engrave both the focal length of the objective and the initial magnification on the barrel of the objective lens. This rating system of magnification measures the enlarged image at the level of the ocular. Therefore, when an objective and an ocular are used together, the total magnification is the product of the two. For example, with a 1.0 mm oil immersion objective with an initial magnification of 95 diameters (or about 1.7 mm), the total magnification with a 5× ocular is 5 × 95 or 475 diameters. Some microscopes offer ranges of magnification attainable in a continuous manner, rather than at discrete intervals as may be obtained by changing objectives or oculars. Such a system is called a zoom lens system. This closes the gaps in the magnification range, making possible any magnification desired for optimum viewing of a specimen. Zoom lens systems do not form an intermediate real image, but simply move the image plane outward. The image is held in constant focus during zoom by accurately cut cams, which control lens motions.

With most microscopes, magnification can be increased in one of two ways—by using a higher power objective lens or a higher power ocular lens. As a rule, changing the objective lens is the best way, because resolving power is thus also increased. It is also the easiest way, because a turret containing several objective lenses can be placed at the lower margin of the microscope barrel, thus permitting rapid interchange of different magnifications with ease. But this has the disadvantage of reducing the size of the field to be viewed as the magnification is increased. Changing the ocular lenses, although simple, has limited usefulness, because resolving power is not also increased, leading to empty magnification. The extent to which magnification can be satisfactorily increased by oculars depends wholly on the resolving power of the objective, and consequently on the numeric aperture. The greatest magnification that will give crisp images can be estimated by multiplying the numeric aperture of an objective by 400. However, the greatest magnification that can be used with light microscopy is about 1,000 times the numeric aperture. For example, if the usual 1.9 mm objective lens has a numeric aperture of 1.30, the greatest useful magnification would be about 520 diameters, which is obtained by using a 5× ocular. Higher power oculars (up to 12.5×) can be used to produce a total magnification of 1,300 diameters, beyond which the image bcomes wholly unsatisfactory.

RESOLVING POWER AND NUMERIC APERTURE[4,5]

The resolving power of a microscope depends generally on the design of the objective. The objective that picks up the larger cone of light coming from the specimen will have the better resolving power. The size of the cone of light transmitted through the lens is dependent upon the numeric aperture of the lens, which designates the amount of light entering the objective from a point in the microscope field. In reality, however, the image of a point object is not a point at all but, because of diffraction phenomena, is a small circular spot of light surrounded by concentric discs of light, a phenomenon investigated by Sir George Airy in 1834, and now known as the Airy disc or Airy phenomenon (Fig. 9–4).

The numeric aperture can be calculated from the radius of the first diffraction ring as follows:

$$NA = \frac{0.61}{h'} \lambda$$

where h′ is the separation of the first diffraction ring and the point (the fineness of detail), λ is the wavelength of light (about 0.005 mm or 0.00002″), and NA is the numeric aperture of the objective. Numeric aperture also can be calculated by the formula:

$$NA = N \sin U$$

where N is the refractive index of the object, and U is the angle formed by the central point of the lens and the cone of light emitted through the objective lens (Fig. 9–4). The higher the NA, the more complex and more expensive the lens system. The angle U cannot be increased entirely to the maximum theoretical 90 degrees with an NA equal to 1.00, but only to the practical limit.

Resolving power actually depends upon two variables—the numeric aperture and the wavelength of light, but the latter can be ignored in practice when speaking of light microscopy, since it is changed only by using other wavelengths of electromagnetic radiation, as the ultraviolet or infrared ranges. The condenser lens also has a numeric aperture, and in microscopic design the numeric aperture of the objective can be reduced nearly to that of the condenser. The condenser lens numeric aperture is indicated by lowercase letters "na." The condenser should have a numeric aperture almost equal to that of the objective with which it is to be used. Lowering the condenser lens below its focal distance and closing the diaphragm beneath it have the effect of reducing its working aperture. A condenser, whatever its numeric aperture, cannot deliver through the air a cone of light greater than a numeric aperture of 1.00.[5] From these considerations, it follows that the proper adjustment of the substage condenser is a matter of great importance when using objectives of high numeric aperture. To gain the full benefit of the resolving power of such objectives, the condenser must be focused on the object under examination and it must be oiled to the undersurface of the slide in the same way that the immersion objective lens is oiled to the glass slide (Fig. 9–5). Also, the substage iris diaphragm must be open to an optimal degree. A wide open substage

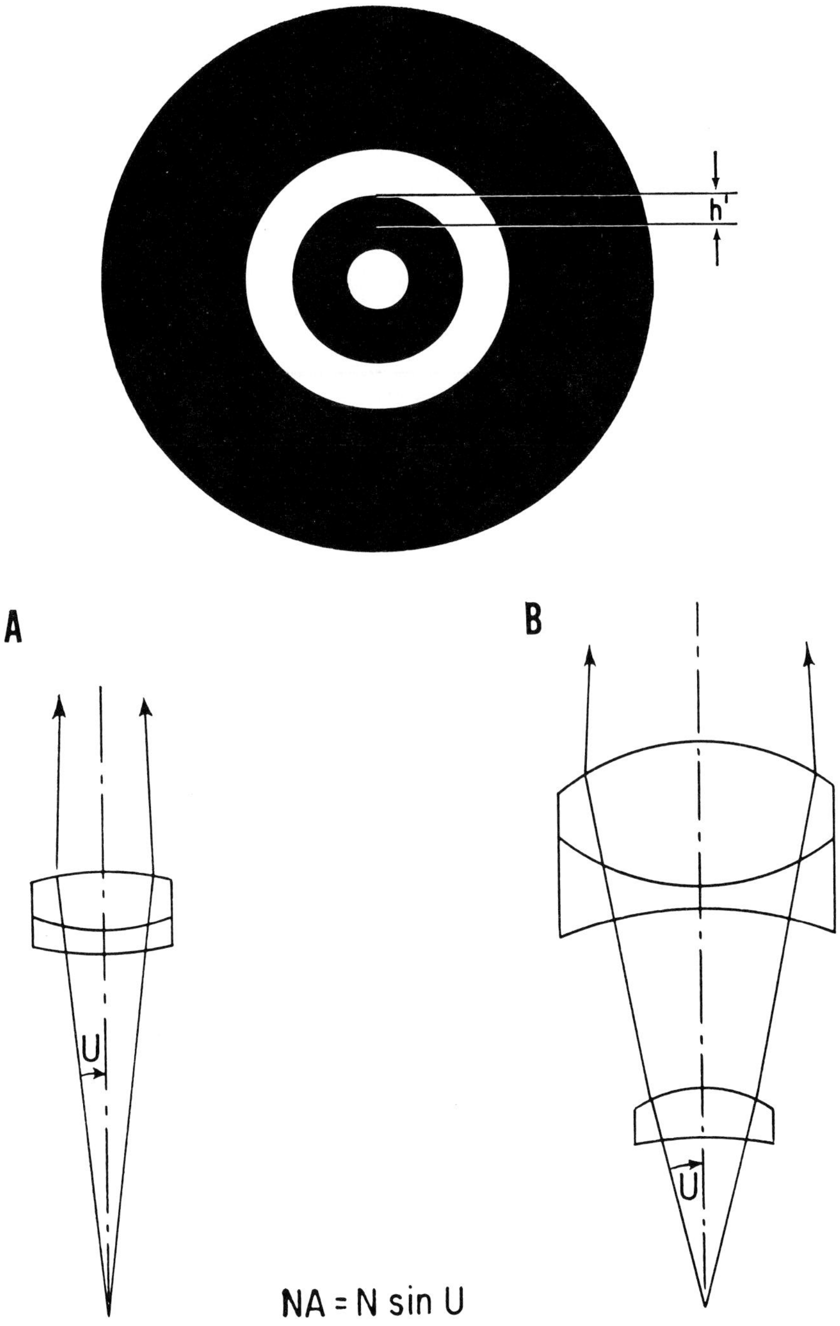

Fig. 9–4. *Above,* Airy phenomenon. Objective lens NA can be calculated by knowing the radius of the first dark ring, h', of the disc. *Below,* Objective lens NA can also be calculated by knowing the angle, U, of the cone of light transmitted through the lens. Lens B, transmitting a larger cone of light than lens A, has a greater NA.

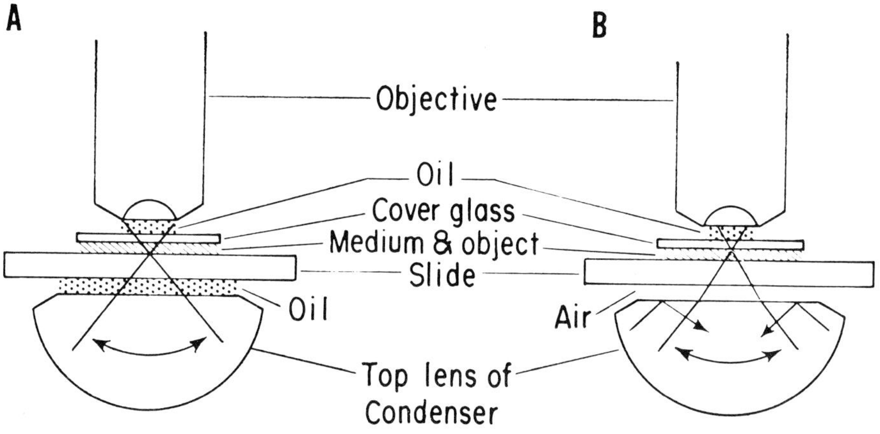

Fig. 9–5. Illuminating cone of light through slide B is smaller than illuminating cone of light through slide A, since the undersurface of slide B is not in oil contact with the condenser lens.

diaphragm will produce an unsatisfactory image fogged by a glare of light. The size of the light source should be so regulated by a diaphragm that its image, thrown on the slide by the condenser, coincides with the real field of the objective. In this manner, it is possible to reduce the glare light and dispel the fog without closing the diaphragm. In practice, this can be achieved by removing the ocular from the barrel and peering down the open barrel end, thus viewing the iris diaphragm, which is opened or closed until the image of the diaphragm is the same size as the diameter of the barrel. The relation of the illuminated central portion to the unilluminated peripheral portion (black zone) indicates roughly the proportion of the numeric aperture in use. The effect of raising and lowering the condenser and of oiling it to the slide can thus be easily seen.

DEPTH OF FOCUS[4,5]

Depth of focus, the capacity of the objective lens to render details in different planes clearly at the same time, is largely a function of numeric aperture. When one focuses a microscope on an object, there is a range above and below the object in which other portions of the same object will also appear in sharp focus. The depth of focus varies markedly with objective numeric apertures, in accordance with the following formula:

$$d = \lambda \sqrt{\frac{N^2 - (NA)^2}{(NA)^2}}$$

where d is the depth of focus for photomicrography, N is the refractive index of the object, NA is the numeric aperture, and λ is the wavelength of the illuminating light. For visual use, one must add further depth, since the eye is capable of a certain amount of accommodation. In this case, the depth becomes:

$$d' = d + \frac{250}{M^2}$$

where d′ is the depth of field, M is the magnification of the microscope in diameters, and d is the depth of focus for photomicrography. (An assumption is made that the eye can accommodate on an image 250 mm from the retina.) The higher the numeric aperture and the greater the magnification, the less the depth of focus. Any two objectives of the same focal length and the same numeric aperture will have the same depth of focus. Depth of focus can be increased somewhat by closing the iris diaphragm of the eye, thus reducing the numeric aperture. Great depth of focus is desirable for certain work done with low-power objectives. When high-power objectives are used, closing the diaphragm does not offer significant advantage to balance the loss of numeric aperture. In some cases, the procedure is disadvantageous.

In general, the depths of focus for the three most common objectives are:

		Depth of Focus	
Objective	*Ocular*	*Photomicro.*	*Visual*
10×, 0.25 NA	10×	0.0080 mm	0.0335 mm
40×, 0.65 NA	10×	0.0010 mm	0.0026 mm
100×, 1.25 NA	10×	0.0003 mm	0.00005 mm

The visual depth of focus of an oil immersion objective is very close to the wavelength of light, indicating how closely and carefully one must focus when using such magnification.

OBJECTIVE AND OCULAR LENSES

Objective lenses, in widest use today, are achromatic, and they fulfill all requirements for ordinary work. Apochromatic objectives are more highly corrected for chromatic and spheric aberrations (see image aberrations) and are the finest microscope lenses produced. They give crisp images with little or no trace of color fringes, and are used in the infinity-corrected lenses, which give a flat field. A compensating *ocular* lens must be used with an apochromatic objective. A third type of objective, which is made of fluorite, requires no special ocular and offers color correction midway between achromatic and apochromatic objectives. This fluorite objective is sometimes designated "semi-apochromat."

Huygenian oculars have long been used with achromatic objectives. They are named after the 17th-century Dutch scientist Christian Huygens. Huygenian oculars work well with low-power achromats, but introduce lateral color (see image aberrations) when used with high-power apochromats. As mentioned, compensating oculars must be used with apochromatic objectives. These are huygenian oculars corrected to overcome certain defects in lateral color. These oculars utilize two separate lens systems to achieve this color correction. The same compensating oculars may be used with oil immersion and high power dry objectives of the achromatic series. The widefield (Greenough type) oculars were first designed for stereomicroscopes, but have subsequently been converted to conventional use. Many persons who wear glasses while using a microscope find that there is a great advantage in using the 10× widefield ocular with binocular microscopes. The widefield oculars are gradually supplanting huygenian oculars because of the larger field and the greater eye comfort. The lateral-color correction of the widefield oculars is close to that of huygenian oculars, and they work well with the flat-field objectives now in general use (Fig. 9–6). Hyperplane oculars have a correction intermediate between that of huygenian and compensating oculars.

For critical work, especially with apochromatic objectives, even the thickness of the coverglass is important, although this seems not to be well understood by clinical laboratory workers (Fig. 9–7). High power (dry) objectives always require a coverglass, but the exact thickness is

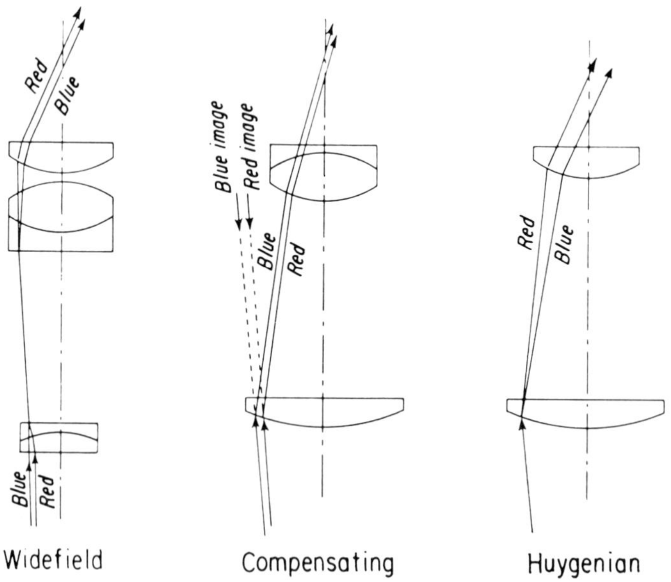

Fig. 9–6. Basic optics of widefield, compensating, and huygenian ocular lenses.

A

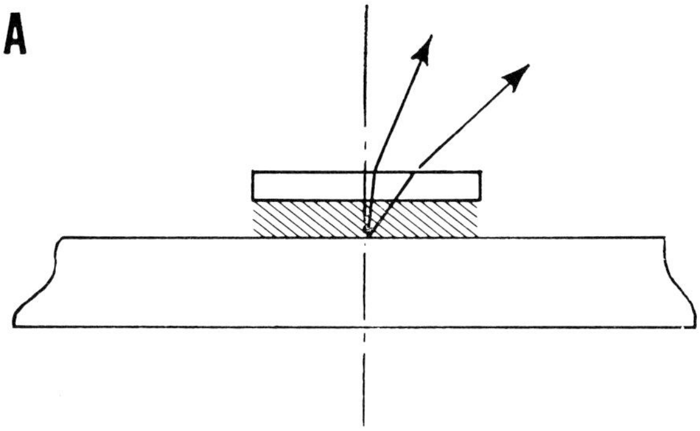

B

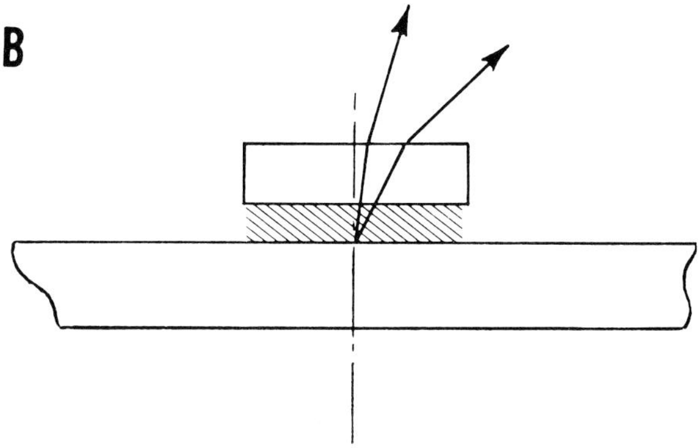

Fig. 9–7. The apparent position of an object on a slide depends on image transmission through the coverglass, which, in turn, is a function of coverglass thickness.

not critical in routine work. Low-power objectives and oil-immersion objectives may be used without coverglasses. Correction for the medium between the objective and the coverglass is also important for critical work. This medium may be air or fluid, and the objective is either a dry or an immersion objective. The immersion fluid generally used is specially prepared cedar oil that has a great optical advantage in that its index of refraction is the same as that of the crown glass. There are other objectives that require use of water for immersion. It is obvious that only objectives with very short working distances, about 2 mm or less, can be used with immersion fluid. Proper use of an oil-immersion objective, in sequence, involves finding a suitable field for study with the low-power objective, placing a drop of immersion oil on the slide, revolving the turret until the oil-immersion lens is in place, and lowering the oil-immersion objective until it almost touches the slide and is in contact with the oil. This can be observed from the side with the eyes at the level of the mechanical stage. It is also good practice to place a drop of oil between the slide and the condenser lens when fine detail is needed. In order to avoid formation of air bubbles, oil should be placed on the slide without introducing much turbulence. Bubbles are a frequent source of trouble and should always be avoided. If bubbles are introduced, the oil should be removed and a new drop applied. Immediately after use, both the objective and the slide should be wiped clean of oil with specially prepared lens paper or soft, lint-free cloth.

SUBSTAGE CONDENSER LENSES

For work in the clinical laboratory, a substage condenser is a necessity. The condenser functions to direct the beam of light of desired numeric aperture and field size onto the specimen. There are several types of condensers. Most common are the Abbé, the variable focus, and the achromatic (Fig. 9–8). The Abbé condenser is a 1.30 na condenser utilizing only two lenses and is the simplest of the three. Because of its simplicity and its good light-gathering property, it has come into wide use. It does not, however, provide correction for spheric or chromatic aberration. The variable focus condenser is a two-lens condenser with a 1.30 na maximum in which the upper lens element is fixed and the lower one focusable. By this means, it is possible to fill the field of the lower power objective without the necessity of removing the top element when the lower lens is raised. This condenser is very similar to the Abbé condenser. The achromatic condenser is 1.40 na condenser, which is corrected for both chromatic and spheric aberrations, and is the one utilized most frequently in research microscopy and color photomicrography.

In order to obtain numeric apertures over 0.95 in the condenser sys-

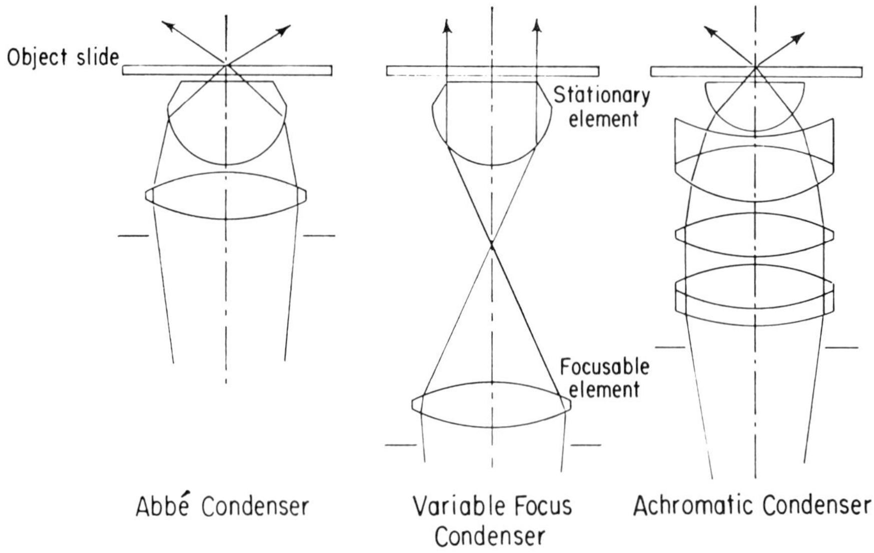

Fig. 9–8. Basic optics of commonly used condenser lens systems.

tem for critical work, it is necessary to bring the condenser and the specimen slide into contact with an oil drop as previously mentioned.

For critical work, the light must be focused on the object by raising or lowering the condenser by means of a screw or knob. The condenser is constructed to receive parallel rays of light. When daylight or artificial light not emitted directly into the condenser from a base illumination system is used, a concave mirror must be employed to convert the convergent rays of light into parallel paths before reflecting them into the condenser. It is very important that the condenser be centered accurately in the optical axis of the instrument, and most instruments have centering screws or adjustment knobs for this purpose. The easiest way to determine if the condenser is centered is to close the iris diaphragm as completely as possible, remove the ocular, and peer down the microscope barrel. If the diaphragm opening does not appear in the center of the field, the condenser is off center.

MICROSCOPE AND IMAGE ABERRATIONS[4]

Since the perfect lens system has yet to be designed, all lenses have some defects depending upon manufacture and instrument design. Because a lens system is composed of spherical surfaces and spherical surfaces cannot form a perfect image, by judicious combinations of lens shapes and sizes, the manufacturer is generally able to counteract the defects of one surface by introducing equal and opposite defects on other surfaces. It is not possible, however, to achieve absolute perfection, and certain defects (aberrations) are inherent in the image.

Spheric aberration is the defect the microscopist should understand and know best how to control. It is manifest as a loss of contrast, imparting a hazy appearance to the image. It expresses the fact that the outer portion of the spheric surface has more power than the central portion. Therefore, the central portion may appear to be in focus while the outer appears hazy. This is, in effect, an extension of the Airy phenomenon. This undesirable diffusion will cause loss in contrast as well. In newer microscopes, the infinity-corrected lenses give a flat-field appearance and are thus compensated for most spheric aberration. Presence of such an aberration and a washed out image of low contrast in these microscopes usually indicates use of wrong coverglass thickness. This is particularly true of high power dry objectives, which are normally designed for coverglasses 0.18 mm in thickness.

Curvature of field is frequently present when spheric aberration is maximum; it is one of the most difficult aberrations with which to contend. Bausch and Lomb's introduction of flat-field objectives to replace the conventional achromatic objectives eliminated much of the difficulty with curvature of field. In essence, with maximum curvature of field, lines will appear narrow and sharply focused in the center of the image, but will appear broad and out of focus at the periphery. In

in the center of the field will appear to sway from side to side when the fine adjustment is turned back and forth. This is frequently a problem with beginners who use oblique illumination without recognizing it.

The amount of light admitted by the illumination system is important and can be regulated by the iris diaphragm, or in the newer microscopes, by a diaphragm within the illuminator itself. As mentioned previously, to obtain the most effective illumination, the condenser system must be capable of delivering as large an angular cone of light as the objective is capable of utilizing. However, in routine use, full numeric aperture illumination is not used because contrast drops as the illuminated numeric aperture of the condenser system approaches the full objective numeric aperture. With regard to illumination, each specimen is unique and requires use of the proper illuminating numeric aperture. With high-contrast specimens having fine detail, one would use nearly full numeric aperture illumination. The converse is true of low-contrast specimens, in order to prevent washing out of the image by low illumination. The old adage, "use the least amount of light that will show the object well" is not good enough for routine work, much less for critical work. It may be necessary to change the illumination many times during the microscopic examination to bring out the best color, outline, contour, or form of the object being studied. For best color renditions, central illumination with strong light is necessary. A stained glass window, for example, shows truest color when the light is streaming directly through it. To study the outline of an object, however, subdued central illumination is best. The diaphragm should be closed to the point that trial and error shows to be best in each case. This type of illumination is required for examination of colorless objects, such as casts in urine sediments, trichomonads in vaginal aspirates, and cholesterol crystals in tissue. Strong light will often render these semitransparent structures entirely invisible.

There are two general forms of illumination utilized in microscopy today—critical, or Nelson illumination, and Koehler illumination (Fig. 9–9). Critical illumination is that form in which the light source is imaged directly on the specimen. It is generally used in photomicrography and microprojection in which an intense beam of light, from a mercury lamp or carbon arc, is necessary. It is impractical to image a filament on the plane of the specimen, however. Although critical illumination has been claimed to permit higher resolving power than other forms of illumination, it gradually has been replaced by another intense form of illumination—Koehler illumination. This form of illumination requires a field diaphragm control. Uneven distribution of energy in the source does not result in uneven brightness in the field of view since the source is imaged in the aperture of the system. These practical advantages have led to the replacement of critical illumination

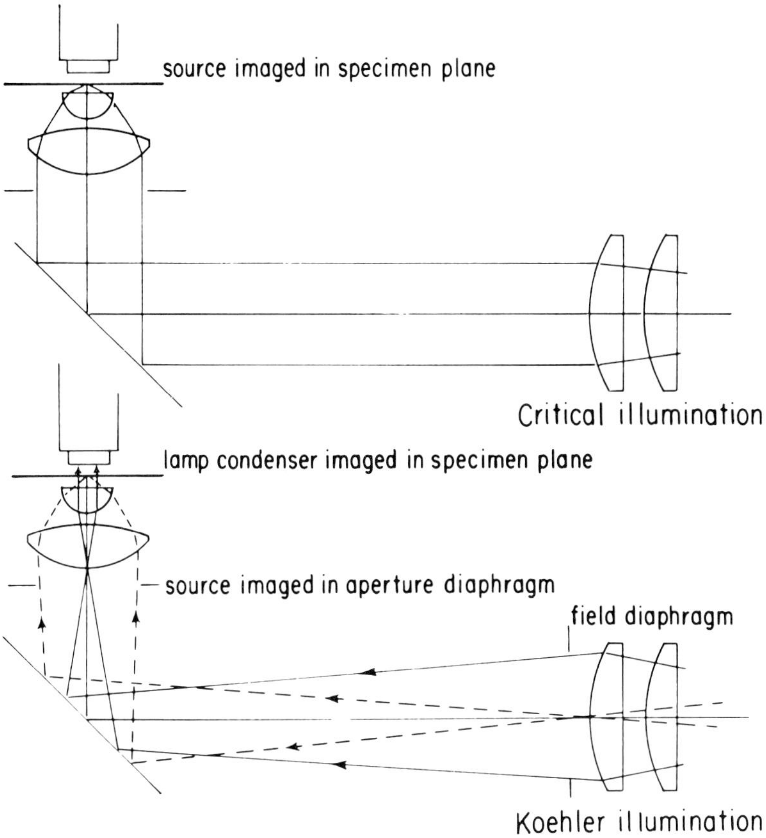

Fig. 9–9. Optical principles of critical (Nelson) and Koehler illumination.

by Koehler illumination. Recently, it has been theorized that the two systems have equivalent resolving powers. Most modern microscopes have built-in illumination systems in the base that are optically equivalent to Koehler systems. The illumination is permanently aligned, so centering need not be performed by the microscopist. Usually, these illuminators employ a low voltage, concentrated filament lamp so that high brightness levels can be obtained, and the frosting of one of the lamp condensers will permit even illumination at all microscope magnifications. When using a separate illuminator, place it 8 to 10 inches in front of the microscope and adjust it so that light falls on the mirror. Focus lamp so that filament image is focused on the condenser iris diaphragm. Adjust condenser until illumination diaphragm is in focus with specimen. Open diaphragm until field is just filled.

Darkfield illumination is achieved by blocking out the central rays of light and directing the peripheral rays against the microscope objective from the side. Only those rays that strike the object and are reflected upward pass into the objective lens. The object that is being examined thus appears bright on a black background. By means of this form of illumination, very minute structures can be seen, just as particles of the dust in the atmosphere become visible when a beam of sunlight enters a darkened room. Darkfield illumination is most frequently used in the clinical laboratory examination of material from ulcers for *Treponema pallidum*. Two types of darkfield condensers generally available are paraboloid condensers and cardioid condensers, which differ from each other only in the different pathways of light entering through the condenser system itself (Fig. 9–10). Darkfield condensers depend upon the use of a high numeric aperture with a hollow cone of light. The condensers must be in contact with the lower face of the object to be viewed in order to obtain the required numeric aperture in the illuminated cone. When using the low-power objective, darkfield illumination can be obtained by means of the ring stops with central discs, which accompany most microscopes. The stop is placed in a special ring beneath the condenser. When the regular stop is not available, one can use the glass disc supplied with the microscope or an extra large round coverglass in the center of which is placed a circular disc of black paper to produce a paraboloid effect. The size of such a black disc would depend on the aperture of the objective with which it is to be used. This size can be ascertained by trial and error. It is necessary to use an objective of numeric aperture somewhat under the illuminated numeric aperture of the darkfield condenser to prevent direct light from getting into the image. Objectives with higher than

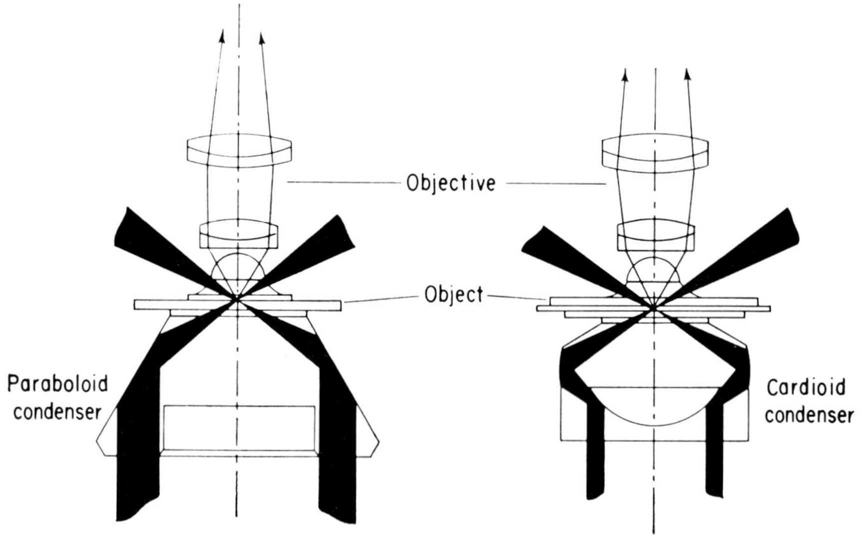

Fig. 9–10. Basic optics of paraboloid and cardioid condensers for darkfield illumination.

1.00 NA must be provided with the appropriate ring stops or funnel stops to reduce their numeric aperture to 1.00. The funnel stop is a small baffle which fits into the back of the objective lens and reduces the aperture at the rear lens surface. When the oil immersion objective is used, special condensers are necessary. These are known as reflecting condensers or darkfield illuminators. The most desirable form of condenser for this purpose is one that is interchangeable with a regular substage condenser. The use of a darkfield system is also dependent on the intense light beam for the lamp condenser and a homogeneous brilliant source of light such as a ribbon filament or arc. Thickness of the slide is important when using the darkfield condenser owing to the need for accurate focusing of the condenser. Slide thickness usually varies between 1.00 and 1.55 mm. Because of the short working distance of oil-immersion objectives, no. 1 coverglasses must be used. The layer of fluid or the tissue to be examined must also be thin. Air bubbles, scratches on the glass, and blood corpuscles may interfere with darkfield visualization.

To facilitate centering, a series of concentric circles is generally ruled on the top of the darkfield condenser. These circles are brought to center of the field of a low-power objective by means of centering screws. A drop of immersion oil is then placed on the apex of the condenser, the slide is placed in position on the stage, and the condenser is raised until the oil is in contact with the undersurface of the slide. The low-power objective is then focused on the slide. If the slide is sufficiently lighted, a spot of light should be seen in the center of the field. Presence of a circle instead of a spot indicates that the condenser is above or below its correct position. The condenser is then focused by raising or lowering it until the circle becomes a spot of light as small and as bright as can be obtained. The high-power objective is then put in place and brought into focus in the usual manner.

The most frequent causes of failure to secure satisfactory darkfield when objects are brilliantly illuminated and appear to be self-luminous are use of an objective with too wide an aperture, failure to focus the center of the condenser accurately, air bubbles in the preparation, or too many microscope structures in the field reflecting the light at too many angles.

Polarized illumination is useful in clinical microscopy.[7] Because light is transmitted in all directions and vibration of the waves is at right angles to the direction of the transmission, light viewed through the microscope will be vibrating in many different directions. Wave vibrations can be made unidirectional by inserting devices called polarizers between the light source and the viewer. If two such polarizers are inserted in the optical beam in such a manner that the second one transmits in a direction at right angles to the first, all light will be extinguished. If the same polarizers are inserted at parallel angles, the light will be transmitted but will be vibrational only in one direction (Fig. 9–11).

Polarized light passes through some materials with unchanged velocity regardless of the direction of the entering light waves. These tissues are designated isotropic and have an index of refraction that is the same in all directions. On the other hand, anisotropic materials alter the velocity of transmitted polarized light waves, depending upon the direction of the light waves. The latter are birefringent because they have different indices of refraction corresponding to the respective velocities of polarized light transmission. Birefringence may be expressed quantitatively as the difference between two indices of refraction:

$$B = Ne - No = \frac{r}{d}$$

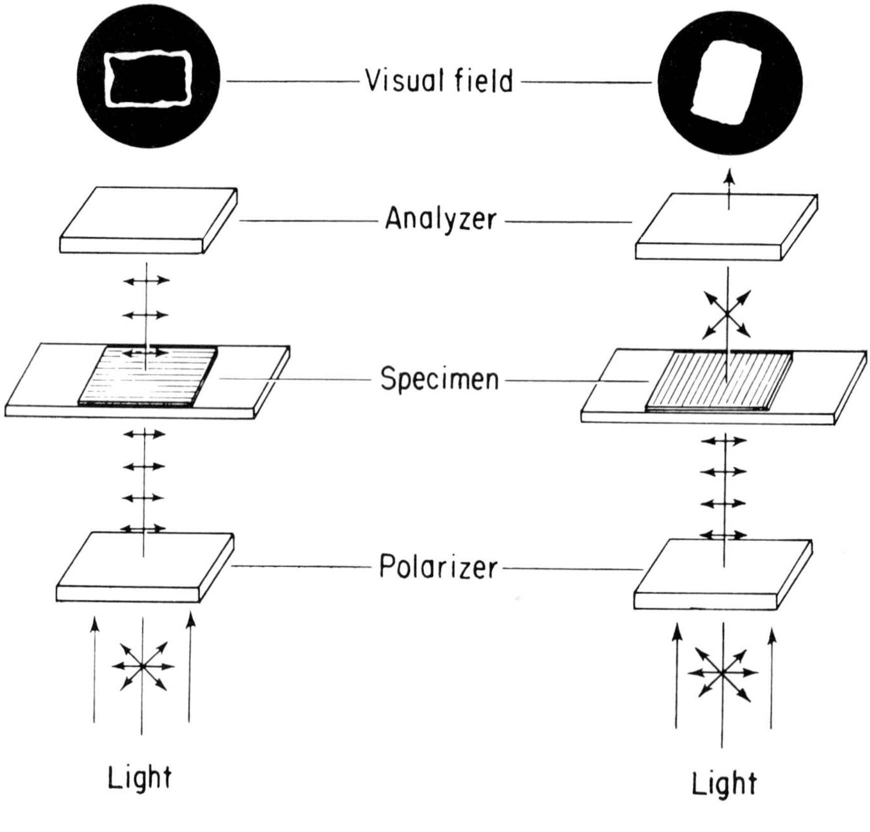

Fig. 9–11. Basic principles of polarizing illumination. With polarizer and analyzer rotated 90° (left), there is no visual image; with polarizer rotated 45° (right), an image is seen.

$$B = Ne - No = \frac{r}{d}$$

where b is the birefringence, Ne and No are the indices of refraction, r is the retardation of wave velocity, and d is the thickness of the specimen. Birefringence of biologic material is generally very small, ranging from about 0.01 to 0.001 units. Measurement of the retardation is carried out by use of compensation introduced into the optical system. The measurement is in nanometers (nm) or in fractions of a wavelength (λ). In practice, one measures the retardation of polarized light in one plane relative to that of light polarized in another, perpendicular to it.

One of the two polarizing devices is called the polarizer, and the other the analyzer. They can be made from a sheet of Polaroid film or from Nicol prisms of calcite. The polarizer is mounted below the substage condenser between the condenser and the illuminator, and the analyzer is located above the objective lens system. When the analyzer is rotated 360°, the visual field alternates between bright and dark at each 180° turn. Maximal light is transmitted when the analyzer is set parallel to the polarizer.

The main types of birefringence are crystalline birefringence, form birefringence, strain birefringence, and dichroism. Crystalline birefringence is independent of the refractive index of the media and is usually found in systems in which there are asymmetric bonds between molecules and ions, such as is the case with proteins or lipids. Form birefringence is produced when asymmetric particles are present in a medium of different refractive index. This type of birefringence is changed when the refractive index of the medium is changed. Strain birefringence is demonstrated when a substance is subjected to tension of pressure, such as with muscle. In dichroism, the wavelength of polarized light changes with orientation of the object, and the changes are actually changes in amplitude (intensity) of the transmitted light. Dichroism is seldom seen with visible light in biologic objects. It can be induced in tissues by staining with congo red or thionine.

Fluorescence illumination is also valuable in microscopy. Fluorescence is the ability of a substance to emit light of longer wavelength when excited by light of a shorter wavelength. Since fluorescence is usually weak, a very intense illuminating source and special filter devices are necessary to accentuate the fluorescent image to the point of usefulness. The source is usually a high pressure mercury arc with an emission near the lower range of ultraviolet (300 *nm*). Various other sources have been used for an intense source of illumination. Of these, the iron arc is most intense, but not most efficient and convenient, since it requires direct current. By insertion of special filters, exciter filters, in the illuminating beam below the substage condenser, the proper wavelength of light can be selected. A second filter, the barrier filter, is inserted into the path of the fluorescent image to remove blue-violet exciting light, while passing the longer wavelengths of fluorescent light emitted by the specimen, thus permitting observation of the image without danger of damage to the eye by ultraviolet irradiation. A special darkfield system can be combined with this system to remove almost completely the blue-violet light inadvertently transmitted.

Fluorescence can be classified as natural (autofluorescence), when it is produced by substances normally present in tissue, and secondary, when it is induced by staining with fluorescent dyes (fluorochromes). Fluorochromes are dilute solutions of organic pigments that will induce more intense fluorescence without damaging the tissue. Because of these properties, many living specimens are accessible to study by fluorescence microscopy. Acridine orange, one such fluorochrome, has been utilized in cytology to study rapidly regenerating cells. Other widely used fluorochromes include rhodamine B, thioflavine S, and uranine yellow. Vitamin A, thiamine, riboflavin, and other substances can be visualized within the cytoplasm of cells by fluorescence. Many cell components normally autofluoresce: cytoplasm, diffuse blue; granules, strong yellow; calcium, yellow-white; free porphyrins, strong red; and unsaturated fatty acids, various colors depending upon the degree of oxidation. Usually the nucleus does not autofluoresce. Skin fluoresces intense blue; teeth, greenish white; nails, vivid bluish white; bone, intense milky blue; and gelatin, intense bluish white. Red blood cells do not ordinarily fluoresce. Hematoporphyrins (hemoglobin precursors), however, fluoresce brilliant orange-red.

The standard fluorescence microscope has quartz optics between the high pressure mercury arc and the specimen, and ordinary glass optics above the specimen.

The best contrast and most vivid fluorescence is obtained when the object to be viewed is mounted dry. Since fluorescence can be obtained from unsaturated fats and oils, it is undesirable to use them to mount specimens. Satisfactory permanent mounts may be made in clarite since this substance is only slightly fluorescent.

Perhaps the most valuable clinical laboratory application of fluorescence is based in the method developed by A.H. Coons to render antigen located within the tissues visible by reacting it with fluorochrome-tagged antibody, thus producing fluorescence at the site of antigen-antibody combination. The most commonly used of these specific immunologic chemical "stains" is fluorescin isothiocyanate. Fluorescin-labeled antibodies have been used to identify bacterial polysaccharides, viruses, rickettsiae, leptospira, protozoa, and many other specific protein antigens. Thus, there are many useful applications of the technique in microbiology. With the fluorescent technique, it is possible to determine whether the antigen is located within the nucleus or the cytoplasm, or is extracellular. Fluorescence has been used to localize hormones in various cells, including ACTH in the basophilic cell of the pituitary, myosin in the A-band of myofibrils, and gamma globulin in plasma cells.

The technique is useful and can readily be utilized in the routine diagnostic laboratory. The most difficult problem has been to obtain satisfactory pure and reactive reagents. Fluorescent microscopy generally requires use of tissues frozen and sectioned in a cryostat. These are then placed on slides and permitted to dry at room temperature. They are then coupled with fluorescin-labeled antibody for subsequent study.

Phase illumination has also been used in clinical microscopy. Although the majority of cell components are transparent to visible light, some organelles and their structures cause minor retardations, phase changes, with transmitted light waves. These phase differences, which result from small differences in the refractive indices and thicknesses of the organelles and tissues, can be accentuated and visualized by use of the microscope (Fig. 9–12). When light traverses a transparent object, its amplitude is not affected, but the velocity of the wave is changed. If the refractive index of the material is higher than that of the surrounding medium, there is a delay or retardation. Obviously, when traversing semiopaque objects, there is also a decrease in amplitude of the light waves. The phase change increases in direct proportion to the difference between the refractive index of the cell organelles or specimen, and the refractive index of the surrounding medium (and also the thickness of the specimen). Although the phase contrast microscope was originally developed by the Dutchman, Fritz Zernicke, in 1935, for testing microscope mirrors, it has been successfully applied to visualization of components of living cells.

In biologic materials, the phase difference is usually about one-quarter of the wavelength ($^1/_4\lambda$) of the light traversing the specimen. The most lateral light passing through the objective of the microscope is either advanced or retarded by one-fourth of the wavelength with respect to the central light traversing the specimen. The effect is achieved by placing an annular phase plate into the rear focal plane of the objective lens and an annular diaphragm below or in the substage condenser. The net result with this combination is that undiffracted rays of light acquire a one-quarter wavelength difference from the diffracted rays; thus, the different rays have different levels of brightness when visualized (Fig. 9–12).

There are basically two types of phase contrast that can be achieved by such a system, bright or negative contrast and dark or positive contrast. In negative contrast, the two sets of wavelengths are additive, and

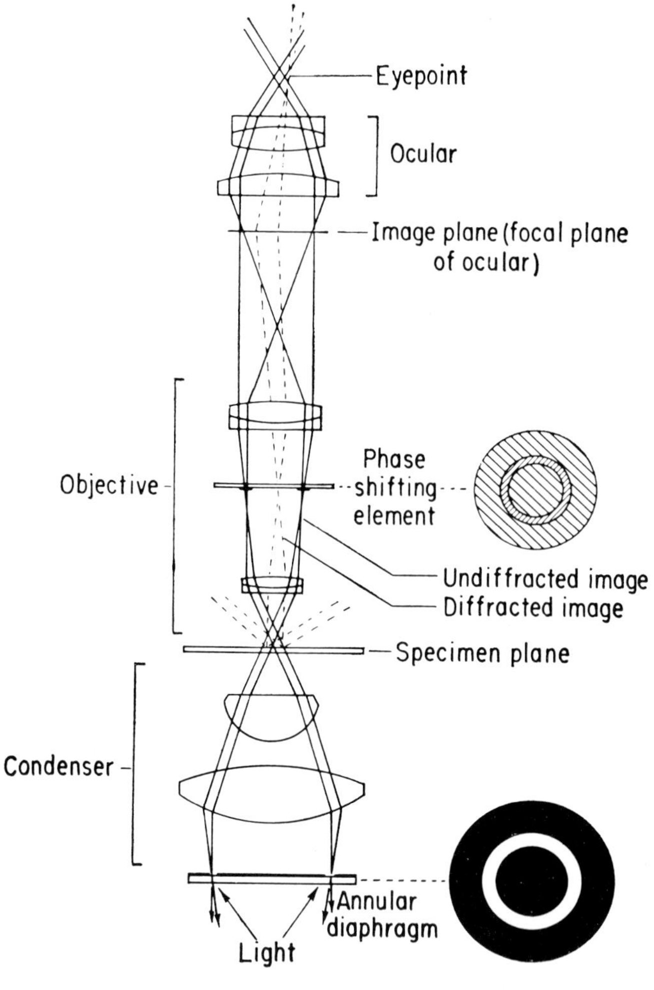

Fig. 9–12. Basic principles of phase contrast illumination. The annular diaphragm controls the illumination, and the phase shifting element creates a one-quarter wavelength retardation of the image.

the specimen appears brighter than the surrounding area. In positive contrast, the two sets of ray are subtracted, and the image appears darker than the surrounding area. Because there is also a change in amplitude, the specimen appears in various shades of gray, depending on the thickness and the refractive indices of the specimen and the medium.

Phase microscopy is particularly valuable for observation of unstained living cells, for cinemicrography, and for demonstration of various organelles and their motion within cells.

Interference illumination is based on principles similar to those of phase illumination. With interference microscopy, however, it is possible to determine the optical-phase difference for various cell structures and to measure the dry weight of these structures. The interference microscope is more sensitive than the phase microscope for detecting minute changes of refractive index. For interference illumination, light emitted from a single source is split into two beams, one of which penetrates the specimen, while the other bypasses the specimen. The two beams are recombined above the specimen. The beam that has penetrated the specimen is retarded, thus giving a phase change. As in phase microscopy, the retardation is a function of the refractive index and the thickness of the specimen. If the refractive indices of the specimen and of the surrounding medium are known, the dry weight of the specimen can be determined by the following formula:

$$C = \frac{100\ (s - m)}{X}$$

where C is the percentage concentration of dry material in the specimen, s is the refractive index of the specimen, m is the refractive index of the medium (usually water), and X is a constant that equals 100α (α being the specific refractive increment of the material in solution. It is about 0.18 units for most substances in the cell). Interference microscopy, therefore, has been used to determine protein, lipid, and nucleic acid content of cells. Dry mass of the tissue is first determined. The components of interest are then extracted from the tissue, and the difference in measurement before and after extraction is determined.

USE AND CARE OF THE OPTICAL MICROSCOPE[3,8]

Optically it is a matter of indifference whether the instrument is used in the vertical or inclined position. However, because much work in the clinical laboratory involves examination of fluids, it is advisable to become accustomed to use of the microscope in a vertical position.

It is best to "focus upward," obviating damage to slides and objectives. This is accomplished by bringing the objective nearer the slide than the proper focus while watching from one side. Then, looking into the oculars, bring the tube up until the object is seen clearly. The fine adjustment should be used only for exact focusing with the higher power objectives, after the instrument is in approximate focus. It should not be turned more than one revolution.

There will be less eye fatigue if both are kept open while using the monocular microscope and if no effort is made to see objects that are not in distinct focus. Fine focusing should be done with the fine adjustment, not with the eye. An experienced microscopist keeps his fingers almost constantly on one of the focusing adjustments.

It is preferable to work with the low-power objective as much as possible. Reserving the high-power objective for detailed study of objects found under low power increases both speed and accuracy. Even such minute objects as nucleated erythrocytes in a stained blood film are found more quickly with an 8 mm, or even a 16 mm, objective combined with a 10× ocular than with the oil immersion lens. It is difficult to realize intuitively how small the "real field" is—that is, the actual area of the slide that is seen through the microscope (Fig. 9–13).

Objects should be centered in the field for clarity. Acuity of observation will be greatly enhanced and fatigue lessened if external illumination is subdued. Strong light should not be allowed to fall directly on the surface of the slide, for this clouds the image, especially if a low-power objective is used.

A useful pointer can be made by placing a straight piece of hair across the opening of the diaphragm of the ocular, cementing one end with a tiny drop of epoxy resin and dividing the hair with small scissors. When the ocular is in place, the hair appears as a black line extending from the periphery to the center of the microscope field. If the pointer does not appear sharply defined, it is out of focus and the diaphragm within the ocular must be raised or lowered slightly.

One often wishes to mark a particular field on a permanent preparation to be able to find it again quickly. If the mechanical stage is permanently fastened to the stage of the microscope, the vernier can be used to mark the position of an object on the slide. There are on the market several "object markers" by which a desired field can be marked with ink or by a circle scratched on the coverglass by a small diamond while the slide is in place on the microscope. The circle is easily located with a low-power objective.

The microscope is a delicate instrument and should be handled accordingly. Even a slight disturbance of its adjustments may cause serious trouble. It seems unnecessary to say that when there is unusual resistance to any manipulation, force should never be used to overcome it until the cause has first been determined.

The microscope should be kept scrupulously clean, and dust must not be allowed to settle on it. When not in use, the instrument should be kept in its case or under a soft cover. A bell jar is particularly liable to strike the mechanical stage and disturb the adjustment. In the absence

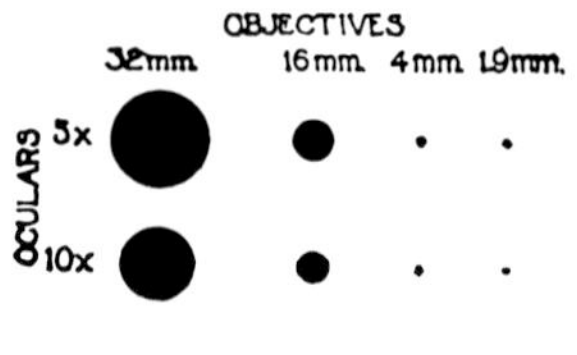

Fig. 9–13. Approximate size of "real fields" (actual areas seen through most microscopes).

of a special cover, a square of lint-free cloth may be draped over the microscope.

Lens surfaces that have been exposed to dust should be cleaned only with a camel's-hair brush or a good grade of lens paper. Surfaces that are exposed to finger marks should be cleaned with lens paper. The rubbing should be done very gently and with a circular motion. Particles of dirt that appear in the field may be on the slide, the ocular, or the condenser. Their site can be determined by moving the slide, rotating the ocular, and lowering the condenser. Dirt on the objective cannot be seen as such; it causes diffuse cloudiness. When the image is hazy, the objective probably needs cleaning; in case of an oil-immersion objective there may be bubbles in the oil.

Oil that has dried upon the lenses—an insult from which even dry objectives are not immune—may be removed with alcohol, xylol, or Windex, but these substances must be used sparingly and carefully because there is danger of softening the cement between the components of the objective. Some manufacturers now claim to use cement that resists xylol.

If the vulcanite stage becomes brown and discolored, the black color can be restored by rubbing well with petrolatum.

MEASUREMENT OF OBJECTS UNDER THE OPTICAL MICROSCOPE[8]

Size is an important clue for identification of microscope structures. Even very rough measurements will often prevent humiliating blunders. Among the objects most frequently measured for clinical diagnosis are animal parasites and their ova, and abnormal blood corpuscles. The metric system is used almost exclusively. For very small objects, the micron (1×10^{-6} meters) is the convenient unit of measurement (represented by the Greek letter μ). For larger objects, if exact measurement is not essential, the diameter of a red blood corpuscle (7 to 8 μ) is sometimes taken as a unit. Of the several methods of measurement, the most convenient and accurate is use of a micrometer ocular. In its simplest form, this is similar to an ordinary ocular, but it has within it a glass disk on which is etched a graduated scale. When this ocular is placed in the tube of the microscope, the ruled lines appear in the microscope field, and the size of an object can be determined readily in terms of divisions of this scale. The value of these divisions (in mm) obviously will vary with different magnifications. Their value must therefore be determined separately for each objective. This is accomplished through use of a stage micrometer—a glass slide with a ruled scale, accurately subdivided into hundredths of a millimeter. A typical example would be a stage micrometer on which a length of 2 mm is ruled into 200 divisions—each division being 10 μ (Fig. 9–14). The stage micrometer is placed upon the stage of the microscope and brought into focus. The tube of the microscope is then lowered or raised until

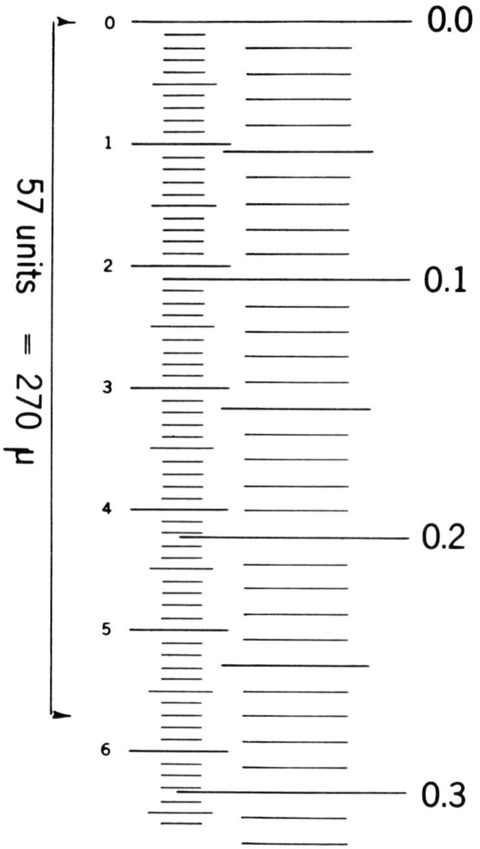

Fig. 9–14. Stage micrometer divided into hundredths of a mm (upper scale) and ocular micrometer (lower scale). The ocular micrometer aligns at 57 units with the stage micrometer at 0.27 mm (270μ), therefore the micrometer value is 4.74 μ/unit with the particular lens system used. (Reproduced from E. Leitz Tech. Info. Bull., *7*[2–3]:3, Oct. 31, 1967.)

two lines of one scale exactly coincide with two lines of the other. From the number of divisions of the ocular scale, which then correspond to each division of the stage micrometer, the value of the former in microns or in fractions of a millimeter can be easily calculated. Both the number of units of the ocular micrometer, and a corresponding number of units on the stage micrometer, when the scales are aligned, are counted. For example, if the ocular micrometer aligns at 57 units with the stage micrometer at 0.27 mm (or 270 μ), the micrometer value (1 unit) is:

$$\frac{270}{57} = 4.74\ \mu$$

Therefore, each scale division of the micrometer with that particular lens is 4.74 μ wide. This procedure should be repeated at least 10 times and the mean value and standard deviation determined. This value, of course, applies only to the objective and the tube length with which it was determined. The counting slide of a hemocytometer may be used in place of a stage micrometer. The lines of the sides of the small squares used in counting erythrocytes are 50 μ apart. When using the counting chamber with an oil-immersion objective, a coverglass must be used; otherwise, the oil will fill the ruled lines and cause them to disappear. Any ocular can be converted into a micrometer ocular by placing a micrometer disc—a small circular glass plate with a ruled scale—ruled side down on its diaphragm. If the lines on this are at all hazy, the disc has probably been inserted upside down or else the diaphragm is out of its proper position. Usually, it can be pushed up or down as required.

REFERENCES

1. Ey, J., Jr. (coordinating editor): The Billings Microscope Collection of the Medical Museum of the Armed Forces Institute of Pathology. Washington, D.C., The American Registry of Pathology, 1967, p. 1.
2. Vollmer, E. (ed.): Leonardo da Vinci. Instituto Geografico De Agostine S.p.A., Italy (original printer). New York, Reynal and Co., 1966, p. 419.
3. Freeman, J.: The microscope. *In* Clinical Diagnosis by Laboratory Methods. 14th Ed. Edited by I. Davidsohn and J. Henry. Philadelphia, W.B. Saunders, 1968.
4. Benford, J.: The Theory of the Microscope. 4th Ed. Rochester, Bausch and Lomb, Inc., 1965 (succinct explanation from which many illustrations for this chapter were modified and reproduced).
5. Gage, S.: The Microscope. 16th Ed. Ithaca, Comstock Publishing Co., 1936.
6. Kay, D. (ed.): Techniques for Electron Microscopy. 2nd Ed. Philadelphia, F.A. Davis, 1965.
7. DeRobertis, E., Nowinski, W., and Saez, F.: Cell Biology. 4th Ed. Philadelphia, W.B. Saunders, 1965, p. 57.
8. Needham, G.: The Practical Use of the Microscope, Including Photomicrography. Springfield, Charles C Thomas, 1958.

Index

Page numbers in *italics* indicate figures; numbers followed by "t" indicate tables.